THE COMPLETE BOOK OF VITAMIN AND MIN-
ERAL COUNTS gives you all the information you need to
plan your meals and evaluate your diet to ensure that you
are getting your RDAs, or more, of essential nutrients. By
scanning the pages for your favorite foods, you'll discover
how to create a vitamin- and mineral-packed meal, which
candy bar is not just empty calories, or what kind of lunch-
eon meat is your best health value, and much, much more.
Or, if you are interested in boosting specific vitamins but
are bored by the same foods, you'll find many tasty options.
For example:

- While we all know orange juice is a good source of vitamin C, red peppers are also loaded with it.

- Mothers always say to eat your peas. Should you? You
  bet; they're high in vitamin A, folacin, phosphorus, and
  potassium.

- If you're lactose sensitive and staying away from milk,
  what other ways can you get your RDA of calcium? Try
  tofu, kale, or broccoli.

- Searching for a good source of vitamin A? Look no further than the humble sweet potato—it's brimming with
  the vitamin A you need for healthy bones, hair, skin, and
  teeth.

# The Complete Book of
# Vitamin and Mineral Counts

Corinne T. Netzer

**A Dell Book**

Published by
Dell Publishing
a division of
Random House, Inc.
1540 Broadway
New York, New York 10036

ISBN: 0-440-22335-0

Printed in the United States of America

Published simultaneously in Canada

February 1997

10  9  8  7  6  5  4  3

RAD

# Vitamins and Minerals

The more nutrition-conscious we become, the more importance we must place on vitamins and minerals and their vital role in forming and maintaining our overall good health. Indeed, any discussion of nutrients and nutrition would be incomplete without including these life-sustaining substances.

I have divided this book into two parts: *Vitamins* (starting on page 5) and *Minerals* (page 209). Preceding each part is a brief description of the major vitamins and minerals, their main functions and sources, recommended dosages, and toxicity. Following this are listings that give the vitamin and mineral content for several hundred foods. The listings will be especially valuable if you, like me, prefer getting these dietary nutrients from natural sources.

Because of space limitations, I could not cover all the vitamins and minerals currently recognized. To determine which nutrients to omit, I used these criteria: when a substance, as in the case of pantothenic acid and Vitamin K, was plentiful and deficiencies extremely rare; when the natural sources of a substance, as with Vitamin D and iodine, were so limited that I was able to cover them within the descriptive text; and when I did not find the data plentiful enough or reliable enough to be of use to the reader. If a vitamin or a mineral is not included, this does not mean it is unimportant. *All vitamins and minerals are essential*, even those whose functions and requirements have not yet been well defined. They are all interrelated and work together to maintain good health—a deficiency in one substance can disrupt the body's entire balance.

My primary source of data for this book is the federal government; however, I have included data from individual food producers and distributors when the actual data, rather than percentages, were available.

As with all nutrients, the values in this book can vary according to seasonal and regional differences. In the case of vitamins, values may vary greatly depending on when a food is harvested and how it is stored and shipped. Mineral values will vary according to the soil in which the food is grown (this affects animal feed and thereby includes food of animal origin).

**A word about recommended dosages:** RDAs (Recommended Dietary Allowances) for several vitamins and minerals have been established by the National Research Council of the Food and Nutrition Board, National Academy of Sciences. Based on these standards, similar recommendations (called USRDAs) have been established by the Food and Drug Administration.

These RDAs are guidelines only, given to help define the safe and adequate intake of specific nutrients needed for optimal health in most individuals. While they are meant to offset nutritional deficiencies, RDAs are not meant as a cure or treatment for physical disorders. Bear in mind that individual requirements may differ and that RDAs do not cover special nutritional needs resulting from physical disorders or the use of specific medications.

For vitamins and minerals that have a designated RDA, I have given the latest information available; for those that do not have an ''official'' RDA at this time, I have given the dosage generally recommended by health professionals.

It's important to note that the RDAs are periodically revised. This is because scientific knowledge of our nutritional requirements is not yet complete and many questions related to our health remain to be solved. The world of nutrition is still being explored, and new essential nutrients may be found as research progresses. These facts emphasize the importance of a balanced and healthy diet.

# Abbreviations and Symbols

| | |
|---|---|
| approx. | approximately |
| diam. | diameter |
| fl. | fluid |
| " | inch(es) |
| IU | International Units |
| < | less than |
| (0) | may contain trace amount |
| Mcg | micrograms |
| Mg | milligrams |
| n.a. | not available |
| oz. | ounce(s) |
| pkg. | package |
| pkt. | packet |
| lb. | pound(s) |
| tbsp. | tablespoon(s) |
| tsp. | teaspoon(s) |
| tr. | trace |
| w/ | with |

# Vitamins

# Vitamins

Vitamins are organic substances found in all living things. With a few exceptions, our bodies cannot manufacture an adequate supply of vitamins, and we must obtain them from dietary sources— in the form of food or dietary supplements. We need only minute quantities to sustain life, but a deficiency in even one vitamin can endanger the entire body.

At this time there are thirteen recognized vitamins, and they are generally distinguished as being *fat-soluble* or *water-soluble*.

Fat-soluble vitamins, which include vitamins A, D, E, and K, are absorbed into the body with the aid of fats in the diet or bile produced by the liver. These vitamins are stored in body fat, and if you are getting adequate amounts it's generally not necessary to consume them daily. On the other hand, because they are stored in the body, they can build up to toxic levels if too many are consumed.

Water-soluble vitamins, including the B-complex group and vitamin C, do not need fat or bile to be absorbed, and generally are not stored in the body. What the body does not use is excreted through urination and perspiration, so they should be replaced daily. These vitamins are fragile and can be destroyed during food processing, storage, or preparation.

The following is an overview of the major vitamins.

### Vitamin A (Carotene and Retinol)

Fat-soluble. Comes in two forms: *preformed vitamin A*, or *retinol*, which is found only in foods of animal origin; and *provitamin A*, or *carotene* (which includes *beta-carotene*), found in foods of both plant and animal origin, but especially of plants. While retinol is absorbed almost instantly, the body must convert carotene into retinol-like vitamin A before it can be utilized. One well-known indicator of a deficiency of this vitamin is night blindness.

*Main Functions:* Aids in the treatment of many eye disorders; promotes bone growth, healthy hair, skin, and teeth; helps protect mucous membranes and boosts resistance to respiratory and other infections; fights acne.

*Best Natural Sources:* Retinol: liver and fish-liver oil. Carotene: yellow and dark-green fruits and vegetables (carrots, apricots, cantaloupe, sweet potatoes, spinach, kale, broccoli, mustard greens), cheese, butter, fortified margarine.

*Recommended Daily Dosage:* 5000 International Units, for adults. This amount increases during illness, trauma, pregnancy, and lactation. Requirements may be higher for people who smoke or who live in areas of high air pollution.

*Toxicity:* Because the body stores vitamin A, daily dosages of over 50,000 International Units may be toxic if there is no deficiency. Symptoms of prolonged excessive intake include blurred vision, hair loss, nausea and vomiting, diarrhea, and skin rash. Symptoms usually disappear in a short time if vitamin A intake is discontinued.

### Thiamine (Vitamin B₁)

Water-soluble; part of the B-complex group, which works together. Vulnerable to heat, air, and water in cooking. Thiamine is sometimes called the ''nerve vitamin'' or ''morale vitamin'' because of its beneficial effect on the nervous system and mental attitude.

*Main Functions:* Maintains muscle tissue and a healthy nervous system and heart; promotes growth; aids in digestion, particularly of carbohydrates.

*Best Natural Sources:* Pork, liver, brewer's yeast, bran, whole grains, enriched breads, cereals and pasta.

*Recommended Daily Dosage:* 1 to 1.5 milligrams for adults. Need increases during illness, stress, pregnancy, and lactation.

*Toxicity:* Nontoxic. However, very large doses may contribute to an imbalance of B complex. This group of vitamins is interrelated and an excess in one might result in a deficiency of other B vitamins.

### Riboflavin (Vitamin B₂)

Water-soluble; part of the B-complex group. Easily absorbed and not vulnerable to heat or air, but can be destroyed by exposure to sunlight.

*Main Functions:* Acts with other substances to utilize carbohydrates, fats, and proteins; helps maintain mucous membranes and cell respiration; promotes good vision and healthy skin, hair, and nails.

*Best Natural Sources:* Liver and other organ meats, poultry, milk, eggs, brewer's yeast, whole grains, enriched bread, cereals and pasta, almonds, dried beans and peas, dark green vegetables.

*Recommended Daily Dosage:* 1.2 to 1.7 milligrams for adults, slightly higher for pregnant and lactating women.

*Toxicity:* Nontoxic. However, as with all B vitamins, it is important to maintain a proper balance within this group (see Thiamine).

### Niacin (Vitamin B₃)

Water-soluble, part of the B-complex group. Very resistant to heat, light, and air. With the amino acid *tryptophan*, the body can manufacture its own niacin, assuming there is no deficiency in the other B vitamins. There are also three synthetic forms: niacinamide, nicotinic acid, and nicotinamide.

*Main Functions:* Promotes a healthy nervous and digestive system and maintains healthy skin and hair; aids circulation and assists in breakdown of carbohydrates, fats, and proteins.

*Best Natural Sources:* Tuna, liver, lean meat, poultry, fish, whole grains, enriched wheat products, and nuts.

*Recommended Daily Dosage:* 20 milligrams for adults.

*Toxicity:* Basically nontoxic, but doses over 100 milligrams may cause temporary burning, tingling, or itching of the skin. These side effects are not present in niacinamide, but excessive doses of this substance have been known to cause depression in some individuals.

### Pantothenic Acid (Vitamin B₅)

Water-soluble, part of the B-complex group. Occurs in all living cells, but can be destroyed with overprocessing.

*Main Functions:* Aids cell building, healing, and the formation and maintenance of adrenal hormones; helps in metabolism of carbohydrates, fats, and proteins.

*Best Natural Sources:* All plants and foods of animal origin, particularly liver and other organ meats, poultry, egg yolks, whole grains, nuts, dark-green vegetables, and brewer's yeast.

*Recommended Daily Dosage:* 10 milligrams for adults. Need may increase with illness, stress, or use of antibiotics.

*Toxicity:* Nontoxic (see Thiamine).

### Pyridoxine, Pyridoxal, and Pyridoxamine (Vitamin B₆)

Water-soluble, part of the B-complex group. Helps maintain the body's sodium-potassium balance; useful in preventing various nerve and skin disorders.

*Main Functions:* Aids in formation of red blood cells and metabolism of proteins and fats; helps regulate body fluids and nervous system; alleviates nausea.

*Best Natural Sources:* Whole grains, liver, beef, avocado, cantaloupe, bananas, nuts, and dark-green leafy vegetables.

*Recommended Daily Dosage:* 1.5 to 2 milligrams for adults. Higher doses are suggested for pregnant and lactating women, and for those on a high-protein diet.

*Toxicity:* Nontoxic (see Thiamine).

## Cobalamin (Vitamin B$_{12}$)

Water-soluble, part of the B-complex group; the only vitamin that contains essential mineral elements. Highly effective in very small doses, B$_{12}$ needs calcium for proper absorption.

*Main Functions:* Forms and regulates red blood cells and prevents anemia; helps maintain a healthy nervous system; alleviates irritability and increases energy.

*Best Natural Sources:* Found only in foods of animal origin, particularly liver, kidneys, beef, pork, fish, eggs, milk, cheese. (*Note:* Strict vegetarians may require supplements.)

*Recommended Daily Dosage:* 6 micrograms for adults, higher during pregnancy and lactation.

*Toxicity:* Nontoxic (see Thiamine).

## Folacin (Folic Acid)

Water-soluble, part of the B-complex group. Easily destroyed by heat, light, and air. Although the body can store folacin, it is one of the vitamins most deficient in our diets.

*Main Functions:* Aids in formation of red blood cells; helps maintain healthy nervous system and promotes mental health; essential for reproduction of all cells.

*Best Natural Sources:* Dark-green leafy vegetables, brewer's yeast, liver, kidneys, dried beans and peas, broccoli, carrots, asparagus.

*Recommended Daily Dosage:* 400 micrograms; increases during pregnancy and lactation. Need also increases with use of alcohol or oral contraceptives and during periods of stress or illness.

*Toxicity:* Nontoxic, but temporary skin rash might occur in some individuals, and an overabundance may mask a deficiency of $B_{12}$ (see Thiamine).

### Ascorbic Acid (Vitamin C)

Water-soluble. Very sensitive to oxygen; its potency can be lost through exposure to air, light, and heat. Vitamin C has been—and continues to be—the subject of a wide range of studies, and has been touted as a cure-all for everything from the common cold to cancer. While most animals synthesize their own supply, man, apes, and a few other animals must rely on dietary sources.

*Main Functions:* Aids production of collagen and red blood cells; maintains healthy blood vessels, bones, teeth, and gums; helps body absorb iron; promotes healing.

*Best Natural Sources:* Fresh fruits and vegetables, especially citrus fruits, leafy green vegetables, tomatoes, strawberries, melon, green peppers, broccoli, brussels sprouts, cabbage, potatoes.

*Recommended Daily Dosage:* 60 milligrams for adults, with increased dosage during illness, stress, pregnancy, or lactation. Smokers require higher doses, and it is believed that the need for vitamin C increases with age. (*Note:* Supplements are best taken in frequent small doses, because the body can absorb only so much at once.)

*Toxicity:* Basically nontoxic, but excessive doses may cause diarrhea, skin rashes, or other temporary side effects in some individuals.

### Cholecalciferol (Vitamin D)

Fat-soluble. Called the "sunshine vitamin" because it can be acquired by exposure to the sun's ultraviolet rays. Best utilized when combined with vitamin A.

*Main Functions:* Aids in formation and maintenance of bones and teeth; helps body absorb and utilize calcium and phosphorus; in adults it also helps maintain the nervous system, heart action, and blood clotting.

*Best Natural Sources:* Sunlight, but pigmentation is a determining factor: the darker the skin—whether natural or tanned—the less vitamin D produced. Adequate absorption can be inhibited by air pollution, clouds, and clothing. Other sources are cod-liver oil and fortified milk and dairy products.

*Recommended Daily Dosage:* 400 International Units.

*Toxicity:* Excessive doses (over 5000 International Units daily) over an extended period can produce temporary toxic effects, such as frequent urination, nausea and vomiting, dizziness, and muscular weakness.

### Tocopherol (Vitamin E)

Fat-soluble. Composed of eight tocopherols (named for letters in the Greek alphabet), with alpha-tocopherol the most potent and effective form. Like vitamin C, E has been the subject of numerous studies and health claims. Vitamin E deficiencies are extremely rare in humans.

*Main Functions:* Supplies oxygen to the body; aids in formation of red blood cells; helps maintain muscles and other tissues; protects vitamin A and fatty acids from oxidation; promotes healing and is effective in preventing raised scar tissue.

*Best Natural Sources:* Cold-pressed vegetable oils, wheat germ, whole grains, liver, raw seeds, and margarine.

*Recommended Daily Dosage:* 8 to 10 International Units for adults. Need increases with a diet high in polyunsaturated fats and exposure to air pollution. (*Note:* Many health professionals consider the official RDA exceedingly low and have recommended dosages of 400 International Units, and even higher.)

*Toxicity:* Basically nontoxic (excessive doses are extracted in the urine); but may have an adverse effect on individuals with high blood pressure or chronic heart disorders.

## Vitamin K

Fat-soluble. There are three K vitamins: two ($K_1$ and $K_2$) can be produced in the body by intestinal bacteria; the third ($K_3$) is a synthetic used when a supplement is needed for a specific purpose, such as during surgery, or when the body is unable to manufacture its own supply.

*Main Functions:* Promotes proper blood clotting and helps prevent internal bleeding; aids normal liver functioning; enhances vitality.

*Best Natural Sources:* Dark-green leafy vegetables, kelp, brussels sprouts, cabbage, cauliflower, peas, liver, fish-liver oils.

*Recommended Daily Dosage:* 55 to 80 micrograms for adults.

*Toxicity:* Basically nontoxic, but possibly toxic when large doses of synthetic ($K_3$) are mixed with anticoagulants; supplements can also build up in the blood and result in symptoms such as flushing and sweating.

# A

| | Vitamin A | Vitamin C | Thiamin | Riboflavin | Niacin | B6 | Folacin | B12 |
|---|---|---|---|---|---|---|---|---|
| | (IU) | (Mg) | (Mg) | (Mg) | (Mg) | (Mg) | (Mcg) | (Mcg) |
| **Acerola,** fresh: | | | | | | | | |
| untrimmed, 1 lb. . . . . . . . | 2782 | 6088 | .07 | .22 | 1.45 | .03 | n.a. | 0 |
| trimmed, ½ cup. . . . . . . . | 376 | 822 | .01 | .03 | .20 | <.01 | n.a. | 0 |
| **Acerola juice,** fresh, | | | | | | | | |
| 6 fl. oz. . . . . . . . . . . . . | 924 | 2899 | .04 | .11 | .73 | .01 | n.a. | 0 |
| **Acorn squash:** | | | | | | | | |
| raw, untrimmed, 1 lb. . . . | 1172 | 38 | .48 | .03 | 2.41 | .53 | 57.7 | 0 |
| raw, trimmed, cubed, | | | | | | | | |
| ½ cup . . . . . . . . . . . . . | 238 | 8 | .10 | .01 | .49 | .11 | 11.7 | 0 |
| baked or boiled, drained, | | | | | | | | |
| cubed, ½ cup . . . . . . . | 437 | 11 | .17 | .01 | .90 | .20 | 19.1 | 0 |
| boiled, drained, mashed, | | | | | | | | |
| ½ cup. . . . . . . . . . . . . | 315 | 8 | .12 | .01 | .65 | .14 | 13.8 | 0 |
| **Adzuki beans,** dried: | | | | | | | | |
| uncooked, 1 lb. . . . . . . . | 75 | 0 | 2.06 | 1.00 | 11.93 | n.a. | n.a. | 0 |
| uncooked, ½ cup. . . . . . . | 33 | 0 | .90 | .43 | 5.18 | n.a. | n.a. | 0 |
| boiled, ½ cup . . . . . . . . | 7 | 0 | .13 | .07 | .83 | n.a. | n.a. | 0 |
| **Agar,** see "Seaweed" | | | | | | | | |
| **Alfalfa seeds, sprouted,** raw: | | | | | | | | |
| raw, 1 lb.. . . . . . . . . . . | 705 | 37 | .35 | .57 | 2.18 | .15 | 163.3 | 0 |
| raw, 1 cup. . . . . . . . . . . | 51 | 3 | .03 | .04 | .16 | .01 | 12.2 | 0 |
| **Allspice,** ground, | | | | | | | | |
| 1 tsp. . . . . . . . . . . . . . | 10 | 1 | <.01 | <.01 | .01 | n.a. | n.a. | 0 |
| **Almond,** shelled, except as noted: | | | | | | | | |
| dried, unblanched: | | | | | | | | |
| in shell, 1 lb. . . . . . . . | 0 | 1 | .38 | 1.41 | 6.01 | .21 | 106.5 | 0 |
| 1 oz. . . . . . . . . . . . . | 0 | <1 | .06 | .22 | .96 | .03 | 16.7 | 0 |
| whole kernels, 1 cup | 0 | 1 | .30 | 1.11 | 4.77 | .16 | 83.3 | 0 |
| dried, blanched, 1 oz. . . . | 0 | <1 | .05 | .19 | .90 | .03 | 10.9 | 0 |
| dried, blanched, whole | | | | | | | | |
| kernels, 1 cup . . . . . . . | 0 | 1 | .23 | .98 | 4.59 | .15 | 55.7 | 0 |
| dry-roasted, 1 oz. . . . . . . | 0 | <1 | .04 | .17 | .80 | .02 | 18.1 | 0 |
| dry-roasted, whole | | | | | | | | |
| kernels, 1 cup . . . . . . . | 0 | 1 | .18 | .83 | 3.89 | .10 | 88.1 | 0 |

| | Vitamin A | Vitamin C | Thiamin | Riboflavin | Niacin | B₆ | Folacin | B₁₂ |
|---|---|---|---|---|---|---|---|---|
| | (IU) | (Mg) | (Mg) | (Mg) | (Mg) | (Mg) | (Mcg) | (Mcg) |
| **Almond,** *continued* | | | | | | | | |
| honey-roasted, 1 oz. | 0 | n.a. | .03 | .27 | .80 | n.a. | 9.0 | 0 |
| oil-roasted: | | | | | | | | |
|    unblanched, 1 oz. . . . | 0 | <1 | .04 | .28 | .99 | .02 | 18.1 | 0 |
|    unblanched, whole | | | | | | | | |
|       kernels, 1 cup . . . . | 0 | 1 | .20 | 1.55 | 5.50 | .13 | 100.1 | 0 |
|    blanched, 1 oz. . . . . . | 0 | <1 | .02 | .08 | 1.11 | .03 | 18.0 | 0 |
|    blanched, whole | | | | | | | | |
|       kernels, 1 cup . . . . | 0 | 1 | .11 | .40 | 5.54 | .13 | 90.2 | 0 |
| toasted, unblanched, | | | | | | | | |
|    1 oz. . . . . . . . . . . . . . | 0 | <1 | .04 | .17 | .80 | .02 | 18.2 | 0 |
| **Almond butter:** | | | | | | | | |
| plain, 1 tbsp. . . . . . . . . . | 0 | <1 | .02 | .10 | .46 | .01 | 10.4 | 0 |
| honey and cinnamon, | | | | | | | | |
|    1 tbsp. | 0 | <1 | .02 | .10 | .46 | .01 | 10.3 | 0 |
| **Almond extract** (*Virginia* | | | | | | | | |
| *Dare*), 1 tsp. . . . . . . . . | 0 | 0 | 0 | 0 | 0 | 0 | 0 | 0 |
| **Almond paste:** | | | | | | | | |
| 1 oz. . . . . . . . . . . . . . . . | 0 | <1 | .06 | .21 | .82 | .03 | 15.8 | 0 |
| ½ cup packed . . . . . . . . | 0 | 1 | .24 | .83 | 3.28 | .11 | 63.2 | 0 |
| **Amaranth,** fresh: | | | | | | | | |
| raw, untrimmed, | | | | | | | | |
|    1 lb. . . . . . . . . . . . | 12,436 | 185 | .16 | .67 | 2.81 | n.a. | 363.7 | 0 |
| raw, trimmed, | | | | | | | | |
|    ½ cup . . . . . . . . . . . | 408 | 6 | <.01 | .02 | .09 | tr. | 11.9 | 0 |
| boiled, drained, | | | | | | | | |
|    ½ cup . . . . . . . . . . . | 1828 | 27 | .01 | .09 | .37 | tr. | n.a. | 0 |
| **Amaranth,** whole grain, | | | | | | | | |
|    1 cup . . . . . . . . . . . | n.a. | 8 | .16 | .41 | 2.51 | .44 | 95.0 | 0 |
| **Anchovy,** European, fresh, | | | | | | | | |
| meat only, raw, 1 lb. . . . . | n.a. | (0) | .25 | 1.61 | 63.6 | .65 | n.a. | 2.81 |
| **Anchovy, canned,** in olive oil: | | | | | | | | |
| drained, yield from | | | | | | | | |
|    2-oz. can . . . . . . . . . . | n.a. | (0) | .04 | .16 | 8.96 | .09 | n.a. | .40 |
|    5 medium . . . . . . . . . . . | n.a. | (0) | .02 | .07 | 3.98 | .04 | n.a. | .18 |

| | Vitamin A | Vitamin C | Thiamin | Riboflavin | Niacin | B6 | Folacin | B12 |
|---|---|---|---|---|---|---|---|---|
| | (IU) | (Mg) | (Mg) | (Mg) | (Mg) | (Mg) | (Mcg) | (Mcg) |
| **Anise extract** (*Virginia Dare*), 1 tsp. . . . . . . . | 0 | 0 | 0 | 0 | 0 | 0 | 0 | 0 |
| **Apple:** | | | | | | | | |
| fresh, cored, unpeeled: | | | | | | | | |
|   raw, untrimmed, | | | | | | | | |
|     1 lb. . . . . . . . . . . | 223 | 24 | .07 | .06 | .32 | .20 | 11.7 | 0 |
|   raw, 1 medium, 2¾" | | | | | | | | |
|   diam., approx. | | | | | | | | |
|     3 per lb. . . . . . . . | 74 | 8 | .02 | .02 | .11 | .07 | 3.9 | 0 |
|   raw, sliced, ½ cup. . . | 30 | 3 | .01 | .01 | .04 | .03 | 1.6 | 0 |
| fresh, cored, peeled: | | | | | | | | |
|   raw, sliced, ½ cup. . . | 24 | 2 | .01 | .01 | .05 | .03 | .2 | 0 |
|   raw, 1 medium, 2¾" | | | | | | | | |
|   diam., approx. | | | | | | | | |
|     3 per lb. . . . . . . . | 56 | 5 | .02 | .01 | .12 | .06 | .5 | 0 |
|   boiled, sliced, ½ cup | 38 | <1 | .01 | .01 | .08 | .04 | .5 | 0 |
|   microwaved, sliced, | | | | | | | | |
|     ½ cup. . . . . . . . . . | 34 | <1 | .01 | .01 | .05 | .04 | .5 | 0 |
| canned, sweetened, | | | | | | | | |
|   sliced: | | | | | | | | |
|     unheated, ½ cup . . . . | 52 | <1 | .01 | .01 | .07 | .05 | .3 | 0 |
|     heated, ½ cup . . . . . . | 57 | <1 | .01 | .01 | .08 | .05 | .1 | 0 |
| dehydrated, sulfured: | | | | | | | | |
|     uncooked, ½ cup. . . . | 24 | 1 | .01 | .04 | .20 | .08 | .3 | 0 |
|     cooked, ½ cup . . . . . | 18 | 1 | .01 | .03 | .14 | .05 | .1 | 0 |
| dried, sulfured: | | | | | | | | |
|     uncooked, ½ cup. . . . | 0 | 2 | 0 | .07 | .40 | .05 | n.a. | 0 |
|   uncooked, 10 rings, | | | | | | | | |
|     2.3 oz. . . . . . . . . . | 0 | 3 | 0 | .10 | .59 | .08 | n.a. | 0 |
|   cooked, unsweetened, | | | | | | | | |
|     ½ cup . . . . . . . . . | 22 | 1 | .01 | .02 | .17 | .06 | 0 | 0 |
|   cooked, sweetened, | | | | | | | | |
|     ½ cup. . . . . . . . . . | 22 | 1 | .01 | .03 | .17 | .07 | n.a. | 0 |
| frozen, unsweetened, sliced: | | | | | | | | |
|     unheated, ½ cup . . . . | 29 | <1 | .01 | .01 | .04 | .03 | .6 | 0 |
|     heated, ½ cup . . . . . . | 21 | <1 | .01 | .01 | .04 | .03 | .6 | 0 |

| | Vitamin A | Vitamin C | Thiamin | Riboflavin | Niacin | B₆ | Folacin | B₁₂ |
|---|---|---|---|---|---|---|---|---|
| | (IU) | (Mg) | (Mg) | (Mg) | (Mg) | (Mg) | (Mcg) | (Mcg) |
| **Apple butter,** 1 tbsp..... | 0 | tr. | tr. | .01 | n.a. | n.a. | 0 | 0 |
| **Apple juice**[1]: | | | | | | | | |
| canned or bottled, | | | | | | | | |
| 6 fl. oz............. | 2 | 2 | .04 | .03 | .19 | .05 | 0 | 0 |
| frozen, undiluted, | | | | | | | | |
| 6-fl.-oz. container..... | n.a. | 4 | .02 | .11 | .29 | .25 | 2.1 | 0 |
| frozen, diluted, 8 fl. oz. | n.a. | 1 | .01 | .04 | .09 | .08 | .7 | 0 |
| **Applesauce,** canned: | | | | | | | | |
| unsweetened[1], ½ cup | 35 | 2 | .02 | .03 | .23 | .03 | .7 | 0 |
| sweetened, ½ cup ...... | 14 | 2 | .02 | .04 | .24 | .03 | .7 | 0 |
| **Apricot:** | | | | | | | | |
| fresh: | | | | | | | | |
| untrimmed, 1 lb. .....11,017 | | 42 | .13 | .17 | 2.53 | .23 | 36.3 | 0 |
| 3 medium, approx. | | | | | | | | |
| 4 oz............ | 2769 | 11 | .03 | .04 | .64 | .06 | 9.1 | 0 |
| pitted, halves, ½ cup | 2024 | 8 | .02 | .03 | .47 | .04 | 6.7 | 0 |
| canned, unpeeled, halves: | | | | | | | | |
| in water, ½ cup..... | 1571 | 4 | .03 | .03 | .48 | .07 | 2.1 | 0 |
| in juice, ½ cup ..... | 2098 | 6 | .02 | .02 | .43 | n.a. | n.a. | 0 |
| in light syrup, ½ cup | 1672 | 4 | .02 | .03 | .38 | .07 | 2.2 | 0 |
| in heavy syrup, | | | | | | | | |
| ½ cup.......... | 1587 | 4 | .03 | .03 | .49 | .07 | 2.2 | 0 |
| canned, peeled, whole: | | | | | | | | |
| in water, ½ cup..... | 2055 | 2 | .02 | .03 | .50 | .06 | 2.0 | 0 |
| in heavy syrup, | | | | | | | | |
| ½ cup.......... | 1600 | 4 | .02 | .03 | .54 | .07 | 2.2 | 0 |
| in extra heavy syrup, | | | | | | | | |
| ½ cup.......... | 1809 | 3 | .02 | .03 | .42 | .07 | 2.0 | 0 |
| dehydrated, sulfured: | | | | | | | | |
| uncooked, ½ cup.... | 7601 | 6 | .03 | .09 | 2.10 | .31 | 2.7 | 0 |
| cooked, ½ cup ..... | 5465 | 9 | .02 | .08 | 2.00 | .20 | 1.9 | 0 |
| dried, sulfured, halves: | | | | | | | | |
| uncooked, 10 halves, | | | | | | | | |
| 1.2 oz........... | 2534 | 1 | tr. | .05 | 1.05 | .06 | 3.6 | 0 |

[1] *Without added ascorbic acid.*

| | Vitamin A | Vitamin C | Thiamin | Riboflavin | Niacin | B6 | Folacin | B12 |
|---|---|---|---|---|---|---|---|---|
| | (IU) | (Mg) | (Mg) | (Mg) | (Mg) | (Mg) | (Mcg) | (Mcg) |
| uncooked, ½ cup.... | 4706 | 2 | .01 | .10 | 1.94 | .10 | 4.5 | 0 |
| cooked, unsweetened, ½ cup......... | 2955 | 2 | .01 | .04 | 1.18 | .14 | 0 | 0 |
| cooked, sweetened, ½ cup......... | 2888 | 2 | .01 | .04 | 1.15 | .14 | 0 | 0 |
| frozen, sweetened, ½ cup........... | 2033 | 11 | .02 | .05 | .97 | .07 | n.a. | 0 |
| **Apricot nectar**[1], canned, 8 fl. oz............ | 3304 | 1 | .02 | .04 | .65 | n.a. | 3.3 | 0 |
| **Arrowroot flour**, 1 cup... | 0 | 0 | <.01 | 0 | 0 | .01 | 9.0 | 0 |
| **Artichoke,** globe: | | | | | | | | |
| fresh: | | | | | | | | |
| raw, untrimmed, 1 lb........... | 335 | 21 | .13 | .12 | 1.90 | .21 | 123.0 | 0 |
| boiled, drained, 1 medium, approx. 10.6 oz.... | 212 | 12 | .08 | .08 | .41 | .13 | 61.0 | 0 |
| hearts, boiled, drained, ½ cup... | 149 | 8 | .06 | .06 | .84 | .09 | 42.0 | 0 |
| frozen, hearts: | | | | | | | | |
| 9-oz. pkg......... | 392 | 13 | .15 | .36 | 2.19 | .48 | 320.2 | 0 |
| boiled, drained, ⅓ of 9-oz. pkg........ | 131 | 4 | .05 | .13 | .73 | .07 | 95.0 | 0 |
| **Arugula**, raw: | | | | | | | | |
| untrimmed, 1 lb........ | 6461 | n.a. | .12 | .23 | .83 | .20 | 265.0 | 0 |
| trimmed, ½ cup........ | 237 | n.a. | <.01 | .01 | .03 | .01 | 10.0 | 0 |
| **Asparagus:** | | | | | | | | |
| fresh: | | | | | | | | |
| raw, untrimmed, 1 lb. | 1401 | 32 | .34 | .31 | 2.81 | .32 | 308.0 | 0 |
| raw, trimmed, 4 spears, ½"-diam. base .... | 338 | 8 | .08 | .07 | .68 | .08 | 74.0 | 0 |
| raw, trimmed, cuts and spears, ½ cup .... | 390 | 9 | .09 | .09 | .78 | .09 | 86.0 | 0 |

[1] *Without added ascorbic acid.*

| | Vitamin A | Vitamin C | Thiamin | Riboflavin | Niacin | B6 | Folacin | B12 |
|---|---|---|---|---|---|---|---|---|
| | (IU) | (Mg) | (Mg) | (Mg) | (Mg) | (Mg) | (Mcg) | (Mcg) |
| **Asparagus, fresh,** *continued* | | | | | | | | |
| boiled, drained, | | | | | | | | |
| 4 spears . . . . . . . . | 323 | 7 | .07 | .08 | .65 | .07 | 88.0 | 0 |
| boiled, drained, | | | | | | | | |
| ½ cup . . . . . . . . . | 485 | 10 | .11 | .11 | .97 | .11 | 132.0 | 0 |
| canned, w/liquid, | | | | | | | | |
| ½ cup . . . . . . . . . . . | 578 | 20 | .07 | .11 | 1.04 | .12 | 104.1 | 0 |
| frozen: | | | | | | | | |
| 10-oz. pkg. . . . . . . . | 2692 | 90 | .34 | .37 | 3.41 | .32 | 541.7 | 0 |
| boiled, drained, ⅓ of | | | | | | | | |
| 10-oz. pkg. . . . . . . | 799 | 24 | .06 | .10 | 1.01 | .02 | 131,5 | 0 |
| boiled, drained, | | | | | | | | |
| 4 spears . . . . . . . . | 491 | 15 | .04 | .06 | .62 | .01 | 80.8 | 0 |
| **Avocado:** | | | | | | | | |
| California: | | | | | | | | |
| untrimmed, 1 lb. . . . . | 2109 | 27 | .37 | .42 | 6.62 | .97 | 225.8 | 0 |
| 1 medium, approx. | | | | | | | | |
| 8 oz. . . . . . . . . . . . | 1059 | 14 | .19 | .21 | 3.32 | .48 | 113.3 | 0 |
| pureed, ½ cup . . . . . . | 704 | 9 | .12 | .14 | 2.20 | .32 | 75.4 | 0 |
| Florida, 1 medium, | | | | | | | | |
| approx. 1 lb. | | | | | | | | |
| untrimmed . . . . . . . . . | 1860 | 24 | .33 | .37 | 5.80 | .85 | 161.9 | 0 |
| Florida, pureed, ½ cup . . . | 704 | 9 | .12 | .14 | 2.20 | .32 | 61.3 | 0 |

# B

| | Vitamin A (IU) | Vitamin C (Mg) | Thiamin (Mg) | Riboflavin (Mg) | Niacin (Mg) | B₆ (Mg) | Folacin (Mcg) | B₁₂ (Mcg) |
|---|---|---|---|---|---|---|---|---|
| **Bacon**[1], cooked, 3 medium slices, 20 per lb. . . . . . . . . | 0 | 6 | .13 | .05 | 1.39 | .05 | 1.0 | .33 |
| **Bacon, Canadian-style**[1]: | | | | | | | | |
| unheated, 1-oz. slice . . . . | 0 | 6 | .21 | .05 | 1.77 | .44 | 4.5 | .76 |
| grilled, 2 slices, yield from 2 unheated 1-oz. slices . . . . . . . . | 0 | 10 | .38 | .09 | 3.22 | .21 | 2.0 | .36 |
| **Bacon, substitute:** | | | | | | | | |
| beef[2], heated, 3 strips, 1.2 oz. . . . . . . . . . . . . | 0 | 12 | .03 | .09 | 2.20 | .11 | n.a. | 1.17 |
| pork[1], cured, heated, 3 strips, 15 per 12-oz. pkg. . . . . . . . . | 0 | 15 | .25 | .13 | 2.58 | .12 | 1.0 | .60 |
| **"Bacon," vegetarian, frozen:** | | | | | | | | |
| .3-oz. strip . . . . . . . . . . . | 7 | 0 | .35 | .04 | .61 | .04 | 3.3 | 0 |
| (*Morningstar Farms* Breakfast Strips), .6-oz. strip . . . . . . . . . . . | 0 | 0 | .75 | .04 | .60 | .07 | n.a. | .39 |
| (*Worthington Stripples*), .6-oz. strip | 0 | 0 | .75 | .04 | .60 | .07 | n.a. | .39 |
| **Bagel,** 3½"-diam. piece, except as noted: | | | | | | | | |
| plain or water . . . . . . . . . | 0 | 0 | .38 | .22 | 3.24 | .04 | 16.0 | 0 |
| plain or water, toasted . . . | 0 | 0 | .31 | .20 | 2.91 | .03 | 11.0 | 0 |
| cinnamon-raisin . . . . . . . . | 52 | 1 | .27 | .20 | 2.19 | n.a. | n.a. | 0 |
| cinnamon-raisin, toasted | 47 | tr. | .22 | .18 | 1.2 | n.a. | n.a. | 0 |
| egg . . . . . . . . . . . . . . . . | 77 | tr. | .38 | .17 | 2.44 | .06 | 16.0 | .11 |
| egg, toasted. . . . . . . . . . | 70 | tr. | .3 | .15 | 2.2 | .06 | 11.0 | .11 |
| oat bran | 3 | tr. | .24 | .24 | 2.1 | n.a. | n.a. | 0 |

[1] *With added ascorbic acid or sodium ascorbate; vitamin C value for product without additives would be negligible.*
[2] *With added sodium ascorbate.*

| | Vitamin A | Vitamin C | Thiamin | Riboflavin | Niacin | B6 | Folacin | B12 |
|---|---|---|---|---|---|---|---|---|
| | (IU) | (Mg) | (Mg) | (Mg) | (Mg) | (Mg) | (Mcg) | (Mcg) |
| **Bagel,** *continued* | | | | | | | | |
| oat bran, toasted . . . . . . . | 3 | tr. | .19 | .22 | 1.89 | n.a. | n.a. | 0 |
| (*Roman Meal* Original), | | | | | | | | |
| 1 piece . . . . . . . . . . . . | 0 | 0 | .48 | .31 | 4.88 | n.a. | n.a. | n.a. |
| **Baked beans,** canned: | | | | | | | | |
| (*Grandma Brown's*), | | | | | | | | |
| ½ cup . . . . . . . . . . . . | 115 | 4 | .06 | .05 | .40 | n.a. | n.a. | n.a. |
| (*Grandma Brown's* | | | | | | | | |
| Saucepan), ½ cup . . . . | 811 | 2 | .06 | .05 | .34 | n.a. | n.a. | n.a. |
| plain or vegetarian, | | | | | | | | |
| 8 oz. . . . . . . . . . . . . . | 388 | n.a. | .35 | .14 | .97 | .22 | 54.2 | 0 |
| plain or vegetarian, | | | | | | | | |
| ½ cup . . . . . . . . . . . . | 217 | n.a. | .19 | .08 | .54 | .17 | 30.4 | 0 |
| w/beef, 8 oz. . . . . . . . . . | 482 | 4 | .12 | .10 | 1.07 | .20 | n.a. | .57 |
| w/beef, ½ cup . . . . . . . . | 283 | 2 | .07 | .60 | 1.25 | .12 | n.a. | .33 |
| w/franks, 8 oz. . . . . . . . . | 349 | 5 | .13 | .13 | 2.04 | .10 | 68.1 | .77 |
| w/franks, ½ cup . . . . . . . | 197 | 3 | .07 | .07 | 1.15 | .06 | 38.4 | .44 |
| w/pork: | | | | | | | | |
| 8 oz. . . . . . . . . . . . . . | 405 | 4 | .12 | .09 | 1.01 | .15 | 82.4 | .05 |
| ½ cup . . . . . . . . . . . . | 225 | 3 | .07 | .05 | .56 | .08 | 45.8 | .03 |
| and sweet sauce, | | | | | | | | |
| 8 oz. . . . . . . . . . . . . | 259 | 7 | .11 | .14 | .80 | .18 | 84.7 | .05 |
| and sweet sauce, | | | | | | | | |
| ½ cup . . . . . . . . . . | 144 | 4 | .06 | .08 | .44 | .11 | 47.1 | .03 |
| and tomato sauce, | | | | | | | | |
| 8 oz. . . . . . . . . . . . . | 281 | 7 | .12 | .10 | 1.13 | .16 | 51.0 | .03 |
| and tomato sauce, | | | | | | | | |
| ½ cup . . . . . . . . . . | 156 | 4 | .07 | .06 | .63 | .09 | 28.3 | .02 |
| **Baking powder,** all types, | | | | | | | | |
| 1 tsp. . . . . . . . . . . . . | 0 | 0 | 0 | 0 | 0 | 0 | 0 | 0 |
| **Baking soda,** 1 tsp. . . . . . | 0 | 0 | 0 | 0 | 0 | 0 | 0 | 0 |
| **Balsam pear,** fresh: | | | | | | | | |
| leafy tips: | | | | | | | | |
| raw, untrimmed, | | | | | | | | |
| 1 lb. . . . . . . . . . . . | 2989 | 152 | .31 | .62 | 1.91 | n.a. | n.a. | 0 |

|  | Vitamin A | Vitamin C | Thiamin | Riboflavin | Niacin | B6 | Folacin | B12 |
|---|---|---|---|---|---|---|---|---|
|  | (IU) | (Mg) | (Mg) | (Mg) | (Mg) | (Mg) | (Mcg) | (Mcg) |
| raw, trimmed, ½ cup | 416 | 21 | .04 | .09 | .27 | n.a. | n.a. | 0 |
| boiled, drained, ½ cup.......... | 503 | 16 | .04 | .08 | .29 | .22 | 25.4 | 0 |
| pods: |  |  |  |  |  |  |  |  |
| raw, untrimmed, 1 lb............ | 1431 | 316 | .15 | .15 | 1.51 | n.a. | 316.3 | 0 |
| raw, trimmed, ½" pieces, ½ cup | 353 | 78 | .04 | .04 | .37 | n.a. | 67.0 | 0 |
| boiled, drained, ½" pieces, ½ cup | 70 | 21 | .03 | .03 | .17 | n.a. | n.a. | 0 |
| **Bamboo shoots:** |  |  |  |  |  |  |  |  |
| fresh: |  |  |  |  |  |  |  |  |
| raw, untrimmed, 1 lb............ | 26 | 5 | .20 | .09 | .79 | n.a. | n.a. | 0 |
| raw, trimmed, ½" slices, ½ cup | 15 | 3 | .11 | .05 | .46 | n.a. | n.a. | 0 |
| boiled, drained, ½" slices, ½ cup | 0 | 0 | .01 | .03 | .18 | n.a. | n.a. | 0 |
| canned, drained, ⅛" slices, ½ cup | 11 | 1 | .03 | .03 | .18 | n.a. | n.a. | 0 |
| **Banana:** |  |  |  |  |  |  |  |  |
| fresh: |  |  |  |  |  |  |  |  |
| untrimmed, 1 lb..... | 239 | 28 | .13 | .30 | 1.59 | 1.70 | 56.4 | 0 |
| 1 medium, 8¾" long, 6.2 oz. untrimmed | 92 | 10 | .05 | .11 | .62 | .66 | 21.8 | 0 |
| peeled, mashed, ½ cup.......... | 91 | 10 | .05 | .11 | .61 | .65 | 21.5 | 0 |
| dehydrated or powdered, 1 oz.............. | 87 | 2 | .05 | .07 | .79 | n.a. | n.a. | 0 |
| dehydrated or powdered, 1 tbsp. ............ | 19 | <1 | .01 | .02 | .17 | n.a. | n.a. | 0 |
| **Banana, baking,** see "Plantain" |  |  |  |  |  |  |  |  |
| **Banana chips,** 1 oz. .... | n.a. | 2 | .02 | .01 | .2 | .07 | 4.0 | 0 |

| | Vitamin A | Vitamin C | Thiamin | Riboflavin | Niacin | B₆ | Folacin | B₁₂ |
|---|---|---|---|---|---|---|---|---|
| | (IU) | (Mg) | (Mg) | (Mg) | (Mg) | (Mg) | (Mcg) | (Mcg) |
| **Barbecue loaf**[1], pork and beef, 1 oz.......... | n.a. | 5 | .10 | .07 | .64 | .07 | n.a. | .48 |
| **Barbecue sauce:** | | | | | | | | |
| 1 cup ............... | 2170 | 18 | .08 | .05 | 2.25 | .19 | n.a. | 0 |
| 1 tbsp. ............. | 139 | 1 | .01 | <.01 | .14 | .01 | n.a. | 0 |
| **Barbecue seasoning** (*Tone's Perc*), ¼ tsp. | 208 | tr. | tr. | .01 | .07 | .02 | .2 | 0 |
| **Barley:** | | | | | | | | |
| uncooked, 1 cup ....... | n.a. | 0 | 1.19 | .53 | n.a. | .59 | 35.0 | 0 |
| pearled, uncooked, 1 cup ............. | 44 | 0 | .38 | .23 | 9.21 | .52 | 46.0 | 0 |
| pearled, cooked, 1 cup... | n.a. | 0 | .13 | .10 | 3.24 | .18 | 26.0 | 0 |
| **Basil,** ground, 1 tsp..... | 131 | 1 | <.01 | <.01 | .10 | n.a. | n.a. | 0 |
| **Bay leaf,** crumbled, 1 tsp. ............. | 37 | <1 | tr. | <.01 | .01 | n.a. | n.a. | 0 |
| **Bean sprouts,** see specific listings | | | | | | | | |
| **Beans,** see specific listings | | | | | | | | |
| **Beef,** retail trim[2], meat only[3], 4 oz.: | | | | | | | | |
| brisket, whole, all grades, braised: | | | | | | | | |
| lean and fat (trimmed to ¼") .......... | 0 | 0 | .07 | .20 | 3.40 | .27 | 6.8 | 2.59 |
| lean and fat (trimmed to 0") .......... | 0 | 0 | .08 | .23 | 3.82 | .31 | 7.9 | 2.78 |
| lean only .......... | 0 | 0 | .08 | .25 | 4.21 | .33 | 9.1 | 2.95 |
| brisket, flat half, all grades, braised: | | | | | | | | |
| lean and fat (trimmed to ¼") .......... | 0 | 0 | .07 | .20 | 3.56 | .29 | 6.8 | 2.63 |

---

[1] *With added sodium ascorbate; vitamin C value for product without additive would be negligible.*
[2] *Meat trimmed to 0" or ¼" fat refers to amount of fat present during cooking. For "lean only" listings, all visible fat is trimmed after cooking. (Bear in mind that a small amount of fat is always present, even in meat trimmed to 0" fat before cooking.)*
[3] *Prepared without added ingredients, except as noted.*

| | Vitamin A | Vitamin C | Thiamin | Riboflavin | Niacin | B6 | Folacin | B12 |
|---|---|---|---|---|---|---|---|---|
| | (IU) | (Mg) | (Mg) | (Mg) | (Mg) | (Mg) | (Mcg) | (Mcg) |
| lean and fat (trimmed to 0")........... | 0 | 0 | .08 | .24 | 4.24 | .34 | 9.1 | 2.93 |
| lean only.......... | 0 | 0 | .08 | .25 | 4.38 | .35 | 9.1 | 2.98 |
| brisket, point half, all grades, braised: | | | | | | | | |
| lean and fat (trimmed to ¼").......... | 0 | 0 | .07 | .20 | 3.27 | .26 | 6.8 | 2.55 |
| lean and fat (trimmed to 0")........... | 0 | 0 | .07 | .22 | 3.45 | .27 | 7.9 | 2.64 |
| lean only.......... | 0 | 0 | .08 | .26 | 4.05 | .32 | 9.1 | 2.93 |
| chuck, arm pot roast, choice grade, braised: | | | | | | | | |
| lean and fat (trimmed to ¼").......... | 0 | 0 | .08 | .27 | 3.55 | .32 | 10.2 | 3.31 |
| lean and fat (trimmed to 0")........... | 0 | 0 | .08 | .29 | 3.82 | .34 | 11.3 | 3.54 |
| lean only.......... | 0 | 0 | .09 | .33 | 4.22 | .37 | 12.5 | 3.85 |
| chuck, arm pot roast, select grade, braised: | | | | | | | | |
| lean and fat (trimmed to ¼").......... | 0 | 0 | .08 | .27 | 3.65 | .33 | 10.2 | 3.39 |
| lean and fat (trimmed to 0")........... | 0 | 0 | .08 | .29 | 3.90 | .35 | 11.3 | 3.59 |
| lean only.......... | 0 | 0 | .09 | .33 | 4.22 | .37 | 12.5 | 3.86 |
| chuck, blade roast, choice grade, braised: | | | | | | | | |
| lean and fat (trimmed to ¼").......... | 0 | 0 | .08 | .27 | 2.72 | .28 | 5.7 | 2.57 |
| lean and fat (trimmed to 0")........... | 0 | 0 | .08 | .28 | 2.77 | .29 | 5.7 | 2.61 |
| lean only.......... | 0 | 0 | .09 | .32 | 3.03 | .33 | 6.8 | 2.80 |
| chuck, blade roast, select grade, braised: | | | | | | | | |
| lean and fat (trimmed to ¼").......... | 0 | 0 | .08 | .28 | 2.77 | .29 | 5.7 | 2.61 |
| lean and fat (trimmed to 0")........... | 0 | 0 | .08 | .28 | 2.81 | .29 | 5.7 | 2.64 |
| lean only.......... | 0 | 0 | .09 | .32 | 3.03 | .33 | 6.8 | 2.80 |

| | Vitamin A | Vitamin C | Thiamin | Riboflavin | Niacin | B6 | Folacin | B12 |
|---|---|---|---|---|---|---|---|---|
| | (IU) | (Mg) | (Mg) | (Mg) | (Mg) | (Mg) | (Mcg) | (Mcg) |

Beef, *continued*
flank, choice grade:
 braised, lean and fat

| | | | | | | | | |
|---|---|---|---|---|---|---|---|---|
| (trimmed to 0") . . . | 0 | 0 | .16 | .20 | 5.01 | .4 | 10.2 | 3.74 |
| braised, lean only. . . . | 0 | 0 | .16 | .22 | 5.22 | .41 | 10.2 | 3.87 |
| broiled, lean and fat | | | | | | | | |
| (trimmed to 0") . . . | 0 | 0 | .11 | .20 | 5.56 | .39 | 9.1 | 3.62 |
| broiled, lean only . . . . | 0 | 0 | .12 | .22 | 5.70 | .39 | 9.1 | 3.69 |
| ground, extra lean: | | | | | | | | |
| baked, medium . . . . . | 0 | 0 | .05 | .27 | 4.72 | .25 | 10.2 | 1.96 |
| baked, well-done . . . . | 0 | 0 | .06 | .35 | 6.13 | .33 | 12.5 | 2.11 |
| broiled, medium. . . . . | 0 | 0 | .07 | .31 | 5.62 | .31 | 10.2 | 2.46 |
| broiled, well-done . . . | 0 | 0 | .08 | .36 | 6.63 | .36 | 12.5 | 2.90 |
| pan-fried, medium . . . | 0 | 0 | .07 | .29 | 5.34 | .31 | 10.2 | 2.27 |
| pan-fried, well-done | 0 | 0 | .08 | .34 | 6.17 | .35 | 11.3 | 2.63 |
| ground, lean: | | | | | | | | |
| baked, medium . . . . . | 0 | 0 | .06 | .22 | 4.85 | .23 | 10.2 | 2.01 |
| baked, well-done . . . . | 0 | 0 | .08 | .27 | 6.19 | .29 | 13.6 | 2.56 |
| broiled, medium. . . . . | 0 | 0 | .06 | .24 | 5.85 | .29 | 10.2 | 2.66 |
| broiled, well-done . . . | 0 | 0 | .07 | .27 | 6.77 | .34 | 12.5 | 3.08 |
| pan-fried, medium . . . | 0 | 0 | .06 | .25 | 5.43 | .32 | 10.2 | 2.57 |
| pan-fried, well-done | 0 | 0 | .07 | .27 | 6.18 | .36 | 11.3 | 2.93 |
| ground, regular: | | | | | | | | |
| baked, medium . . . . . | 0 | 0 | .03 | .18 | 5.39 | .26 | 10.2 | 2.65 |
| baked, well-done . . . . | 0 | 0 | .05 | .23 | 6.68 | .33 | 12.5 | 3.29 |
| broiled, medium. . . . . | 0 | 0 | .03 | .22 | 6.54 | .31 | 10.2 | 3.32 |
| broiled, well-done . . . | 0 | 0 | .05 | .24 | 7.34 | .34 | 11.3 | 3.72 |
| pan-fried, medium . . . | 0 | 0 | .03 | .23 | 6.61 | .27 | 10.2 | 3.07 |
| pan-fried, well-done | 0 | 0 | .05 | .24 | 7.33 | .31 | 11.3 | 3.40 |
| ground, frozen patties, | | | | | | | | |
| broiled, medium. . . . . . | 0 | 0 | .06 | .23 | 5.98 | .29 | 10.2 | 2.80 |
| porterhouse steak (short loin), choice grade, broiled: | | | | | | | | |
| lean and fat | | | | | | | | |
| (trimmed to ¼") . . . | 0 | 0 | .11 | .25 | 4.59 | .40 | 7.9 | 2.44 |
| lean only . . . . . . . . . . | 0 | 0 | .12 | .28 | 5.25 | .45 | 9.1 | 2.57 |

| | Vitamin A | Vitamin C | Thiamin | Riboflavin | Niacin | B₆ | Folacin | B₁₂ |
|---|---|---|---|---|---|---|---|---|
| | (IU) | (Mg) | (Mg) | (Mg) | (Mg) | (Mg) | (Mcg) | (Mcg) |

| | | | | | | | | |
|---|---|---|---|---|---|---|---|---|
| rib, whole (ribs 6–12), choice grade: | | | | | | | | |
| broiled, lean and fat | | | | | | | | |
|   (trimmed to ¼")... | 0 | 0 | .09 | .19 | 3.64 | .31 | 6.8 | 3.22 |
| broiled, lean only.... | 0 | 0 | .10 | .23 | 4.35 | .36 | 7.9 | 3.76 |
| roasted, lean and fat | | | | | | | | |
|   (trimmed to ¼")... | 0 | 0 | .08 | .19 | 3.81 | .26 | 7.9 | 2.86 |
| roasted, lean only ... | 0 | 0 | .09 | .24 | 4.72 | .31 | 9.1 | 3.30 |
| rib, whole (ribs 6–12), prime grade: | | | | | | | | |
| broiled, lean and fat | | | | | | | | |
|   (trimmed to ¼")... | 0 | 0 | .09 | .19 | 3.57 | .33 | 6.8 | 3.20 |
| broiled, lean only.... | 0 | 0 | .10 | .24 | 4.29 | .40 | 7.9 | 3.72 |
| roasted, lean and fat | | | | | | | | |
|   (trimmed to ¼")... | 0 | 0 | .08 | .19 | 3.79 | .29 | 7.9 | 2.87 |
| roasted, lean only ... | 0 | 0 | .09 | .24 | 4.66 | .34 | 10.2 | 3.31 |
| rib, whole (ribs 6–12), select grade: | | | | | | | | |
| broiled, lean and fat | | | | | | | | |
|   (trimmed to ¼")... | 0 | 0 | .09 | .19 | 3.73 | .31 | 6.8 | 3.29 |
| broiled, lean only.... | 0 | 0 | .10 | .23 | 4.35 | .36 | 7.9 | 3.76 |
| roasted, lean and fat | | | | | | | | |
|   (trimmed to ¼")... | 0 | 0 | .08 | .20 | 3.93 | .26 | 7.9 | 2.91 |
| roasted, lean only ... | 0 | 0 | .09 | .24 | 4.72 | .31 | 9.1 | 3.29 |
| rib, large end (ribs 6–9), choice grade: | | | | | | | | |
| broiled, lean and fat | | | | | | | | |
|   (trimmed to ¼")... | 0 | 0 | .08 | .18 | 3.07 | .26 | 6.8 | 3.20 |
| broiled, lean only.... | 0 | 0 | .09 | .22 | 3.61 | .29 | 7.9 | 3.75 |
| roasted, lean and fat | | | | | | | | |
|   (trimmed to ¼")... | 0 | 0 | .08 | .20 | 4.03 | .25 | 7.9 | 2.61 |
| roasted, lean and fat | | | | | | | | |
|   (trimmed to 0")... | 0 | 0 | .08 | .22 | 4.13 | .26 | 7.9 | 2.64 |
| roasted, lean only ... | 0 | 0 | .10 | .25 | 5.05 | .29 | 10.2 | 2.96 |
| rib, large end (ribs 6–9), prime grade: | | | | | | | | |
| broiled, lean and fat | | | | | | | | |
|   (trimmed to ¼")... | 0 | 0 | .08 | .19 | 2.95 | .29 | 6.8 | 3.12 |
| broiled, lean only.... | 0 | 0 | .10 | .23 | 3.48 | .36 | 7.9 | 3.70 |
| roasted, lean and fat | | | | | | | | |
|   (trimmed to ¼")... | 0 | 0 | .08 | .20 | 4.06 | .25 | 7.9 | 2.62 |

| | Vitamin A | Vitamin C | Thiamin | Riboflavin | Niacin | B6 | Folacin | B12 |
|---|---|---|---|---|---|---|---|---|
| | (IU) | (Mg) | (Mg) | (Mg) | (Mg) | (Mg) | (Mcg) | (Mcg) |

Beef, rib, large end, prime grade, *continued*
| roasted, lean only . . . | 0 | 0 | .10 | .25 | 5.05 | .29 | 10.2 | 2.96 |

rib, large end (ribs 6–9), select grade:
broiled, lean and fat
| (trimmed to ¼") . . . | 0 | 0 | .08 | .18 | 3.15 | .26 | 6.8 | 3.28 |
| broiled, lean only . . . . | 0 | 0 | .09 | .22 | 3.61 | .29 | 7.9 | 3.75 |
roasted, lean and fat
| (trimmed to ¼") . . . | 0 | 0 | .08 | .22 | 4.20 | .26 | 7.9 | 2.66 |
roasted, lean and fat
| (trimmed to 0") . . . | 0 | 0 | .08 | .22 | 4.25 | .26 | 9.1 | 2.69 |
| roasted, lean only . . . | 0 | 0 | .10 | .25 | 5.05 | .29 | 10.2 | 2.96 |

rib, shortrib, choice grade:
| braised, lean and fat | 0 | 0 | .06 | .17 | 2.78 | .25 | 5.7 | 2.97 |
| braised, lean only . . . . | 0 | 0 | .07 | .23 | 3.64 | .32 | 7.9 | 3.92 |

rib, small end (ribs 10–12), choice grade:
broiled, lean and fat
| (trimmed to ¼") . . . | 0 | 0 | .10 | .20 | 4.49 | .37 | 7.9 | 3.27 |
broiled, lean and fat
| (trimmed to 0") . . . | 0 | 0 | .10 | .22 | 4.74 | .40 | 7.9 | 3.40 |
| broiled, lean only . . . . | 0 | 0 | .11 | .25 | 5.44 | .45 | 9.1 | 3.76 |
roasted, lean and fat
| (trimmed to ¼") . . . | 0 | 0 | .07 | .18 | 3.50 | .27 | 6.8 | 3.20 |
| roasted, lean only . . . | 0 | 0 | .08 | .22 | 4.24 | .32 | 9.1 | 3.78 |

rib, small end (ribs 10–12), prime grade:
broiled, lean and fat
| (trimmed to ¼") . . . | 0 | 0 | .10 | .22 | .4.56 | .39 | 7.9 | 3.30 |
| broiled, lean only . . . . | 0 | 0 | .11 | .25 | 5.44 | .45 | 9.1 | 3.76 |
roasted, lean and fat
| (trimmed to ¼") . . . | 0 | 0 | .07 | .18 | 3.41 | .34 | 6.8 | 3.22 |
| roasted, lean only . . . | 0 | 0 | .09 | .22 | 4.12 | .42 | 9.1 | 3.82 |

rib, small end (ribs 10–12), select grade:
broiled, lean and fat
| (trimmed to ¼") . . . | 0 | 0 | .10 | .22 | 4.56 | .39 | 7.9 | 3.30 |
broiled, lean and fat
| (trimmed to 0") . . . | 0 | 0 | .10 | .22 | 4.79 | .40 | 7.9 | 3.41 |
| broiled, lean only . . . . | 0 | 0 | .11 | .25 | 5.44 | .45 | 9.1 | 3.76 |

| | Vitamin A | Vitamin C | Thiamin | Riboflavin | Niacin | B6 | Folacin | B12 |
|---|---|---|---|---|---|---|---|---|
| | (IU) | (Mg) | (Mg) | (Mg) | (Mg) | (Mg) | (Mcg) | (Mcg) |
| roasted, lean and fat | | | | | | | | |
| (trimmed to ¼")... | 0 | 0 | .07 | .18 | 3.57 | .27 | 6.8 | 3.25 |
| roasted, lean only ... | 0 | 0 | .08 | .22 | 4.24 | .32 | 9.1 | 3.78 |
| rib eye, small end (ribs 10–12), choice grade, broiled: | | | | | | | | |
| lean and fat (trimmed | | | | | | | | |
| to 0")........... | 0 | 0 | .10 | .22 | 4.79 | .40 | 7.9 | 3.41 |
| lean only .......... | 0 | 0 | .11 | .25 | 5.44 | .45 | 9.1 | 3.76 |
| round, full cut, choice grade: | | | | | | | | |
| broiled, lean and fat | | | | | | | | |
| (trimmed to ¼")... | 0 | 0 | .10 | .24 | 4.52 | .43 | 10.2 | 3.41 |
| broiled, lean only.... | 0 | 0 | .11 | .25 | 4.83 | .45 | 11.3 | 3.59 |
| round, full cut, select grade: | | | | | | | | |
| broiled, lean and fat | | | | | | | | |
| (trimmed to ¼")... | 0 | 0 | .10 | .24 | 4.54 | .43 | 10.2 | 3.42 |
| broiled, lean only.... | 0 | 0 | .11 | .25 | 4.84 | .46 | 11.3 | 3.59 |
| round, bottom, choice grade: | | | | | | | | |
| braised, lean and fat | | | | | | | | |
| (trimmed to ¼")... | 0 | 0 | .08 | .27 | 4.23 | .37 | 11.3 | 2.66 |
| braised, lean and fat | | | | | | | | |
| (trimmed to 0") ... | 0 | 0 | .08 | .28 | 4.55 | .40 | 12.5 | 2.77 |
| braised, lean only.... | 0 | 0 | .08 | .29 | 4.63 | .41 | 12.5 | 2.80 |
| roasted, lean and fat | | | | | | | | |
| (trimmed to ¼")... | 0 | 0 | .09 | .25 | 4.25 | .39 | 12.5 | 2.90 |
| roasted, lean and fat | | | | | | | | |
| (trimmed to 0") ... | 0 | 0 | .09 | .27 | 4.56 | .42 | 13.6 | 3.04 |
| roasted, lean only ... | 0 | 0 | .09 | .27 | 4.62 | .42 | 13.6 | 3.06 |
| round, bottom, select grade: | | | | | | | | |
| braised, lean and fat | | | | | | | | |
| (trimmed to ¼")... | 0 | 0 | .08 | .27 | 4.25 | .37 | 11.3 | 2.68 |
| braised, lean and fat | | | | | | | | |
| (trimmed to 0") ... | 0 | 0 | .08 | .29 | 4.57 | .41 | 12.5 | 2.78 |
| braised, lean only.... | 0 | 0 | .08 | .29 | 4.63 | .41 | 12.5 | 2.80 |
| roasted, lean and fat | | | | | | | | |
| (trimmed to ¼")... | 0 | 0 | .09 | .26 | 4.31 | .40 | 12.5 | 2.93 |
| roasted, lean and fat | | | | | | | | |
| (trimmed to 0") ... | 0 | 0 | .09 | .27 | 4.59 | .42 | 13.6 | 3.05 |

| | Vitamin A | Vitamin C | Thiamin | Riboflavin | Niacin | B₆ | Folacin | B₁₂ |
|---|---|---|---|---|---|---|---|---|
| | (IU) | (Mg) | (Mg) | (Mg) | (Mg) | (Mg) | (Mcg) | (Mcg) |

Beef, round, bottom, select grade, *continued*

| | Vitamin A | Vitamin C | Thiamin | Riboflavin | Niacin | B₆ | Folacin | B₁₂ |
|---|---|---|---|---|---|---|---|---|
| roasted, lean only . . . | 0 | 0 | .09 | .27 | 4.62 | .42 | 13.6 | 3.06 |
| round, eye of, choice grade, roasted: | | | | | | | | |
| lean and fat (trimmed to ¼") . . . . . . . . . | 0 | 0 | .09 | .18 | 3.93 | .40 | 6.8 | 2.38 |
| lean and fat (trimmed to 0") . . . . . . . . . . | 0 | 0 | .10 | .19 | 4.23 | .43 | 7.9 | 2.45 |
| lean only . . . . . . . . . . | 0 | 0 | .10 | .19 | 4.25 | .43 | 7.9 | 2.46 |
| round, eye of, select grade, roasted: | | | | | | | | |
| lean and fat (trimmed to ¼") . . . . . . . . . | 0 | 0 | .09 | .18 | 3.98 | .40 | 7.9 | 2.39 |
| lean and fat (trimmed to 0") . . . . . . . . . . | 0 | 0 | .10 | .19 | 4.23 | .43 | 7.9 | 2.45 |
| lean only . . . . . . . . . . | 0 | 0 | .10 | .19 | 4.25 | .43 | 7.9 | 2.46 |
| round, tip, choice grade, roasted: | | | | | | | | |
| lean and fat (trimmed to ¼") . . . . . . . . . . | 0 | 0 | .10 | .28 | 3.95 | .42 | 7.9 | 3.11 |
| lean and fat (trimmed to 0") . . . . . . . . . . | 0 | 0 | .11 | .29 | 4.14 | .44 | 9.1 | 3.22 |
| lean only . . . . . . . . . . | 0 | 0 | .11 | .31 | 4.24 | .45 | 9.1 | 3.28 |
| round, tip, prime grade, roasted: | | | | | | | | |
| lean and fat (trimmed to ¼") . . . . . . . . . . | 0 | 0 | .10 | .27 | 3.92 | .42 | 7.9 | 3.08 |
| lean only . . . . . . . . . . | 0 | 0 | .11 | .31 | 4.24 | .45 | 9.1 | 3.28 |
| round, tip, select grade, roasted: | | | | | | | | |
| lean and fat (trimmed to ¼") . . . . . . . . . . | 0 | 0 | .10 | .28 | 4.01 | .43 | 9.1 | 3.15 |
| lean and fat (trimmed to 0") . . . . . . . . . . | 0 | 0 | .11 | .29 | 4.16 | .44 | 9.1 | 3.23 |
| lean only . . . . . . . . . . | 0 | 0 | .11 | .31 | 4.24 | .45 | 9.1 | 3.28 |
| round, top, choice grade: | | | | | | | | |
| braised, lean and fat (trimmed to ¼") . . . | 0 | 0 | .08 | .27 | 4.06 | .31 | 10.2 | 2.94 |
| braised, lean and fat (trimmed to 0") . . . | 0 | 0 | .08 | .28 | 4.26 | .32 | 10.2 | 3.04 |
| braised, lean only. . . . | 0 | 0 | .08 | .28 | 4.32 | .32 | 10.2 | 3.06 |

| | Vitamin A | Vitamin C | Thiamin | Riboflavin | Niacin | B6 | Folacin | B12 |
|---|---|---|---|---|---|---|---|---|
| | (IU) | (Mg) | (Mg) | (Mg) | (Mg) | (Mg) | (Mcg) | (Mcg) |
| broiled, lean and fat (trimmed to ¼")... | 0 | 0 | .12 | .29 | 6.48 | .60 | 12.5 | 2.74 |
| broiled, lean only.... | 0 | 0 | .14 | .31 | 6.85 | .64 | 13.6 | 2.81 |
| pan-fried in vegetable oil, lean and fat (trimmed to ¼")... | 0 | 0 | .11 | .29 | 5.73 | .64 | 13.6 | 3.66 |
| pan-fried in vegetable oil, lean only..... | 0 | 0 | .12 | .32 | 6.21 | .69 | 14.7 | 3.89 |
| round, top, prime grade: | | | | | | | | |
| broiled, lean and fat (trimmed to ¼")... | 0 | 0 | .14 | .29 | 6.69 | .62 | 13.6 | 2.78 |
| broiled, lean only.... | 0 | 0 | .14 | .31 | 6.85 | .64 | 13.6 | 2.81 |
| round, top, select grade: | | | | | | | | |
| braised, lean and fat (trimmed to ¼")... | 0 | 0 | .08 | .27 | 4.12 | .31 | 10.2 | 2.96 |
| braised, lean and fat (trimmed to 0")... | 0 | 0 | .08 | .28 | 4.26 | .32 | 10.2 | 3.04 |
| braised, lean only.... | 0 | 0 | .08 | .28 | 4.32 | .32 | 10.2 | 3.06 |
| broiled, lean and fat (trimmed to ¼")... | 0 | 0 | .12 | .29 | 6.48 | .60 | 12.5 | 2.74 |
| broiled, lean only.... | 0 | 0 | .14 | .31 | 6.85 | .64 | 13.6 | 2.81 |
| shank, crosscuts, choice grade: | | | | | | | | |
| simmered, lean and fat (trimmed to ¼") | 0 | 0 | .14 | .23 | 6.04 | .39 | 10.2 | 3.98 |
| simmered, lean only | 0 | 0 | .16 | .24 | 6.68 | .42 | 11.3 | 4.30 |
| short loin, see "porterhouse steak," above, and "T-bone steak" and "top loin," below | | | | | | | | |
| sirloin, top, choice grade: | | | | | | | | |
| broiled, lean and fat (trimmed to ¼")... | 0 | 0 | .12 | .31 | 4.42 | .46 | 10.2 | 3.04 |
| broiled, lean and fat (trimmed to 0")... | 0 | 0 | .14 | .32 | 4.67 | .49 | 11.3 | 3.15 |
| broiled, lean only.... | 0 | 0 | .15 | .33 | 4.85 | .51 | 11.3 | 3.23 |
| pan-fried in vegetable oil, lean and fat (trimmed to ¼")... | 0 | 0 | .14 | .32 | 4.25 | .49 | 10.2 | 3.72 |

| | Vitamin A | Vitamin C | Thiamin | Riboflavin | Niacin | B6 | Folacin | B12 |
|---|---|---|---|---|---|---|---|---|
| | (IU) | (Mg) | (Mg) | (Mg) | (Mg) | (Mg) | (Mcg) | (Mcg) |
| Beef, *continued* | | | | | | | | |
| pan-fried in vegetable | | | | | | | | |
| oil, lean only . . . . . | 0 | 0 | .16 | .37 | 4.88 | .57 | 11.3 | 4.18 |
| sirloin, top, select grade, broiled: | | | | | | | | |
| lean and fat (trimmed | | | | | | | | |
| to ¼") . . . . . . . . . | 0 | 0 | .12 | .31 | 4.48 | .46 | 10.2 | 3.06 |
| lean and fat (trimmed | | | | | | | | |
| to 0") . . . . . . . . . . | 0 | 0 | .14 | .33 | 4.76 | .50 | 11.3 | 3.19 |
| lean only . . . . . . . . . | 0 | 0 | .15 | .33 | 4.85 | .51 | 11.3 | 3.23 |
| T-bone steak (short loin), choice grade: | | | | | | | | |
| broiled, lean and fat | | | | | | | | |
| (trimmed to ¼") . . . | 0 | 0 | .11 | .25 | 4.63 | .39 | 7.9 | 2.44 |
| broiled, lean only . . . . | 0 | 0 | .12 | .28 | 5.25 | .44 | 9.1 | 2.57 |
| tenderloin, choice grade: | | | | | | | | |
| broiled, lean and fat | | | | | | | | |
| (trimmed to ¼") . . . | 0 | 0 | .12 | .29 | 3.97 | .44 | 6.8 | 2.72 |
| broiled, lean and fat | | | | | | | | |
| (trimmed to 0") . . . | 0 | 0 | .14 | .32 | 4.26 | .48 | 7.9 | 2.84 |
| broiled, lean only . . . . | 0 | 0 | .15 | .34 | 4.45 | .50 | 7.9 | 2.91 |
| roasted, lean and fat | | | | | | | | |
| (trimmed to ¼") . . . | 0 | 0 | .17 | .31 | 4.34 | .53 | 9.1 | 3.78 |
| roasted, lean only . . . | 0 | 0 | .20 | .37 | 5.16 | .65 | 10.2 | 4.39 |
| tenderlon, prime grade: | | | | | | | | |
| broiled, lean and fat | | | | | | | | |
| (trimmed to ¼") . . . | 0 | 0 | .12 | .29 | 3.93 | .43 | 6.8 | 2.71 |
| broiled, lean only . . . . | 0 | 0 | .15 | .34 | 4.45 | .50 | 7.9 | 2.91 |
| roasted, lean and fat | | | | | | | | |
| (trimmed to ¼") . . . | 0 | 0 | .10 | .31 | 3.37 | .37 | 7.9 | 2.85 |
| roasted, lean only . . . | 0 | 0 | .11 | .36 | 3.84 | .43 | 9.1 | 3.14 |
| tenderloin, select grade: | | | | | | | | |
| broiled, lean and fat | | | | | | | | |
| (trimmed to ¼") . . . | 0 | 0 | .14 | .31 | 4.05 | .44 | 6.8 | 2.76 |
| broiled, lean and fat | | | | | | | | |
| (trimmed to 0") . . . | 0 | 0 | .14 | .33 | 4.29 | .48 | 7.9 | 2.85 |
| broiled, lean only . . . . | 0 | 0 | .15 | .34 | 4.45 | .50 | 7.9 | 2.91 |

| | Vitamin A | Vitamin C | Thiamin | Riboflavin | Niacin | $B_6$ | Folacin | $B_{12}$ |
|---|---|---|---|---|---|---|---|---|
| | (IU) | (Mg) | (Mg) | (Mg) | (Mg) | (Mg) | (Mcg) | (Mcg) |
| roasted, lean and fat (trimmed to ¼")... | 0 | 0 | .09 | .29 | 3.37 | .28 | 7.9 | 2.78 |
| roasted, lean only ... | 0 | 0 | .11 | .35 | 3.87 | .33 | 10.2 | 3.07 |
| **top loin (short loin), choice grade, broiled:** | | | | | | | | |
| lean and fat (trimmed to ¼") .......... | 0 | 0 | .09 | .20 | 5.28 | .42 | 7.9 | 2.19 |
| lean and fat (trimmed to 0").......... | 0 | 0 | .10 | .22 | 5.89 | .46 | 9.1 | 2.25 |
| lean only .......... | 0 | 0 | .10 | .23 | 6.06 | .48 | 9.1 | 2.27 |
| **top loin (short loin), prime grade:** | | | | | | | | |
| broiled, lean and fat (trimmed to ¼")... | 0 | 0 | .09 | .20 | 5.28 | .42 | 7.9 | 2.19 |
| broiled, lean only.... | 0 | 0 | .10 | .23 | 6.06 | .48 | 9.1 | 2.27 |
| **top loin (short loin), select grade, broiled:** | | | | | | | | |
| lean and fat (trimmed to ¼") .......... | 0 | 0 | .09 | .20 | 5.41 | .43 | 7.9 | 2.20 |
| lean and fat (trimmed to 0").......... | 0 | 0 | .10 | .22 | 5.93 | .46 | 9.1 | 2.26 |
| lean only .......... | 0 | 0 | .10 | .23 | 6.06 | .48 | 9.1 | 2.27 |
| **Beef, corned:** | | | | | | | | |
| brisket, cured[1], cooked, 4 oz. .............. | 0 | 18 | .03 | .19 | 3.44 | .26 | n.a. | 1.85 |
| loaf[2], jellied, 1-oz. slice | n.a. | 2 | 0 | .03 | .50 | .03 | n.a. | .36 |
| **"Beef," vegetarian** (see also "'Hamburger,' vegetarian"): | | | | | | | | |
| canned: | | | | | | | | |
| (*Worthington* Savory Slices), 3 slices, 3 oz. ........... | 0 | 0 | .24 | .17 | 1.44 | .31 | n.a. | 1.53 |
| steak (*Worthington* Prime Stakes), 3.25-oz. piece .... | 0 | 0 | .12 | .13 | 1.98 | .38 | n.a. | 1.03 |

---

[1] *Contains added sodium ascorbate.*
[2] *With added ascorbic acid or sodium ascorbate; vitamin C value for product without additives would be negligible.*

| | Vitamin A | Vitamin C | Thiamin | Riboflavin | Niacin | B6 | Folacin | B12 |
|---|---|---|---|---|---|---|---|---|
| | (IU) | (Mg) | (Mg) | (Mg) | (Mg) | (Mg) | (Mcg) | (Mcg) |
| "Beef," vegetarian, canned, *continued* | | | | | | | | |
| steak (*Worthington Vegetable Steaks*), 2.5 oz. | 0 | 0 | .53 | .12 | 4.47 | .23 | n.a. | 3.27 |
| stew (*Worthington Country Stew*), 1 cup, 8.5 oz. | 2158 | 0 | 1.84 | .29 | 4.21 | .86 | n.a. | 3.67 |
| Swiss steak (*Loma Linda Swiss Stake*), w/gravy, 3.2 oz. | 0 | 0 | 1.25 | .65 | 5.41 | 1.0 | n.a. | 5.26 |
| frozen: | | | | | | | | |
| (*Worthington* Beef Style Meatless), 1.9 oz. | 0 | 0 | .89 | .34 | 6.46 | .56 | n.a. | 4.03 |
| (*Worthington Stakelets*), 2.5-oz. piece | 0 | 0 | 1.51 | .12 | 3.10 | .26 | n.a. | 1.58 |
| corned (*Worthington*), 4 slices, 2 oz. | 0 | 0 | 10.61 | .07 | 1.36 | .30 | n.a. | 1.73 |
| pie (*Worthington*), 8-oz. pie | 830 | 0 | .36 | .10 | 0 | .39 | n.a. | .46 |
| smoked (*Worthington*), 6 slices, 2 oz. | 0 | 0 | 2.12 | .14 | 3.15 | .30 | n.a. | 1.73 |
| steak (*Loma Linda Griddle Steaks*), 1.9-oz. piece | 0 | 0 | .55 | .44 | .87 | .35 | n.a. | 2.48 |
| **Beef gravy,** canned, ¼ cup | 0 | 0 | .02 | .02 | .38 | .01 | n.a. | .06 |
| **Beef jerky,** chopped, formed, 1 oz. | n.a. | n.a. | n.a. | .258 | 2.61 | n.a. | n.a. | n.a. |
| **Beef luncheon meat[1]:** | | | | | | | | |
| loaf, 1-oz. slice | 0 | 4 | .03 | .06 | 1.04 | .05 | n.a. | 1.10 |

[1] *With added ascorbic acid or sodium ascorbate; vitamin C value for product without additives would be negligible.*

| | Vitamin A | Vitamin C | Thiamin | Riboflavin | Niacin | B$_6$ | Folacin | B$_{12}$ |
|---|---|---|---|---|---|---|---|---|
| | (IU) | (Mg) | (Mg) | (Mg) | (Mg) | (Mg) | (Mcg) | (Mcg) |
| thin-sliced, 5 slices, approx. ¾ oz. . . . . . . | 0 | 3 | .02 | .04 | 1.11 | .07 | n.a. | .54 |
| **Beef seasoning** (*Tone's Perc*), ¼ tsp. . . . . . . . . | 10 | <1 | tr. | tr. | .01 | .03 | .9 | 0 |
| **Beer,** alcoholic: | | | | | | | | |
| regular, 12 fl. oz. . . . . . . . | 0 | 0 | .02 | .09 | 1.60 | .18 | 21.4 | .06 |
| light, 12 fl. oz. . . . . . . . . . | 0 | 0 | .03 | .11 | 1.40 | .12 | 14.7 | .02 |
| **Beet,** root: | | | | | | | | |
| fresh: | | | | | | | | |
|     raw, untrimmed, 1 lb.. . . | 114 | 15 | .09 | .12 | 1.02 | .21 | 332.0 | 0 |
|     raw, 2 beets, 2" diam., 8.5 oz. . . . | 61 | 8 | .05 | .07 | .54 | .11 | 178.0 | 0 |
|     raw, sliced, ½ cup. . . | 26 | 3 | .02 | .03 | .23 | .05 | 74.0 | 0 |
|     boiled, drained, 2 beets, 2" diam. | 35 | 4 | .03 | .04 | .33 | .07 | 80.0 | 0 |
|     boiled, drained, sliced, ½ cup. . . . . | 30 | 3 | .02 | .03 | .28 | .06 | 68.0 | 0 |
| canned, w/liquid: | | | | | | | | |
|     sliced, ½ cup. . . . . . | 14 | 5 | .01 | .05 | .19 | .07 | 35.7 | 0 |
|     Harvard, sliced, ½ cup. . . . . . . . . | n.a. | 3 | n.a. | .06 | .10 | n.a. | n.a. | 0 |
|     pickled, sliced, ½ cup. . . . . . . . . | 7 | 3 | .03 | .06 | .29 | n.a. | n.a. | 0 |
| **Beet greens:** | | | | | | | | |
| raw, untrimmed, 1 lb. . . . | 15,494 | 76 | .25 | .56 | 1.02 | .27 | n.a. | 0 |
| raw, trimmed, 1" pieces, ½ cup . . . . . | 1159 | 6 | .02 | .04 | .08 | .02 | n.a. | 0 |
| boiled, drained, 1" pieces, ½ cup . . . . . | 3672 | 18 | .08 | .21 | .36 | .10 | n.a. | 0 |
| **Berliner**[1], pork and beef, 1 oz. . . . . . . . . . . . . . | 0 | 2 | .11 | .06 | .88 | .06 | n.a. | .76 |

---

[1] *With added ascorbic acid or sodium ascorbate; vitamin C value for product without additives would be negligible.*

| | Vitamin A | Vitamin C | Thiamin | Riboflavin | Niacin | B6 | Folacin | B12 |
|---|---|---|---|---|---|---|---|---|
| | (IU) | (Mg) | (Mg) | (Mg) | (Mg) | (Mg) | (Mcg) | (Mcg) |
| **Biscuit,** ready-to-eat, plain or buttermilk, 1 piece | n.a. | 0 | .15 | .10 | 1.17 | .02 | 3.0 | .05 |
| **Biscuit, refrigerated dough:** | | | | | | | | |
| plain or buttermilk, baked, 1 piece | 0 | 0 | .09 | .06 | .83 | .01 | n.a. | 0 |
| mixed grain, 1 piece | 0 | 0 | .17 | .09 | 1.5 | n.a. | n.a. | 0 |
| **Black beans,** dried: | | | | | | | | |
| uncooked, 1 lb. | 77 | 0 | 4.08 | .88 | 8.87 | .30 | 2015.1 | 0 |
| uncooked, ½ cup | 16 | 0 | .87 | .19 | 1.90 | .28 | 430.9 | 0 |
| boiled, ½ cup | 5 | 0 | .21 | .05 | .43 | .06 | 127.9 | 0 |
| **Black turtle soup beans,** dried: | | | | | | | | |
| uncooked, 1 lb. | 77 | 0 | 4.08 | .88 | 8.87 | 1.30 | 2015.5 | 0 |
| uncooked, ½ cup | 16 | 0 | .83 | .18 | 1.80 | .26 | 408.8 | 0 |
| boiled, ½ cup | 5 | 0 | .21 | .52 | .49 | .07 | 78.7 | 0 |
| canned, w/liquid, 8 oz. | 10 | 6 | .32 | .27 | 1.41 | .12 | 137.9 | 0 |
| canned, w/liquid, ½ cup | 5 | 3 | .17 | .14 | .74 | .07 | 73.0 | 0 |
| **Blackberry:** | | | | | | | | |
| fresh, untrimmed, 1 lb. | 717 | 92 | .13 | .17 | 1.74 | .25 | n.a. | 0 |
| fresh, trimmed, ½ cup | 119 | 15 | .02 | .03 | .29 | .04 | n.a. | 0 |
| canned, in heavy syrup, ½ cup | 280 | 4 | .04 | .05 | .37 | .05 | 33.9 | 0 |
| frozen, unsweetened, ½ cup | 86 | 2 | .02 | .03 | .31 | .05 | 25.7 | 0 |
| **Black-eyed peas,** see "Cowpeas" | | | | | | | | |
| **Blueberry:** | | | | | | | | |
| fresh, untrimmed, 1 lb. | 445 | 58 | .21 | .22 | 1.60 | .41 | 28.4 | 0 |
| fresh, trimmed, ½ cup | 73 | 10 | .04 | .04 | .26 | .03 | 4.7 | 0 |
| canned, in heavy syrup, ½ cup | 82 | 1 | .04 | .07 | .15 | .05 | 2.1 | 0 |
| frozen: | | | | | | | | |
| unsweetened, ½ cup | 63 | 2 | .03 | .03 | .40 | .05 | 5.2 | 0 |
| sweetened, ⅓ of 10-oz. pkg. | 42 | 9 | .02 | .05 | .24 | .06 | 6.4 | 0 |
| sweetened, ½ cup | 51 | 1 | .02 | .06 | .29 | .07 | 7.8 | 0 |

| | Vitamin A | Vitamin C | Thiamin | Riboflavin | Niacin | B6 | Folacin | B12 |
|---|---|---|---|---|---|---|---|---|
| | (IU) | (Mg) | (Mg) | (Mg) | (Mg) | (Mg) | (Mcg) | (Mcg) |

**Bluefish,** meat only:

| | | | | | | | | |
|---|---|---|---|---|---|---|---|---|
| raw, 1 lb.............. | 1805 | (0) | .26 | .36 | 26.9 | 1.82 | 7.2 | 24.45 |
| baked, broiled, or | | | | | | | | |
|   microwaved[1], 4 oz. ... | 540 | (0) | .07 | .11 | 8.23 | .53 | 2.3 | 7.05 |

**Bologna**[2]:

| | | | | | | | | |
|---|---|---|---|---|---|---|---|---|
| beef, 1-oz. slice........ | n.a. | 6 | .01 | .03 | .68 | .04 | 1.0 | .40 |
| beef and pork, | | | | | | | | |
|   1-oz. slice .......... | 0 | 6 | .05 | .04 | .73 | .05 | 1.0 | .38 |
| Lebanon, beef, | | | | | | | | |
|   1-oz. slice .......... | n.a. | 6 | .02 | .05 | 1.24 | .07 | 1.0 | .72 |
| pork, 1-oz. slice........ | 0 | 10 | .15 | .05 | 1.11 | .08 | 1.0 | .26 |

**"Bologna," vegetarian,** frozen (*Worthington*

| | | | | | | | | |
|---|---|---|---|---|---|---|---|---|
|   *Bolono*), 2 oz. ....... | 0 | 0 | .58 | .13 | .34 | .36 | n.a. | .86 |

**Borage,** raw, untrimmed,

| | | | | | | | | |
|---|---|---|---|---|---|---|---|---|
|   1 lb. .............. | 19,889 | 147 | .27 | .75 | 4.26 | n.a. | n.a. | 0 |

**Boysenberry:**

fresh, see "Blackberry"

| | | | | | | | | |
|---|---|---|---|---|---|---|---|---|
| canned, in heavy syrup, | | | | | | | | |
|   ½ cup............. | 51 | 8 | .03 | .04 | .29 | .05 | 44.1 | 0 |
| frozen, unsweetened, | | | | | | | | |
|   ½ cup............. | 45 | 4 | .08 | .02 | .51 | .04 | 41.8 | 0 |

**Brain**[3]:

| | | | | | | | | |
|---|---|---|---|---|---|---|---|---|
| beef, pan-fried in | | | | | | | | |
|   vegetable oil, 4 oz..... | 0 | 4 | .15 | .29 | 4.29 | .44 | 6.8 | 17.24 |
| beef, simmered, 4 oz. | 0 | 1 | .09 | .19 | 2.47 | .27 | 7.9 | 9.75 |
| lamb, braised, 4 oz...... | 0 | 14 | .12 | .27 | 2.80 | .12 | 5.7 | 10.49 |
| lamb, pan-fried in | | | | | | | | |
|   vegetable oil, 4 oz..... | 0 | 26 | .19 | .42 | 5.16 | .26 | 7.9 | 27.33 |
| pork, braised, 4 oz. ..... | 0 | 16 | .09 | .25 | 3.78 | .16 | n.a. | 1.61 |

---

[1] *Prepared without added ingredients.*

[2] *With added ascorbic acid or sodium ascorbate; vitamin C value for product without additives would be negligible.*

[3] *Prepared without added ingredients, except as noted.*

| | Vitamin A | Vitamin C | Thiamin | Riboflavin | Niacin | B6 | Folacin | B12 |
|---|---|---|---|---|---|---|---|---|
| | (IU) | (Mg) | (Mg) | (Mg) | (Mg) | (Mg) | (Mcg) | (Mcg) |

**Brain,** *continued*

| | | | | | | | | |
|---|---|---|---|---|---|---|---|---|
| veal, braised, 4 oz...... | 0 | 15 | .09 | .23 | 2.76 | .19 | 3.4 | 10.94 |
| veal, pan-fried in | | | | | | | | |
| vegetable oil, 4 oz..... | 0 | 17 | .17 | .41 | 6.37 | .37 | 6.8 | 24.15 |

**Bran,** see "Cereal, ready-to-eat" and specific bran listings

**Bratwurst:**

| | | | | | | | | |
|---|---|---|---|---|---|---|---|---|
| pork, cooked, 1 oz. ..... | n.a. | 0 | .14 | .05 | .91 | .06 | n.a. | .27 |
| pork and beef[1], 1 oz..... | n.a. | 8 | .07 | .06 | .94 | .04 | n.a. | .58 |

**Braunschweiger**[1] (see also "Liverwurst"),

| | | | | | | | | |
|---|---|---|---|---|---|---|---|---|
| pork, 1 oz.......... | 3984 | 3 | .07 | .43 | 2.37 | .09 | n.a. | 5.69 |

**Brazil nut,** dried:

| | | | | | | | | |
|---|---|---|---|---|---|---|---|---|
| in shell, 1 lb.......... | 0 | 2 | 2.17 | .27 | 3.53 | .55 | 8.7 | 0 |
| shelled, 1 oz., | | | | | | | | |
| 8 medium or 6 large ... | 0 | <1 | .28 | .04 | .46 | .07 | 1.1 | 0 |
| shelled, 1 cup, approx. 32 | | | | | | | | |
| large ............. | 0 | 1 | 1.40 | .17 | 2.27 | .35 | 5.6 | 0 |

**Bread,** 1 slice or piece, except as noted:

| | | | | | | | | |
|---|---|---|---|---|---|---|---|---|
| Boston brown[2], canned, | | | | | | | | |
| 1.6-oz slice.......... | 25 | 0 | tr. | .03 | .32 | .02 | 2.0 | 0 |
| egg................. | 30 | 0 | .18 | .18 | 1.93 | .03 | 28.0 | .04 |
| egg, toasted........... | 28 | 0 | .14 | .16 | 1.78 | .02 | 20.0 | .04 |
| French............... | 0 | 0 | .13 | .08 | 1.19 | .01 | 8.0 | 0 |
| French, toasted ........ | 0 | 0 | .10 | .07 | 1.1 | .01 | 5.0 | 0 |
| hazelnut poppyseed | | | | | | | | |
| (*Roman Meal* | | | | | | | | |
| Premium) .......... | tr. | 0 | .18 | .10 | 1.35 | n.a. | n.a. | n.a. |
| high calcium: | | | | | | | | |
| dark ............. | n.a. | n.a. | .08 | .07 | .72 | n.a. | n.a. | n.a. |
| dark, toasted ....... | n.a. | n.a. | .06 | .06 | .64 | n.a. | n.a. | n.a. |
| light ............. | n.a. | n.a. | .08 | .06 | .74 | .01 | 4.0 | n.a. |
| light, toasted ....... | n.a. | n.a. | .06 | .05 | .66 | .01 | 3.0 | n.a. |

---

[1] *With added ascorbic acid or sodium ascorbate. Nonfat dry milk added.*

[2] *Made with white cornmeal.*

| | Vitamin A | Vitamin C | Thiamin | Riboflavin | Niacin | B6 | Folacin | B12 |
|---|---|---|---|---|---|---|---|---|
| | (IU) | (Mg) | (Mg) | (Mg) | (Mg) | (Mg) | (Mcg) | (Mcg) |
| Indian (Navajo) fry, 5"-diam. piece . . . . . . . | 0 | 0 | .39 | .27 | 3.27 | .02 | 11.0 | 0 |
| Italian . . . . . . . . . . . . . . | 0 | 0 | .14 | .09 | 1.31 | .01 | 9.0 | 0 |
| Italian, toasted . . . . . . . . | 0 | 0 | .11 | .08 | 1.17 | .01 | 6.0 | 0 |
| mixed grain: | | | | | | | | |
| regular. . . . . . . . . . . | 0 | tr. | .11 | .09 | 1.14 | .09 | 12.0 | .02 |
| regular, toasted . . . . . | 0 | tr. | .09 | .08 | 1.03 | .08 | 9.0 | .02 |
| 7-grain (*Roman Meal* Premium) . . . . . . . | 0 | 0 | .11 | .07 | 1.09 | n.a. | n.a. | n.a. |
| 7-grain, light (*Roman Meal*), 2 slices . . . . | 0 | 0 | .15 | .10 | 1.48 | n.a. | n.a. | n.a. |
| 12-grain (*Roman Meal* Premium) . . . | tr. | 0 | .14 | .08 | 1.18 | n.a. | n.a. | n.a. |
| oat (*Roman Meal* Premium) . . . . . . . . . | 0 | 0 | .14 | .08 | 1.13 | n.a. | n.a. | n.a. |
| oat bran: | | | | | | | | |
| regular. . . . . . . . . . . | n.a. | n.a. | .15 | .1 | 1.45 | n.a. | n.a. | 0 |
| regular, toasted . . . . . | n.a. | n.a. | .12 | .09 | 1.30 | n.a. | n.a. | 0 |
| light . . . . . . . . . . . . | n.a. | n.a. | .08 | .05 | .87 | n.a. | n.a. | 0 |
| light, toasted . . . . . . . | n.a. | 0 | .06 | .04 | .77 | n.a. | n.a. | 0 |
| (*Roman Meal*) . . . . . . | 0 | 0 | .13 | .09 | 1.24 | n.a. | n.a. | n.a. |
| (*Roman Meal* Honey) | 0 | 0 | .14 | .08 | .92 | n.a. | n.a. | n.a. |
| (*Roman Meal* Honey Nut). . . . . . . . . . . | 0 | 0 | .13 | .08 | .90 | n.a. | n.a. | n.a. |
| (*Roman Meal* Light), 2 slices . . . . . . . . | 0 | 0 | .15 | .10 | 1.34 | n.a. | n.a. | n.a. |
| oatmeal: | | | | | | | | |
| regular. . . . . . . . . . . | n.a. | n.a. | .11 | .07 | .85 | .02 | 7.0 | n.a. |
| regular, toasted . . . . . | n.a. | n.a. | .09 | .06 | .77 | .02 | 5.0 | n.a. |
| light . . . . . . . . . . . . | n.a. | n.a. | .08 | .07 | .70 | n.a. | n.a. | n.a. |
| light, toasted . . . . . . . | n.a. | n.a. | .06 | .06 | .62 | n.a. | n.a. | n.a. |
| pita, enriched, 6½"-diam. piece. . . . . . | 0 | 0 | .36 | .20 | 2.78 | .02 | 14.0 | 0 |
| pita, whole wheat, 6½"-diam. piece. . . . . . | 0 | 0 | .22 | .05 | 1.82 | n.a. | n.a. | 0 |

| | Vitamin A | Vitamin C | Thiamin | Riboflavin | Niacin | B6 | Folacin | B12 |
|---|---|---|---|---|---|---|---|---|
| | (IU) | (Mg) | (Mg) | (Mg) | (Mg) | (Mg) | (Mcg) | (Mcg) |
| Bread, *continued* | | | | | | | | |
| protein.............. | n.a. | 0 | .07 | .08 | .82 | .01 | 7.0 | 0 |
| protein, toasted ........ | 0 | 0 | .05 | .07 | .72 | .01 | 5.0 | 0 |
| pumpernickel, 1.1 oz..... | 0 | 0 | .11 | .10 | .99 | .04 | 11.0 | 0 |
| pumpernickel, 1.1 oz., | | | | | | | | |
|   toasted ............ | 0 | 0 | .08 | .09 | .89 | .04 | 7.0 | 0 |
| raisin, enriched ........ | n.a. | n.a. | .09 | .10 | .90 | .02 | 9.0 | 0 |
| raisin, enriched, toasted | n.a. | n.a. | .07 | .09 | .81 | .02 | 6.0 | 0 |
| rice bran ............. | n.a. | n.a. | .18 | .08 | 1.84 | n.a. | n.a. | 0 |
| rice bran, toasted....... | n.a. | n.a. | .14 | .07 | 1.67 | n.a. | n.a. | 0 |
| rye: | | | | | | | | |
|   seeded or unseeded | n.a. | n.a. | .14 | .11 | 1.22 | .02 | 16.0 | 0 |
|   seeded or unseeded, | | | | | | | | |
|     toasted ......... | n.a. | n.a. | .11 | .10 | 1.09 | .02 | 11.0 | 0 |
|   light, .9 oz. ........ | n.a. | n.a. | .08 | .06 | .58 | n.a. | n.a. | n.a. |
|   light, .9 oz., toasted | n.a. | n.a. | .07 | .05 | .51 | n.a. | n.a. | n.a. |
|   (*Roman Meal* Round | | | | | | | | |
|     Top) ........... | 0 | 0 | .13 | .09 | 1.34 | n.a. | n.a. | n.a. |
|   (*Roman Meal* | | | | | | | | |
|     Sandwich), 2 slices | 0 | 0 | .21 | .15 | 2.18 | n.a. | n.a. | n.a. |
|   (*Roman Meal* | | | | | | | | |
|     Sungrain) ....... | tr. | 0 | .14 | .08 | 1.10 | n.a. | n.a. | n.a. |
|   (*Roman Meal* Whole | | | | | | | | |
|     Grain) .......... | 0 | 0 | .14 | .10 | 1.40 | n.a. | n.a. | n.a. |
| Vienna, enriched, .9 oz. | tr. | tr. | .12 | .09 | 1.00 | n.a. | n.a. | 0 |
| wheat: | | | | | | | | |
|   plain, .9 oz......... | 0 | 0 | .10 | .07 | 1.03 | .02 | n.a. | 0 |
|   plain, .9 oz., toasted | 0 | 0 | .08 | .06 | .93 | .02 | n.a. | 0 |
|   bran, 1.3 oz. ........ | 0 | n.a. | .14 | .10 | 1.59 | .06 | n.a. | 0 |
|   bran, 1.3 oz., toasted | 0 | n.a. | .12 | .09 | 1.44 | .06 | n.a. | 0 |
|   cracked (18 slices | | | | | | | | |
|     per lb.) ......... | n.a. | 0 | .09 | .06 | .92 | .08 | 10.0 | n.a. |
|   cracked, toasted..... | n.a. | n.a. | .07 | .05 | .83 | .07 | 7.0 | n.a. |
|   hearty (*Roman Meal* | | | | | | | | |
|     Light), 2 slices.... | 0 | 0 | .15 | .10 | 1.53 | n.a. | n.a. | n.a. |

| | Vitamin A | Vitamin C | Thiamin | Riboflavin | Niacin | B6 | Folacin | B12 |
|---|---|---|---|---|---|---|---|---|
| | (IU) | (Mg) | (Mg) | (Mg) | (Mg) | (Mg) | (Mcg) | (Mcg) |
| light, .8 oz. . . . . . . . . | n.a. | n.a. | .10 | .07 | .89 | .03 | n.a. | n.a. |
| light (*Roman Meal*), 2 slices . . . . . . . . | 0 | 0 | .15 | .11 | 1.59 | n.a. | n.a. | n.a. |
| light, toasted, .8 oz. | n.a. | n.a. | .08 | .06 | .79 | .03 | n.a. | n.a. |
| natural (*Roman Meal Premium*) . . . . . . . | 0 | 0 | .18 | .11 | 2.00 | n.a. | n.a. | n.a. |
| whole . . . . . . . . . . . | n.a. | n.a. | .10 | .06 | 1.09 | .05 | 14.0 | n.a. |
| whole (*Roman Meal Premium*) . . . . . . . | 0 | 0 | .08 | .04 | 1.07 | n.a. | n.a. | n.a. |
| whole, light (*Roman Meal*), 2 slices . . . . | 0 | 0 | .09 | .06 | 1.32 | n.a. | n.a. | n.a. |
| whole, toasted . . . . . . | n.a. | n.a. | .08 | .05 | .97 | .05 | 10.0 | n.a. |
| wheat germ . . . . . . . . . . | n.a. | n.a. | .11 | .11 | 1.28 | n.a. | 16.0 | n.a. |
| wheat germ, toasted . . . . | n.a. | n.a. | .08 | .10 | 1.14 | n.a. | 11.0 | n.a. |
| wheatberry, honey (*Roman Meal Premium*) . . . . . . . . . . | 0 | 0 | .11 | .08 | 1.22 | n.a. | n.a. | n.a. |
| wheatberry, light (*Roman Meal*), 2 slices . . . . . . . | 0 | 0 | .15 | .10 | 1.56 | n.a. | n.a. | n.a. |
| white, enriched: | | | | | | | | |
| regular, .9 oz. . . . . . . | 0 | 0 | .12 | .09 | .99 | .02 | 8.0 | n.a. |
| regular, .9 oz., toasted . . . . . . . . . | 0 | 0 | .10 | .08 | .90 | .01 | 6.0 | n.a. |
| light, .8 oz. . . . . . . . . | n.a. | n.a. | .09 | .07 | .84 | .01 | n.a. | n.a. |
| light (*Roman Meal*), 2 slices . . . . . . . . | 0 | 0 | .16 | .11 | 1.51 | n.a. | n.a. | n.a. |
| light, .8 oz., toasted | n.a. | n.a. | .07 | .06 | .74 | .01 | n.a. | n.a. |
| whole grain (*Roman Meal*). . . . . . . . . . . . . | 0 | 0 | .18 | .12 | 1.88 | n.a. | n.a. | n.a. |
| **Bread, sweet, mix**[1], corn bread, 2½"-square piece . . . . . . . . . . . . . | 130 | tr. | .10 | .10 | .80 | n.a. | n.a. | (0) |

[1] *Prepared according to package directions, with eggs and milk.*

| | Vitamin A | Vitamin C | Thiamin | Riboflavin | Niacin | B6 | Folacin | B12 |
|---|---|---|---|---|---|---|---|---|
| | (IU) | (Mg) | (Mg) | (Mg) | (Mg) | (Mg) | (Mcg) | (Mcg) |
| **Bread crumbs,** enriched: | | | | | | | | |
| dry, grated, plain, | | | | | | | | |
| 1 cup .............. | n.a. | n.a. | .22 | .12 | 1.94 | .03 | n.a. | n.a. |
| dry, grated, seasoned, | | | | | | | | |
| 1 cup .............. | n.a. | n.a. | .19 | .20 | 3.28 | n.a. | n.a. | n.a. |
| soft, 1 cup............ | tr. | tr. | .21 | .14 | 1.70 | n.a. | n.a. | n.a. |
| **Bread cubes,** white, | | | | | | | | |
| 1 cup .............. | tr. | tr. | .14 | .09 | 1.10 | n.a. | n.a. | (0) |
| **Bread stick,** plain, | | | | | | | | |
| 1 stick, 9¼" x ⅜".... | 0 | 0 | .04 | .03 | .32 | tr. | n.a. | 0 |
| **Breadfruit:** | | | | | | | | |
| untrimmed, 1 lb....... | 142 | 103 | .39 | .11 | 3.18 | n.a. | n.a. | 0 |
| trimmed, ½ cup........ | 44 | 32 | .12 | .03 | .99 | n.a. | n.a. | 0 |
| **Breadfruit seeds,** raw, | | | | | | | | |
| 1 oz............... | 73 | 2 | .14 | .09 | .12 | n.a. | n.a. | 0 |
| **Broad beans,** fresh: | | | | | | | | |
| raw, untrimmed, 1 lb.... | 1540 | 145 | .75 | .48 | 6.60 | n.a. | n.a. | 0 |
| raw, trimmed, ½ cup.... | 191 | 18 | .09 | .06 | .82 | n.a. | n.a. | 0 |
| **Broad beans,** dried: | | | | | | | | |
| uncooked, 1 lb........ | 240 | 6 | 2.52 | 1.51 | 12.85 | 1.66 | 1918.2 | 0 |
| uncooked, ½ cup....... | 40 | 1 | .42 | .25 | 2.12 | .28 | 317.2 | 0 |
| boiled, ½ cup ......... | 13 | <1 | .08 | .08 | .60 | .06 | 88.5 | 0 |
| canned, w/liquid, 8 oz.... | 23 | 4 | .46 | .11 | 2.18 | .10 | 74.2 | 0 |
| canned, w/liquid, | | | | | | | | |
| ½ cup............. | 13 | 2 | .03 | .06 | 1.23 | .06 | 41.9 | 0 |
| **Broccoli:** | | | | | | | | |
| fresh: | | | | | | | | |
| raw, untrimmed, | | | | | | | | |
| 1 lb............ | 4267 | 258 | .18 | .33 | 1.77 | .44 | 196.5 | 0 |
| raw, trimmed, | | | | | | | | |
| 1 spear, 5.3 oz.... | 2328 | 141 | .10 | .18 | .96 | .24 | 107.2 | 0 |
| raw, trimmed, | | | | | | | | |
| chopped, ½ cup .. | 678 | 41 | .03 | .05 | .28 | .07 | 31.2 | 0 |
| boiled, drained, | | | | | | | | |
| 1 spear, 6.3 oz.... | 2498 | 134 | .10 | .20 | 1.03 | .26 | 89.0 | 0 |

| | Vitamin A | Vitamin C | Thiamin | Riboflavin | Niacin | B6 | Folacin | B12 |
|---|---|---|---|---|---|---|---|---|
| | (IU) | (Mg) | (Mg) | (Mg) | (Mg) | (Mg) | (Mcg) | (Mcg) |
| boiled, drained, chopped, ½ cup . . | 1082 | 58 | .04 | .09 | .45 | .11 | 39.0 | 0 |
| frozen: | | | | | | | | |
| chopped, 10-oz. pkg. | 5866 | 160 | .15 | .27 | 1.34 | .37 | 190.2 | 0 |
| chopped, boiled, drained, ½ cup . . . | 1741 | 37 | .05 | .75 | .42 | .12 | 51.9 | 0 |
| spears, 10-oz. pkg. | 4059 | 194 | .20 | .32 | 1.31 | .50 | 267.8 | 0 |
| spears, boiled, drained, ⅓ of 10-oz. pkg. . . . . . . | 1577 | 33 | .05 | .07 | .38 | .11 | 25.3 | 0 |
| spears, boiled, drained, ½ cup . . . | 1741 | 37 | .05 | .08 | .42 | .12 | 28.0 | 0 |
| **Brown gravy mix,** vegetarian (*Loma Linda*), .2 oz. . . . . . . . | 0 | 0 | .44 | .01 | 0 | tr. | n.a. | 0 |
| **Brownie:** | | | | | | | | |
| 1-oz. piece, 1¾" × ¾" . . . | 20 | n.a. | .07 | .06 | .49 | .01 | n.a. | (0) |
| w/nuts, .9-oz. piece . . . . . | 70 | tr. | .08 | .07 | .30 | n.a. | n.a. | (0) |
| frozen, w/chocolate icing, .9-oz. piece . . . . . . . . . | 50 | tr. | .02 | .02 | .10 | n.a. | n.a. | (0) |
| mix[1], .7-oz. piece. . . . . . . | 20 | tr. | .03 | .02 | .10 | n.a. | n.a. | (0) |
| **Brussels sprouts:** | | | | | | | | |
| fresh: | | | | | | | | |
| raw, untrimmed, 1 lb. . . . . . . . . . . | 3604 | 347 | .57 | .37 | 3.04 | .89 | 249.4 | 0 |
| raw, 1 sprout, .75 oz. . . . . . . . . | 168 | 16 | .03 | .02 | .14 | .04 | 11.6 | 0 |
| boiled, drained, 1 sprout, .75 oz. . . . | 151 | 13 | .02 | .02 | .13 | .04 | 12.6 | 0 |
| boiled, drained, ½ cup . . . . . . . . . . | 561 | 48 | .08 | .06 | .47 | .14 | 46.8 | 0 |
| frozen, 10-oz. pkg. . . . . . . | 2314 | 210 | .30 | .35 | 1.81 | .57 | 350.6 | 0 |
| frozen, boiled, drained, ½ cup . . . . . . . . . . . . . | 459 | 36 | .08 | .09 | .42 | .23 | 79.0 | 0 |

[1] *Prepared according to package directions, with eggs, water, and nuts.*

| | Vitamin A | Vitamin C | Thiamin | Riboflavin | Niacin | B6 | Folacin | B12 |
|---|---|---|---|---|---|---|---|---|
| | (IU) | (Mg) | (Mg) | (Mg) | (Mg) | (Mg) | (Mcg) | (Mcg) |
| **Buckwheat,** whole grain, | | | | | | | | |
| 1 cup . . . . . . . . . . . . | (0) | 0 | .17 | .72 | 11.93 | .36 | 51.0 | 0 |
| **Buckwheat flour,** 1 cup | (0) | 0 | .50 | .23 | 7.38 | .70 | 64.0 | 0 |
| **Buckwheat groats,** roasted: | | | | | | | | |
| uncooked, 1 oz. . . . . . . . | (0) | 0 | .06 | .08 | 1.46 | .10 | 11.9 | 0 |
| uncooked, ½ cup. . . . . . . | (0) | 0 | .18 | .22 | 4.21 | .29 | 35.0 | 0 |
| cooked, 1 cup . . . . . . . . . | (0) | 0 | .08 | .08 | 1.86 | .15 | 27.0 | 0 |
| **Bulgar:** | | | | | | | | |
| uncooked, 1 oz. . . . . . . . . | (0) | 0 | .07 | .03 | 1.45 | .10 | 7.7 | 0 |
| uncooked, ½ cup. . . . . . . | (0) | 0 | .16 | .08 | 3.58 | .24 | 19.0 | 0 |
| cooked, 1 cup . . . . . . . . . | (0) | 0 | .10 | .05 | 1.82 | .15 | 33.0 | 0 |
| **Burdock root,** raw: | | | | | | | | |
| untrimmed, 1 lb. . . . . . . . | 0 | 10 | .03 | .10 | 1.02 | n.a. | n.a. | 0 |
| trimmed, 1 root, 5.5 oz. . . . | 0 | 5 | .02 | .05 | .47 | n.a. | n.a. | 0 |
| **Butter:** | | | | | | | | |
| regular, 1 stick . . . . . . . . | 3468 | 0 | .01 | .04 | .05 | <.01 | 3.0 | (0) |
| regular, 1 tbsp. . . . . . . . | 434 | 0 | tr. | <.01 | .01 | tr. | .4 | (0) |
| whipped, 1 stick . . . . . . . | 2312 | 0 | <.01 | .03 | .03 | <.01 | 2.0 | (0) |
| whipped, 1 tbsp. . . . . . . . | 287 | 0 | tr. | tr. | tr. | tr. | .3 | (0) |
| **Butter beans,** see "Lima beans" | | | | | | | | |
| **Butterbur:** | | | | | | | | |
| raw, untrimmed, 1 lb. . . . | 200 | 126 | .08 | .08 | .80 | n.a. | n.a. | 0 |
| raw, trimmed, 1 cup . . . . | 46 | 30 | .02 | .02 | .19 | n.a. | n.a. | 0 |
| canned, chopped, 1 cup . . . | 0 | 15 | .01 | .01 | .17 | n.a. | n.a. | 0 |
| **Butternut squash:** | | | | | | | | |
| fresh: | | | | | | | | |
| raw, untrimmed, 1 lb. | 29,718 | 80 | .38 | .08 | 4.57 | .59 | 101.7 | 0 |
| raw, trimmed, cubed, | | | | | | | | |
| ½ cup . . . . . . . . . | 5460 | 15 | .07 | .01 | .84 | .11 | 18.7 | 0 |
| boiled, drained, | | | | | | | | |
| cubed, ½ cup . . . . | 7141 | 15 | .07 | .02 | .99 | .13 | 19.6 | 0 |
| frozen, 12-oz. pkg. . . . . . . | 16,286 | 21 | .31 | .20 | 2.52 | .37 | n.a. | 0 |
| frozen, boiled, mashed, | | | | | | | | |
| ½ cup . . . . . . . . . . . . | 4007 | 4 | .06 | .05 | .56 | .08 | n.a. | 0 |
| **Butterscotch,** see "Candy" | | | | | | | | |
| **Butterscotch topping,** | | | | | | | | |
| 2 tbsp. . . . . . . . . . . . | n.a. | n.a. | n.a. | .04 | n.a. | n.a. | n.a. | 0 |

# C

| | Vitamin A | Vitamin C | Thiamin | Riboflavin | Niacin | B6 | Folacin | B12 |
|---|---|---|---|---|---|---|---|---|
| | (IU) | (Mg) | (Mg) | (Mg) | (Mg) | (Mg) | (Mcg) | (Mcg) |
| **Cabbage:** | | | | | | | | |
| raw: | | | | | | | | |
| untrimmed, 1 lb. . . . . | 483 | 117 | .18 | .15 | 1.09 | .35 | 157.0 | 0 |
| trimmed, 1 head, | | | | | | | | |
| 5⅜"-diam. . . . . . . | 1143 | 429 | .45 | .27 | 2.72 | .86 | 514.8 | 0 |
| trimmed, shredded, | | | | | | | | |
| ½ cup . . . . . . . . . | 47 | 11 | .02 | .01 | .05 | .03 | 15.0 | 0 |
| boiled, drained, shredded, | | | | | | | | |
| ½ cup . . . . . . . . . . . | 99 | 15 | .04 | .04 | .21 | .09 | 15.0 | 0 |
| **Cabbage, Chinese:** | | | | | | | | |
| bok-choy: | | | | | | | | |
| raw, untrimmed, | | | | | | | | |
| 1 lb. . . . . . . . . . . | 11,976 | 180 | .16 | .28 | 2.00 | n.a. | n.a. | 0 |
| raw, trimmed, | | | | | | | | |
| shredded, ½ cup | 1050 | 16 | .01 | .03 | .18 | n.a. | n.a. | 0 |
| boiled, drained, | | | | | | | | |
| shredded, ½ cup | 2183 | 22 | .03 | .05 | .36 | n.a. | n.a. | 0 |
| pe-tsai: | | | | | | | | |
| raw, untrimmed, | | | | | | | | |
| 1 lb. . . . . . . . . . . | 5062 | 114 | .17 | .21 | 1.69 | .98 | 331.8 | 0 |
| raw, trimmed, | | | | | | | | |
| shredded, ½ cup | 456 | 10 | .02 | .02 | .15 | .09 | 29.9 | 0 |
| boiled, drained, | | | | | | | | |
| .5-oz. leaf . . . . . . . | 135 | 2 | .01 | .01 | .07 | .02 | 7.5 | 0 |
| boiled, drained, | | | | | | | | |
| shredded, ½ cup | 576 | 9 | .03 | .03 | .30 | .11 | 63.5 | 0 |
| **Cabbage, red:** | | | | | | | | |
| raw, untrimmed, 1 lb. | 145 | 207 | .18 | .11 | 1.09 | 1.18 | 75.2 | 0 |
| raw, trimmed, shredded, | | | | | | | | |
| ½ cup . . . . . . . . . . . | 14 | 20 | .02 | .01 | .11 | .07 | 7.3 | 0 |
| boiled, drained, | | | | | | | | |
| .75-oz. leaf . . . . . . . | 6 | 8 | .01 | <.01 | .04 | .03 | 2.8 | 0 |
| boiled, drained, shredded, | | | | | | | | |
| ½ cup . . . . . . . . . . . | 20 | 26 | .03 | .02 | .15 | .11 | 9.4 | 0 |

| | Vitamin A | Vitamin C | Thiamin | Riboflavin | Niacin | B6 | Folacin | B12 |
|---|---|---|---|---|---|---|---|---|
| | (IU) | (Mg) | (Mg) | (Mg) | (Mg) | (Mg) | (Mcg) | (Mcg) |

**Cabbage, savoy:**

| | | | | | | | | |
|---|---|---|---|---|---|---|---|---|
| raw, untrimmed, 1 lb. | 3629 | 113 | .25 | .11 | 1.09 | .69 | n.a. | 0 |
| raw, trimmed, shredded, ½ cup . . . . . . . . . . . . | 350 | 11 | .03 | .01 | .11 | .07 | n.a. | 0 |
| boiled, drained, shredded, ½ cup . . . . . . . . . . . . | 649 | 12 | .04 | .02 | .02 | .11 | n.a. | 0 |

**Cabbage, swamp,** see "Swamp cabbage"

**Cake:**

| | | | | | | | | |
|---|---|---|---|---|---|---|---|---|
| angel food, 1/12 of 9" cake . . . . . . . . . . . | 0 | 0 | .03 | .14 | .25 | .01 | n.a. | n.a. |
| Boston creme pie, 1/8 of 19.5-oz. cake. . . . | 74 | n.a. | .38 | .25 | .18 | .02 | 7 | .15 |
| cheesecake, 1 oz. . . . . . . . | n.a. | n.a. | .01 | .06 | .06 | .02 | 4.0 | .05 |
| chocolate, w/chocolate frosting, 1/8 of 18-oz. cake . . . . . . . . . . . . . | n.a. | n.a. | .02 | .09 | .37 | n.a. | n.a. | n.a. |
| coffee cake: | | | | | | | | |
| cheese, 1 oz. . . . . . . . | n.a. | n.a. | .03 | .04 | .19 | n.a. | n.a. | n.a. |
| cinnamon, w/crumb topping, 1 oz. . . . . | n.a. | n.a. | .06 | .07 | .48 | .01 | 9 | n.a. |
| creme-filled, w/chocolate frosting, 1 oz. . . . . . . . | n.a. | n.a. | .02 | .02 | .24 | n.a. | n.a. | n.a. |
| fruit, 1 oz. . . . . . . . . . . . | 40 | tr. | .01 | .05 | .73 | .01 | 5.0 | n.a. |
| fruitcake, 1.5-oz. piece | n.a. | n.a. | .02 | .04 | .34 | .02 | 1.0 | n.a. |
| pound, 1-oz. slice . . . . . . | 172 | n.a. | .04 | .07 | .37 | n.a. | n.a. | n.a. |
| pound, fat-free, 1-oz. slice . . . . . . . . . | 27 | 0 | .04 | .09 | .19 | tr. | 1.0 | 0 |
| sponge, 1/12 of 16-oz. cake . . . . . . . . . . . . . | 59 | 0 | .09 | .10 | .73 | .02 | 5.0 | .09 |
| white, w/white frosting, 2.3-oz. slice. . . . . . . . | 40 | 0 | .06 | .05 | .32 | n.a. | n.a. | n.a. |
| yellow, w/chocolate frosting, 2.3-oz. slice | n.a. | n.a. | .08 | .1 | .8 | n.a. | n.a. | n.a. |

**Cake, frozen,** devil's food:

| | | | | | | | | |
|---|---|---|---|---|---|---|---|---|
| w/chocolate frosting, 1/8 of 7½" cake. . . . . . . | 370 | tr. | .02 | .07 | .20 | n.a. | n.a. | n.a. |

| | Vitamin A | Vitamin C | Thiamin | Riboflavin | Niacin | B6 | Folacin | B12 |
|---|---|---|---|---|---|---|---|---|
| | (IU) | (Mg) | (Mg) | (Mg) | (Mg) | (Mg) | (Mcg) | (Mcg) |
| w/whipped cream filling and chocolate frosting, 2 layer, ⅙ of 7¼" cake . . . . . . . . . . | 230 | tr. | .02 | .07 | .20 | n.a. | n.a. | n.a. |
| **Cake, snack:** | | | | | | | | |
| chocolate, cupcake, w/frosting, low fat, 1.5-oz. piece . . . . . . . . | 0 | 0 | .02 | .06 | .31 | tr. | 2.0 | 0 |
| devil's food, w/creme filling, 1.8-oz. piece . . . | 8 | n.a. | .11 | .15 | 1.21 | n.a. | n.a. | n.a. |
| sponge, w/creme filling, 1.5-oz. piece . . . . . . . . | n.a. | n.a. | .07 | .06 | .52 | n.a. | n.a. | n.a. |
| **Cake mix[1], 1 piece:** | | | | | | | | |
| angel food, 1/12 of 9¾" tube . . . . . . . . . . | 0 | 0 | .32 | 1.27 | 1.60 | n.a. | n.a. | n.a. |
| brownie, see "Brownie" | | | | | | | | |
| coffee cake, crumb, 2.5 oz. . . . . . . . . . . . . | 120 | tr. | .14 | .15 | 1.30 | n.a. | n.a. | n.a. |
| devil's food, w/chocolate frosting, 2 layer, 2.4 oz. . . . . . . | 100 | tr. | .07 | .10 | .60 | n.a. | n.a. | n.a. |
| gingerbread, ⅑ of 8" square . . . . . . . . . . | 0 | tr. | .09 | .11 | .80 | n.a. | n.a. | n.a. |
| yellow, w/chocolate frosting, 2 layer, 2.4 oz. . . . . . . . . . . . . | 100 | tr. | .08 | .10 | .70 | n.a. | n.a. | n.a. |
| **Candy:** | | | | | | | | |
| almond, chocolate coated, 1 oz. . . . . . . . . . . . . | tr. | tr. | .03 | .15 | .50 | n.a. | n.a. | n.a. |
| almond, sugar coated, 1 oz. . . . . . . . . . . . . | 0 | 0 | .01 | .08 | .30 | n.a. | n.a. | n.a. |
| (*Baby Ruth*), 2.1-oz. bar . . . | n.a. | n.a. | n.a. | .05 | 2.1 | n.a. | n.a. | n.a. |

[1] Prepared according to package directions.

| | Vitamin A | Vitamin C | Thiamin | Riboflavin | Niacin | B₆ | Folacin | B₁₂ |
|---|---|---|---|---|---|---|---|---|
| | (IU) | (Mg) | (Mg) | (Mg) | (Mg) | (Mg) | (Mcg) | (Mcg) |

Candy, *continued*

| | | | | | | | | |
|---|---|---|---|---|---|---|---|---|
| (*Bar None*), 1.5-oz. bar | n.a. | n.a. | .03 | .12 | .68 | n.a. | n.a. | n.a. |
| (*Butterfinger*), 2.16-oz. bar | 40 | n.a. | n.a. | .03 | 2.01 | .04 | 19.0 | n.a. |
| butterscotch, 1 oz. | 39 | 0 | tr. | .01 | tr. | tr. | 0 | 0 |
| candy corn, 1 oz. | 0 | 0 | tr. | tr. | tr. | n.a. | n.a. | 0 |
| caramel, plain, .3-oz. piece | 3 | n.a. | tr. | n.a. | .02 | tr. | 0 | 0 |
| caramel, chocolate coated: | | | | | | | | |
| w/cookie (*Twix*), 2-oz. pkg. | n.a. | n.a. | .03 | .11 | .21 | n.a. | n.a. | n.a. |
| milk chocolate coated (*Rolo*), 1.93-oz. pkg. | 33 | n.a. | .03 | .14 | .05 | n.a. | n.a. | n.a. |
| w/peanut, chocolate coated (*Oh! Henry*), 2-oz. bar | 27 | n.a. | .01 | .09 | 1.6 | n.a. | n.a. | n.a. |
| carob, 1 oz. | 13 | n.a. | .01 | n.a. | .34 | .05 | 9.0 | 0 |
| chocolate, w/almonds: | | | | | | | | |
| (*Hershey's* Golden Almond), 3-oz. bar | 125 | n.a. | .05 | .45 | .90 | n.a. | n.a. | n.a. |
| (*Hershey's Solitaires*), 3-oz. pkg. | 42 | n.a. | .05 | .43 | .92 | n.a. | n.a. | n.a. |
| chocolate, candy coated (*M&M's*), 1.69-oz. pkg. | 50 | n.a. | .03 | .12 | .26 | .03 | 4.0 | n.a. |
| chocolate, w/caramel (*Caramello*), 1.6-oz. bar | n.a. | n.a. | .02 | .18 | .52 | n.a. | n.a. | n.a. |
| chocolate, dark, sweet (*Hershey's Special Dark*), 1.45 oz. | 8 | n.a. | .01 | .1 | .26 | n.a. | n.a. | n.a. |
| chocolate, milk: | | | | | | | | |
| 1 oz. | 30 | tr. | .02 | .10 | .10 | n.a. | n.a. | n.a. |

| | Vitamin A | Vitamin C | Thiamin | Riboflavin | Niacin | B6 | Folacin | B12 |
|---|---|---|---|---|---|---|---|---|
| | (IU) | (Mg) | (Mg) | (Mg) | (Mg) | (Mg) | (Mcg) | (Mcg) |
| 1.55-oz. bar | 82 | tr. | .04 | .13 | .14 | .02 | 4.0 | .17 |
| w/almonds, 1.55-oz. bar | 33 | tr. | .03 | .19 | .33 | n.a. | n.a. | n.a. |
| creamy (*Hershey's Symphony*), 1.4-oz. bar | 28 | n.a. | .04 | .15 | .13 | n.a. | n.a. | n.a. |
| w/crisps (*Krackel*), 1.6-oz. bar | 23 | n.a. | .02 | .14 | .21 | .02 | 4.0 | n.a. |
| w/crisps (*Nestlé Crunch*), 1.4-oz. bar | 23 | tr. | .02 | .11 | .2 | .03 | 4.0 | n.a. |
| w/crisps and peanuts (*Nestlé 100 Grand*), 1.5-oz. bar | 33 | 0 | .02 | .10 | .10 | n.a. | n.a. | n.a. |
| w/fruit and nuts (*Chunky*), 1.4-oz. bar | 25 | .01 | .04 | .16 | .76 | n.a. | n.a. | n.a. |
| w/peanuts (*Mr. Goodbar*),1.75-oz. bar | 20 | n.a. | .03 | .14 | 2.4 | n.a. | n.a. | .22 |
| w/pecan and caramel (*Demet's Turtles*), .6-oz. piece | 26 | n.a. | .03 | .04 | .06 | n.a. | n.a. | n.a. |
| w/peanuts, candy coated (*M&M's*), 1.74-oz. pkg. | n.a. | n.a. | .03 | .10 | 1.6 | .09 | 27.0 | n.a. |
| chocolate, semisweet, 1 oz. | 6 | 0 | .02 | .03 | .12 | .01 | 1.0 | 0 |
| chocolate, white, w/ almonds (*Nestlé Alpine*), 1.25-oz. bar | 29 | tr. | .03 | .15 | .03 | n.a. | n.a. | n.a. |
| chocolate chips, see "Chocolate, baking" | | | | | | | | |
| coconut, chocolate coated: (*Mound's*), 1.9-oz. bar | n.a. | n.a. | .01 | .03 | .02 | n.a. | n.a. | n.a. |
| w/almonds (*Almond Joy*), 1.76-oz. bar | n.a. | n.a. | .02 | .08 | .24 | n.a. | n.a. | n.a. |
| (*5th Avenue*), 2.6-oz. bar | 18 | n.a. | .01 | .13 | 2.0 | n.a. | n.a. | n.a. |

|  | Vitamin A | Vitamin C | Thiamin | Riboflavin | Niacin | B₆ | Folacin | B₁₂ |
|---|---|---|---|---|---|---|---|---|
|  | (IU) | (Mg) | (Mg) | (Mg) | (Mg) | (Mg) | (Mcg) | (Mcg) |
| Candy, *continued* | | | | | | | | |
| fondant, mint, 1 oz...... | 0 | 0 | tr. | tr. | tr. | n.a. | n.a. | 0 |
| fruit-flavored chews (*Starburst*), 2.07-oz. pkg................ | n.a. | 31 | tr. | tr. | tr. | 0 | 0 | 0 |
| fudge: | | | | | | | | |
| chocolate or chocolate w/nuts, 1 oz........ | tr. | tr. | .01 | .03 | .10 | n.a. | n.a. | n.a. |
| vanilla or vanilla w/nuts, 1 oz...... | tr. | tr. | .01 | .04 | tr. | n.a. | n.a. | n.a. |
| fudge, chocolate coated: | | | | | | | | |
| chocolate, 1 oz...... | tr. | tr. | .04 | .10 | 0 | n.a. | n.a. | n.a. |
| chocolate w/nuts, 1 oz................ | tr. | tr. | .04 | .10 | tr. | n.a. | n.a. | n.a. |
| w/caramel and peanuts, 1 oz..... | tr. | tr. | .05 | .06 | .50 | n.a. | n.a. | n.a. |
| w/peanuts and caramel, 1 oz..... | tr. | tr. | .07 | .04 | 1.00 | n.a. | n.a. | n.a. |
| gum, chewing, 1 stick ... | 0 | 0 | 0 | 0 | 0 | n.a. | n.a. | 0 |
| hard, 1 oz............. | 0 | n.a. | n.a. | n.a. | n.a. | n.a. | n.a. | 0 |
| honey (*Bit-O-Honey*), 1.7-oz. bar......... | 0 | 0 | 0 | .12 | .03 | n.a. | n.a. | n.a. |
| honeycomb, w/peanut butter, chocolate coated, 1 oz......... | tr. | tr. | .01 | .03 | .80 | n.a. | n.a. | n.a. |
| jelly beans, 10 large..... | 0 | 0 | 0 | 0 | 0 | n.a. | n.a. | 0 |
| licorice: | | | | | | | | |
| cherry (*Y&S Nibs*), 1 oz............. | 6 | n.a. | .01 | .01 | .03 | n.a. | n.a. | 0 |
| strawberry (*Y&S Twizzlers*), 2.5-oz. pkg............. | n.a. | n.a. | .01 | .03 | .07 | n.a. | n.a. | 0 |
| (*Mars*), 1.76-oz. bar..... | n.a. | n.a. | .02 | .16 | .47 | n.a. | n.a. | n.a. |
| marshmallow, ¼-oz. piece.............. | 0 | 0 | 0 | 0 | 0 | n.a. | 0 | 0 |

| | Vitamin A | Vitamin C | Thiamin | Riboflavin | Niacin | B₆ | Folacin | B₁₂ |
|---|---|---|---|---|---|---|---|---|
| | (IU) | (Mg) | (Mg) | (Mg) | (Mg) | (Mg) | (Mcg) | (Mcg) |
| (*Milky Way*), 2.15-oz. bar | 127 | 1 | .02 | .14 | .21 | .03 | 5.0 | .27 |
| mint, chocolate coated: | | | | | | | | |
| (*York* Peppermint Pattie), | | | | | | | | |
| 1.5-oz. piece . . . . . | n.a. | n.a. | .01 | .04 | .37 | n.a. | n.a. | n.a. |
| dark (*After Eight*), | | | | | | | | |
| 2 pieces . . . . . . . . | 2 | n.a. | tr. | tr. | .02 | n.a. | n.a. | n.a. |
| nougat and caramel, | | | | | | | | |
| chocolate coated, 1 oz. | 10 | tr. | .02 | .05 | .10 | n.a. | n.a. | n.a. |
| peanut, chocolate coated: | | | | | | | | |
| 1 oz. . . . . . . . . . . . . . | tr. | tr. | .10 | .05 | 2.10 | n.a. | n.a. | n.a. |
| (*Goobers*), 1.38-oz. | | | | | | | | |
| pkg. . . . . . . . . . . . | 0 | 0 | .05 | .08 | 2.03 | .08 | 3.0 | n.a. |
| peanut bar, 1 oz. . . . . . . | 0 | 0 | .12 | .02 | 2.70 | n.a. | n.a. | n.a. |
| peanut brittle, 1 oz. . . . . . | 0 | 0 | .05 | .01 | 1.00 | n.a. | n.a. | n.a. |
| peanut butter: | | | | | | | | |
| candy coated | | | | | | | | |
| (*Reese's Pieces*), | | | | | | | | |
| 1.95 oz. pkg. . . . . . | 11 | n.a. | .03 | .13 | 3.14 | n.a. | n.a. | n.a. |
| chocolate coated, w/cookies | | | | | | | | |
| (*Twix*), 2-oz. pkg. | 87 | tr. | .03 | .11 | .21 | .02 | 4.0 | .16 |
| cup, chocolate coated | | | | | | | | |
| (*Reese's*), 1.6-oz. pkg. | 31 | tr. | .02 | .09 | 1.79 | .04 | 12.0 | .21 |
| raisins, chocolate coated | | | | | | | | |
| (*Raisinets*), 1.56 oz. . . . | 17 | tr. | .04 | .09 | .18 | n.a. | n.a. | n.a. |
| raisins, milk chocolate | | | | | | | | |
| coated, 10 pieces, | | | | | | | | |
| .35 oz. . . . . . . . . . . . . | 4 | 0 | .01 | .02 | .04 | n.a. | n.a. | 0 |
| sesame crunch, 1 oz. . . . . | n.a. | n.a. | n.a. | n.a. | 1.05 | n.a. | n.a. | 0 |
| (*Snickers*), 2.16-oz. bar . . | 72 | n.a. | .03 | .11 | 1.82 | .11 | 24.0 | .25 |
| (*3 Musketeers*), | | | | | | | | |
| 2.13-oz. bar. . . . . . . . . | n.a. | tr. | .02 | .08 | .14 | .01 | 0 | n.a. |
| toffee (*Skor*), | | | | | | | | |
| 1.4-oz. bar. . . . . . . . . | 112 | n.a. | .01 | .14 | .04 | n.a. | n.a. | n.a. |

| | Vitamin A | Vitamin C | Thiamin | Riboflavin | Niacin | B6 | Folacin | B12 |
|---|---|---|---|---|---|---|---|---|
| | (IU) | (Mg) | (Mg) | (Mg) | (Mg) | (Mg) | (Mcg) | (Mcg) |

Candy, *continued*
wafer, bar, chocolate
coated (*Kit Kat*),

| | | | | | | | | |
|---|---|---|---|---|---|---|---|---|
| 2.8-oz. pkg. . . . . . . . . | 85 | 1 | .05 | .20 | .32 | .04 | 0 | .49 |
| (*Whatchamacallit*), | | | | | | | | |
| 1.8-oz. bar. . . . . . . . . | 36 | n.a. | .31 | .14 | 1.06 | n.a. | n.a. | n.a. |
| **Cantaloupe:** | | | | | | | | |
| untrimmed, 1 lb. . . . . . . | 7457 | 98 | .08 | .05 | 1.32 | .27 | 39.4 | 0 |
| ½ of 5"-diam. melon . . . . | 8608 | 113 | .10 | .06 | 1.53 | .31 | 45.5 | 0 |
| pulp, cubed, ½ cup . . . . . | 2579 | 34 | .03 | .02 | .46 | .09 | 13.7 | 0 |
| **Capon,** see "Chicken" | | | | | | | | |
| **Carambola:** | | | | | | | | |
| untrimmed, 1 lb. . . . . . . . | 2125 | 91 | .12 | .12 | 1.77 | n.a. | n.a. | 0 |
| 1 medium, approx. | | | | | | | | |
| 4.5 oz. . . . . . . . . . . . . | 626 | 27 | .04 | .03 | .52 | n.a. | n.a. | 0 |
| trimmed, cubed, | | | | | | | | |
| ½ cup . . . . . . . . . . . . | 338 | 15 | .02 | .02 | .28 | n.a. | n.a. | 0 |
| **Caramel,** see "Candy" | | | | | | | | |
| **Caramel topping,** 2 tbsp. | n.a. | n.a. | n.a. | .04 | n.a. | n.a. | n.a. | 0 |
| **Caraway seed,** 1 tsp. . . . | 8 | n.a. | .01 | .01 | .08 | n.a. | n.a. | 0 |
| **Cardamom,** ground, | | | | | | | | |
| 1 tsp. . . . . . . . . . . . . | 0 | n.a. | <.01 | .01 | .02 | n.a. | n.a. | 0 |
| **Cardoon,** raw: | | | | | | | | |
| untrimmed, 1 lb. . . . . . . . | 267 | 4 | .04 | .07 | .68 | n.a. | n.a. | 0 |
| trimmed, shredded, | | | | | | | | |
| ½ cup . . . . . . . . . . . . | 107 | 2 | .02 | .03 | .27 | n.a. | n.a. | 0 |
| **Carissa:** | | | | | | | | |
| untrimmed, 1 lb. . . . . . . . | 156 | 148 | .16 | .23 | .78 | n.a. | n.a. | 0 |
| 1 medium, approx. | | | | | | | | |
| ¾ oz. . . . . . . . . . . . . | 8 | 8 | .01 | .01 | .04 | n.a. | n.a. | 0 |
| trimmed, sliced, ½ cup | 30 | 29 | .03 | .05 | .15 | n.a. | n.a. | 0 |
| **Carob flour,** 1 cup . . . . . | 15 | <1 | .06 | .48 | 1.95 | .38 | 29.9 | 0 |
| **Carp,** meat only: | | | | | | | | |
| raw, 1 lb. . . . . . . . . . . . | 132 | 7 | n.a. | n.a. | n.a. | .86 | n.a. | 6.94 |

| | Vitamin A | Vitamin C | Thiamin | Riboflavin | Niacin | B6 | Folacin | B12 |
|---|---|---|---|---|---|---|---|---|
| | (IU) | (Mg) | (Mg) | (Mg) | (Mg) | (Mg) | (Mcg) | (Mcg) |
| baked, broiled, or microwaved[1], 4 oz. . . . | 36 | 2 | n.a. | n.a. | n.a. | .25 | n.a. | 1.67 |
| **Carrot:** | | | | | | | | |
| fresh: | | | | | | | | |
| raw, untrimmed, 1 lb. . . | 113,557 | 38 | .39 | .24 | 3.75 | .59 | 56.4 | 0 |
| raw, 7½"-long carrot, 2.8 oz. . . . . . . . . . | 20,253 | 7 | .07 | .04 | .67 | .11 | 10.1 | 0 |
| raw, shredded, ½ cup . . . . . . . . . | 15,471 | 5 | .05 | .03 | .51 | .08 | 7.7 | 0 |
| boiled, drained, sliced, ½ cup. . . . . | 19,152 | 2 | .03 | .04 | .40 | .19 | 10.8 | 0 |
| fresh, baby, raw: | | | | | | | | |
| trimmed, 1 lb. . . . . . . | 8944 | 38 | .014 | n.a. | 4.01 | .35 | 150.0 | 0 |
| 1 large, 3¼" long, .5 oz. . . . . . . . . . | 296 | 1 | .01 | n.a. | .13 | .01 | 5.0 | 0 |
| 1 medium, 2¾" long, .4 oz. . . . . . . . . . | 197 | 1 | tr. | n.a. | .09 | .01 | 3.0 | 0 |
| canned, w/liquid, sliced, ½ cup . . . . . . . . . . . . | 16,196 | 3 | .02 | .03 | .52 | .14 | 10.0 | 0 |
| canned, drained, sliced, ½ cup . . . . . . . . . . . . | 10,055 | 2 | .01 | .02 | .40 | .08 | 6.7 | 0 |
| frozen, sliced, 10-oz. pkg. . . . . . . . . | 60,441 | 12 | .11 | .13 | 1.80 | .51 | 27.2 | 0 |
| frozen, boiled, drained, sliced, ½ cup. . . . . . . | 12,922 | 2 | .02 | .03 | .32 | .09 | 7.9 | 0 |
| **Carrot juice,** canned, 6 fl. oz. . . . . . . . . . . . . | 47,381 | 16 | .17 | .10 | .71 | .40 | 7.0 | 0 |
| **Casaba melon:** | | | | | | | | |
| untrimmed, 1 lb. . . . . . . . | 82 | 44 | .16 | .05 | 1.09 | n.a. | n.a. | 0 |
| pulp, cubed, ½ cup . . . . . | 26 | 14 | .05 | .02 | .34 | n.a. | n.a. | 0 |
| **Cashew:** | | | | | | | | |
| dry-roasted, 1 oz. . . . . . . | 0 | 0 | .06 | .06 | .40 | .07 | 19.7 | 0 |
| dry-roasted, wholes and halves, 1 cup. . . . . . . . | 0 | 0 | .27 | .27 | 1.92 | .35 | 94.8 | 0 |

[1] *Prepared without added ingredients.*

| | Vitamin A | Vitamin C | Thiamin | Riboflavin | Niacin | B6 | Folacin | B12 |
|---|---|---|---|---|---|---|---|---|
| | (IU) | (Mg) | (Mg) | (Mg) | (Mg) | (Mg) | (Mcg) | (Mcg) |
| Cashew, *continued* | | | | | | | | |
| oil-roasted, 1 oz........ | 0 | 0 | .12 | .05 | .51 | .07 | 19.2 | 0 |
| oil-roasted, wholes and | | | | | | | | |
| halves, 1 cup........ | 0 | 0 | .55 | .23 | 2.34 | .33 | 88.0 | 0 |
| **Cashew butter:** | | | | | | | | |
| 1 oz................. | 0 | 0 | .09 | .05 | .45 | .07 | 19.4 | 0 |
| 1 tbsp. ............. | 0 | 0 | .05 | .03 | .26 | .04 | 10.9 | 0 |
| **Catfish,** channel, meat only: | | | | | | | | |
| wild, raw, lb.......... | 227 | 3 | .95 | .33 | 8.65 | .53 | 45.0 | 10.12 |
| wild, baked, broiled, or | | | | | | | | |
| microwaved[1], 4 oz. .... | 57 | 1 | .26 | .08 | 2.70 | .12 | 11.3 | 3.29 |
| farmed, raw, 1 lb........ | 227 | 3 | 1.64 | .34 | 10.45 | .85 | 45.0 | 11.19 |
| farmed, baked, broiled, or | | | | | | | | |
| microwaved[1], 4 oz. | 57 | 1 | .48 | .08 | 2.85 | .18 | 7.9 | 3.18 |
| **Catfish, ocean,** see "Wolffish" | | | | | | | | |
| **Catsup,** 1 tbsp......... | 152 | 2 | .01 | .01 | .21 | .03 | 2.0 | 0 |
| **Cauliflower:** | | | | | | | | |
| fresh: | | | | | | | | |
| raw, untrimmed, | | | | | | | | |
| 1 lb. ........... | 34 | 82 | .10 | .11 | .93 | .39 | 101.0 | 0 |
| raw, trimmed, | | | | | | | | |
| 3 florets, 2 oz..... | 11 | 26 | .03 | .04 | .37 | .12 | 32.0 | 0 |
| raw, trimmed, | | | | | | | | |
| 1" pieces, ½ cup .. | 10 | 23 | .03 | .03 | .26 | .11 | 28.0 | 0 |
| boiled, drained, | | | | | | | | |
| 3 florets ........ | 9 | 24 | .02 | .03 | .22 | .09 | 24.0 | 0 |
| boiled, drained, | | | | | | | | |
| 1" pieces, ½ cup .. | 10 | 28 | .03 | .03 | .25 | .11 | 27.0 | 0 |
| frozen, 10-oz. pkg....... | 87 | 139 | .15 | .20 | 1.22 | .35 | 181.5 | 0 |
| frozen, boiled, drained, | | | | | | | | |
| 1" pieces, ½ cup ..... | 20 | 28 | .03 | .05 | .28 | .08 | 36.9 | 0 |
| **Cauliflower, green:** | | | | | | | | |
| raw: | | | | | | | | |
| untrimmed, 1 lb..... | 421 | 244 | .22 | .28 | 2.03 | .61 | 159 | 0 |

[1] *Prepared without added ingredients.*

| | Vitamin A | Vitamin C | Thiamin | Riboflavin | Niacin | B6 | Folacin | B12 |
|---|---|---|---|---|---|---|---|---|
| | (IU) | (Mg) | (Mg) | (Mg) | (Mg) | (Mg) | (Mcg) | (Mcg) |
| trimmed, ⅕ head, 3.3 oz.......... | 141 | 82 | .07 | .10 | .68 | .21 | 53.0 | 0 |
| trimmed, 1" pieces, ½ cup.......... | 76 | 44 | .04 | .05 | .37 | .11 | 29 | 0 |
| boiled, drained, ⅕ head............ | 127 | 65 | .06 | .09 | .62 | .19 | 37.0 | 0 |
| boiled, drained, 1" pieces, ½ cup............. | 87 | 45 | .04 | .06 | .42 | .13 | 26 | 0 |
| **Celeriac,** raw: | | | | | | | | |
| untrimmed, 1 lb........ | 0 | 31 | .20 | .23 | 2.73 | .64 | n.a. | 0 |
| trimmed, ½ cup........ | 0 | 6 | .04 | .05 | .55 | .13 | n.a. | 0 |
| **Celery:** | | | | | | | | |
| raw: | | | | | | | | |
| untrimmed, 1 lb..... | 541 | 28 | .19 | .18 | 1.30 | .35 | 113.0 | 0 |
| trimmed, 7½"-long stalk, 1.6 oz...... | 54 | 3 | .02 | .02 | .13 | .04 | 11.0 | 0 |
| diced, ½ cup....... | 80 | 4 | .03 | .03 | .19 | .05 | 17.0 | 0 |
| boiled, drained, diced, ½ cup............. | 99 | 5 | .03 | .04 | .24 | .07 | 16.0 | 0 |
| **Celtuce,** raw, trimmed, .3-oz. leaf .......... | 280 | 2 | <.01 | .01 | .04 | n.a. | n.a. | 0 |
| **Cereal, ready-to-eat:** | | | | | | | | |
| bran (see also "oat bran" and "wheat bran," below, and "Rice bran"): | | | | | | | | |
| (*All Bran*), ½ cup.... | 750 | 15 | .38 | .43 | 5.00 | .50 | n.a. | 1.50 |
| (*All Bran* Extra Fiber), ½ cup .......... | 750 | 15 | .38 | .43 | 5.00 | .50 | n.a. | 1.50 |
| (*Bran Buds*), ⅓ cup | 750 | 15 | .38 | .43 | 5.00 | .50 | n.a. | 0 |
| (*Frosted Bran*), ¾ cup.......... | 750 | 15 | .38 | .43 | 5.00 | .50 | n.a. | 1.50 |
| (*Fruitful Bran*), 1¼ cup.......... | 750 | 0 | .38 | .43 | 5.00 | .50 | n.a. | 1.50 |
| (*Kellogg's* Raisin Bran), 1 cup ..... | 750 | 0 | .38 | .43 | 5.00 | .50 | n.a. | 1.50 |
| corn: | | | | | | | | |
| (*Corn Pops*), 1 cup .. | 750 | 15 | .38 | .43 | 5.00 | .50 | n.a. | 0 |

| | Vitamin A | Vitamin C | Thiamin | Riboflavin | Niacin | B6 | Folacin | B12 |
|---|---|---|---|---|---|---|---|---|
| | (IU) | (Mg) | (Mg) | (Mg) | (Mg) | (Mg) | (Mcg) | (Mcg) |

Cereal, ready-to-eat, corn, *continued*
  (*Kellogg's Corn*
    *Flakes*), 1 cup . . . .

| | | | | | | | | |
|---|---|---|---|---|---|---|---|---|
| (*Kellogg's Corn Flakes*), 1 cup . . . . | 750 | 15 | .38 | .43 | 5.00 | .50 | n.a. | 0 |
| (*Kellogg's Frosted Flakes*), ¾ cup . . . . | 750 | 15 | .38 | .43 | 5.00 | .50 | n.a. | 0 |
| (*Nut & Honey Crunch*), 1¼ cup . . . . . . . . | 750 | 15 | .38 | .43 | 5.00 | .50 | n.a. | 0 |
| (*Nut & Honey Crunch O's* ), ¾ cup . . . . . | 750 | 15 | .38 | .43 | 5.00 | .50 | n.a. | 0 |
| (*Nutri-Grain Corn*), 1 oz. . . . . . . . . . . . | n.a. | 15 | .38 | .43 | 5.00 | .50 | n.a. | 2.00 |

granola, see "mixed grain" below
mixed grain:

| | | | | | | | | |
|---|---|---|---|---|---|---|---|---|
| (*Apple Jacks*), 1 cup | 750 | 15 | .38 | .43 | 5.00 | .50 | n.a. | 0 |
| (*Cinnamon Mini Buns*), ¾ cup . . . . | 750 | 15 | .38 | .43 | 5.00 | .50 | n.a. | 0 |
| (*Crispix*), 1 cup . . . . . | 750 | 15 | .38 | .43 | 5.00 | .50 | n.a. | 0 |
| (*Double Dip Crunch*), ¾ cup . . . . . . . . | 750 | 15 | .38 | .43 | 5.00 | .50 | n.a. | 0 |
| (*Froot Loops*), 1 cup | 750 | 15 | .38 | .43 | 5.00 | .50 | n.a. | 0 |
| (*Healthy Choice Flakes*), 1 cup . . . . | 500 | 0 | .53 | .60 | 7.00 | .70 | n.a. | 2.10 |
| (*Healthy Choice Squares*), 1¼ cup . . | 500 | 0 | .53 | .60 | 7.00 | .70 | n.a. | 2.10 |
| (*Kellogg's Low Fat Granola*), ½ cup . . | 750 | 0 | .38 | .43 | 5.00 | .50 | n.a. | 1.50 |
| (*Kellogg's Mueslix Crispy Blend*), ⅔ cup | 200 | 0 | .38 | .43 | 5.00 | .50 | n.a. | 1.50 |
| (*Kellogg's Mueslix Golden Crunch*), ¾ cup . . . . . . . . | 750 | 0 | .38 | .43 | 5.00 | .50 | n.a. | 1.20 |
| (*King Vitamin*), 1 oz. | 1500 | 24 | .60 | .68 | 8.00 | .60 | 160.0 | 2.40 |
| (*Pop-Tarts Crunch*), all flavors, ¾ cup | 750 | 15 | .38 | .43 | 5.00 | .50 | n.a. | n.a. |
| (*Product 19*), 1 cup | 750 | 60 | 1.50 | 1.70 | 20.00 | 2.00 | n.a. | 6.00 |

| | Vitamin A | Vitamin C | Thiamin | Riboflavin | Niacin | B₆ | Folacin | B₁₂ |
|---|---|---|---|---|---|---|---|---|
| | (IU) | (Mg) | (Mg) | (Mg) | (Mg) | (Mg) | (Mcg) | (Mcg) |
| (*Special K*), 1 cup . . . | 750 | 15 | .53 | .60 | 7.00 | .70 | n.a. | 0 |
| w/almonds (*Kellogg's Temptations*), ¾ cup | 750 | 15 | .38 | .43 | 5.00 | .50 | n.a. | n.a. |
| almond raisin (*Nutri-Grain*), 1¼ cup . . . | 0 | 0 | .38 | .43 | 5.00 | .50 | n.a. | 1.50 |
| w/fiber nuggets or fruit and nuts (*Just Right*), 1 cup . . . . . | 1250 | 0 | .38 | .43 | 5.00 | .50 | n.a. | 1.50 |
| w/pecans (*Kellogg's Temptations*), 1 cup | 750 | 15 | .38 | .43 | 5.00 | .50 | n.a. | n.a. |
| w/raisins (*Kellogg's Low Fat Granola*), ⅔ cup . . . . . . . . . | 750 | 0 | .38 | .43 | 5.00 | .50 | n.a. | 1.50 |
| w/raisins, oat clusters, and almonds (*Healthy Choice*), 1 cup . . . . | 500 | 0 | .53 | .60 | 7.00 | .70 | n.a. | 2.10 |
| oat (*Life*), 1 oz. . . . . . . . . | 0 | 0 | .46 | .45 | 5.58 | .04 | 19.0 | n.a. |
| oat, cinnamon (*Life*), 1 oz. . . . . . . . . . . . . . | 0 | 0 | .50 | .51 | 6.84 | .05 | 19.0 | n.a. |
| oat bran (*Common Sense*), ¾ cup . . . . . . . | 750 | 0 | .38 | .43 | 5.00 | .50 | n.a. | 1.50 |
| oat bran (*Cracklin' Oat Bran*), ¾ cup . . . . . . . . | 750 | 15 | .38 | .43 | 5.00 | .50 | n.a. | 0 |
| rice: | | | | | | | | |
| (*Cocoa Krispies*), ¾ cup . . . . . . . . . | 750 | 15 | .38 | .43 | 5.00 | .50 | n.a. | 0 |
| (*Frosted Krispies*), ¾ cup . . . . . . . . . | 750 | 15 | .38 | .43 | 5.00 | .50 | n.a. | 0 |
| (*Fruity Marshmallow Krispies*), ¾ cup . . | 750 | 15 | .38 | .43 | 5.00 | .50 | n.a. | 0 |
| (*Rice Krispies*), 1¼ cup . . . . . . . . | 750 | 15 | .38 | .43 | 5.00 | .50 | n.a. | 0 |
| (*Rice Krispie Treats*), ¾ cup . . . . . . . . . | 750 | 15 | .38 | .43 | 5.00 | .50 | n.a. | 1.50 |

|  | Vitamin A | Vitamin C | Thiamin | Riboflavin | Niacin | B6 | Folacin | B12 |
|---|---|---|---|---|---|---|---|---|
|  | (IU) | (Mg) | (Mg) | (Mg) | (Mg) | (Mg) | (Mcg) | (Mcg) |

Cereal, ready-to-eat, rice, *continued*

| w/apple (*Apple Raisin Crisp*), 1 cup . . . . . | 750 | 0 | .38 | .43 | 5.00 | .50 | n.a. | 1.50 |
|---|---|---|---|---|---|---|---|---|
| w/apple cinnamon (*Rice Krispies*), ¾ cup . . . . . . . . . | 750 | 15 | .38 | .43 | 5.00 | .50 | n.a. | 0 |

wheat:

| (*Apple Cinnamon Squares*), ¾ cup . . | 0 | 0 | .38 | .43 | 5.00 | .50 | n.a. | 1.50 |
|---|---|---|---|---|---|---|---|---|
| (*Blueberry Squares*), ¾ cup . . . . . . . . . | 0 | 0 | .38 | .43 | 5.00 | .50 | n.a. | 1.50 |
| (*Frosted Mini-Wheats* Regular/Bite Size), 1 cup . . . . . . . . . | 0 | 0 | .38 | .43 | 5.00 | .50 | n.a. | 1.50 |
| (*Kellogg's Smacks*), ¾ cup . . . . . . . . . | 750 | 15 | .38 | .43 | 5.00 | .50 | n.a. | 0 |
| (*Nutri-Grain* Wheat), ¾ cup . . . . . . . . . | 0 | 0 | .38 | .43 | 5.00 | .50 | n.a. | 1.50 |
| (*Nutri-Grain* Wheat & Raisins), 1¼ cup | 0 | 0 | .38 | .43 | 5.00 | .50 | .10 | 1.50 |
| (*Raisin Squares*), ¾ cup . . . . . . . . . | 0 | 0 | .38 | .43 | 5.00 | .50 | n.a. | 1.50 |
| (*Strawberry Squares*), ¾ cup . . . . . . . . . | 0 | 0 | .38 | .43 | 5.00 | .50 | n.a. | 1.50 |
| w/wheat bran (*Kellogg's Complete*), ¾ cup | 1250 | 15 | .38 | .43 | 5.00 | .50 | n.a. | 1.50 |

**Cereal, cooking,** uncooked, except as noted:

corn grits, yellow, enriched, regular or

| quick[1], 1 pkt. . . . . . . . . | 125 | n.a. | .18 | .11 | 1.41 | .04 | 1.4 | n.a. |
|---|---|---|---|---|---|---|---|---|
| (*Roman Meal* Original), 1 oz. . . . . . . . . . . . . . | 0 | 0 | .13 | .05 | 1.47 | n.a. | n.a. | n.a. |

---

[1] *White corn grits contain only a trace of Vitamin A.*

| | Vitamin A | Vitamin C | Thiamin | Riboflavin | Niacin | B6 | Folacin | B12 |
|---|---|---|---|---|---|---|---|---|
| | (IU) | (Mg) | (Mg) | (Mg) | (Mg) | (Mg) | (Mcg) | (Mcg) |
| oat and oatmeal: | | | | | | | | |
| (*Instant Quaker*), 1 pkt. . . . . . . . . . | 1237 | 0 | .44 | .21 | 3.64 | .47 | 122.0 | n.a. |
| (*Quaker* Quick/Old Fashioned), ⅓ cup or ⅔ cup cooked | 26 | 0 | .14 | .03 | .22 | .03 | 7.0 | n.a. |
| (*Roman Meal*), 1.2 oz. . . . . . . . . . | 0 | 0 | .20 | .06 | 1.09 | n.a. | n.a. | n.a. |
| apple and cinnamon (*Instant Quaker*), 1 pkt. . . . . . . . . . | 1233 | <1 | .37 | .21 | 3.69 | .43 | 113.0 | 0 |
| apple and cinnamon (*Roman Meal*), 1.2 oz. . . . . . . . . . | tr. | tr. | .22 | .05 | 1.99 | n.a. | n.a. | n.a. |
| cinnamon and spice (*Instant Quaker*), 1 pkt. . . . . . . . . . | 1309 | 0 | .39 | .23 | 3.72 | .46 | 120.0 | n.a. |
| maple and brown sugar (*Instant Quaker*), 1 pkt.. . . . | 1380 | 0 | .40 | .23 | 3.77 | .44 | 116.0 | n.a. |
| raisins and spice (*Instant Quaker*), 1 pkt. . . . . . . . . . | 1298 | 0 | .36 | .23 | 3.68 | .44 | 103.0 | .08 |
| wheat, dates, raisins, and almonds (*Roman Meal*), 1.3 oz. . . . . . | tr. | tr. | .18 | .05 | .74 | n.a. | n.a. | n.a. |
| wheat, honey, coconut, and almonds (*Roman Meal*), 1.3 oz. . . . . | tr. | tr. | .16 | .06 | .58 | n.a. | n.a. | n.a. |
| rye, cream of (*Roman Meal*), 1.3 oz. . . . . . . . | 0 | 0 | .16 | .08 | .59 | n.a. | n.a. | n.a. |
| wheat, farina, enriched, 1 pkt. . . . . . . . . . . . | n.a. | n.a. | .16 | .10 | 1.15 | .02 | 6.8 | n.a. |

**Cervelat,** see "Thuringer cervelat"
**Chard,** see "Swiss chard"

| | Vitamin A | Vitamin C | Thiamin | Riboflavin | Niacin | B6 | Folacin | B12 |
|---|---|---|---|---|---|---|---|---|
| | (IU) | (Mg) | (Mg) | (Mg) | (Mg) | (Mg) | (Mcg) | (Mcg) |

**Chayote:**

| | | | | | | | | |
|---|---|---|---|---|---|---|---|---|
| raw, untrimmed, 1 lb. ... | 251 | 49 | .14 | .18 | 2.25 | n.a. | n.a. | 0 |
| raw, trimmed, 1 medium, 7.2 oz............. | 114 | 22 | .06 | .08 | 1.02 | n.a. | n.a. | 0 |
| boiled, drained, 1" pieces, ½ cup............. | 37 | 6 | .02 | .03 | .34 | n.a. | n.a. | 0 |

**Cheese:**

| | | | | | | | | |
|---|---|---|---|---|---|---|---|---|
| American, pasteurized processed, 1 oz. ...... | 343 | 0 | .01 | .10 | .02 | .02 | 2.0 | .20 |
| blue, 1 oz............. | 204 | 0 | .01 | .11 | .29 | .05 | 10.0 | .35 |
| brick, 1 oz. ........... | 307 | 0 | <.01 | .10 | .03 | .02 | 6.0 | .36 |
| Brie, 1 oz............. | 189 | 0 | .02 | .15 | .11 | .07 | 18.0 | .47 |
| Camembert, 1 oz. ...... | 262 | 0 | .01 | .14 | .18 | .06 | 18.0 | .37 |
| cheddar, 1 oz......... | 300 | 0 | .01 | .11 | .02 | .02 | 5.0 | .23 |
| cheddar, low fat, 1 oz. | 66 | 0 | tr. | .06 | .01 | .01 | 3.0 | .14 |
| cheddar, low sodium, 1 oz............. | 297 | 0 | .01 | .11 | .03 | .02 | 5.0 | .23 |
| Colby, 1 oz............ | 293 | 0 | <.01 | .11 | .03 | .02 | n.a. | .23 |
| cottage, ½ cup not packed: | | | | | | | | |
| creamed, large curd | 183 | tr. | .02 | .18 | .14 | .08 | 13.5 | .70 |
| creamed, small curd | 171 | tr. | .02 | .17 | .13 | .07 | 12.6 | .65 |
| creamed, w/fruit | 139 | tr. | .02 | .15 | .11 | .06 | 11.0 | .56 |
| dry curd .......... | 22 | 0 | .02 | .10 | .11 | .06 | 10.9 | .60 |
| low fat 2% ........ | 79 | tr. | .03 | .21 | .16 | .09 | 15.0 | .81 |
| low fat 1% ........ | 42 | tr. | .02 | .19 | .15 | .08 | 14.0 | .72 |
| cream, 1 oz. .......... | 405 | 0 | .01 | .06 | .03 | .01 | 4.0 | .12 |
| Edam, 1 oz............ | 260 | 0 | .01 | .11 | .02 | .02 | 5.0 | .44 |
| fontina, 1 oz........... | 333 | 0 | .01 | .06 | .04 | n.a. | n.a. | n.a. |
| goat, hard, 1 oz. ....... | n.a. | n.a. | .04 | .34 | .68 | n.a. | n.a. | n.a. |
| goat, semisoft, 1 oz. | n.a. | n.a. | .02 | .19 | .33 | n.a. | n.a. | n.a. |
| goat, soft, 1 oz......... | n.a. | n.a. | .02 | .11 | .12 | n.a. | n.a. | n.a. |
| Gouda, 1 oz. ......... | 183 | 0 | .01 | .10 | .02 | .02 | 6.0 | n.a. |
| Gruyère, 1 oz. ......... | 346 | 0 | .02 | .08 | .03 | .02 | 3.0 | .45 |
| Limburger, 1 oz. ....... | 363 | 0 | .02 | .14 | .05 | .02 | 16.0 | .30 |
| Mexican, queso anejo, 1 oz............. | 63 | 0 | .01 | .06 | .01 | .01 | 0 | .39 |

| | Vitamin A | Vitamin C | Thiamin | Riboflavin | Niacin | B6 | Folacin | B12 |
|---|---|---|---|---|---|---|---|---|
| | (IU) | (Mg) | (Mg) | (Mg) | (Mg) | (Mg) | (Mcg) | (Mcg) |
| Mexican, queso asadero, 1 oz.............. | 63 | 0 | .01 | .06 | .05 | .02 | 2.0 | .28 |
| Mexican, queso chihuahua, 1 oz. ..... | 64 | 0 | .01 | .06 | .04 | .02 | 1.0 | .29 |
| mozzarella: | | | | | | | | |
| whole milk, 1 oz..... | 225 | 0 | <.01 | .07 | .02 | .02 | 2.0 | .19 |
| whole milk, low moisture, 1 oz. .... | 256 | 0 | .01 | .08 | .03 | .02 | 2.0 | .21 |
| part skim, 1 oz...... | 166 | 0 | .01 | .09 | .03 | .02 | 2.0 | .23 |
| part skim, low moisture, 1 oz. .... | 178 | 0 | .01 | .10 | .03 | .02 | 3.0 | .26 |
| Muenster, 1 oz......... | 318 | 0 | <.01 | .09 | .03 | .02 | 3.0 | .42 |
| Neufchâtel, 1 oz........ | 321 | 0 | <.01 | .06 | .04 | .01 | 3.0 | .08 |
| Parmesan: | | | | | | | | |
| grated, 1 oz. ....... | 199 | 0 | .01 | .11 | .09 | .03 | 2.0 | n.a. |
| grated, 1 tbsp....... | 35 | 0 | <.01 | .02 | .02 | .01 | tr. | n.a. |
| hard, 1 oz.......... | 171 | 0 | .01 | .09 | .08 | .03 | 2.0 | n.a. |
| pimiento, pasteurized processed, 1 oz. ..... | 358 | 0 | .01 | .10 | .02 | .02 | 2.0 | .20 |
| Port du Salut, 1 oz...... | 378 | 0 | 0 | .07 | .02 | .02 | 5.0 | .43 |
| provolone, 1 oz......... | 231 | 0 | .01 | .09 | .04 | .02 | 3.0 | .42 |
| ricotta: | | | | | | | | |
| whole milk, ½ cup... | 608 | 0 | .02 | .24 | .13 | .05 | n.a. | .41 |
| part skim, ½ cup.... | 536 | 0 | .03 | .23 | .10 | .03 | n.a. | .36 |
| Romano, 1 oz.......... | 162 | 0 | n.a. | .11 | .02 | n.a. | 2.0 | n.a. |
| Roquefort, 1 oz........ | 297 | 0 | .01 | .17 | .21 | .04 | 14.0 | .18 |
| Swiss, 1 oz........... | 240 | 0 | .01 | .10 | .03 | .02 | 2.0 | .48 |
| Swiss, pasteurized processed, 1 oz. ..... | 229 | 0 | <.01 | .08 | .01 | .01 | n.a. | .35 |
| Tilsit, 1 oz. ........... | 296 | 0 | .02 | .10 | .06 | n.a. | n.a. | .60 |
| **Cheese food:** | | | | | | | | |
| American, cold pack, 1 oz............... | 200 | 0 | .01 | .13 | .02 | .04 | 2.0 | .36 |
| American, pasteurized processed, 1 oz. ..... | 259 | 0 | .01 | .13 | .04 | n.a. | n.a. | .32 |

| | Vitamin A | Vitamin C | Thiamin | Riboflavin | Niacin | B6 | Folacin | B12 |
|---|---|---|---|---|---|---|---|---|
| | (IU) | (Mg) | (Mg) | (Mg) | (Mg) | (Mg) | (Mcg) | (Mcg) |
| **Cheese food,** *continued* | | | | | | | | |
| Swiss, pasteurized | | | | | | | | |
| processed, 1 oz. . . . . . | 243 | 0 | tr. | .11 | .03 | n.a. | n.a. | .65 |
| **Cheese spread,** American | | | | | | | | |
| pasteurized processed, | | | | | | | | |
| 1 oz. . . . . . . . . . . . . . | 223 | 0 | .01 | .12 | .04 | .03 | 2.0 | .11 |
| **Cheese stick or straw,** 5" | | | | | | | | |
| long, 10 pieces, 2.1 oz. | 230 | 0 | .01 | .10 | .20 | n.a. | n.a. | n.a. |
| **Cheese substitute,** | | | | | | | | |
| mozzarella, 1 oz. . . . . . | 413 | 0 | .01 | .13 | .09 | .02 | 3.0 | .23 |
| **Cherimoya,** trimmed, | | | | | | | | |
| 1 oz. . . . . . . . . . . . . . | 3 | 3 | .03 | .03 | .37 | n.a. | n.a. | 0 |
| **Cherry:** | | | | | | | | |
| fresh, sour, red: | | | | | | | | |
| untrimmed, 1 lb. . . . . | 5237 | 41 | .12 | .16 | 1.63 | .18 | 30.6 | 0 |
| pitted, ½ cup. . . . . . . | 995 | 8 | .02 | .03 | .31 | .03 | 5.8 | 0 |
| w/pits, ½ cup . . . . . . | 661 | 5 | .02 | .02 | .21 | .02 | 3.9 | 0 |
| fresh, sweet: | | | | | | | | |
| untrimmed, 1 lb. . . . . | 874 | 29 | .20 | .25 | 1.63 | .15 | 17.1 | 0 |
| w/pits, ½ cup . . . . . . | 155 | 5 | .04 | .04 | .29 | .03 | 3.1 | 0 |
| 10 medium, approx. | | | | | | | | |
| 2.6 oz. . . . . . . . . . | 146 | 5 | .03 | .04 | .27 | .02 | 2.8 | 0 |
| canned, sour, red: | | | | | | | | |
| in water, ½ cup. . . . . | 920 | 3 | .02 | .05 | .22 | .05 | 9.8 | 0 |
| in light syrup, ½ cup | 914 | 3 | .02 | .05 | .21 | .06 | 9.7 | 0 |
| in heavy syrup, | | | | | | | | |
| ½ cup . . . . . . . . . . | 914 | 3 | .02 | .05 | .22 | .06 | 9.7 | 0 |
| canned, sweet: | | | | | | | | |
| in water, ½ cup. . . . . | 198 | 3 | .03 | .05 | .51 | .04 | n.a. | 0 |
| in juice, ½ cup . . . . . | 156 | 3 | .02 | .03 | .51 | n.a. | n.a. | 0 |
| in light syrup, ½ cup | 197 | 5 | .03 | .05 | .51 | .04 | n.a. | 0 |
| in heavy syrup, | | | | | | | | |
| ½ cup . . . . . . . . . . | 199 | 5 | .03 | .05 | .51 | .04 | n.a. | 0 |
| frozen: | | | | | | | | |
| sour, red, unsweetened, | | | | | | | | |
| ½ cup. . . . . . . . . . | 675 | 1 | .03 | .03 | .11 | .05 | 3.5 | 0 |

| | Vitamin A | Vitamin C | Thiamin | Riboflavin | Niacin | B6 | Folacin | B12 |
|---|---|---|---|---|---|---|---|---|
| | (IU) | (Mg) | (Mg) | (Mg) | (Mg) | (Mg) | (Mcg) | (Mcg) |
| sweet, sweetened, 10-oz. pkg. . . . . . . | 536 | 3 | .08 | .13 | .50 | n.a. | n.a. | 0 |
| sweet, sweetened, ½ cup . . . . . . . . . . | 245 | 1 | .04 | .06 | .23 | n.a. | n.a. | 0 |
| **Chestnut, Chinese,** shelled, except as noted: | | | | | | | | |
| raw, in shell, 1 lb. . . . . . . | 770 | 137 | .61 | .69 | 3.05 | n.a. | n.a. | 0 |
| raw, 1 oz. . . . . . . . . . . . . | 57 | 10 | .05 | .05 | .23 | n.a. | n.a. | 0 |
| roasted, 1 oz. . . . . . . . . . | 1 | n.a. | .04 | .03 | .43 | n.a. | n.a. | 0 |
| **Chestnut, European,** shelled, except as noted: | | | | | | | | |
| raw, in shell, 1 lb. . . . . . . | 94 | 144.3 | .80 | .56 | 3.96 | 1.26 | 208.1 | 0 |
| raw, unpeeled, 1 oz. . . . . | 8 | 12 | .07 | .05 | .34 | .11 | 17.6 | 0 |
| dried, unpeeled, 1 oz. . . . | 0 | 4 | .08 | .10 | .24 | .19 | 31.0 | 0 |
| roasted: | | | | | | | | |
| in shell, 1 lb. . . . . . . . . | 70 | 74 | .69 | .50 | 3.83 | 1.42 | 200.0 | 0 |
| peeled, 1 oz. . . . . . . . . | 7 | 7 | .07 | .05 | .38 | .14 | 19.9 | 0 |
| peeled, 1 cup, approx. 17 kernels . . . . . . . | 35 | 37.2 | .35 | .25 | 1.92 | .71 | 100.1 | 0 |
| **Chestnut, Japanese,** shelled, except as noted: | | | | | | | | |
| raw, in shell, 1 lb. . . . . . . | 110 | 79 | 1.03 | .49 | 4.49 | n.a. | n.a. | 0 |
| raw, 1 oz. . . . . . . . . . . . . | 10 | 8 | .10 | .05 | .43 | n.a. | n.a. | 0 |
| boiled or steamed, 1 oz. . . . . . . . . . . . . . | 4 | 3 | .04 | .02 | .15 | n.a. | n.a. | 0 |
| dried, in shell, 1 lb. . . . . . . | 256 | 184 | 2.40 | 1.14 | 10.48 | n.a. | n.a. | 0 |
| dried, 1 oz. . . . . . . . . . . . | 24 | 17 | .23 | .11 | .99 | n.a. | n.a. | 0 |
| roasted, 1 oz. . . . . . . . . . | 21 | 8 | .13 | .07 | .20 | n.a. | n.a. | 0 |
| **Chia seeds,** dried, 1 oz. | 10 | n.a. | .25 | .05 | 1.65 | n.a. | n.a. | 0 |
| **Chicken**[1], fresh, 4 oz., except as noted: | | | | | | | | |
| broiler-fryer, flour-coated, fried: | | | | | | | | |
| meat w/skin . . . . . . . . | 101 | 0 | .10 | .22 | 10.20 | .46 | 6.8 | .35 |
| dark meat w/skin . . . . | 118 | 0 | .11 | .27 | 7.76 | .36 | 9.1 | .34 |
| light meat w/skin . . . . | 77 | 0 | .09 | .15 | 13.65 | .61 | 4.5 | .37 |
| back meat w/skin . . . . | 139 | 0 | .12 | .27 | 8.27 | .34 | 9.1 | .32 |
| breast meat w/skin . . . | 57 | 0 | .09 | .15 | 15.58 | .66 | 4.5 | .39 |

[1] *Prepared without added ingredients, except as noted.*

|  | Vitamin A | Vitamin C | Thiamin | Riboflavin | Niacin | B₆ | Folacin | B₁₂ |
|---|---|---|---|---|---|---|---|---|
|  | (IU) | (Mg) | (Mg) | (Mg) | (Mg) | (Mg) | (Mcg) | (Mcg) |

**Chicken, broiler-fryer, flour-coated, fried,** *continued*

| | Vitamin A | Vitamin C | Thiamin | Riboflavin | Niacin | B₆ | Folacin | B₁₂ |
|---|---|---|---|---|---|---|---|---|
| drumstick, meat w/skin, 1.7 oz. (2.6 oz. raw w/bone) | 41 | 0 | .04 | .11 | 2.96 | .17 | .4 | .16 |
| leg, meat w/skin, 4 oz. (5.5 oz. raw w/bone) | 103 | 0 | .10 | .26 | 7.33 | .38 | 9.0 | .35 |
| thigh, meat w/skin, 2.2 oz. (2.9 oz. raw w/bone) | 61 | 0 | .06 | .15 | 4.31 | .21 | 5.0 | .19 |
| wing, meat w/skin, 1.1 oz. (2.2 oz. raw w/bone) | 40 | 0 | .02 | .04 | 2.14 | .13 | 1.0 | .09 |
| broiler-fryer, roasted: | | | | | | | | |
| meat w/skin | 183 | 0 | .07 | .19 | 9.62 | .45 | 5.7 | .34 |
| meat only | 60 | 0 | .08 | .20 | 10.40 | .53 | 6.8 | .37 |
| skin only, 1 oz. | 74 | 0 | .01 | .04 | 1.58 | .03 | .6 | .06 |
| dark meat w/skin | 228 | 0 | .07 | .23 | 7.21 | .35 | 7.9 | .33 |
| dark meat only | 82 | 0 | .08 | .26 | 7.43 | .41 | 9.1 | .36 |
| light meat w/skin | 125 | 0 | .07 | .13 | 12.63 | .59 | 3.4 | .36 |
| light meat only | 33 | 0 | .07 | .13 | 14.09 | .68 | 4.5 | .39 |
| roaster, roasted: | | | | | | | | |
| meat w/skin | 94 | 0 | .06 | .16 | 8.41 | .40 | 5.7 | .31 |
| meat only | 46 | 0 | .07 | .17 | 8.94 | .46 | 5.7 | .32 |
| dark meat only | 61 | 0 | .07 | .22 | 6.50 | .35 | 7.9 | .31 |
| light meat only | 28 | 0 | .07 | .11 | 11.87 | .61 | 3.4 | .35 |
| stewing, stewed: | | | | | | | | |
| meat w/skin | 149 | 0 | .11 | .27 | 6.57 | .28 | 5.7 | .26 |
| meat only | 127 | 0 | .13 | .31 | 7.27 | .35 | 6.8 | .29 |
| dark meat only | 164 | 0 | .15 | .39 | 5.17 | .27 | 9.1 | .28 |
| light meat only | 83 | 0 | .11 | .22 | 9.68 | .44 | 4.5 | .31 |
| capon, roasted, meat w/skin | 77 | 0 | .08 | .19 | 10.15 | .49 | 6.8 | .37 |
| Cornish hen, see "Cornish game hen" | | | | | | | | |
| **Chicken, canned,** boned, w/broth, 5-oz. can | n.a. | 3 | .02 | .18 | 8.99 | .50 | n.a. | .42 |

| | Vitamin A | Vitamin C | Thiamin | Riboflavin | Niacin | B₆ | Folacin | B₁₂ |
|---|---|---|---|---|---|---|---|---|
| | (IU) | (Mg) | (Mg) | (Mg) | (Mg) | (Mg) | (Mcg) | (Mcg) |
| **Chicken giblets,** | | | | | | | | |
| simmered[1], 4 oz..... | 8427 | 9 | .10 | 1.08 | 4.65 | .39 | 426.4 | 11.50 |
| **Chicken gizzard,** | | | | | | | | |
| simmered[1], 4 oz...... | 213 | 2 | .03 | .28 | 4.51 | .14 | 60.1 | 2.20 |
| **"Chicken," vegetarian:** | | | | | | | | |
| canned: | | | | | | | | |
| (*Worthington Fri-Chik*), 2 pieces, 3.2 oz.......... | 0 | 0 | .08 | .14 | .61 | .15 | n.a. | 2.16 |
| diced (*Worthington*), ¼ cup, 1.9 oz..... | 0 | 0 | .06 | .05 | .34 | .08 | n.a. | .27 |
| fried, w/gravy (*Loma Linda*), 2 pieces, 5.2 oz.......... | 0 | 0 | 1.49 | .69 | 3.06 | .35 | n.a. | 2.93 |
| sliced (*Worthington*), 3 slices, 3.2 oz.... | 0 | 0 | .09 | .08 | .55 | .13 | n.a. | .44 |
| frozen: | | | | | | | | |
| (*Worthington Chicketts*), 2 slices, 1.9 oz.......... | 0 | 0 | .36 | .12 | .75 | .11 | n.a. | 1.26 |
| (*Worthington Chik-Stiks*), 1.7-oz. piece........... | 0 | 0 | .32 | .03 | 2.47 | .34 | n.a. | 2.06 |
| fried (*Loma Linda Chik'n*), 2-oz. piece | 0 | 0 | .98 | .46 | 2.09 | .35 | n.a. | .82 |
| nuggets (*Loma Linda*), 5 pieces, 3 oz............ | 0 | 0 | .67 | .30 | 2.89 | .45 | n.a. | 4.50 |
| patty (*Morningstar Farms*), 2.5-oz. patty........... | 0 | 0 | 2.15 | .16 | 1.51 | .14 | n.a. | .95 |
| patty (*Worthington Crispy Chik*), 2.5-oz. patty ..... | 0 | 0 | 1.14 | .13 | .57 | .18 | n.a. | .74 |

[1] *Prepared without added ingredients.*

| | Vitamin A | Vitamin C | Thiamin | Riboflavin | Niacin | B6 | Folacin | B12 |
|---|---|---|---|---|---|---|---|---|
| | (IU) | (Mg) | (Mg) | (Mg) | (Mg) | (Mg) | (Mcg) | (Mcg) |
| **"Chicken," frozen, vegetarian,** *continued* | | | | | | | | |
| pie (*Worthington*), | | | | | | | | |
| 8-oz. pie . . . . . . . . | 1318 | 0 | .23 | .14 | 0 | .20 | n.a. | 1.16 |
| sliced (*Worthington*), | | | | | | | | |
| 2 slices, 2 oz. . . . . | 0 | 0 | .32 | .13 | 1.23 | .21 | n.a. | .91 |
| mix, supreme (*Loma* | | | | | | | | |
| *Linda*), ⅓ cup, .9 oz. | 0 | 0 | .55 | .42 | 2.45 | .30 | n.a. | 1.75 |
| **Chicken gravy,** canned, | | | | | | | | |
| ¼ cup . . . . . . . . . . . . | 220 | 0 | .01 | .03 | .26 | .01 | n.a. | n.a. |
| **"Chicken" gravy mix,** | | | | | | | | |
| vegetarian, (*Loma* | | | | | | | | |
| *Linda*), 2 tbsp., .2 oz. | 0 | 0 | .32 | .01 | 0 | .01 | n.a. | 0 |
| **Chicken heart,** see "Heart" | | | | | | | | |
| **Chicken liver,** see "Liver" | | | | | | | | |
| **Chicken seasoning** | | | | | | | | |
| (*Tone's Perc*), ¼ tsp. | 2 | <1 | tr. | tr. | .02 | .03 | .8 | 0 |
| **Chickpeas:** | | | | | | | | |
| uncooked, 1 lb. . . . . . . . | 304 | 18 | 2.16 | .96 | 6.99 | 2.43 | 2524.9 | 0 |
| uncooked, ½ cup. . . . . . . | 67 | 4 | .48 | .21 | 1.54 | .54 | 556.6 | 0 |
| boiled, ½ cup . . . . . . | 22 | 1 | .10 | .05 | .43 | .11 | 141.0 | 0 |
| canned, w/liquid, 8 oz. | 55 | 9 | .07 | .08 | .31 | 1.07 | 151.4 | 0 |
| canned, w/liquid, | | | | | | | | |
| ½ cup . . . . . . . . . . . . | 29 | 5 | .04 | .04 | .17 | .57 | 80.1 | 0 |
| **Chicory, witloof,** raw: | | | | | | | | |
| untrimmed, 1 lb. . . . . . . | 118 | 11.5 | .25 | .11 | .65 | .17 | 149.0 | 0 |
| 1 head, 5" to 7" long, | | | | | | | | |
| approx. 2 oz. . . . . . . . . | 15 | 2 | .03 | .01 | .09 | .02 | 20.0 | 0 |
| trimmed, chopped, | | | | | | | | |
| ½ cup . . . . . . . . . . . . | 13 | 1 | .03 | .01 | .07 | .02 | 17.0 | 0 |
| **Chicory greens,** fresh: | | | | | | | | |
| untrimmed, 1 lb. . . . . . . . | 14,880 | 89 | .22 | .37 | 1.86 | n.a. | n.a. | 0 |
| trimmed, chopped, | | | | | | | | |
| ½ cup . . . . . . . . . . . . | 3600 | 22 | .05 | .09 | .45 | n.a. | n.a. | 0 |
| **Chicory root,** raw: | | | | | | | | |
| untrimmed, 1 lb. . . . . . . | 22 | 19 | .15 | .11 | 1.49 | n.a. | n.a. | 0 |

| | Vitamin A | Vitamin C | Thiamin | Riboflavin | Niacin | B6 | Folacin | B12 |
|---|---|---|---|---|---|---|---|---|
| | (IU) | (Mg) | (Mg) | (Mg) | (Mg) | (Mg) | (Mcg) | (Mcg) |
| trimmed, 1" pieces, ½ cup | 3 | 2 | .02 | .01 | .18 | n.a. | n.a. | 0 |
| **Chili, canned:** | | | | | | | | |
| w/beans, 8 oz | 765 | 4 | .11 | .24 | .81 | .30 | n.a. | .02 |
| w/beans, ½ cup | 432 | 2 | .06 | .13 | .46 | .17 | n.a. | .01 |
| vegetarian (*Natural Touch*), 8.1 oz | 469 | 0 | .64 | .21 | 0 | .30 | n.a. | 0 |
| vegetarian (*Worthington*), 8.1 oz | 0 | 0 | .05 | .07 | 2.25 | .67 | n.a. | 1.61 |
| **Chili powder,** 1 tsp | 908 | 2 | .01 | .02 | .21 | n.a. | n.a. | 0 |
| **Chitterlings,** pork, simmered[1], 4 oz | 0 | 0 | 0 | .09 | .11 | n.a. | n.a. | n.a. |
| **Chives:** | | | | | | | | |
| fresh, untrimmed, 1 lb | 19,744 | 263.6 | .35 | .52 | 2.93 | .63 | 475.0 | 0 |
| fresh, chopped, 1 tbsp | 131 | 2 | tr. | tr. | .02 | tr. | 3.0 | 0 |
| freeze-dried, 1 tbsp | 137 | 1 | tr. | tr. | .01 | n.a. | n.a. | 0 |
| **Chocolate,** see "Candy" | | | | | | | | |
| **Chocolate, baking:** | | | | | | | | |
| chips, semisweet, ¼ cup | 8 | tr. | .03 | .04 | .23 | n.a. | n.a. | n.a. |
| unsweetened, 1-oz. square | 28 | 0 | .02 | .05 | .32 | .027 | 2.0 | 0 |
| **Chocolate flavor drink mix,** powder: | | | | | | | | |
| 2–3 heaping tsp. or ¾ oz. | 4 | <1 | .01 | .03 | .11 | <.01 | n.a. | 0 |
| regular or malt (*Carnation* Instant Breakfast), 1 pkt. | 1750 | 27 | .30 | .17 | 5.00 | .40 | 100.0 | .60 |
| **Chocolate milk:** | | | | | | | | |
| whole, 1 cup | 302 | 2 | .09 | .41 | .31 | .10 | 12.0 | .84 |
| low fat[2], 2%, 1 cup | 500 | 2 | .09 | .41 | .32 | .10 | 12.0 | .85 |
| low fat[2], 1%, 1 cup | 500 | 2 | .10 | .42 | .32 | .10 | 12.0 | .86 |

[1] *Prepared without added ingredients.*
[2] *Vitamin A added.*

| | Vitamin A | Vitamin C | Thiamin | Riboflavin | Niacin | B6 | Folacin | B12 |
|---|---|---|---|---|---|---|---|---|
| | (IU) | (Mg) | (Mg) | (Mg) | (Mg) | (Mg) | (Mcg) | (Mcg) |

**Chocolate syrup** (see also "Chocolate topping"):

| | | | | | | | | |
|---|---|---|---|---|---|---|---|---|
| thin type, w/out added nutrients, 2 tbsp. or 1 fl. oz. . . . . . . . . . . . | 11 | <1 | <.01 | .02 | .12 | <.01 | 1.5 | 0 |
| thin type, w/added nutrients, 1 tbsp. . . . . . | 817 | <1 | <.01 | .16 | 6.31 | <.01 | n.a. | 0 |
| **Chocolate topping,** fudge type, 1 tbsp. . . . . . . . . | 19 | tr. | .05 | .04 | n.a. | n.a. | n.a. | (0) |
| **Chrysanthemum garland:** | | | | | | | | |
| raw: | | | | | | | | |
| untrimmed, 1 lb. . . . . | 63,910 | 161 | .14 | .97 | 3.75 | n.a. | 333.2 | 0 |
| trimmed, .5-oz. stem | 2055 | 5 | <.01 | .03 | .12 | n.a. | 10.7 | 0 |
| trimmed, 1" pieces, 1 cup . . . . . . . . . | 3669 | 9 | .01 | .06 | .22 | n.a. | 19.1 | 0 |
| boiled, drained, 1" pieces, ½ cup. . . . . . . . . . . . | 2525 | 12 | .01 | .08 | .36 | n.a. | n.a. | 0 |
| **Cilantro,** see "Coriander" | | | | | | | | |
| **Cinnamon,** ground, 1 tsp. | 6 | 1 | <.01 | <.01 | .03 | n.a. | n.a. | 0 |
| **Cisco,** smoked, 4 oz. . . . . | 1069 | tr. | .05 | .18 | 2.62 | .30 | 2.4 | 4.83 |
| **Citrus fruit juice drink,** frozen, diluted, 6 fl. oz. | 78 | 50 | .03 | n.a. | .33 | .04 | 3.7 | 0 |
| **Clam,** mixed species, meat only: | | | | | | | | |
| raw, 1 lb. . . . . . . . . . . . | 1361 | n.a. | n.a. | 1.00 | 8.01 | n.a. | n.a. | 224.28 |
| raw, 9 large or 20 small, 6.3 oz. . . . . . . . . . . | 540 | tr. | n.a. | .38 | 3.18 | n.a. | n.a. | 89.00 |
| boiled, poached, or steamed[1], 4 oz. . . . . . . | 646 | n.a. | n.a. | .48 | 3.80 | n.a. | n.a. | 112.14 |
| boiled, poached, or steamed[1], 20 small . . . | 513 | n.a. | na. | .38 | 3.02 | n.a. | n.a. | 89.00 |
| breaded, fried, 20 small . . . . . . . . . . | 568 | n.a. | n.a. | .46 | 3.88 | n.a. | n.a. | 75.71 |
| **Clam, canned,** drained, 4 oz. . . . . . . . . . . . . . | 646 | tr. | n.a. | .48 | 3.80 | n.a. | n.a. | 112.14 |
| **Clove,** ground, 1 tsp. . . . . | 11 | 2 | <.01 | .01 | .03 | n.a. | n.a. | 0 |

---

[1] *Prepared without added ingredients.*

|  | Vitamin A | Vitamin C | Thiamin | Riboflavin | Niacin | B6 | Folacin | B12 |
|---|---|---|---|---|---|---|---|---|
|  | (IU) | (Mg) | (Mg) | (Mg) | (Mg) | (Mg) | (Mcg) | (Mcg) |
| **Cocoa mix,** powder: |  |  |  |  |  |  |  |  |
| unsweetened, 1 tbsp. | 1 | 0 | tr. | .02 | .11 | .01 | 2.0 | 0 |
| (*Carnation* 70 Calorie), 1 pkt. | 3 | <1 | .03 | .11 | .07 | .03 | 4.0 | .30 |
| (*Hershey's* European Style), 1 tbsp. | n.a. | n.a. | tr. | .01 | .17 | n.a. | n.a. | n.a. |
| w/out added nutrients, 1-oz. pkt. or 3–4 heaping tsp. | 4 | 1 | .03 | .16 | .17 | .03 | 0 | .38 |
| w/added nutrients, 1.1-oz. pkt. | 500 | 6 | .15 | .17 | 2.00 | n.a. | n.a. | n.a. |
| chocolate, 1 pkt.: |  |  |  |  |  |  |  |  |
| fudge (*Carnation*) | 5 | <1 | .03 | .11 | .12 | <.01 | 3.2 | .12 |
| milk (*Carnation*) | 3 | <1 | .04 | .15 | .12 | .04 | 2.0 | .23 |
| rich (*Carnation*) | 3 | <1 | .04 | .15 | .12 | .04 | 1.0 | .17 |
| w/marshmallows (*Carnation*), 1 pkt. or 4 heaping tsp. | 3 | <1 | .03 | .14 | .12 | .04 | 1.0 | .16 |
| reduced calorie, .53-oz. pkt. | n.a. | 0 | .04 | .21 | .16 | .05 | 2.2 | n.a. |
| **Coconut,** shelled, except as noted: |  |  |  |  |  |  |  |  |
| raw: |  |  |  |  |  |  |  |  |
| in shell, 1 lb. | 0 | 8 | .16 | .05 | 1.27 | .13 | 62.3 | 0 |
| 1 piece, 2" × 2" × ½", 1.6 oz. | 0 | 2 | .03 | .01 | .24 | .02 | 11.9 | 0 |
| shredded or grated, 1 cup | 0 | 3 | .05 | .02 | .43 | .04 | 21.1 | 0 |
| dried: |  |  |  |  |  |  |  |  |
| unsweetened, 1 oz. | 0 | <1 | .02 | .03 | .17 | .09 | 2.6 | 0 |
| sweetened, shredded, 1 oz. | 0 | <1 | .01 | .01 | .13 | n.a. | n.a. | 0 |
| sweetened, shredded, 1 cup | 0 | 1 | .03 | .02 | .44 | n.a. | n.a. | 0 |

| | Vitamin A | Vitamin C | Thiamin | Riboflavin | Niacin | B₆ | Folacin | B₁₂ |
|---|---|---|---|---|---|---|---|---|
| | (IU) | (Mg) | (Mg) | (Mg) | (Mg) | (Mg) | (Mcg) | (Mcg) |
| **Coconut milk**[1], 1 cup.... | 0 | 7 | .06 | 0 | 1.82 | n.a. | n.a. | 0 |
| **Coconut water**[2], 1 cup... | 0 | 6 | .07 | .14 | .19 | .08 | n.a. | 0 |
| **Cod,** meat only: | | | | | | | | |
| Atlantic: | | | | | | | | |
| raw, 1 lb.......... | 181 | 5 | .34 | .30 | 9.35 | 1.11 | n.a. | 4.12 |
| baked, broiled, or | | | | | | | | |
| microwaved[3], 4 oz. | 52 | 1 | .10 | .09 | 2.85 | .32 | n.a. | 1.19 |
| dried, salted, 1 oz.... | 40 | 1 | .08 | .07 | 2.10 | .24 | n.a. | 2.80 |
| Pacific: | | | | | | | | |
| raw, 1 lb.......... | 127 | n.a. | .10 | .19 | 9.25 | n.a. | n.a. | n.a. |
| baked, broiled, or | | | | | | | | |
| microwaved[3], 4 oz. | 36 | n.a. | .03 | .05 | 2.81 | n.a. | n.a. | n.a. |
| **Cod, canned,** Atlantic: | | | | | | | | |
| w/liquid, 11-oz. can ..... | 144 | 3 | .27 | .25 | 7.82 | .88 | n.a. | 3.26 |
| w/liquid, 4 oz.......... | 52 | 1 | .10 | .09 | 2.84 | .32 | n.a. | 1.19 |
| **Cod liver oil,** 1 tbsp.....| 13,600 | n.a. | n.a. | n.a. | n.a. | n.a. | n.a. | n.a. |
| **Coffee,** brewed, 6 fl. oz. | 0 | 0 | 0 | 0 | .39 | 0 | .3 | 0 |
| **Coffee, flavored,** instant, prepared: | | | | | | | | |
| cappuccino flavor, | | | | | | | | |
| 6 fl. oz............. | 0 | 0 | .02 | .01 | .32 | 0 | 0 | 0 |
| mocha flavor, 6 fl. oz. ... | 0 | 0 | <.01 | <.01 | .26 | 0 | 0 | 0 |
| **Coffee flavor drink mix** (*Carnation* Instant Breakfast), 1 pkt...... | 1750 | 27 | .30 | .17 | 5.00 | .40 | 100.0 | .60 |
| **Coffee substitute,** cereal grain (*Kaffree Roma*), 1 tsp. ............. | 0 | 0 | n.a. | n.a. | n.a. | n.a. | n.a. | n.a. |
| **Collards:** | | | | | | | | |
| fresh: | | | | | | | | |
| raw, untrimmed, 1 lb. ........... | 8611 | 60 | .08 | .17 | .99 | .17 | 30.0 | 0 |

[1] *Liquid expressed from mixture of grated coconut and water.*

[2] *Liquid from coconuts.*

[3] *Prepared without added ingredients.*

| | Vitamin A | Vitamin C | Thiamin | Riboflavin | Niacin | B6 | Folacin | B12 |
|---|---|---|---|---|---|---|---|---|
| | (IU) | (Mg) | (Mg) | (Mg) | (Mg) | (Mg) | (Mcg) | (Mcg) |
| raw, trimmed, chopped, ½ cup .. | 599 | 4 | .01 | .01 | .07 | .01 | 2.0 | 0 |
| boiled, drained, chopped, ½ cup .. | 1745 | 8 | .01 | .03 | .19 | .03 | 4.0 | 0 |
| frozen, chopped, 10-oz. pkg. ......... | 16,226 | 113.5 | .14 | .31 | 1.82 | .33 | 207.5 | 0 |
| frozen, boiled, drained, chopped, ½ cup ..... | 5084 | 23 | .04 | .10 | .54 | .10 | 64.7 | 0 |
| **Cookie:** | | | | | | | | |
| animal crackers, 1 oz., about 11 pieces...... | n.a. | 0 | .10 | .09 | .98 | .01 | 4.0 | .01 |
| butter, 2"-diam. piece.... | n.a. | 0 | .02 | .02 | .16 | tr. | 0 | n.a. |
| chocolate chip, 2¼"-diam. piece, .4 oz.......... | n.a. | 0 | .02 | .03 | .27 | .01 | 1.0 | n.a. |
| chocolate chip, soft type, .5-oz. piece ......... | n.a. | 0 | .02 | .03 | .24 | .02 | 1.0 | 0 |
| coconut bar, 10 pieces, 3.2 oz.............. | 140 | 0 | .04 | .05 | .4 | n.a. | n.a. | n.a. |
| fig bar, square, .6-oz. piece.............. | n.a. | n.a. | .03 | .04 | .3 | .01 | 2.0 | n.a. |
| fortune, .3-oz. piece..... | n.a. | 0 | .02 | .01 | .15 | tr. | 1.0 | n.a. |
| fudge, cake-type, .7-oz. piece.............. | n.a. | n.a. | .05 | .04 | .25 | n.a. | n.a. | n.a. |
| gingersnap, .2-oz. piece.............. | n.a. | 0 | .01 | .02 | .23 | n.a. | n.a. | 0 |
| graham cracker: | | | | | | | | |
| chocolate coated, 2½"-square piece | n.a. | 0 | .02 | .03 | .31 | n.a. | n.a. | 0 |
| sugar honey, 2 square pieces ... | n.a. | (0) | tr. | .02 | .10 | n.a. | n.a. | n.a. |
| ladyfinger, .4-oz. piece | 61 | tr. | .03 | .05 | .23 | .01 | 4.0 | .08 |
| macaroon, 2 pieces or 1.3 oz.............. | 0 | 0 | .02 | .06 | .20 | n.a. | n.a. | n.a. |
| marshmallow, chocolate coated, .5-oz. piece ... | n.a. | n.a. | .01 | .03 | .10 | n.a. | n.a. | n.a. |

| | Vitamin A | Vitamin C | Thiamin | Riboflavin | Niacin | B₆ | Folacin | B₁₂ |
|---|---|---|---|---|---|---|---|---|
| | (IU) | (Mg) | (Mg) | (Mg) | (Mg) | (Mg) | (Mcg) | (Mcg) |

| | Vitamin A (IU) | Vitamin C (Mg) | Thiamin (Mg) | Riboflavin (Mg) | Niacin (Mg) | $B_6$ (Mg) | Folacin (Mcg) | $B_{12}$ (Mcg) |
|---|---|---|---|---|---|---|---|---|
| Cookie, _continued_ | | | | | | | | |
| molasses, .5-oz. piece ... | n.a. | 0 | .05 | .04 | .46 | n.a. | n.a. | 0 |
| oatmeal raisin: | | | | | | | | |
| regular, .6-oz. piece | n.a. | n.a. | .05 | .04 | .4 | n.a. | n.a. | 0 |
| light, 2 pieces, 1 oz. | 0 | 0 | .04 | .07 | .34 | .02 | 2.0 | 0 |
| soft type, .5-oz. | | | | | | | | |
| piece . . . . . . . . . . | n.a. | n.a. | .03 | .03 | .27 | n.a. | n.a. | n.a. |
| peanut butter: | | | | | | | | |
| regular, .5-oz. piece | n.a. | 0 | .03 | .03 | .64 | n.a. | n.a. | n.a. |
| soft type, .5-oz. | | | | | | | | |
| piece . . . . . . . . . . | 0 | 0 | .04 | .03 | .32 | n.a. | 1.0 | 0 |
| sandwich, .5-oz. | | | | | | | | |
| piece . . . . . . . . . . | 1 | 0 | .05 | .04 | .52 | n.a. | n.a. | n.a. |
| raisin, soft type, .5-oz. | | | | | | | | |
| piece . . . . . . . . . . . . . | n.a. | n.a. | .03 | .03 | .30 | n.a. | n.a. | n.a. |
| sandwich, chocolate: | | | | | | | | |
| regular, .4-oz. piece | n.a. | 0 | .01 | .02 | .21 | tr. | 0 | n.a. |
| chocolate coated, | | | | | | | | |
| .6-oz. piece . . . . . . | n.a. | n.a. | .02 | .04 | .23 | n.a. | n.a. | n.a. |
| w/extra creme, | | | | | | | | |
| .5-oz. piece . . . . . . | n.a. | 0 | .01 | .02 | .20 | n.a. | n.a. | n.a. |
| sandwich, vanilla, | | | | | | | | |
| .4-oz. piece . . . . . . . . | 0 | 0 | .03 | .02 | .27 | n.a. | 0 | 0 |
| shortbread: | | | | | | | | |
| plain, .3-oz. piece. . . . | n.a. | 0 | .03 | .03 | .27 | n.a. | 1.0 | n.a. |
| w/pecan, .5-oz. piece | n.a. | n.a. | .04 | .03 | .35 | tr. | 1.0 | n.a. |
| sugar, .5-oz. piece . . . . . | 13 | n.a. | .04 | .03 | .4 | .01 | n.a. | n.a. |
| sugar wafer, creme-filled, | | | | | | | | |
| .1-oz. piece. . . . . . . . | n.a. | 0 | tr. | .01 | .09 | n.a. | n.a. | 0 |
| tofu (_The Great Tofu_ | | | | | | | | |
| _Cookie_), 2 pieces . . . . . | 99 | 3 | .04 | .05 | .46 | 0 | 1.1 | 0 |
| wafer: | | | | | | | | |
| chocolate, | | | | | | | | |
| .2-oz. piece . . . . . . | n.a. | n.a. | .01 | .02 | .17 | n.a. | n.a. | n.a. |

| | Vitamin A | Vitamin C | Thiamin | Riboflavin | Niacin | B<sub>6</sub> | Folacin | B<sub>12</sub> |
|---|---|---|---|---|---|---|---|---|
| | (IU) | (Mg) | (Mg) | (Mg) | (Mg) | (Mg) | (Mcg) | (Mcg) |
| vanilla, regular, .2-oz. piece . . . . . . | n.a. | n.a. | .02 | .01 | .18 | n.a. | n.a. | n.a. |
| vanilla, light, .1-oz. piece . . . . . . | n.a. | 0 | .01 | .01 | .12 | tr. | n.a. | n.a. |
| vanilla, brown-edge, 10 pieces, 2 oz. . . . | 80 | 0 | .01 | .04 | .20 | n.a. | n.a. | n.a. |
| wheat free (*The Great Wheat Free Cookie*), 4 pieces . . . . . . . . . . | 3 | 4 | .07 | .08 | .39 | 0 | 1.3 | 0 |
| **Cookie, refrigerated dough:** | | | | | | | | |
| chocolate chip, 1 oz. . . . . | 17 | 0 | .05 | .05 | .56 | n.a. | n.a. | n.a. |
| oatmeal, 1 oz. . . . . . . . . | 20 | n.a. | .07 | .04 | .53 | n.a. | n.a. | n.a. |
| peanut butter, 1 oz. . . . . . | 13 | 0 | .05 | .05 | 1.18 | n.a. | n.a. | n.a. |
| sugar, 1 oz. . . . . . . . . . . | 10 | 0 | .06 | .04 | .68 | n.a. | n.a. | n.a. |
| **Coriander,** fresh: | | | | | | | | |
| untrimmed, 1 lb. . . . . . . . | 10,670 | 40.5 | .29 | .46 | 2.82 | n.a. | n.a. | 0 |
| trimmed, 9 plants, .75 oz. . . . . . . . . . . . . | 553 | 2 | .02 | .02 | .15 | n.a. | n.a. | 0 |
| trimmed, ¼ cup. . . . . . . | 111 | <1 | <.01 | .01 | .03 | n.a. | n.a. | 0 |
| **Coriander seeds,** 1 tsp. | tr. | tr. | <.01 | .01 | .04 | n.a. | n.a. | 0 |
| **Corn,** yellow or white: | | | | | | | | |
| fresh: | | | | | | | | |
| raw, untrimmed (in husk), 1 lb. . . . . . . . | 458 | 11 | .33 | .10 | 2.78 | .09 | 74.8 | 0 |
| raw, trimmed, 1 ear, 3.2 oz. . . . . . . . . . . . . | 253 | 6 | .18 | .05 | 1.53 | .05 | 41.2 | 0 |
| raw, kernels, ½ cup | 216 | 5 | .15 | .05 | 1.31 | .04 | 35.3 | 0 |
| boiled, drained, 1 ear | 167 | 5 | .17 | .06 | 1.24 | .05 | 35.7 | 0 |
| boiled, drained, kernels, ½ cup. . . . | 178 | 5 | .18 | .06 | 1.32 | .05 | 38.1 | 0 |
| canned, kernels: | | | | | | | | |
| w/liquid, ½ cup . . . . . | 153 | 9 | .03 | .08 | 1.20 | .05 | 48.8 | 0 |
| cream style, ½ cup | 124 | 6 | .03 | .07 | 1.23 | .08 | 57.3 | 0 |

| | Vitamin A | Vitamin C | Thiamin | Riboflavin | Niacin | B6 | Folacin | B12 |
|---|---|---|---|---|---|---|---|---|
| | (IU) | (Mg) | (Mg) | (Mg) | (Mg) | (Mg) | (Mcg) | (Mcg) |

| | | | | | | | | |
|---|---|---|---|---|---|---|---|---|
| Corn, canned, *continued* | | | | | | | | |
| vacuum pack, ½ cup | 253 | 9 | .04 | .08 | 1.23 | .06 | 51.8 | 0 |
| w/red and green | | | | | | | | |
| peppers, ½ cup ... | 265 | 10 | .03 | .09 | 1.08 | n.a. | n.a. | 0 |
| frozen, kernels, except as noted: | | | | | | | | |
| 10-oz. pkg. ........ | 368 | 18 | .24 | .20 | 4.90 | .51 | 101.4 | 0 |
| ½ cup ........... | 106 | 5 | .07 | .06 | 1.41 | .15 | 29.3 | 0 |
| boiled, 4-oz. ear..... | 133 | 3 | .11 | .04 | .96 | .14 | 19.2 | 0 |
| boiled, drained, ⅓ of | | | | | | | | |
| 10-oz. pkg. ...... | 208 | 3 | .08 | .07 | 1.23 | .12 | 29.7 | 0 |
| boiled, drained, | | | | | | | | |
| ½ cup ......... | 180 | 3 | .07 | .06 | 1.07 | .11 | 26.0 | 0 |
| **Corn, whole grain,** 1 cup | n.a. | 0 | .64 | .33 | 6.02 | 1.03 | n.a. | 0 |
| **Corn bran,** crude, 1 cup | 54 | 0 | .01 | .08 | 2.08 | .12 | 3.0 | 0 |
| **Corn bread,** see "Bread, sweet, mix" | | | | | | | | |
| **Corn chips and similar snacks:** | | | | | | | | |
| plain, 1 oz. ........... | 27 | 0 | .01 | .04 | .34 | .07 | 6.0 | 0 |
| barbecue, 1 oz. ........ | 173 | 1 | .02 | .06 | .47 | .07 | n.a. | 0 |
| onion flavor, 1 oz....... | 34 | 1 | .06 | .09 | .9 | .04 | n.a. | 0 |
| puffs/twists, cheese, | | | | | | | | |
| 1 oz.............. | 75 | 0 | .08 | .1 | .9 | .03 | 34.0 | .04 |
| tortilla, see "Tortilla chips" | | | | | | | | |
| **Corn flour:** | | | | | | | | |
| whole grain, 1 cup...... | n.a. | 0 | .29 | .09 | 2.22 | n.a. | 30.0 | 0 |
| masa, enriched, 1 cup ... | n.a. | 0 | 1.63 | .86 | 11.22 | .42 | 28.0 | 0 |
| **Corn grits:** | | | | | | | | |
| uncooked, 1 cup ....... | n.a. | n.a. | 1.00 | .59 | 7.73 | .23 | 7.0 | 0 |
| cooked, white, enriched, | | | | | | | | |
| 1 cup ............. | tr. | n.a. | .24 | .15 | 1.96 | .06 | 1.0 | 0 |
| cooked, yellow, enriched, | | | | | | | | |
| 1 cup ............. | 145 | n.a. | .24 | .15 | 1.96 | .06 | 1.0 | 0 |
| **Corn syrup:** | | | | | | | | |
| dark, 1 tbsp. .......... | 0 | 0 | tr. | tr. | .00 | tr. | 0 | 0 |
| high fructose, 1 tbsp..... | n.a. | 0 | n.a. | tr. | 0 | tr. | 0 | 0 |
| light, 1 tbsp. .......... | 0 | 0 | tr. | tr. | tr. | tr. | 0 | 0 |

| | Vitamin A | Vitamin C | Thiamin | Riboflavin | Niacin | B6 | Folacin | B12 |
|---|---|---|---|---|---|---|---|---|
| | (IU) | (Mg) | (Mg) | (Mg) | (Mg) | (Mg) | (Mcg) | (Mcg) |
| malt, 1 tbsp. . . . . . . . . . | 0 | 0 | n.a. | .09 | 2.0 | .12 | 3.0 | 0 |
| **Cornish game hen:** | | | | | | | | |
| raw, meat w/skin, 1 bird, 11.8 oz. . . . . . . . . . . . | 363 | 2 | .25 | .57 | 19.01 | .99 | 9.0 | 1.12 |
| raw, meat only, 1 bird, 8.4 oz. . . . . . . . . . . . | 178 | 2 | .22 | .52 | 16.13 | .92 | 7.0 | .95 |
| roasted[1], meat w/skin, 1 bird, 8.1 oz. . . . . . . . | 241 | 1 | .15 | .45 | 13.49 | .70 | 5.0 | .64 |
| roasted[1], meat only, 1 bird, 3.8 oz. . . . . . . . | 70 | 1 | .08 | .24 | 6.7 | .38 | 2.0 | .32 |
| **Cornmeal:** | | | | | | | | |
| whole grain, white, 1 cup . . . . . . . . . . . . | tr. | 0 | .47 | .25 | 4.43 | .37 | n.a. | 0 |
| whole grain, yellow, 1 cup . . . . . . . . . . . . | 573 | 0 | .47 | .25 | 4.43 | .37 | n.a. | 0 |
| degermed, enriched, white, 1 cup . . . . . . . . | tr. | 0 | .99 | .56 | 6.95 | .35 | 66.0 | 0 |
| degermed, enriched, yellow, 1 cup. . . . . . . . | 570 | 0 | .99 | .56 | 6.95 | .35 | 66.0 | 0 |
| self-rising, enriched[2]: bolted, 1 cup. . . . . . . | n.a. | 0 | .81 | .49 | 6.46 | .66 | 70.0 | 0 |
| bolted, w/wheat flour, white, 1 cup . . . . . . . . | tr. | 0 | 1.21 | .74 | 8.84 | .65 | 112.0 | 0 |
| bolted, w/wheat flour, yellow, 1 cup. . . . . | 488 | 0 | 1.21 | .74 | 8.84 | .65 | 112.0 | 0 |
| degermed, 1 cup . . . . | n.a. | 0 | .94 | .54 | 6.30 | .54 | 43.0 | 0 |
| **Cornstarch,** stirred, 1 tbsp. . . . . . . . . . . . | (0) | (0) | (0) | (0) | (0) | n.a. | n.a. | 0 |
| **Cottonseed flour,** low fat, 1 oz. . . . . . . . . . . . | 123 | 1 | .59 | .11 | 1.15 | .22 | n.a. | 0 |
| **Cottonseed kernels,** roasted, 1 tbsp. . . . . . . | n.a. | 1 | .08 | .03 | .30 | n.a. | n.a. | 0 |

[1] Prepared without added ingredients.

[2] With added nutrients.

| | Vitamin A | Vitamin C | Thiamin | Riboflavin | Niacin | B6 | Folacin | B12 |
|---|---|---|---|---|---|---|---|---|
| | (IU) | (Mg) | (Mg) | (Mg) | (Mg) | (Mg) | (Mcg) | (Mcg) |
| **Country gravy mix,** vegetarian (*Loma Linda*), 1 tbsp., .2 oz. | 0 | 0 | 0 | .01 | 0 | .01 | n.a. | .01 |
| **Couscous:** | | | | | | | | |
| uncooked: | | | | | | | | |
| 1 cup . . . . . . . . . . . | 0 | 0 | .30 | .14 | 6.42 | .20 | 37.0 | 0 |
| (*Casbah*), 3.5 oz. . . . . | 0 | 0 | .43 | .11 | 4.30 | n.a. | n.a. | 0 |
| whole wheat (*Casbah*), 3.5 oz. | 0 | 0 | .66 | .12 | 4.40 | n.a. | n.a. | 0 |
| cooked, 1 cup . . . . . . . . | 0 | 0 | .11 | .05 | 1.76 | .09 | 26.1 | 0 |
| **Cowpeas:** | | | | | | | | |
| fresh: | | | | | | | | |
| raw, untrimmed (in pods), 1 lb. . . . . . . | 1890 | 6 | .25 | .34 | 3.35 | .16 | 389.0 | 0 |
| raw, trimmed, ½ cup | 588 | 2 | .08 | .10 | 1.04 | .05 | 121.0 | 0 |
| boiled, drained, ½ cup . . . . . . . . . | 648 | 2 | .08 | .12 | 1.15 | .05 | 104.0 | 0 |
| fresh, leafy tips: | | | | | | | | |
| raw, untrimmed, 1 lb. . . . . . . . . . . | 1680 | 85 | .84 | .41 | 2.64 | n.a. | n.a. | 0 |
| raw, trimmed, chopped, 1 cup . . . | 256 | 13 | .13 | .06 | 40 | n.a. | n.a. | 0 |
| boiled, drained, chopped, ½ cup . . | 150 | 5 | .07 | .04 | .26 | n.a. | n.a. | 0 |
| fresh, young pods, w/seeds: | | | | | | | | |
| raw, untrimmed, 1 lb. . . . . . . . . . . | 6605 | 136 | .62 | .58 | 4.95 | n.a. | n.a. | 0 |
| raw, trimmed, ½ cup | 752 | 16 | .07 | .07 | .56 | n.a. | n.a. | 0 |
| boiled, drained, ½ cup . . . . . . . . . | 658 | 8 | .04 | .04 | .38 | n.a. | n.a. | 0 |
| frozen, 10-oz. pkg. . . . . . . | 238 | 11 | .70 | .20 | 2.30 | .30 | 530.6 | 0 |
| frozen, boiled, drained, ½ cup . . . . . . . . . . . . | 64 | 2 | .22 | .05 | .62 | .08 | 120.1 | 0 |
| **Cowpeas, dried:** | | | | | | | | |
| uncooked, 1 lb. . . . . . . . . | 227 | 7 | 3.87 | 1.03 | 9.41 | 1.62 | 2869.3 | 0 |

| | Vitamin A | Vitamin C | Thiamin | Riboflavin | Niacin | B6 | Folacin | B12 |
|---|---|---|---|---|---|---|---|---|
| | (IU) | (Mg) | (Mg) | (Mg) | (Mg) | (Mg) | (Mcg) | (Mcg) |
| uncooked, ½ cup....... | 42 | 1 | .72 | .19 | 1.74 | .30 | 531.3 | 0 |
| boiled, ½ cup ......... | 13 | <1 | .17 | .05 | .43 | .09 | 178.8 | 0 |
| canned, w/liquid, 8 oz. | 30 | 6 | .17 | .17 | .80 | .10 | 116.2 | 0 |
| canned, w/liquid, | | | | | | | | |
| ½ cup............. | 16 | 3 | .09 | .09 | .43 | .05 | 61.5 | 0 |
| canned, w/pork, ½ cup | 0 | <1 | .08 | .06 | .52 | n.a. | 61.5 | 0 |
| **Cowpeas, Catjang,** dried: | | | | | | | | |
| uncooked, 1 lb........ | 150 | 7 | 3.08 | .77 | 12.68 | 1.64 | 2898.6 | 0 |
| uncooked, ½ cup....... | 28 | 1 | .57 | .14 | 2.35 | 1.27 | 536.8 | 0 |
| boiled, ½ cup ......... | 9 | tr. | .14 | .04 | .61 | .08 | 121.7 | 0 |
| **Crab,** Alaska king, meat only: | | | | | | | | |
| raw, 1 lb.............. | 109 | (0) | .20 | .20 | 4.99 | n.a. | n.a. | n.a. |
| raw, in shell, 6 oz., yield | | | | | | | | |
| from 1-lb. leg ....... | 41 | (0) | .07 | .07 | 1.82 | n.a. | n.a. | n.a. |
| boiled or steamed[1], | | | | | | | | |
| 4 oz............... | 33 | (0) | .06 | .06 | 1.52 | n.a. | n.a. | n.a. |
| boiled or steamed[1], | | | | | | | | |
| 4.7 oz. (1-lb. raw leg ) | 39 | (0) | .07 | .07 | 1.80 | n.a. | n.a. | n.a. |
| **Crabapple:** | | | | | | | | |
| untrimmed, 1 lb........ | 167 | 33 | .12 | .08 | .41 | n.a. | n.a. | 0 |
| w/skin, sliced, ½ cup.... | 22 | 4 | .02 | .01 | .06 | n.a. | n.a. | 0 |
| **Cracker:** | | | | | | | | |
| butter, 10 round, | | | | | | | | |
| 1.2 oz.............. | 70 | (0) | tr. | .01 | .30 | n.a. | n.a. | n.a. |
| cheese, plain, | | | | | | | | |
| 1"- square piece...... | 2 | 0 | .01 | tr. | .05 | .01 | 0 | 0 |
| cheese–peanut butter | | | | | | | | |
| sandwich, .3-oz. piece | n.a. | 0 | .03 | .02 | .46 | .10 | 2.0 | n.a. |
| crispbread, rye, | | | | | | | | |
| 1 piece, .4 oz. ....... | 0 | 0 | .02 | .01 | .10 | .02 | 2.0 | 0 |
| graham, see "Cookie" | | | | | | | | |
| matzo, 1-oz. piece: | | | | | | | | |
| plain ............. | 0 | 0 | .11 | .08 | 1.10 | .03 | 4.0 | 0 |

[1] *Prepared without added ingredients.*

| | Vitamin A | Vitamin C | Thiamin | Riboflavin | Niacin | B6 | Folacin | B12 |
|---|---|---|---|---|---|---|---|---|
| | (IU) | (Mg) | (Mg) | (Mg) | (Mg) | (Mg) | (Mcg) | (Mcg) |
| Cracker, matzo, *continued* | | | | | | | | |
| egg . . . . . . . . . . . . . . | 12 | n.a. | n.a. | .18 | 1.44 | .02 | n.a. | n.a. |
| egg and onion . . . . . . | n.a. | n.a. | .16 | .12 | 1.39 | .03 | 3.0 | .06 |
| whole wheat . . . . . . . | 0 | 0 | .10 | .08 | 1.53 | .05 | 10.0 | 0 |
| melba toast: | | | | | | | | |
| plain, .2-oz. piece. . . . | 0 | 0 | .02 | .01 | .21 | .01 | 1.0 | 0 |
| rye, .2-oz. piece . . . . . | n.a. | n.a. | .02 | .01 | .24 | tr. | 1.0 | 0 |
| wheat, .2-oz. piece . . . | 0 | 0 | .02 | .02 | .25 | .01 | 1.0 | 0 |
| milk, .4-oz. piece . . . . . . . | n.a. | n.a. | .07 | .05 | .53 | n.a. | n.a. | n.a. |
| rusk toast, .4-oz. piece | n.a. | 0 | .04 | .04 | .46 | n.a. | n.a. | n.a. |
| rye: | | | | | | | | |
| plain, 1 triple cracker, .9 oz. . . . . . . . . . . . | n.a. | n.a. | .11 | .07 | .40 | .07 | 11.0 | 0 |
| sandwich type, w/cheese filling, .3-oz. piece . . . . . . | n.a. | n.a. | .04 | .04 | .25 | .01 | n.a. | n.a. |
| seasoned, 1 triple cracker, .8 oz. . . . . | n.a. | n.a. | .07 | .05 | .54 | .04 | 12.0 | 0 |
| saltine, 1 piece, .1 oz. . . . | 0 | 0 | .02 | .01 | .16 | tr. | 1.0 | 0 |
| saltine, no fat, low sodium, 3 pieces, .5 oz. . . . . . . . . . . . . . . | 0 | 0 | .08 | .09 | .86 | .01 | 2.0 | 0 |
| snack type: | | | | | | | | |
| 1 round piece, .1 oz. | 0 | 0 | .01 | .01 | .12 | tr. | 0 | 0 |
| sandwich, w/cheese filling, .3-oz. piece . . . . . . | n.a. | n.a. | .03 | .05 | .26 | n.a. | n.a. | n.a. |
| soda biscuit, 10 pieces, 1.8 oz. . . . . . . . . . . . . . | (0) | (0) | .01 | .03 | .50 | n.a. | n.a. | n.a. |
| soup or oyster, 10 pieces. . . . . . . . . . . | (0) | (0) | tr. | tr. | .10 | n.a. | n.a. | n.a. |
| wheat: | | | | | | | | |
| plain, .1-oz. piece. . . . | 0 | 0 | .01 | .01 | .10 | tr. | 0 | 0 |

| | Vitamin A | Vitamin C | Thiamin | Riboflavin | Niacin | B6 | Folacin | B12 |
|---|---|---|---|---|---|---|---|---|
| | (IU) | (Mg) | (Mg) | (Mg) | (Mg) | (Mg) | (Mcg) | (Mcg) |
| sandwich type, w/cheese filling, .3-oz. piece | 5 | tr. | .03 | .03 | .22 | .02 | n.a. | n.a. |
| sandwich type, w/peanut butter filling, .3-oz. piece | n.a. | 0 | .03 | .02 | .41 | .01 | n.a. | 0 |
| thin, 4 pieces, .3 oz. | tr. | 0 | .04 | .03 | .40 | n.a. | n.a. | 0 |
| whole, .1-oz. piece... | 0 | 0 | .01 | tr. | .18 | .01 | 1.0 | 0 |
| **Cracker crumbs and meal:** | | | | | | | | |
| 1 cup | 0 | 0 | .80 | .54 | 6.56 | n.a. | n.a. | 0 |
| (*Kellogg's* Corn Flake Crumbs), 1 oz. | 0 | 15 | .38 | .43 | 5.00 | .50 | n.a. | n.a. |
| **Cranberry,** fresh: | | | | | | | | |
| untrimmed, 1 lb. | 197 | 58 | .13 | .09 | .43 | .28 | 7.3 | 0 |
| whole, ½ cup | 22 | 6 | .01 | .01 | .05 | .03 | .8 | 0 |
| chopped, ½ cup | 25 | 7 | .02 | .01 | .06 | .04 | 1.0 | 0 |
| **Cranberry beans,** dried: | | | | | | | | |
| uncooked, 1 lb. | 9 | 0 | 3.39 | .97 | 6.60 | 1.40 | 2741.4 | 0 |
| uncooked, ½ cup | 2 | 0 | .73 | .21 | 1.43 | .30 | 592.3 | 0 |
| boiled, ½ cup | 0 | 0 | .19 | .06 | .45 | .07 | 181.9 | 0 |
| canned, w/liquid, 8 oz. | 0 | 2 | .03 | .03 | 1.14 | .12 | 175.6 | 0 |
| canned, w/liquid, ½ cup | 0 | 1 | .05 | .05 | .66 | .06 | 100.6 | 0 |
| **Cranberry juice cocktail[1]:** | | | | | | | | |
| bottled, 6 fl. oz. | 7 | 68 | .02 | .02 | .07 | .04 | .5 | 0 |
| frozen, diluted, 6 fl. oz. | 18 | 18 | .01 | .02 | .02 | .03 | 0 | 0 |
| **Cranberry sauce,** canned, sweetened, ½ cup | 28 | 3 | .02 | .03 | .14 | .02 | n.a. | 0 |
| **Cranberry-apple juice drink[1],** bottled, 6 fl. oz. | n.a. | 59 | .01 | .04 | .11 | n.a. | n.a. | 0 |
| **Cranberry-apricot juice drink,** bottled, 6 fl. oz. | n.a. | 0 | .01 | .02 | .22 | n.a. | n.a. | 0 |

[1] With added ascorbic acid.

| | Vitamin A | Vitamin C | Thiamin | Riboflavin | Niacin | B₆ | Folacin | B₁₂ |
|---|---|---|---|---|---|---|---|---|
| | (IU) | (Mg) | (Mg) | (Mg) | (Mg) | (Mg) | (Mcg) | (Mcg) |
| **Cranberry-grape juice** | | | | | | | | |
| **drink**[1], bottled, 6 fl. oz. | n.a. | 59 | .02 | .03 | .22 | n.a. | n.a. | 0 |
| **Cranberry-orange relish,** | | | | | | | | |
| canned, ½ cup ...... | 97 | 25 | .04 | .03 | .14 | n.a. | n.a. | 0 |
| **Crayfish,** mixed species, meat only: | | | | | | | | |
| wild: | | | | | | | | |
| raw, 1 lb.......... | 236 | 6 | .32 | .15 | 10.02 | .49 | 168.0 | 9.07 |
| raw, 8 crayfish, | | | | | | | | |
| approx. 1 oz...... | 14 | <1 | .02 | .01 | .60 | .03 | 10.0 | .54 |
| boiled or steamed[2], | | | | | | | | |
| 4 oz............ | 57 | 1 | .06 | .10 | 2.59 | .09 | 49.9 | 2.44 |
| farmed: | | | | | | | | |
| raw, 1 lb.......... | 227 | 2 | .20 | .15 | 8.47 | .35 | 136.0 | 9.53 |
| raw, 8 crayfish, | | | | | | | | |
| approx. 1 oz...... | 13 | <1 | .01 | .01 | .50 | .03 | 8.0 | .57 |
| boiled or steamed[2], | | | | | | | | |
| 4 oz............ | 57 | <1 | .05 | .09 | 1.89 | .15 | 12.5 | 3.52 |
| **Cream:** | | | | | | | | |
| half and half, 1 cup ..... | 1050 | 2 | .09 | .36 | .19 | .09 | 6.0 | .80 |
| half and half, 1 tbsp..... | 65 | <1 | .01 | .02 | .01 | .01 | tr. | .05 |
| light, coffee or table, | | | | | | | | |
| 1 cup ............. | 1728 | 2 | .08 | .36 | .14 | .08 | 6.0 | .53 |
| light, coffee or table, | | | | | | | | |
| 1 tbsp. ........... | 108 | <1 | .01 | .02 | .01 | .01 | tr. | .03 |
| medium (25% fat), | | | | | | | | |
| 1 cup ............. | 2251 | 2 | .07 | .33 | .12 | .07 | 6.0 | .52 |
| medium, (25% fat), | | | | | | | | |
| 1 tbsp. ........... | 141 | <1 | <1 | .02 | .01 | .01 | tr. | .03 |
| whipping: | | | | | | | | |
| light, 1 cup, approx. | | | | | | | | |
| 2 cups whipped... | 2694 | 2 | .06 | .30 | .10 | .07 | 9.0 | .47 |
| light, 1 tbsp. ....... | 169 | <1 | <.01 | .02 | .01 | <.01 | 1.0 | .03 |

[1] *With added ascorbic acid.*
[2] *Prepared without added ingredients.*

| | Vitamin A | Vitamin C | Thiamin | Riboflavin | Niacin | B6 | Folacin | B12 |
|---|---|---|---|---|---|---|---|---|
| | (IU) | (Mg) | (Mg) | (Mg) | (Mg) | (Mg) | (Mcg) | (Mcg) |
| heavy, 1 cup, approx. 2 cups whipped . . . | 3499 | 1 | .05 | .26 | .09 | .06 | 9.0 | .43 |
| heavy, 1 tbsp. . . . . . . | 220 | <1 | <.01 | .02 | .01 | <.01 | 1.0 | .03 |
| whipped topping, pressurized, 1 cup . . . . | 548 | 0 | .02 | .03 | .04 | .03 | n.a. | .18 |
| whipped topping, pressurized, 1 tbsp. . . . | 27 | 0 | <.01 | <.01 | <.01 | <.01 | n.a. | .01 |
| **Cream, sour, cultured:** | | | | | | | | |
| 1 cup . . . . . . . . . . . . . . | 1817 | 2 | .08 | .34 | .15 | .04 | 25.0 | .69 |
| 1 tbsp. . . . . . . . . . . . . | 95 | <1 | <.01 | .02 | .01 | <.01 | 1.0 | .04 |
| half and half, 1 tbsp. . . . . | 68 | <1 | .01 | .02 | .01 | <.01 | 2.0 | .05 |
| **Cream, sour, nondairy,** | | | | | | | | |
| 1 oz. . . . . . . . . . . . . . | 0 | 0 | 0 | 0 | 0 | 0 | 0 | 0 |
| **Cream of tartar, 1 tsp.** . . . | 0 | 0 | 0 | 0 | 0 | 0 | 0 | 0 |
| **Cream topping, nondairy:** | | | | | | | | |
| frozen: | | | | | | | | |
| semisolid, 1 tbsp. . . . | 34 | 0 | 0 | 0 | 0 | 0 | 0 | 0 |
| (*Rich's*), 3.5 oz. . . . . . | 0 | 0 | 0 | 0 | 0 | 0 | 0 | 0 |
| powdered[1], 1½ oz. dry | 458 | 0 | 0 | 0 | 0 | 0 | 0 | 0 |
| powdered[1], prepared w/whole milk, 1 tbsp. | 14 | <1 | <.01 | .01 | <.01 | <.01 | tr. | .01 |
| pressurized, 1 tbsp. . . . . . | 19 | 0 | 0 | 0 | 0 | 0 | 0 | 0 |
| **Creamer, nondairy:** | | | | | | | | |
| (*Rich's Coffee Rich*), 3.5 oz. . . . . . . . . . . . | 0 | 0 | 0 | 0 | 0 | 0 | 0 | 0 |
| (*Rich's Farm Rich*), 3.5 oz. . . . . . . . . . . . | 0 | 0 | 0 | 0 | 0 | 0 | 0 | 0 |
| liquid (*Coffee-mate*), ½ fl. oz. . . . . . . . . . . | 18 | 0 | 0 | 0 | 0 | 0 | 0 | 0 |
| powdered[1], 1 tsp. . . . . . . | 13 | 0 | 0 | 0 | 0 | 0 | 0 | 0 |
| **Cress, garden:** | | | | | | | | |
| raw, untrimmed, 1 lb. | 29,955 | 222 | .26 | .84 | 3.22 | .80 | n.a. | 0 |

[1] Includes vitamin A contributed from beta-carotene used for coloring.

| | Vitamin A | Vitamin C | Thiamin | Riboflavin | Niacin | B6 | Folacin | B12 |
|---|---|---|---|---|---|---|---|---|
| | (IU) | (Mg) | (Mg) | (Mg) | (Mg) | (Mg) | (Mcg) | (Mcg) |
| Cress, garden, *continued* | | | | | | | | |
| raw, trimmed, ½ cup.... | 2325 | 17 | .02 | .07 | 25 | .06 | n.a. | 0 |
| boiled, drained, ½ cup | 5236 | 16 | .04 | .11 | .54 | n.a. | n.a. | 0 |
| **Croissant:** | | | | | | | | |
| plain, 2-oz. piece....... | n.a. | n.a. | .22 | .14 | 1.25 | .03 | 16.0 | n.a. |
| apple filled, 2-oz. piece | n.a. | n.a. | .13 | .09 | .91 | .02 | 7.0 | n.a. |
| cheese filled, | | | | | | | | |
| 2-oz. piece.......... | n.a. | n.a. | .3 | .19 | 1.23 | .04 | 19.0 | .18 |
| **Crookneck squash:** | | | | | | | | |
| fresh: | | | | | | | | |
| raw, untrimmed, 1 lb. | 1519 | 38 | .23 | .19 | 2.04 | .49 | 102.6 | 0 |
| raw, trimmed, sliced, | | | | | | | | |
| ½ cup.......... | 220 | 5 | .03 | .03 | .30 | .07 | 14.9 | 0 |
| boiled, drained, | | | | | | | | |
| sliced, ½ cup..... | 259 | 5 | .04 | .04 | .46 | .09 | 18.1 | 0 |
| canned, drained, sliced, | | | | | | | | |
| ½ cup............. | 130 | 3 | .02 | .03 | .45 | .05 | 11.3 | 0 |
| frozen, boiled, drained, | | | | | | | | |
| sliced, ½ cup....... | 187 | 7 | .04 | .05 | .42 | .10 | 12.2 | 0 |
| **Croutons:** | | | | | | | | |
| plain, 1 cup........... | 0 | 0 | .19 | .08 | 1.63 | .01 | 7.0 | 0 |
| seasoned, 1 cup ....... | n.a. | n.a. | .20 | .17 | 1.86 | .03 | .16 | n.a. |
| (*Kellogg's Croutettes*), | | | | | | | | |
| 1 cup ............. | 0 | tr. | .13 | .20 | 2.00 | .03 | 0 | n.a. |
| **Cucumber,** w/peel: | | | | | | | | |
| untrimmed, 1 lb....... | 946 | 24 | .10 | .10 | .97 | .18 | 56.0 | 0 |
| 1 medium, 8¼" long, | | | | | | | | |
| 10.6 oz........... | 647 | 16 | .07 | .07 | .67 | .13 | 38.0 | 0 |
| sliced, ½ cup ........ | 112 | 3 | .01 | .01 | .12 | .02 | 7.0 | 0 |
| **Cumin seed,** 1 tsp...... | 27 | <1 | .01 | .01 | .10 | n.a. | n.a. | 0 |
| **Cupcake mix[1],** devil's | | | | | | | | |
| food, w/chocolate | | | | | | | | |
| frosting, 2½"-diam. | | | | | | | | |
| piece.............. | 50 | tr. | .04 | .05 | .30 | n.a. | n.a | n.a. |

[1] *Prepared according to package directions.*

|  | Vitamin A (IU) | Vitamin C (Mg) | Thiamin (Mg) | Riboflavin (Mg) | Niacin (Mg) | B6 (Mg) | Folacin (Mcg) | B12 (Mcg) |
|---|---|---|---|---|---|---|---|---|
| **Currant:** | | | | | | | | |
| fresh: | | | | | | | | |
| black, untrimmed, 1 lb. . . . . . . . . . . | 1022 | 804 | .22 | .22 | .33 | .29 | n.a. | 0 |
| black, fresh, trimmed, ½ cup . . . . . . . . . | 129 | 101 | .03 | .03 | .17 | .04 | n.a. | 0 |
| red[1] or white, untrimmed, 1 lb. . . . | 533 | 182 | .18 | .22 | .45 | .31 | n.a. | 0 |
| red[1] or white, trimmed, ½ cup . . . | 67 | 23 | .02 | .03 | .06 | .04 | n.a. | 0 |
| dried, Zante, ½ cup . . . . . | 52 | 3 | .12 | .10 | 1.16 | .21 | 7.3 | 0 |
| **Curry powder,** 1 tsp. . . . . | 20 | <1 | .01 | .01 | .07 | n.a. | n.a. | 0 |
| **Cusk,** meat only, baked, broiled, or microwaved[2], 4 oz. . . . | n.a. | (0) | n.a. | .18 | 3.71 | .51 | n.a. | 1.36 |
| **Custard mix,** dry: | | | | | | | | |
| egg, 3-oz. pkg. . . . . . . . . | 185 | .2 | .12 | .35 | .22 | .15 | 21.0 | 1.02 |
| flan/caramel, 3-oz. pkg. | 0 | 0 | 0 | 0 | 0 | 0 | 0 | 0 |
| **Custard mix, rennet,** see "Pudding mix" | | | | | | | | |
| **Custard apple:** | | | | | | | | |
| untrimmed, 1 lb. . . . . . . . | n.a. | 51 | .21 | .26 | 1.32 | .58 | n.a. | 0 |
| trimmed, 1 oz. . . . . . . . . . | n.a. | 5 | .02 | .03 | .14 | .06 | n.a. | 0 |
| **Cuttlefish,** mixed species, meat only: | | | | | | | | |
| raw, 1 lb. . . . . . . . . . . . . | n.a. | 24 | .04 | 4.13 | 5.52 | n.a. | n.a. | 13.61 |
| baked, broiled, or microwaved[2], 4 oz. . . . | n.a. | 10 | .02 | 1.96 | 2.48 | n.a. | n.a. | 6.12 |

[1] *Vitamin A figure applies to red currant only.*
[2] *Prepared without added ingredients.*

# D

| | Vitamin A | Vitamin C | Thiamin | Riboflavin | Niacin | B6 | Folacin | B12 |
|---|---|---|---|---|---|---|---|---|
| | (IU) | (Mg) | (Mg) | (Mg) | (Mg) | (Mg) | (Mcg) | (Mcg) |

**Daikon,** see "Radish, Oriental"

**Dandelion greens:**

| | | | | | | | | |
|---|---|---|---|---|---|---|---|---|
| raw, untrimmed, 1 lb. | 63,504 | 159 | .86 | 1.18 | n.a. | n.a. | n.a. | 0 |
| raw, trimmed, chopped, ½ cup . . . . . . . . . . . . | 3920 | 10 | .05 | .07 | n.a. | n.a. | n.a. | 0 |
| boiled, drained, chopped, ½ cup . . . . . . . . . . . . | 6084 | 9 | .07 | .09 | n.a. | n.a. | n.a. | 0 |

**Danish pastry:**

| | | | | | | | | |
|---|---|---|---|---|---|---|---|---|
| plain, round, 2-oz. piece | 60 | tr. | .16 | .17 | 1.40 | n.a. | n.a. | n.a. |
| cheese, 2.5-oz. piece . . . . | n.a. | n.a. | .14 | .19 | 1.42 | n.a. | n.a. | n.a. |
| cinnamon, 2.3-oz. piece | n.a. | n.a. | .2 | .17 | 1.86 | n.a. | n.a. | n.a. |
| w/fruit, 2.5-oz. piece . . . . | 37 | 3 | .19 | .16 | 1.41 | n.a. | 12.0 | n.a. |
| w/nut, 2.3-oz. piece . . . . . | 34 | 1 | .14 | .16 | 1.5 | n.a. | n.a. | n.a. |

**Date,** domestic, natural or dry:

| | | | | | | | | |
|---|---|---|---|---|---|---|---|---|
| w/pits, 1 lb. . . . . . . . . . . . | 204 | 0 | .37 | .41 | 8.98 | .78 | 51.3 | 0 |
| 10 dates, 2.9 oz. . . . . . . . | 42 | 0 | .08 | .08 | 1.83 | .16 | 10.4 | 0 |
| pitted, chopped, ½ cup | 45 | 0 | .08 | .09 | 1.96 | .17 | 11.1 | 0 |

**Dill,** dried:

| | | | | | | | | |
|---|---|---|---|---|---|---|---|---|
| seeds, 1 tsp. . . . . . . . . . | 1 | n.a. | .01 | .01 | .06 | n.a. | n.a. | 0 |
| weed, 1 cup sprigs . . . . . | 0 | n.a. | .01 | .03 | .14 | .02 | 13 | 0 |

**Dock,** raw:

| | | | | | | | | |
|---|---|---|---|---|---|---|---|---|
| untrimmed, 1 lb. . . . . . . . | 12,700 | 152 | .13 | .32 | 1.59 | n.a. | n.a. | 0 |
| trimmed, chopped, ½ cup . . . . . . . . . . . . | 2680 | 32 | .03 | .07 | .34 | n.a. | n.a. | 0 |

**Donut:**

cake type:

| | | | | | | | | |
|---|---|---|---|---|---|---|---|---|
| plain, 1.7-oz. piece. . . | 27 | n.a. | .10 | .11 | .87 | .03 | 4.0 | n.a. |
| plain, chocolate coated, 1.5-oz. piece . . . . . . . . . . | n.a. | n.a. | .05 | .05 | .56 | n.a. | n.a. | n.a. |
| plain, sugared or glazed, 1.6-oz. piece . . . . . . . . . . | 4 | n.a. | .11 | .09 | .68 | .01 | n.a. | n.a. |

| | Vitamin A | Vitamin C | Thiamin | Riboflavin | Niacin | B6 | Folacin | B12 |
|---|---|---|---|---|---|---|---|---|
| | (IU) | (Mg) | (Mg) | (Mg) | (Mg) | (Mg) | (Mcg) | (Mcg) |
| chocolate, sugared or glazed, 1.5-oz. piece . . . . . . . . . . | n.a. | n.a. | .02 | .03 | .20 | n.a. | n.a. | n.a. |
| wheat, sugared or glazed, 1.6-oz. piece . . . . . . . . . . | n.a. | n.a. | .10 | .11 | .83 | n.a. | n.a. | n.a. |
| French cruller, glazed, 1.4-oz. piece . . . . . . . . | n.a. | n.a. | .07 | .09 | n.a. | n.a. | n.a. | n.a. |
| yeast type: glazed, 2.1-oz. piece | n.a. | n.a. | .22 | .13 | 1.71 | .03 | 13.0 | n.a. |
| creme filled, 3-oz. piece . . . . . . . . . . | n.a. | n.a. | .29 | .13 | 1.91 | n.a. | n.a. | n.a. |
| jelly filled, 3-oz. piece . . . . . . . . . . | n.a. | n.a. | .27 | .12 | 1.82 | n.a. | n.a. | n.a. |
| **Duck, domesticated:** roasted[1], meat w/skin, 4 oz. . . . . . . . . . . . . . | 238 | 0 | .20 | .31 | 5.47 | .20 | 6.8 | .34 |
| roasted[1], meat only, 4 oz. . . . . . . . . . . . . . | 87 | 0 | .29 | .53 | 5.78 | .28 | 11.3 | .45 |
| **Duck, wild,** raw, meat w/skin, 1 oz. . . . . . . . . | n.a. | 1 | .10 | .08 | .94 | .15 | n.a. | .18 |
| **Dutch brand loaf[2],** pork and beef, 1-oz. slice. . . | 0 | 5 | .09 | .08 | .68 | .06 | n.a. | .37 |

[1] *Prepared without added ingredients.*
[2] *With added ascorbic acid or sodium ascorbate; vitamin C value for product without additives would be negligible.*

# E

| | Vitamin A (IU) | Vitamin C (Mg) | Thiamin (Mg) | Riboflavin (Mg) | Niacin (Mg) | B6 (Mg) | Folacin (Mcg) | B12 (Mcg) |
|---|---|---|---|---|---|---|---|---|
| **Eclair,** chocolate, frozen: | | | | | | | | |
| (*Rich's*), 3.5 oz........ | 103 | 0 | .08 | .12 | .56 | .02 | 10.7 | 0 |
| **Eel,** mixed species, meat only: | | | | | | | | |
| raw, 1 lb.............. | 15,763 | (0) | .68 | .18 | 15.88 | .30 | n.a. | 13.61 |
| baked, broiled, or | | | | | | | | |
| microwaved[1], 4 oz. ... | 4294 | (0) | .21 | .06 | 5.09 | .09 | n.a. | 3.27 |
| **Egg,** chicken: | | | | | | | | |
| raw, fresh: | | | | | | | | |
| whole, 1 large, | | | | | | | | |
| approx. 1.75 oz.... | 317 | 0 | .03 | .25 | .04 | .07 | 23.0 | .50 |
| white, from 1 large | | | | | | | | |
| egg ........... | n.a. | 0 | <.01 | .15 | .03 | <.01 | 1.0 | .07 |
| yolk, from 1 large | | | | | | | | |
| egg ........... | 323 | 0 | .03 | .11 | <.01 | .07 | 24.0 | .52 |
| cooked, 1 large egg: | | | | | | | | |
| fried[2] ............ | 394 | 0 | .03 | .24 | .04 | .07 | 18.0 | .42 |
| hard boiled ........ | 280 | 0 | .03 | .26 | .03 | .06 | 22.0 | .56 |
| omelet[3] ........... | 399 | 0 | .03 | .24 | .04 | .07 | 18.0 | .43 |
| poached .......... | 316 | 0 | .03 | .22 | .03 | .06 | 18.0 | .40 |
| scrambled[4] ........ | 416 | <1 | .03 | .27 | .05 | .07 | 18.0 | .47 |
| yolk, frozen[5], 1 oz....... | 465 | 0 | .04 | .17 | .01 | .09 | 34.9 | .74 |
| yolk, frozen, sugared, | | | | | | | | |
| 1 oz............... | 419 | 0 | .04 | .16 | .01 | .09 | 31.3 | .67 |
| dried, whole, 1 oz....... | 553 | 0 | .09 | .33 | .07 | .11 | 52.2 | 2.84 |
| dried, stabilized[6]: | | | | | | | | |
| whole, 1 oz........ | 581 | 0 | .09 | .35 | .07 | .12 | 54.7 | 2.98 |
| white, flakes, 1 oz. | 0 | 0 | .01 | .61 | .19 | .01 | 25.2 | .14 |
| white, powder, 1 oz. | 0 | 0 | .01 | .66 | .20 | .01 | 27.2 | .15 |

[1] *Prepared without added ingredients.*
[2] *Recipe: 95% egg, 5% margarine, and salt.*
[3] *Recipe: 74% egg, 22% water, 4% margarine, and salt.*
[4] *Recipe: 74% egg, 22% whole milk, 4% margarine, and salt.*
[5] *Includes approximately 17% white.*
[6] *Glucose reduced.*

| | Vitamin A | Vitamin C | Thiamin | Riboflavin | Niacin | B₆ | Folacin | B₁₂ |
|---|---|---|---|---|---|---|---|---|
| | (IU) | (Mg) | (Mg) | (Mg) | (Mg) | (Mg) | (Mcg) | (Mcg) |
| dried, yolk, 1 oz. . . . . . . | 970 | 0 | .12 | .23 | .04 | .16 | 60.4 | 2.01 |
| **Egg, chicken, substitute or imitation:** | | | | | | | | |
| frozen[1], 1 oz. . . . . . . . . . | 383 | 0 | .03 | .11 | n.a. | .04 | n.a. | n.a. |
| frozen (*Morningstar Farms Better'n Eggs*), ¼ cup, 2 oz. . . . . . . . | 640 | 0 | .01 | .26 | 0 | .11 | n.a. | .60 |
| liquid[1], 1 oz. . . . . . . . . . | 612 | 0 | .03 | .09 | .03 | n.a. | n.a. | .08 |
| **Egg, duck,** fresh, whole, raw, 1 egg, approx. 2.5 oz. . . . . . | 930 | 0 | .11 | .28 | .14 | .18 | 56.0 | 3.78 |
| **Egg, quail,** fresh, whole, raw, 1 egg, approx. .3 oz. . . . . . . . . . . . . | 27 | 0 | .01 | .07 | .01 | .01 | n.a. | n.a. |
| **"Egg," breakfast, vegetarian,** frozen (*Morningstar Farms Scramblers*), 2 oz. . . . . | 311 | 0 | .29 | .39 | 0 | .13 | n.a. | 1.77 |
| **Egg roll,** frozen, vegetarian (*Worthington*), 3-oz. roll. . . . . | 0 | 0 | 1.22 | .19 | 0 | .03 | n.a. | .12 |
| **Eggnog,** dairy, nonalcoholic, 1 cup . . . | 894 | 4 | .09 | .48 | .27 | .13 | 2.0 | 1.14 |
| **Eggplant:** | | | | | | | | |
| raw: | | | | | | | | |
| untrimmed, 1 lb. . . . . | 310 | 6 | .19 | .13 | 2.20 | .31 | 70.0 | 0 |
| trimmed, peeled, 1 eggplant, 1.9 lbs. untrimmed. . . . . . . | 387 | 8 | .24 | .16 | 2.74 | .39 | 87.0 | 0 |
| trimmed, peeled, 1" pieces, ½ cup . . | 35 | 1 | .02 | .01 | .25 | .03 | 8.0 | 0 |
| boiled, drained, 1" cubes, ½ cup . . . . . . . . . . . . | 31 | 1 | .04 | .01 | .29 | .04 | 6.9 | 0 |

---

[1] *Vitamin A contributed largely from beta-carotene used for coloring.*

| | Vitamin A | Vitamin C | Thiamin | Riboflavin | Niacin | B₆ | Folacin | B₁₂ |
|---|---|---|---|---|---|---|---|---|
| | (IU) | (Mg) | (Mg) | (Mg) | (Mg) | (Mg) | (Mcg) | (Mcg) |
| **Elderberry:** | | | | | | | | |
| 1 lb. . . . . . . . . . . . . . . | 2722 | 163 | .32 | .27 | 2.27 | 1.04 | n.a. | 0 |
| ½ cup . . . . . . . . . . . . . | 435 | 26 | .05 | .04 | .36 | .17 | n.a. | 0 |
| **Endive:** | | | | | | | | |
| untrimmed, 1 lb. . . . . . . | 7997 | 25 | .31 | .29 | 1.56 | .08 | 554.0 | 0 |
| trimmed, 1 head, | | | | | | | | |
|   1.3 lbs. . . . . . . . . . . . | 10,517 | 33 | .41 | .39 | 2.05 | .10 | 728.5 | 0 |
| trimmed, chopped, | | | | | | | | |
|   ½ cup . . . . . . . . . . . . . | 513 | 2 | .02 | .02 | .10 | .01 | 35.5 | 0 |
| **Endive, Belgian,** see "Chicory, witloof" | | | | | | | | |
| **Eppaw,** raw, ½ cup . . . . . | 0 | 7 | .06 | .06 | 15 | n.a. | n.a. | 0 |

# F

| | Vitamin A | Vitamin C | Thiamin | Riboflavin | Niacin | B₆ | Folacin | B₁₂ |
|---|---|---|---|---|---|---|---|---|
| | (IU) | (Mg) | (Mg) | (Mg) | (Mg) | (Mg) | (Mcg) | (Mcg) |
| **Falafel**[1]: | | | | | | | | |
| 4 oz. . . . . . . . . . . . . . | 15 | 2 | .17 | .19 | 1.19 | .14 | 88.0 | 0 |
| 2¼"-diam. patty, .6 oz. . . . | 2 | tr. | .03 | .03 | .18 | .02 | 13.2 | 0 |
| **Farina**, whole grain: | | | | | | | | |
| enriched, uncooked, | | | | | | | | |
| 1 cup . . . . . . . . . . . . | n.a. | n.a. | 1.01 | .63 | 7.12 | .10 | 42.0 | n.a. |
| enriched, cooked, | | | | | | | | |
| 1 cup . . . . . . . . . . . . | 0 | 0 | .19 | .12 | 1.28 | .02 | 6.0 | 0 |
| **Fast foods** (unspecified), 1 serving: | | | | | | | | |
| breakfast: | | | | | | | | |
| biscuit, plain, 2.6 oz. | 98 | 0 | .26 | .17 | 1.62 | .03 | 6.0 | .10 |
| biscuit, w/egg: | | | | | | | | |
| 4.8 oz. . . . . . . . . . | 649 | 0 | .34 | .33 | .71 | .08 | 29.0 | .75 |
| and bacon, 5.3 oz. . . . | 191 | 3 | .13 | .22 | 2.41 | .13 | 29.0 | 1.03 |
| and ham, 6.8 oz. . . . . | 874 | <1 | .68 | .60 | 2.00 | .26 | 32.0 | 1.20 |
| and sausage, 6.3 oz. . . | 635 | <1 | .50 | .46 | 3.60 | .20 | 40.0 | 1.37 |
| and steak, 5.2 oz. . . . | 704 | <1 | .36 | .53 | 3.06 | .18 | 28.0 | 1.41 |
| cheese and bacon, | | | | | | | | |
| 5.1 oz. . . . . . . . . . | 648 | 2 | .30 | .43 | 2.30 | .11 | 37.0 | 1.05 |
| biscuit, w/ham, 4 oz. | 133 | <1 | .51 | .31 | 3.48 | .14 | 8.0 | .03 |
| biscuit, w/sausage, | | | | | | | | |
| 4.4 oz. . . . . . . . . . | 56 | <1 | .40 | .28 | 3.28 | .12 | 9.0 | .51 |
| biscuit, w/steak, | | | | | | | | |
| 5 oz. . . . . . . . . . . | 65 | <1 | .35 | .40 | 4.16 | .16 | 11.0 | .95 |
| croissant, w/egg and cheese: | | | | | | | | |
| 4.5 oz. . . . . . . . . . | 1000 | <1 | .19 | .38 | 1.51 | .10 | 36.0 | .78 |
| and bacon, 4.6 oz. | 472 | 2 | .35 | .34 | 2.19 | .12 | 35.0 | .86 |
| and ham, 5.4 oz. . . . | 451 | 11 | .52 | .30 | 3.19 | .23 | 36.0 | 1.01 |
| and sausage, 5.6 oz. | 422 | <1 | .99 | .32 | 4.00 | .12 | 38.0 | .90 |
| danish pastry: | | | | | | | | |
| cheese, 3.2 oz. . . . . | 155 | 3 | .27 | .21 | 2.55 | .06 | 15.0 | .23 |

[1] Recipe: water, broad beans, soybean oil, onions, flour, salt, garlic, coriander, and cumin.

| | Vitamin A | Vitamin C | Thiamin | Riboflavin | Niacin | B6 | Folacin | B12 |
|---|---|---|---|---|---|---|---|---|
| | (IU) | (Mg) | (Mg) | (Mg) | (Mg) | (Mg) | (Mcg) | (Mcg) |

Fast foods, breakfast, danish pastry, *continued*

| | | | | | | | | |
|---|---|---|---|---|---|---|---|---|
| cinnamon, 3.1 oz. | 18 | 3 | .26 | .19 | 2.20 | .06 | 14.0 | .22 |
| fruit, 3.3 oz........ | 86 | 2 | .29 | .21 | 1.79 | .06 | 15.0 | .23 |
| eggs, scrambled, | | | | | | | | |
| 2 eggs.......... | 835 | 3 | .08 | .49 | .19 | .18 | 52.0 | .95 |
| English muffin: | | | | | | | | |
| w/butter, 2.2 oz. ... | 136 | 1 | .25 | .32 | 2.61 | .04 | 17.0 | .02 |
| w/cheese and | | | | | | | | |
| sausage, 4.1 oz. | 379 | 1 | .70 | .25 | 4.14 | .15 | 18.0 | .68 |
| w/egg, cheese, and | | | | | | | | |
| Canadian bacon, | | | | | | | | |
| 5.1 oz.......... | 594 | 1 | .49 | .53 | 3.93 | .16 | 44.0 | .80 |
| w/egg, cheese, and | | | | | | | | |
| sausage, 5.8 oz. | 660 | 1 | .84 | .49 | 4.45 | .20 | 54.0 | 1.37 |
| French toast, | | | | | | | | |
| w/butter, 2 slices, | | | | | | | | |
| 4.8 oz........... | 472 | <1 | .58 | .50 | 3.91 | .05 | 30.0 | .36 |
| French toast sticks, | | | | | | | | |
| 5 sticks, 5 oz. .... | 45 | 0 | .23 | .25 | 2.96 | .26 | 134.0 | .06 |
| pancakes, w/butter | | | | | | | | |
| and syrup, | | | | | | | | |
| 3 cakes, 8.2 oz.... | 281 | 3 | .40 | .56 | 3.39 | .12 | 34.0 | .22 |
| potatoes, hashed | | | | | | | | |
| brown, ½ cup .... | 18 | 6 | .08 | .01 | 1.07 | .17 | 8.0 | .02 |
| sausage, 1-oz. patty | tr. | 0 | .20 | .07 | 1.22 | .09 | n.a. | .47 |
| sausage, .5-oz. link | tr. | 0 | .10 | .03 | .59 | .04 | n.a. | .22 |
| entrees: | | | | | | | | |
| chicken, breaded, fried: | | | | | | | | |
| dark meat, 1 thigh | | | | | | | | |
| and 1 drumstick, | | | | | | | | |
| 5.2 oz.......... | 222 | 0 | .14 | .43 | 7.21 | .33 | 10.0 | .83 |
| light meat, 2 pieces, | | | | | | | | |
| 5.7 oz.......... | 192 | 0 | .14 | .30 | 11.98 | .57 | 9.0 | .67 |
| chicken nuggets, breaded, fried, 6 pieces: | | | | | | | | |
| plain, 3.6 oz....... | 102 | <1 | .09 | .15 | 6.86 | .31 | 11.0 | .30 |

| | Vitamin A | Vitamin C | Thiamin | Riboflavin | Niacin | B6 | Folacin | B12 |
|---|---|---|---|---|---|---|---|---|
| | (IU) | (Mg) | (Mg) | (Mg) | (Mg) | (Mg) | (Mcg) | (Mcg) |
| w/barbecue sauce, 4.6 oz......... | 342 | 1 | .10 | .16 | 7.02 | .33 | 28.0 | .30 |
| w/honey, 4.1 oz. ... | 101 | <1 | .09 | .15 | 6.81 | .31 | 11.0 | .30 |
| w/mustard sauce, 4.6 oz......... | 110 | <1 | .11 | .15 | 6.94 | .32 | 12.0 | .32 |
| w/sweet and sour sauce, 4.6 oz. ... | 242 | 1 | .10 | .20 | 6.86 | .32 | 12.0 | .36 |
| chili con carne, 1 cup .......... | 1663 | 2 | .14 | 1.13 | 2.49 | .32 | 30.0 | 1.15 |
| clams, breaded, fried, ¾ cup .......... | 122 | 0 | .20 | .27 | 2.87 | .04 | 9.0 | 1.11 |
| crab, baked, 3.8 oz. | 78 | 3 | .28 | .16 | 4.49 | .45 | 20.0 | 15.75 |
| crab, soft shell, breaded, fried, 4.4-oz. crab...... | 15 | 1 | .10 | .08 | 1.75 | .15 | 20.0 | 4.47 |
| crab cake, 2.1-oz. cake...... | 313 | tr. | .06 | .07 | 1.17 | .15 | 10.0 | 4.40 |
| fish, battered or breaded, fried, 3.2-oz. fillet...... | 35 | 0 | .10 | .10 | 1.91 | .09 | 12.0 | 1.01 |
| oysters, battered or breaded, fried, 6 pieces, 4.9 oz. ... | 363 | 4 | .31 | .35 | 4.42 | .03 | 13.0 | 1.01 |
| scallops, breaded, fried, 6 pieces, 5.1 oz........... | 139 | 0 | .20 | .85 | 0 | .07 | 40.0 | .43 |
| shrimp, breaded, fried, 6–8 pieces, 5.8 oz........... | 119 | 0 | .21 | .90 | 0 | .06 | 48.0 | .15 |
| Mexican foods: | | | | | | | | |
| burrito, w/beans, 2 pieces: | | | | | | | | |
| 7.7 oz............ | 332 | 2 | .62 | .62 | 4.06 | .31 | 118.0 | 1.09 |
| and cheese, 6.6 oz. | 1250 | 2 | .22 | .71 | 3.57 | .25 | 81.0 | .90 |
| and chilies, 7.2 oz. | 205 | 1 | .45 | .71 | 4.38 | .29 | 118.0 | 1.16 |

| | Vitamin A | Vitamin C | Thiamin | Riboflavin | Niacin | B6 | Folacin | B12 |
|---|---|---|---|---|---|---|---|---|
| | (IU) | (Mg) | (Mg) | (Mg) | (Mg) | (Mg) | (Mcg) | (Mcg) |

Mexican foods, burrito, with beans, *continued*

| | | | | | | | | |
|---|---|---|---|---|---|---|---|---|
| and meat, 8.1 oz. | 636 | 2 | .53 | .83 | 5.41 | .37 | 73.0 | 1.74 |
| cheese and beef, | | | | | | | | |
| 7.2 oz.......... | 799 | 5 | .30 | .71 | 3.86 | .23 | 61.0 | 1.10 |
| cheese and chilies, | | | | | | | | |
| 11.9 oz........ | 1596 | 7 | .55 | 1.20 | 7.71 | .41 | 146.0 | 1.99 |
| burrito, w/beef, 2 pieces: | | | | | | | | |
| 7.8 oz........... | 277 | 1 | .23 | .92 | 6.45 | .32 | 39.0 | 1.97 |
| and chilies, 7.1 oz. | 463 | 2 | .39 | .80 | 5.08 | .29 | 37.0 | 1.30 |
| cheese and chilies, | | | | | | | | |
| 10.7 oz........ | 972 | 4 | .62 | 1.24 | 8.34 | .38 | 58.0 | 2.07 |
| chimichanga, w/beef, 1 piece: | | | | | | | | |
| 6.1 oz........... | 147 | 5 | .48 | .64 | 5.77 | .27 | 31.0 | 1.52 |
| and cheese, 6.5 oz. | 540 | 3 | .39 | .85 | 4.68 | .22 | 34.0 | 1.31 |
| and red chilies, | | | | | | | | |
| 6.7 oz......... | 262 | <1 | .29 | .66 | 5.34 | .24 | 34.0 | 1.09 |
| cheese and red | | | | | | | | |
| chilies, 6.3 oz.... | 702 | 2 | .24 | .96 | 3.46 | .16 | 33.0 | 1.28 |
| enchilada, w/cheese, 1 piece: | | | | | | | | |
| 5.7 oz........... | 1160 | 1 | .09 | .42 | 1.91 | .39 | 34.0 | .74 |
| and beef, 6.8 oz.... | 1135 | 1 | .11 | .40 | 2.51 | .26 | 192.0 | 1.02 |
| enchirito, w/cheese, | | | | | | | | |
| beef and beans, | | | | | | | | |
| 1 piece, 6.8 oz.... | 1015 | 5 | .18 | .69 | 2.99 | .21 | 254.0 | 1.63 |
| frijoles, w/cheese, | | | | | | | | |
| 1 cup .......... | 457 | 2 | .14 | .33 | 1.48 | .19 | 111.0 | .68 |
| nachos, w/cheese, 6–8 pieces: | | | | | | | | |
| 4 oz............ | 559 | 1 | .19 | .37 | 1.53 | .20 | 10.0 | .82 |
| and jalapeños, | | | | | | | | |
| 7.2 oz......... | 4061 | 1 | .13 | .49 | 2.84 | .38 | 19.0 | 1.02 |
| and beans, ground | | | | | | | | |
| beef, and | | | | | | | | |
| peppers, 9 oz.... | 3401 | 5 | .24 | .69 | 3.35 | .41 | 39.0 | 1.01 |
| taco, small, 6 oz..... | 855 | 2 | 15 | .45 | 3.22 | .24 | 23.0 | 1.04 |
| taco, large, 9.3 oz.... | 1315 | 3 | .23 | .69 | 4.96 | .36 | 36.0 | 1.61 |

| | Vitamin A | Vitamin C | Thiamin | Riboflavin | Niacin | B6 | Folacin | B12 |
|---|---|---|---|---|---|---|---|---|
| | (IU) | (Mg) | (Mg) | (Mg) | (Mg) | (Mg) | (Mcg) | (Mcg) |
| taco salad[1], 1½ cups | 589 | 4 | .10 | .35 | 2.46 | .21 | 40.0 | .64 |
| taco salad, w/chili[2], 1½ cups ........ | 1573 | 3 | .16 | .49 | 2.54 | .53 | 64.0 | .73 |
| tostado, 1 piece: | | | | | | | | |
| w/beans and cheese, 5.1 oz.......... | 622 | 1 | .10 | .33 | 1.33 | .17 | 75.0 | .68 |
| w/beans, beef, and cheese, 7.9 oz. ... | 1275 | 4 | .09 | .50 | 2.85 | .26 | 97.0 | 1.13 |
| w/beef and cheese, 5.7 oz.......... | 713 | 3 | .10 | .55 | 3.14 | .22 | 15.0 | 1.17 |
| w/guacamole, 2.3 oz. | 876 | 2 | .07 | .30 | 1.00 | .13 | 55.0 | .49 |
| pizza, ⅛ of 12" pie: | | | | | | | | |
| w/cheese .......... | 382 | 1 | .18 | .16 | 2.48 | .04 | 59.0 | .33 |
| w/cheese, meat, vegetables ....... | 524 | 2 | .21 | .17 | 1.96 | .09 | 27.0 | .36 |
| w/pepperoni. ....... | 282 | 2 | .14 | .23 | 3.05 | .05 | 53.0 | .19 |
| sandwiches, 1 piece: | | | | | | | | |
| cheeseburger, single meat patty: | | | | | | | | |
| plain, 3.6 oz....... | 153 | 0 | .40 | .40 | 3.70 | .10 | 26.0 | .97 |
| w/condiments[3], 4 oz. .......... | 462 | 2 | .25 | .23 | 3.72 | .12 | 18.0 | .94 |
| w/condiments and vegetables[4], 5.4 oz......... | 431 | 2 | .32 | .23 | 6.38 | .15 | 22.0 | 1.23 |
| cheeseburger, double meat patty: | | | | | | | | |
| plain, 5.5. oz....... | 332 | 0 | .25 | .37 | 6.01 | .25 | 29.0 | 2.31 |
| w/condiments and vegetables[4], 5.9 oz.......... | 398 | 2 | .35 | .28 | 8.05 | .18 | 23.0 | 1.93 |
| double-decker bun, plain, 5.6 oz. .... | 276 | 0 | .33 | .38 | 6.02 | .22 | 36.0 | 1.92 |

[1] Recipe: lettuce, tomato, chili sauce, ground beef, cheese, and taco shell.
[2] Recipe: chili con carne, lettuce, tomato, cheese, and taco shell.
[3] Condiments include catsup, mustard, pickles, and onions.
[4] Condiments and vegetables include catsup, mustard, mayonnaise-style dressing, pickles, onions, lettuce, and tomatoes.

|  | Vitamin A | Vitamin C | Thiamin | Riboflavin | Niacin | $B_6$ | Folacin | $B_{12}$ |
|---|---|---|---|---|---|---|---|---|
|  | (IU) | (Mg) | (Mg) | (Mg) | (Mg) | (Mg) | (Mcg) | (Mcg) |

Fast foods, cheeseburger, double meat patty, *continued*

double-decker bun, w/
  condiments and

|  | Vitamin A | Vitamin C | Thiamin | Riboflavin | Niacin | $B_6$ | Folacin | $B_{12}$ |
|---|---|---|---|---|---|---|---|---|
| vegetables[1], 8 oz. | 371 | 3 | .57 | .44 | 8.34 | .26 | 34.0 | 2.07 |
| cheeseburger, large, single meat patty: | | | | | | | | |
| plain, 6.5 oz. . . . . . . | 615 | 0 | .48 | .57 | 11.17 | .28 | 38.0 | 2.53 |
| w/bacon and condiments[2], 6.9 oz. . . . . . . . . . | 406 | 2 | .32 | .42 | 6.63 | .31 | 33.0 | 2.34 |
| w/condiments and vegetables[1], 9 oz. . . . . . . . . . . | 614 | 8 | .40 | .46 | 7.37 | .29 | 28.0 | 2.56 |
| w/ham, condiments, and vegetables[1], 9 oz. | 505 | 7 | .54 | .56 | 9.18 | .39 | 50.0 | 2.88 |
| cheeseburger, large, double meat patty, w/condiments and vegetables[1], 9.1 oz. | 348 | 1 | .37 | .50 | 7.24 | .41 | 48.0 | 3.40 |
| chicken fillet sandwich: | | | | | | | | |
| plain, 6.4 oz. . . . . . . | 100 | 9 | .34 | .24 | 6.80 | .19 | 28.0 | .38 |
| w/cheese, 8 oz. . . . . | 620 | 3 | .42 | .46 | 9.08 | .41 | 46.0 | .46 |
| fish sandwich, w/tartar sauce: | | | | | | | | |
| 5.6 oz. . . . . . . . . . . . | 110 | 3 | .33 | .22 | 3.40 | .11 | 44.0 | 1.07 |
| and cheese, 6.5 oz. | 432 | 3 | .45 | .42 | 4.23 | .12 | 32.0 | 1.08 |
| hamburger, single meat patty: | | | | | | | | |
| plain, 3.2 oz. . . . . . . | 0 | 0 | .33 | .27 | 3.72 | .06 | 25.0 | .89 |
| w/condiments[2], 3.8 oz. . . . . . . . . . | 126 | 3 | .26 | .32 | 4.70 | .12 | 17.0 | .84 |
| w/condiments and vegetables[1], 3.9 oz. . . . . . . . . . | 82 | 2 | .23 | .20 | 3.68 | .12 | 18.0 | .89 |
| hamburger, double meat patty: | | | | | | | | |
| plain, 6.2 oz. . . . . . . | 0 | 0 | .33 | .37 | 8.26 | .32 | 38.0 | 2.92 |

---

[1] *Condiments and vegetables include catsup, mustard, mayonnaise-style dressing, pickles, onions, lettuce, and tomatoes.*
[2] *Condiments include catsup, mustard, pickles, and onions.*

| | Vitamin A | Vitamin C | Thiamin | Riboflavin | Niacin | B6 | Folacin | B12 |
|---|---|---|---|---|---|---|---|---|
| | (IU) | (Mg) | (Mg) | (Mg) | (Mg) | (Mg) | (Mcg) | (Mcg) |
| w/condiments[1], 7.6 oz. | 53 | 1 | .35 | .42 | 6.73 | .37 | 45.0 | 3.33 |
| hamburger, large, single meat patty: | | | | | | | | |
| plain, 4.8 oz...... | 0 | 0 | .28 | .29 | 6.24 | .23 | 32.0 | 2.05 |
| w/condiments and vegetables[2], 7.7 oz. | 311 | 3 | .42 | .38 | 7.28 | .33 | 36.0 | 2.38 |
| hamburger, large, double meat patty, w/condiments and vegetables[2], 8 oz. | 102 | 1 | .36 | .39 | 7.57 | .54 | 27.0 | 4.07 |
| ham and cheese, 5.1 oz.......... | 319 | 3 | .31 | .49 | 2.69 | .20 | 71.0 | .54 |
| ham, egg, and cheese, 5 oz...... | 561 | 3 | .43 | .56 | 4.21 | .16 | 43.0 | 1.24 |
| hot dog: | | | | | | | | |
| plain, 3.5 oz...... | 0 | <1 | .24 | .27 | 3.65 | .05 | 30.0 | .51 |
| w/chili, 4 oz....... | 58 | 3 | .21 | .40 | 3.74 | .05 | 50.0 | .29 |
| coated (corn dog), 6.2 oz.......... | 207 | 0 | .29 | .71 | 4.16 | .10 | 60.0 | .44 |
| roast beef, plain, 4.9 oz........... | 210 | 2 | .38 | .31 | 5.86 | .27 | 40.0 | 1.22 |
| roast beef, w/cheese, 6.2 oz........... | 193 | 0 | .38 | .46 | 5.90 | .34 | 41.0 | 2.05 |
| steak, chopped, w/lettuce, tomato, and mayonnaise, 7.2 oz........... | 367 | 6 | .40 | .37 | 7.30 | .37 | 89.0 | 1.57 |
| submarine: | | | | | | | | |
| w/cold cuts[3], 8 oz. | 425 | 12 | 1.00 | .80 | 5.50 | .13 | 54.0 | 1.09 |
| w/roast beef[4], 7.6 oz.......... | 412 | 6 | .42 | .42 | 5.97 | .32 | 45.0 | 1.82 |

---

[1] Condiments include catsup, mustard, pickles and onions.
[2] Condiments and vegetables include catsup, mustard, mayonnaise-style dressing, pickles, onions, lettuce, and tomatoes.
[3] Recipe: bread, lettuce, cheese, salami, ham, tomato, onion, and oil.
[4] Recipe: bread, beef, tomato, lettuce, and mayonnaise.

| | Vitamin A | Vitamin C | Thiamin | Riboflavin | Niacin | B6 | Folacin | B12 |
|---|---|---|---|---|---|---|---|---|
| | (IU) | (Mg) | (Mg) | (Mg) | (Mg) | (Mg) | (Mcg) | (Mcg) |

Fast foods, sandwiches, submarine, *continued*

w/tuna salad[1],

| | | | | | | | | |
|---|---|---|---|---|---|---|---|---|
| 9 oz. . . . . . . . . . | 188 | 4 | .46 | .35 | 11.33 | .23 | 58.0 | 1.61 |
| salad, w/out dressing, 1½ cups: | | | | | | | | |
| plain[2]. . . . . . . . . . . | 2352 | 48 | .06 | .10 | 1.15 | .16 | 77.0 | 0 |
| w/added cheese and | | | | | | | | |
| eggs[3]. . . . . . . . . | 822 | 10 | .10 | .17 | .98 | .11 | 85.0 | .31 |
| w/added chicken[4] | 935 | 17 | .11 | .13 | 5.89 | .43 | 67.0 | .20 |
| w/added pasta and | | | | | | | | |
| seafood[5] . . . . . . . | 6245 | 38 | .30 | .21 | 3.56 | .35 | 100.0 | 1.73 |
| w/added shrimp[6] . . . | 791 | 9 | .12 | .16 | 1.17 | .15 | 87.0 | 3.78 |
| chef, w/added turkey, | | | | | | | | |
| ham, and cheese[7] | 1053 | 17 | .41 | .39 | 5.97 | .43 | 100.0 | .84 |
| side dishes: | | | | | | | | |
| coleslaw, ¾ cup . . . . | 337 | 8 | .04 | .03 | .08 | .11 | 39.0 | .18 |
| corn on the cob, | | | | | | | | |
| w/butter, 1 ear. . . . | 391 | 7 | .25 | .10 | 2.17 | .32 | 44.0 | 0 |
| hush puppies, | | | | | | | | |
| 5 pieces, 2.8 oz. . . | 94 | 0 | 0 | .02 | 2.03 | .10 | 21.0 | .18 |
| onion rings, | | | | | | | | |
| 8–9 rings, 2.9 oz. . . | 8 | 1 | .09 | .10 | .92 | .06 | 11.0 | .12 |
| potato, baked, w/cheese sauce: | | | | | | | | |
| 10.4 oz. . . . . . . . . . | 834 | 26 | .22 | .22 | 3.35 | .72 | 28.0 | .18 |
| and bacon, | | | | | | | | |
| 10.5 oz. . . . . . . . . | 627 | 29 | .28 | .24 | 3.96 | .74 | 28.0 | .33 |
| and broccoli, | | | | | | | | |
| 12 oz. . . . . . . . . . | 1695 | 49 | .26 | .26 | 3.58 | .80 | 61.0 | .33 |

---

[1] *Recipe: tuna salad, bread, lettuce, oil.*

[2] *Recipe: lettuce, cabbage, cucumber, green pepper, tomato, radish, and carrot.*

[3] *Recipe: lettuce, tomato, egg, cheese, celery, cucumber, and radish.*

[4] *Recipe: lettuce, chicken, celery, tomato, green pepper, and carrot.*

[5] *Recipe: lettuce, macaroni, salad dressing, pollock, sweet pepper, carrot, celery, crab, turbot, olives, and onion.*

[6] *Recipe: lettuce, shrimp, celery, tomato, green pepper, and carrot.*

[7] *Recipe: lettuce, tomato, turkey, ham, cheese, egg, celery, cucumber, radish, and carrot.*

| | Vitamin A | Vitamin C | Thiamin | Riboflavin | Niacin | B6 | Folacin | B12 |
|---|---|---|---|---|---|---|---|---|
| | (IU) | (Mg) | (Mg) | (Mg) | (Mg) | (Mg) | (Mcg) | (Mcg) |
| and chili, 13.9 oz. | 768 | 32 | .30 | .34 | 4.17 | .94 | 50.0 | .22 |
| potato, baked, w/sour cream and chives, 10.1 oz.......... | 1346 | 34 | .27 | .18 | 3.70 | .79 | 32.0 | .20 |
| potato, french fried: | | | | | | | | |
| regular, 2.7 oz. .... | 22 | 4 | .10 | .03 | 1.72 | .20 | 25.0 | .09 |
| large, 4.1 oz....... | 33 | 6 | .16 | .04 | 2.60 | .30 | 38.0 | .14 |
| potato, mashed, w/milk and margarine, ⅓ cup | 33 | <1 | .07 | .04 | .96 | .19 | 7.0 | .04 |
| potato chips, 1 oz. | 0 | 9 | .05 | .01 | 1.10 | .19 | 13.0 | 0 |
| potato salad, ⅓ cup | 95 | 1 | .06 | .11 | .26 | .14 | 24.0 | .12 |
| desserts: | | | | | | | | |
| animal crackers, 2.4-oz. box ...... | 27 | 1 | .25 | .24 | 2.46 | .02 | 22.0 | .05 |
| brownie, 2-oz. piece | 39 | n.a. | .14 | .12 | .96 | .02 | n.a. | n.a. |
| chocolate chip cookies, 1.9-oz. box ...... | 52 | 1 | .09 | .19 | 1.39 | .03 | 16.0 | .11 |
| fruit pie[1], fried, 3-oz. pie ........ | 148 | 1 | .10 | .08 | .98 | .03 | 4.0 | .08 |
| ice milk cone, vanilla, soft serve, 3.6 oz. ... | 211 | 1 | .05 | .26 | .31 | .06 | 5.0 | .21 |
| sundae: | | | | | | | | |
| caramel, 5.5 oz..... | 263 | 3 | .06 | .29 | .95 | .05 | 12.0 | .60 |
| hot fudge, 5.6 oz. ... | 221 | 2 | .06 | .30 | 1.07 | .13 | 9.0 | .65 |
| strawberry, 5.4 oz. | 222 | 2 | .06 | .28 | .91 | .07 | 18.0 | .64 |
| beverages: | | | | | | | | |
| beer, regular, 12 fl. oz. ........ | 0 | 0 | .02 | .09 | 1.61 | .18 | 21.4 | .06 |
| beer, light, 12 fl. oz. .... | 0 | 0 | .03 | .11 | 1.39 | .12 | 14.7 | .02 |
| coffee, brewed, 6 fl. oz.......... | 0 | 0 | 0 | 0 | .07 | 0 | 0 | 0 |

[1] *Apple, cherry, or lemon.*

| | Vitamin A | Vitamin C | Thiamin | Riboflavin | Niacin | B6 | Folacin | B12 |
|---|---|---|---|---|---|---|---|---|
| | (IU) | (Mg) | (Mg) | (Mg) | (Mg) | (Mg) | (Mcg) | (Mcg) |

**Fast foods beverages,** *continued*

| | | | | | | | | |
|---|---|---|---|---|---|---|---|---|
| coffee, instant, decaffeinated, 6 fl. oz. . . . . . . . . . | 0 | 0 | .03 | .51 | <.01 | 0 | 0 | 0 |
| hot chocolate, 6 fl. oz. . . . . . . . . | 4 | 1 | .03 | .16 | .17 | .03 | 0 | .37 |
| juice, 6 fl. oz.: | | | | | | | | |
| grapefruit. . . . . . . . | 17 | 62 | .08 | .04 | .40 | .08 | 6.7 | 0 |
| orange. . . . . . . . . . | 146 | 73 | .15 | .03 | .38 | .08 | 81.7 | 0 |
| tomato. . . . . . . . . | 1012 | 33 | .09 | .06 | 1.23 | .20 | 36.1 | 0 |
| lemonade, 8 fl. oz. . . . | 53 | 10 | .02 | .05 | .04 | .02 | 5.5 | 0 |
| milk, whole, 8 fl. oz. | 307 | 2 | .09 | .40 | .21 | .10 | 12.0 | .87 |
| milk, low fat 2%, 8 fl. oz. . . . . . . . . | 500 | 2 | .10 | .40 | .21 | .11 | 12.0 | .89 |
| orange drink, 6 fl. oz. . . . . . . . . | 33 | 64 | .01 | .01 | .06 | .02 | n.a. | 0 |
| shake, 10 fl. oz.: | | | | | | | | |
| chocolate. . . . . . . . | 263 | 1 | .16 | .69 | .46 | .14 | 9.9 | .97 |
| strawberry . . . . . . . | 340 | 2 | .13 | .55 | .50 | .13 | 8.5 | .88 |
| vanilla . . . . . . . . . . | 368 | 2 | .13 | .52 | .52 | .15 | 9.2 | 1.01 |
| soda, 12-fl.-oz. can: | | | | | | | | |
| cola (pepper type), ginger ale or root beer. . . . . . . . . . | 0 | 0 | 0 | 0 | 0 | 0 | 0 | 0 |
| cola, low-calorie[1] . . . | 0 | 0 | .02 | .08 | 0 | 0 | 0 | 0 |
| lemon-lime . . . . . . . | 0 | 0 | 0 | 0 | .06 | 0 | 0 | 0 |
| orange. . . . . . . . . . | 0 | 0 | 0 | 0 | n.a. | 0 | 0 | 0 |
| tea, brewed, 6 fl. oz. | 0 | 0 | 0 | .03 | 0 | 0 | 9.2 | 0 |
| tea, iced, instant, sugar sweetened, lemon flavor, 12 fl. oz. . . . . . . . . | 0 | 0 | 0 | .07 | .14 | 0 | 14.4 | 0 |

**Fat,** see specific listings

**Fava beans,** see "Broad beans"

---

[1] *Aspartame sweetened.*

| | Vitamin A | Vitamin C | Thiamin | Riboflavin | Niacin | B6 | Folacin | B12 |
|---|---|---|---|---|---|---|---|---|
| | (IU) | (Mg) | (Mg) | (Mg) | (Mg) | (Mg) | (Mcg) | (Mcg) |
| **Feijoa:** | | | | | | | | |
| untrimmed, 1 lb. . . . . . . | 0 | 45 | .03 | .11 | .99 | .17 | 130.0 | 0 |
| 1 fruit, approx. 1.8 oz. . . . | 0 | 7 | tr. | .02 | .15 | .03 | 19.0 | 0 |
| pureed, ½ cup. . . . . . . . | 0 | 16 | .01 | .04 | .35 | .06 | 46.5 | 0 |
| **Fennel,** fresh, raw: | | | | | | | | |
| untrimmed, 1 lb. . . . . . . | n.a. | 39 | .03 | .11 | 2.09 | .16 | 87.0 | 0 |
| trimmed, 1 medium, 2¼" × 2½", 8.3 oz. . . . . . . | n.a. | 28 | .02 | .08 | 1.50 | .11 | 62.0 | 0 |
| trimmed, sliced, 1 cup . . . | 0 | 11 | .01 | .03 | .56 | .04 | 23.0 | 0 |
| **Fennel seeds,** 1 tsp. . . . . | 3 | n.a. | .01 | .01 | .12 | n.a. | n.a. | 0 |
| **Fenugreek seeds,** 1 tsp. | n.a. | <1 | .01 | .01 | .06 | n.a. | 2.1 | 0 |
| **Fig:** | | | | | | | | |
| fresh: | | | | | | | | |
| untrimmed, 1 lb. . . . . | 638 | 9 | .27 | .23 | 1.80 | .51 | n.a. | 0 |
| 1 medium, 1.8 oz. . . . | 71 | 1 | .03 | .03 | .20 | .06 | n.a. | 0 |
| 1 large, 2.3 oz. . . . . . | 91 | 1 | .04 | .03 | .26 | .07 | n.a. | 0 |
| canned: | | | | | | | | |
| in water or heavy syrup, ½ cup. . . . . | 48 | 1 | .03 | .05 | .55 | n.a. | n.a. | 0 |
| in light or extra heavy syrup, ½ cup. . . . . | 47 | 1 | .03 | .05 | .55 | n.a. | n.a. | 0 |
| dried: | | | | | | | | |
| uncooked, 1 lb. . . . . . | 1051 | 4 | .32 | .40 | 3.12 | 1.01 | 33.8 | 0 |
| uncooked, 10 figs, 6.6 oz. . . . . . . . . | 248 | 2 | .13 | .17 | 1.30 | .42 | 14.1 | 0 |
| uncooked, ½ cup. . . . | 132 | 1 | .07 | .09 | .69 | .22 | 7.5 | 0 |
| cooked, ½ cup . . . . . | 207 | 6 | .01 | .14 | .83 | .17 | 1.3 | 0 |
| **Filbert,** dried, unblanched: | | | | | | | | |
| in shell, 1 lb. . . . . . . . . . | 139 | 2 | 1.04 | .23 | 2.37 | 1.28 | 149.9 | 0 |
| shelled, 1 oz. . . . . . . . . . | 10 | <1 | .14 | .03 | .32 | .17 | 20.4 | 0 |
| shelled, chopped, 1 cup . . . . . . . . . . . . | 77 | 1 | .58 | .13 | 1.31 | .70 | 82.6 | 0 |
| **Fish,** see specific listings | | | | | | | | |
| **"Fish,"** vegetarian: | | | | | | | | |
| frozen (*Worthington* Fillets), 2 pieces, 3 oz. | 0 | 0 | .65 | .14 | .96 | .36 | n.a. | 2.75 |

| | Vitamin A | Vitamin C | Thiamin | Riboflavin | Niacin | B6 | Folacin | B12 |
|---|---|---|---|---|---|---|---|---|
| | (IU) | (Mg) | (Mg) | (Mg) | (Mg) | (Mg) | (Mcg) | (Mcg) |

**"Fish," vegetarian,** *continued*
mix (*Loma Linda* Ocean

| | | | | | | | | |
|---|---|---|---|---|---|---|---|---|
| Platter), ⅓ cup, .9 oz. | 0 | 0 | 1.76 | .44 | .93 | .39 | n.a. | 1.61 |

**Fish fillet or portion,**
breaded, fried, frozen,
2-oz. piece, 4" × 2" x

| | | | | | | | | |
|---|---|---|---|---|---|---|---|---|
| ½"................ | 60 | n.a. | .07 | .10 | 1.21 | .03 | 10.4 | 1.02 |

**Fish stick,** breaded, fried,
frozen, 1-oz. stick,

| | | | | | | | | |
|---|---|---|---|---|---|---|---|---|
| 4" × 1" × ½"........ | 30 | n.a. | .04 | .05 | .60 | .02 | 5.1 | .50 |

**Flatfish,** meat only:

| | | | | | | | | |
|---|---|---|---|---|---|---|---|---|
| raw, 1 lb.............. | 147 | (0) | .40 | .35 | 13.15 | .94 | n.a. | 6.90 |
| baked, broiled, or | | | | | | | | |
| microwaved[1], 4 oz. ... | 43 | (0) | .09 | .13 | 2.47 | .27 | n.a. | 2.85 |

**Flounder,** see "Flatfish"
**Flour,** see "Wheat flour" and other specific listings
**Frankfurter** [2]:
beef, 1 link, 5" long ×

| | | | | | | | | |
|---|---|---|---|---|---|---|---|---|
| ⅞", approx. 2 oz...... | n.a. | 14 | .03 | .06 | 1.38 | .07 | 2.0 | .88 |
| beef and pork, 1 link, | | | | | | | | |
| 5" long × ⅞", approx. | | | | | | | | |
| 2 oz.............. | n.a. | 12 | .09 | .05 | 1.19 | .06 | 2.0 | .58 |
| cheese (cheesefurter or | | | | | | | | |
| smokie), 1 oz........ | n.a. | 6 | .07 | .05 | .82 | .04 | n.a. | .49 |

**"Frankfurter," vegetarian,** 1 piece:
canned:
(*Loma Linda* Big
Franks),

| | | | | | | | | |
|---|---|---|---|---|---|---|---|---|
| 1.8-oz. link ...... | 0 | 0 | .26 | .46 | 1.98 | .14 | n.a. | 1.14 |
| (*Loma Linda* | | | | | | | | |
| Linketts), | | | | | | | | |
| 1.2-oz. link ...... | 0 | 0 | .13 | .22 | .64 | .29 | n.a. | 1.04 |

---

[1] *Prepared without added ingredients.*
[2] *With added sodium ascorbate; vitamin C value for product without additive would be negligible.*

| | Vitamin A | Vitamin C | Thiamin | Riboflavin | Niacin | B6 | Folacin | B12 |
|---|---|---|---|---|---|---|---|---|
| | (IU) | (Mg) | (Mg) | (Mg) | (Mg) | (Mg) | (Mcg) | (Mcg) |
| (*Worthington Super Links*), 1.7-oz. link.. | 0 | 0 | .09 | .11 | .82 | .13 | n.a. | 1.08 |
| (*Worthington Veja-Links*), 1.1-oz. link.. | 0 | 0 | .12 | .11 | 1.47 | .15 | n.a. | .48 |
| frozen: | | | | | | | | |
| (*Morningstar Farms* Deli Franks), 1.6-oz. link . . . . . . | 0 | 0 | .14 | .02 | 0 | n.a. | n.a. | n.a. |
| (*Worthington Leanies*), 1.4-oz. link . . . . . . | 0 | 0 | .20 | .12 | .99 | .18 | n.a. | .84 |
| corn battered (*Loma Linda* Corn Dogs), 2.5-oz. link . . . . . . | 0 | 0 | .72 | .61 | 1.47 | .87 | n.a. | 2.19 |
| **French beans,** dried: | | | | | | | | |
| uncooked, 1 lb. . . . . . . . . | 36 | 21 | 2.43 | 1.00 | 9.45 | 1.82 | 1807.6 | 0 |
| uncooked, ½ cup. . . . . . | 7 | 4 | .49 | .20 | 1.92 | .37 | 366.6 | 0 |
| boiled, ½ cup . . . . . . . . . | 2 | 1 | .11 | .05 | .47 | .09 | 64.2 | 0 |
| **French-cut beans,** see "Green beans" | | | | | | | | |
| **French toast,** frozen, 2.1-oz. piece . . . . . . . . | 110 | n.a. | .16 | .23 | 1.61 | .29 | 14.0 | .99 |
| **Frosting mix,** dry: | | | | | | | | |
| chocolate, creamy, | | | | | | | | |
| ¹⁄₁₂ pkg. . . . . . . . . . . . | 0 | n.a. | n.a. | n.a. | n.a. | n.a. | n.a. | 0 |
| vanilla, creamy, ¹⁄₁₂ pkg. | 0 | n.a. | n.a. | n.a. | n.a. | n.a. | n.a. | 0 |
| white, fluffy, ¹⁄₁₂ pkg. . . . . | n.a. | n.a. | n.a. | .01 | .17 | n.a. | n.a. | 0 |
| **Frosting mix,** prepared: | | | | | | | | |
| chocolate: | | | | | | | | |
| 1 cup . . . . . . . . . . . | 840 | 0 | .03 | .12 | .60 | n.a. | n.a. | n.a. |
| creamy, ¹⁄₁₂ pkg. . . . . | 249 | n.a. | .01 | .01 | .05 | tr. | 0 | 0 |
| creamy¹, 1 cup . . . . . | tr. | tr. | .05 | .20 | .70 | n.a. | n.a. | n.a. |
| creamy², 1 cup . . . . . | 960 | tr. | .05 | .17 | .70 | n.a. | n.a. | n.a. |

¹ *Prepared with water.*
² *Prepared with water and vegetable table fat.*

| | Vitamin A | Vitamin C | Thiamin | Riboflavin | Niacin | B6 | Folacin | B12 |
|---|---|---|---|---|---|---|---|---|
| | (IU) | (Mg) | (Mg) | (Mg) | (Mg) | (Mg) | (Mcg) | (Mcg) |

| | | | | | | | | |
|---|---|---|---|---|---|---|---|---|
| Frosting mix, prepared, *continued* | | | | | | | | |
| cream cheese, ¹⁄₁₂ pkg. | 146 | n.a. | 0 | tr. | tr. | 0 | 0 | 0 |
| sour cream, ¹⁄₁₂ pkg. . . . . | 152 | n.a. | tr. | .01 | .25 | n.a. | n.a. | n.a. |
| vanilla, creamy, | | | | | | | | |
| ¹⁄₁₂ pkg. . . . . . . . . . . . . | 284 | 0 | 0 | tr. | tr. | 0 | 0 | 0 |
| **Fruit,** see specific listings | | | | | | | | |
| **Fruit, mixed** (see also "Fruit cocktail" and "Fruit salad"): | | | | | | | | |
| canned, in heavy syrup, | | | | | | | | |
| ½ cup[1] . . . . . . . . . . . . | 248 | 88 | .02 | .05 | .77 | n.a. | n.a. | 0 |
| dried, pitted, 1 oz. . . . . . . | 692 | 1 | .01 | .04 | .55 | .05 | n.a. | 0 |
| frozen, sweetened, | | | | | | | | |
| ½ cup[1] . . . . . . . . . . . . | 403 | 94 | .02 | .04 | .50 | n.a. | n.a. | 0 |
| **Fruit cocktail,** canned: | | | | | | | | |
| in water, ½ cup. . . . . . . . | 305 | 3 | .02 | .01 | .44 | .06 | n.a. | 0 |
| in juice, ½ cup . . . . . . . . | 378 | 3 | .02 | .02 | .50 | n.a. | n.a. | 0 |
| in light or heavy syrup, | | | | | | | | |
| ½ cup . . . . . . . . . . . . . | 262 | 2 | .02 | .02 | .48 | .06 | n.a. | 0 |
| **Fruit and juice bar,** | | | | | | | | |
| 1 bar, 2.5 fl. oz. . . . . . . | 23 | 7 | .01 | .01 | .12 | .02 | 4.0 | 0 |
| **Fruit leather:** | | | | | | | | |
| plain, .8-oz. bar . . . . . . . . | 27 | 16 | .01 | .01 | .02 | .69 | n.a. | 0 |
| w/cream, .8-oz. bar . . . . . | n.a. | 15 | n.a. | .01 | n.a. | n.a. | n.a. | n.a. |
| roll, .5-oz. roll . . . . . . . . . | 16 | 1 | .01 | tr. | .01 | .04 | n.a. | 0 |
| **Fruit punch drink**[1]: | | | | | | | | |
| canned, 8 fl. oz. . . . . . . . | 32 | 74 | .06 | .06 | .06 | 0 | 3.2 | 0 |
| frozen, diluted, 8 fl. oz. | 27 | 108 | .03 | .03 | .05 | .02 | 2.3 | 0 |
| **Fruit punch flavor drink** | | | | | | | | |
| **mix**[1], 2 rounded tsp. . . . | 1 | 31 | <.01 | .01 | <.01 | 0 | .2 | 0 |
| **Fruit punch juice drink**[1], | | | | | | | | |
| frozen, 1 cup . . . . . . . . | 15 | 14 | <.01 | .16 | .15 | .03 | 0 | 0 |
| **Fruit salad,** canned: | | | | | | | | |
| in water, ½ cup. . . . . . . . | 536 | 2 | .02 | .03 | .46 | .04 | n.a. | 0 |
| in juice, ½ cup . . . . . . . . | 744 | 4 | .01 | .02 | .44 | n.a. | n.a. | 0 |

---

[1] *With added ascorbic acid.*

| | Vitamin A | Vitamin C | Thiamin | Riboflavin | Niacin | B6 | Folacin | B12 |
|---|---|---|---|---|---|---|---|---|
| | (IU) | (Mg) | (Mg) | (Mg) | (Mg) | (Mg) | (Mcg) | (Mcg) |
| in light syrup, ½ cup.... | 541 | 3 | .02 | .03 | .46 | .04 | n.a. | 0 |
| in heavy syrup, ½ cup | 646 | 3 | .02 | .03 | .44 | .04 | n.a. | 0 |
| tropical[1], in heavy syrup, ½ cup............. | 162 | 22 | .07 | .06 | .72 | n.a. | n.a. | 0 |

**Fuki,** see "Butterbur"

---

[1] With added ascorbic acid.

# G

| | Vitamin A | Vitamin C | Thiamin | Riboflavin | Niacin | B6 | Folacin | B12 |
|---|---|---|---|---|---|---|---|---|
| | (IU) | (Mg) | (Mg) | (Mg) | (Mg) | (Mg) | (Mcg) | (Mcg) |
| **Garbanzo beans,** see "Chickpeas" | | | | | | | | |
| **Garlic,** raw: | | | | | | | | |
| 1 oz. . . . . . . . . . . . . . . | 0 | 9 | .06 | .03 | .20 | (0) | .88 | 0 |
| 3 cloves . . . . . . . . . . . . | 0 | 3 | .02 | .01 | .06 | (0) | .3 | 0 |
| **Garlic herb seasoning** | | | | | | | | |
| (*Tone's Perc*), ¼ tsp. | 7 | <1 | tr. | tr. | tr. | .13 | .4 | 0 |
| **Garlic powder,** 1 tsp. . . . | tr. | tr. | .01 | <.01 | .02 | n.a. | n.a. | 0 |
| **Gefilte fish,** in jars, w/broth: | | | | | | | | |
| sweet, 4 oz. . . . . . . . . . . | 101 | n.a. | .07 | .07 | n.a. | n.a. | 3.2 | .96 |
| sweet, 1.5-oz. piece . . . . . | 37 | n.a. | .03 | .03 | n.a. | n.a. | 1.2 | .35 |
| **Gelatin,** unflavored, dry, | | | | | | | | |
| .2-oz. pkt. . . . . . . . . . . | 0 | 0 | 0 | 0 | 0 | n.a. | n.a. | 0 |
| **Gelatin bar,** 1 piece . . . . | 0 | n.a. | 0 | 0 | 0 | 0 | 0 | 0 |
| **Ginger,** ground, 1 tsp. . . . | 3 | tr. | <.01 | <.01 | .09 | n.a. | n.a. | 0 |
| **Ginger root,** raw: | | | | | | | | |
| untrimmed, 4 oz. . . . . . . . | 0 | 5 | .02 | .03 | .74 | .17 | n.a. | 0 |
| trimmed, sliced, ¼ cup . . | 0 | 1 | .01 | .01 | .17 | .05 | n.a. | 0 |
| **Ginkgo nut,** shelled, except as noted: | | | | | | | | |
| raw, in shell, 1 lb. . . . . . . | 1923 | 52 | .76 | .31 | 20.68 | n.a. | n.a. | 0 |
| raw, 1 oz. . . . . . . . . . . . | 158 | 4 | .06 | .03 | 1.70 | n.a. | n.a. | 0 |
| dried, in shell, 1 lb. . . . . . | 3761 | 101 | 1.48 | .61 | 40.44 | n.a. | n.a. | 0 |
| dried, 1 oz. . . . . . . . . . . | 310 | 8 | .12 | .05 | 3.33 | n.a. | n.a. | 0 |
| **Goose,** domesticated: | | | | | | | | |
| roasted[1], meat w/skin, | | | | | | | | |
| 4 oz. . . . . . . . . . . . . . | 79 | 0 | .09 | .37 | 4.73 | .42 | 2.3 | n.a. |
| roasted[1], meat only, 4 oz. . | n.a. | 0 | .10 | .44 | 4.63 | .53 | n.a. | n.a. |
| **Gooseberry:** | | | | | | | | |
| fresh, 1 lb. . . . . . . . . . . | 1315 | 126 | .18 | .14 | 1.36 | .36 | n.a. | 0 |
| fresh, ½ cup . . . . . . . . . | 218 | 21 | .03 | .02 | .22 | .06 | n.a. | 0 |
| canned, in light syrup, | | | | | | | | |
| ½ cup . . . . . . . . . . . . | 174 | 13 | .03 | .07 | .19 | .02 | 4.0 | 0 |

[1] *Prepared without added ingredients.*

| | Vitamin A | Vitamin C | Thiamin | Riboflavin | Niacin | B6 | Folacin | B12 |
|---|---|---|---|---|---|---|---|---|
| | (IU) | (Mg) | (Mg) | (Mg) | (Mg) | (Mg) | (Mcg) | (Mcg) |
| **Gourd** (see also "Waxgourd"): | | | | | | | | |
| dishcloth: | | | | | | | | |
| raw, untrimmed, 1 lb... | 1358 | 40 | .17 | .20 | 1.32 | n.a. | n.a. | 0 |
| raw, trimmed, 1" slices, ½ cup... | 195 | 6 | .02 | .03 | .19 | n.a. | n.a. | 0 |
| boiled, drained, 1" slices, ½ cup... | 463 | 10 | .08 | .08 | .46 | n.a. | n.a. | 0 |
| white-flowered: | | | | | | | | |
| raw, untrimmed, 1 lb. | 0 | 32 | .09 | .07 | 1.06 | .12 | 18.7 | 0 |
| raw, 1" cubes, ½ cup | 0 | 6 | .02 | .01 | .19 | .02 | 3.4 | 0 |
| boiled, drained, 1" cubes, ½ cup .. | 0 | 6 | .02 | .02 | .29 | n.a. | n.a. | 0 |
| **Gourd, dried,** strips, see "Kanpyo" | | | | | | | | |
| **Grain,** see specific listings | | | | | | | | |
| **Granola and cereal bars:** | | | | | | | | |
| plain, hard, 1-oz. bar | 43 | tr. | .08 | .03 | .45 | .02 | 7.0 | 0 |
| plain, soft, uncoated, 1-oz. bar .......... | 0 | 0 | .08 | .05 | .15 | .03 | 7.0 | .11 |
| all flavors (*Kellogg's Nutri-Grain*), 1 bar .... | 750 | tr. | .38 | .43 | 5.0 | .50 | n.a. | n.a. |
| almond, hard, 1-oz. bar | n.a. | n.a. | .08 | .02 | .17 | n.a. | n.a. | 0 |
| chocolate chip, hard, 1-oz. bar .......... | n.a. | n.a. | .05 | .03 | n.a. | n.a. | n.a. | n.a. |
| chocolate chip, soft, uncoated, 1-oz. bar ... | n.a. | 0 | .07 | .04 | .27 | .03 | 6.0 | .05 |
| milk chocolate coated, soft, 1-oz. bar ....... | n.a. | 0 | .03 | .07 | .20 | .03 | 7.0 | .16 |
| milk chocolate coated, soft, w/peanut butter, 1-oz. bar .......... | 37 | n.a. | .03 | .06 | .93 | n.a. | n.a. | n.a. |
| nut and raisin, soft, uncoated, 1-oz. bar ... | n.a. | 0 | .05 | .05 | .74 | .03 | 9.0 | .07 |
| peanut, hard, 1-oz. bar | n.a. | n.a. | .05 | .02 | .41 | n.a. | n.a. | 0 |
| peanut butter, hard, 1-oz. bar .......... | n.a. | n.a. | .06 | .03 | .56 | n.a. | n.a. | 0 |

| | Vitamin A | Vitamin C | Thiamin | Riboflavin | Niacin | B6 | Folacin | B12 |
|---|---|---|---|---|---|---|---|---|
| | (IU) | (Mg) | (Mg) | (Mg) | (Mg) | (Mg) | (Mcg) | (Mcg) |

**Granola and cereal bars,** *continued*

peanut butter, soft,

| uncoated, 1-oz. bar . . . | n.a. | 0 | .07 | .04 | .89 | .03 | 9.0 | .06 |

raisin, soft, uncoated,

| 1-oz. bar . . . . . . . . . . . | 0 | 0 | .07 | .05 | .31 | .03 | 6.0 | .05 |

**Grape:**

fresh, American type (slip skin):

| untrimmed, 1 lb. . . . . | 263 | 11 | .24 | .15 | .79 | .28 | 10.3 | 0 |
| 10 medium, approx. | | | | | | | | |
| 1.4 oz. | 24 | 1 | .02 | .01 | .07 | .27 | .9 | 0 |
| peeled and seeded, | | | | | | | | |
| ½ cup . . . . . . . . . | 46 | 2 | .04 | .03 | .14 | .05 | 1.8 | 0 |

fresh, European type (adherent skin):

| untrimmed, 1 lb. . . . . | 318 | 47 | .40 | .25 | 1.31 | .48 | 17.1 | 0 |
| seedless or seeded, | | | | | | | | |
| 10 medium, 1.75 oz. | 36 | 5 | .05 | .03 | .15 | .06 | 2.0 | 0 |
| seedless or seeded, | | | | | | | | |
| ½ cup . . . . . . . . . | 59 | 9 | .07 | .05 | .24 | .09 | 3.2 | 0 |

canned, Thompson

seedless, in water or

| heavy syrup, ½ cup. . . | 81 | 1 | .04 | .03 | .16 | n.a. | n.a. | 0 |

**Grape drink[1], canned,**

| 1 fl. oz. . . . . . . . . . . . . | tr. | 11 | <.01 | <.01 | .01 | <.01 | .1 | 0 |

**Grape juice:**

canned or bottled,

| 6 fl. oz. . . . . . . . . . . . . | 12 | <1 | .05 | .07 | .50 | .13 | 4.8 | 0 |
| frozen, diluted, 6 fl. oz. . . | 12 | 45 | .03 | .05 | .23 | .08 | 2.4 | 0 |

**Grape juice drink[1],**

| canned, 1 fl. oz. . . . . . . | 1 | 5 | <.01 | <.01 | .03 | .01 | .3 | 0 |

**Grapefruit:**

fresh, pink and red, all areas:

| untrimmed[2], 1 lb. . . . . | 598 | 88 | .08 | .05 | .44 | .10 | 28.3 | 0 |

---

[1] *With added ascorbic acid.*
[2] *Vitamin A for Texas red grapefruit is 2742 IU.*

|  | Vitamin A | Vitamin C | Thiamin | Riboflavin | Niacin | B6 | Folacin | B12 |
|---|---|---|---|---|---|---|---|---|
|  | (IU) | (Mg) | (Mg) | (Mg) | (Mg) | (Mg) | (Mcg) | (Mcg) |
| ½ of 3¾"-diam. fruit[1], approx. 8.5 oz. . . . | 318 | 47 | .04 | .03 | .24 | .05 | 15.0 | 0 |
| sections[2], w/juice, ½ cup . . . . . . . . . | 298 | 44 | .04 | .02 | .22 | .05 | 14.1 | 0 |
| fresh, white, all areas: |  |  |  |  |  |  |  |  |
| untrimmed, 1 lb. . . . . | 22 | 74 | .08 | .04 | .60 | .10 | 22.2 | 0 |
| ½ of 3¾"-diam. fruit, approx. 8.5 oz. . . . | 12 | 39 | .04 | .02 | .32 | .05 | 11.8 | 0 |
| sections, w/juice, ½ cup . . . | 12 | 38 | .04 | .02 | .31 | .05 | 11.5 | 0 |
| canned or in jars: |  |  |  |  |  |  |  |  |
| in water, ½ cup. . . . . | 0 | 27 | .05 | .03 | .30 | .02 | 10.7 | 0 |
| in juice, ½ cup . . . . . | 0 | 42 | .04 | .02 | n.a. | n.a. | n.a. | 0 |
| in light syrup, ½ cup | 0 | 27 | .05 | .03 | .31 | .03 | 10.8 | 0 |
| **Grapefruit juice:** |  |  |  |  |  |  |  |  |
| fresh, juice from |  |  |  |  |  |  |  |  |
| 1 average grapefruit. . . | n.a. | 75 | .08 | .04 | .39 | n.a. | n.a. | 0 |
| fresh, 6 fl. oz. . . . . . . . . | n.a. | 70 | .07 | .04 | .37 | n.a. | n.a. | 0 |
| canned, unsweetened, |  |  |  |  |  |  |  |  |
| 6 fl. oz. . . . . . . . . . . . | 12 | 54 | .08 | .04 | .43 | .04 | 19.2 | 0 |
| canned, sweetened, |  |  |  |  |  |  |  |  |
| 6 fl. oz. . . . . . . . . . . . | 0 | 50 | .07 | .04 | .60 | .04 | 19.2 | 0 |
| frozen, diluted, 6 fl. oz. . . | 18 | 62 | .08 | .04 | .40 | .08 | 6.6 | 0 |
| **Great northern beans,** dried: |  |  |  |  |  |  |  |  |
| uncooked, 1 lb. . . . . . . . | 14 | 24 | 2.96 | 1.08 | 8.87 | 2.03 | 2186.5 | 0 |
| uncooked, ½ cup. . . . . . . | 3 | 5 | .69 | .22 | 1.78 | .41 | 438.6 | 0 |
| boiled, ½ cup . . . . . . . . . | 1 | 1 | .14 | .05 | .60 | .10 | 89.9 | 0 |
| canned, w/liquid, 8 oz. . . . | 2 | 3 | .32 | .14 | 1.05 | .24 | 184.4 | 0 |
| canned, w/liquid, ½ cup . . . | 1 | 2 | .19 | .08 | .60 | .36 | 106.5 | 0 |
| **Green beans:** |  |  |  |  |  |  |  |  |
| fresh: |  |  |  |  |  |  |  |  |
| raw, untrimmed, 1 lb. . . | 2668 | 65 | .35 | .42 | 3.00 | .30 | 145.6 | 0 |
| raw, ½ cup . . . . . . . . | 368 | 9 | .05 | .06 | .41 | .04 | 20.1 | 0 |
| boiled, drained, ½ cup | 413 | 6 | .05 | .06 | .38 | .04 | 20.6 | 0 |

[1] *Vitamin A for Texas red grapefruit is 743 IU.*
[2] *Vitamin A for Texas red grapefruit is 695 IU.*

| | Vitamin A | Vitamin C | Thiamin | Riboflavin | Niacin | B6 | Folacin | B12 |
|---|---|---|---|---|---|---|---|---|
| | (IU) | (Mg) | (Mg) | (Mg) | (Mg) | (Mg) | (Mcg) | (Mcg) |
| Green beans, *continued* | | | | | | | | |
| canned: | | | | | | | | |
| w/liquid, ½ cup . . . . . | 389 | 5 | .03 | .06 | .24 | .04 | 21.8 | 0 |
| drained, ½ cup . . . . . | 237 | 3 | .01 | .04 | .14 | n.a. | 21.6 | 0 |
| w/onion and red peppers, seasoned, w/liquid, ½ cup . . . | 599 | 4 | .03 | .06 | .27 | n.a. | n.a. | 0 |
| frozen, 10-oz. pkg. . . . . . . | 1363 | 37 | .28 | .26 | 1.42 | .12 | 41.7 | 0 |
| frozen, boiled, drained, ½ cup . . . . . . . . . . . . | 359 | 6 | .03 | .05 | .28 | .04 | n.a. | 0 |
| **Ground cherry:** | | | | | | | | |
| untrimmed, 1 lb. . . . . . . . | 3070 | 47 | .47 | .17 | 11.94 | n.a. | n.a. | 0 |
| trimmed, ½ cup. . . . . . . . | 504 | 8 | .08 | .03 | 1.96 | n.a. | n.a. | 0 |
| **Grouper,** mixed species, meat only: | | | | | | | | |
| raw, 1 lb. . . . . . . . . . . . . | n.a. | (0) | .32 | .02 | 1.42 | n.a. | n.a. | 2.72 |
| baked, broiled, or microwaved[1], 4 oz. . . . | n.a. | (0) | .09 | .01 | .43 | n.a. | n.a. | .78 |
| **Guava:** | | | | | | | | |
| common: | | | | | | | | |
| untrimmed, 1 lb. . . . . . | 2876 | 667 | .18 | .18 | 4.36 | .52 | n.a. | 0 |
| 1 fruit, approx. 4 oz. | 713 | 165 | .05 | .05 | 1.08 | .13 | n.a. | 0 |
| trimmed, ½ cup. . . . . | 654 | 151 | .04 | .04 | .99 | .12 | n.a. | 0 |
| strawberry, untrimmed, 1 lb. . . . . . . . . . . . . | 347 | 143 | .12 | .12 | 2.31 | n.a. | n.a. | 0 |
| strawberry, trimmed, ½ cup . . . . . . . . . . . . | 110 | 45 | .04 | .04 | .73 | n.a. | n.a. | 0 |
| **Guava sauce,** cooked, ½ cup . . . . . . . . . . . . | 337 | 174 | .03 | .02 | .50 | n.a. | n.a. | 0 |

[1] *Prepared without added ingredients.*

# H

| | Vitamin A | Vitamin C | Thiamin | Riboflavin | Niacin | B₆ | Folacin | B₁₂ |
|---|---|---|---|---|---|---|---|---|
| | (IU) | (Mg) | (Mg) | (Mg) | (Mg) | (Mg) | (Mcg) | (Mcg) |
| **Haddock,** meat only: | | | | | | | | |
| raw, 1 lb. . . . . . . . . . . . . | 249 | (0) | .16 | .17 | 17.25 | 1.36 | n.a. | 5.45 |
| baked, broiled, or | | | | | | | | |
|   microwaved[1], 4 oz. . . . | 71 | (0) | .05 | .05 | 5.25 | .39 | n.a. | 1.57 |
| smoked, 4 oz. . . . . . . . . | 83 | (0) | .05 | .06 | 5.75 | .45 | n.a. | 1.82 |
| **Hake,** see "Whiting" | | | | | | | | |
| **Halibut,** meat only: | | | | | | | | |
| Atlantic and Pacific: | | | | | | | | |
|   raw, 1 lb. . . . . . . . . . | 703 | (0) | .27 | .34 | 26.53 | 1.56 | n.a. | 5.37 |
|   baked, broiled, or | | | | | | | | |
|     microwaved[1], 4 oz. | 203 | (0) | .08 | .10 | 8.08 | .45 | n.a. | 1.55 |
| Greenland: | | | | | | | | |
|   raw, 1 lb. . . . . . . . . . | 249 | (0) | .27 | .36 | 6.80 | n.a. | 5.0 | 4.54 |
|   baked, broiled, or | | | | | | | | |
|     microwaved[1], 4 oz. | 68 | (0) | .08 | .12 | 2.18 | n.a. | 20.0 | 1.09 |
| **Ham, canned**[2]: | | | | | | | | |
| regular (approx. 13% fat): | | | | | | | | |
|   unheated, 1 oz. . . . . . | 0 | 6 | .27 | .07 | .91 | .14 | 2.0 | .22 |
|   roasted[1], 4 oz. . . . . . . | 0 | 16 | .93 | .29 | 6.01 | .34 | 5.7 | 1.20 |
| extra lean and regular: | | | | | | | | |
|   unheated, 1 oz. . . . . . | 0 | 7 | .25 | .07 | 1.30 | .13 | 2.0 | .23 |
|   roasted[1], 4 oz. . . . . . . | 0 | 26 | 1.09 | .28 | 5.71 | .45 | 5.7 | .94 |
| extra lean (approx. 4% fat): | | | | | | | | |
|   unheated, 1 oz. . . . . . | 0 | 8 | .24 | .07 | 1.50 | .13 | 2.0 | .23 |
|   roasted[1], 4 oz. . . . . . . | 0 | 32 | 1.17 | .28 | 5.55 | .51 | 5.7 | .81 |
| chopped, 1 oz. . . . . . . . . | 0 | 0 | .15 | .05 | .91 | .09 | n.a. | .20 |
| **Ham, cured,** whole: | | | | | | | | |
| lean and fat, unheated, | | | | | | | | |
|   1 oz. . . . . . . . . . . . . . | n.a. | n.a. | .22 | .05 | 1.27 | .12 | 1.0 | .21 |

[1] Prepared without added ingredients.
[2] With added ascorbic acid or sodium ascorbate; vitamin C for product without additives would be negligible.

|  | Vitamin A | Vitamin C | Thiamin | Riboflavin | Niacin | B6 | Folacin | B12 |
|---|---|---|---|---|---|---|---|---|
|  | (IU) | (Mg) | (Mg) | (Mg) | (Mg) | (Mg) | (Mcg) | (Mcg) |
| **Ham, cured,** *continued* | | | | | | | | |
| lean and fat, roasted[1], 4 oz. | n.a. | n.a. | .68 | .25 | 5.06 | .43 | 3.4 | .73 |
| lean only, unheated, 1 oz. | n.a. | n.a. | .26 | .06 | 1.49 | .15 | 1.0 | .25 |
| lean only, roasted[1], 4 oz. | n.a. | n.a. | .77 | .29 | 5.69 | .53 | 4.5 | .79 |
| **Ham, cured, boneless[2]:** | | | | | | | | |
| regular (approx. 11% fat): | | | | | | | | |
| unheated, 1-oz. slice | 0 | 8 | .25 | .07 | 1.49 | .10 | 1.0 | .23 |
| roasted[1], 4 oz. | 0 | 26 | .83 | .37 | 6.97 | .35 | n.a. | .79 |
| extra lean and regular: | | | | | | | | |
| unheated, 1-oz. slice | 0 | 8 | .25 | .07 | 1.44 | .11 | 1.0 | .23 |
| roasted[1], 4 oz. | 0 | 25 | .84 | .32 | 6.04 | .40 | 3.4 | .77 |
| extra lean (approx. 5% fat): | | | | | | | | |
| unheated, 1-oz. slice | 0 | 7 | .26 | .06 | 1.37 | .13 | 1.0 | .21 |
| roasted[1], 4 oz. | 0 | 24 | .86 | .23 | 4.56 | .45 | 3.4 | .74 |
| steak, extra lean, unheated, 1 oz. | 0 | 9 | .23 | .06 | 1.44 | .10 | 1.0 | .22 |
| **Ham,** fresh, roasted[1] (see also "Ham, cured"), 4 oz.: | | | | | | | | |
| whole leg, lean and fat | 9 | <1 | .72 | .35 | 5.18 | .44 | 11.3 | .79 |
| whole leg, lean only | 8 | <1 | .78 | .40 | 5.60 | .51 | 13.6 | .82 |
| rump half, lean and fat | 11 | <1 | .81 | .37 | 5.38 | .31 | 6.8 | .81 |
| rump half, lean only | 10 | <1 | .86 | .40 | 5.69 | .34 | 6.8 | .83 |
| shank half, lean and fat | 9 | <1 | .65 | .34 | 5.05 | .44 | 5.7 | .78 |
| shank half, lean only | 8 | <1 | .72 | .39 | 5.54 | .52 | 6.8 | .81 |
| **"Ham," vegetarian,** frozen (*Worthington Wham*), 2 slices, 1.6 oz. | 0 | 0 | 2.79 | .15 | 1.43 | .18 | n.a. | 1.18 |
| **Ham luncheon meat[2]:** | | | | | | | | |
| chopped, 1-oz. slice | 0 | 6 | .18 | .06 | 1.10 | .10 | 0 | .26 |

[1] *Prepared without added ingredients.*
[2] *With added ascorbic acid or sodium ascorbate; vitamin C for product without additives would be negligible.*

| | Vitamin A | Vitamin C | Thiamin | Riboflavin | Niacin | B₆ | Folacin | B₁₂ |
|---|---|---|---|---|---|---|---|---|
| | (IU) | (Mg) | (Mg) | (Mg) | (Mg) | (Mg) | (Mcg) | (Mcg) |
| cooked, sliced, extra lean (5% fat), 1-oz. slice . . . | 0 | 7 | .26 | .06 | 1.37 | .13 | 1.0 | .21 |
| cooked, sliced, regular (11% fat), 1-oz. slice | 0 | 8 | .25 | .07 | 1.49 | .10 | 1.0 | .23 |
| minced, 1 oz.. . . . . . . . . | 0 | 8 | .20 | .05 | 1.18 | .07 | n.a. | .27 |
| **Ham patty**[1], grilled, 4 oz. | 0 | 0 | .40 | .21 | 3.68 | .18 | n.a. | .79 |
| **Ham salad spread**[2], 1 tbsp. . . . . . . . . . . . | n.a. | 1 | .07 | .02 | .31 | .02 | n.a. | .11 |
| **Ham and cheese spread**[2], 1 tbsp. . . . . . . | n.a. | 1 | .05 | .03 | .32 | .02 | n.a. | .11 |
| **"Hamburger," vegetarian:** | | | | | | | | |
| canned: | | | | | | | | |
| (*Loma Linda Redi-Burger*), ⅝" slice, 3 oz. . . . . . . . . . | 0 | 0 | .14 | .30 | 1.90 | .51 | n.a. | 1.51 |
| (*Loma Linda Vege-Burger*), ¼ cup, 1.9 oz.. . . . . . . . . | 0 | 0 | .20 | .25 | .78 | .31 | n.a. | .87 |
| (*Worthington* Vegetarian Burger), ¼ cup, 1.9 oz.. . . . | 0 | 0 | .13 | .10 | 1.96 | .24 | n.a. | 1.14 |
| frozen, patty: | | | | | | | | |
| (*Loma Linda* Sizzle Burger), 2.5 oz. . . . | 0 | 0 | .38 | .67 | 4.54 | 1.11 | n.a. | 4.70 |
| (*Morningstar Farms* Grillers), 2.3 oz. . . . | 0 | 0 | 11.74 | .24 | 2.99 | .37 | n.a. | 4.85 |
| (*Morningstar Farms* Prime), 2.3 oz.. . . . | 0 | 0 | .51 | .25 | .92 | .41 | n.a. | 3.63 |
| (*Worthington Fri-Pats*), 2.3 oz.. . . . . | 0 | 0 | 2.70 | .15 | 3.39 | .65 | n.a. | 1.08 |

---

[1] *Fully cooked as purchased.*
[2] *With added ascorbic acid or sodium ascorbate; vitamin C for product without additives would be negligible.*

|  | Vitamin A | Vitamin C | Thiamin | Riboflavin | Niacin | B6 | Folacin | B12 |
|---|---|---|---|---|---|---|---|---|
|  | (IU) | (Mg) | (Mg) | (Mg) | (Mg) | (Mg) | (Mcg) | (Mcg) |

**"Hamburger," vegetarian, frozen patty,** *continued*
   garden vegetable
     (*Morningstar*
      *Farms*), 2.4 oz. . . . | 201 | 0 | 6.47 | .10 | 0 | 0 | n.a. | 0 |

**"Hamburger" mix,** vegetarian, dry:

| (*Loma Linda* Patty Mix), | | | | | | | | |
|---|---|---|---|---|---|---|---|---|
| ⅓ cup, .9 oz. . . . . . . . | 0 | 0 | .43 | .38 | 2.52 | .31 | n.a. | 1.55 |
| (*Worthington Gran-* | | | | | | | | |
| *Burger*), 3 tbsp. .6 oz. . . . | 0 | 0 | .10 | .14 | 2.97 | .09 | n.a. | .37 |
| chunk/granules (*Loma* | | | | | | | | |
| *Linda Vita-Burger*), | | | | | | | | |
| .7 oz. . . . . . . . . . . . . . | 0 | 0 | 1.23 | .17 | 3.06 | .12 | n.a. | .36 |

**Hazelnut,** see "Filbert"

**Head cheese[1],** pork,

| 1-oz. slice . . . . . . . . . | n.a. | 6 | .01 | .05 | .32 | .05 | 1.0 | .30 |

**Heart,** 4 oz.[2]:

| beef, simmered . . . . . . . . | 0 | 2 | .16 | 1.75 | 4.62 | .24 | 2.3 | 16.22 |
|---|---|---|---|---|---|---|---|---|
| chicken, simmered. . . . . . | 32 | 2 | .08 | .84 | 3.18 | .36 | 90.7 | 8.27 |
| lamb, braised. . . . . . . . . | 0 | 8 | .19 | 1.35 | 4.94 | .34 | 2.3 | 12.70 |
| pork, braised . . . . . . . . . | 25 | 2 | .63 | 1.93 | 6.86 | .44 | 4.5 | 4.30 |
| turkey, simmered . . . . . . . | 32 | 2 | .08 | 1.00 | 3.69 | .36 | 89.6 | 8.10 |
| veal, braised . . . . . . . . . | 0 | 11 | .40 | 1.05 | 5.53 | n.a. | n.a. | n.a. |

**Hearts of palm,** see "Palm, hearts of"

**Herring,** Atlantic, meat only:

| raw, 1 lb.. . . . . . . . . . . . | 426 | 3 | .42 | 1.06 | 14.59 | 1.37 | n.a. | 61.99 |
|---|---|---|---|---|---|---|---|---|
| baked, broiled, or | | | | | | | | |
| microwaved[2], 4 oz. . . . | 116 | 1 | .13 | .34 | 4.68 | .39 | n.a. | 14.90 |
| kippered, 4 oz.. . . . . . . . | 145 | 1 | .14 | .36 | 4.99 | .47 | n.a. | 21.21 |
| kippered, 4⅜" fillet, | | | | | | | | |
| 1.4 oz.. . . . . . . . . . . . . | 51 | <1 | .05 | .13 | 1.76 | .16 | n.a. | 7.48 |

[1] *With added ascorbic acid or sodium ascorbate; vitamin C value for product without additives would be negliglible.*
[2] *Prepared without added ingredients.*

| | Vitamin A | Vitamin C | Thiamin | Riboflavin | Niacin | B6 | Folacin | B12 |
|---|---|---|---|---|---|---|---|---|
| | (IU) | (Mg) | (Mg) | (Mg) | (Mg) | (Mg) | (Mcg) | (Mcg) |
| pickled, 4 oz.......... | 1153 | n.a. | .04 | .16 | n.a. | n.a. | 2.7 | 4.84 |
| pickled, 1¾" fillet, | | | | | | | | |
| .5 oz............... | 129 | n.a. | .01 | .02 | n.a. | n.a. | .4 | .64 |
| **Herring, canned,** see "Sardines" | | | | | | | | |
| **Hominy, canned:** | | | | | | | | |
| white, ½ cup.......... | 0 | 0 | <.01 | .01 | .03 | <.01 | 1.0 | 0 |
| yellow, ½ cup ........ | 88 | 0 | <.01 | .01 | .03 | <.01 | 1.0 | 0 |
| **Hominy grits,** see "Corn grits" | | | | | | | | |
| **Honey:** | | | | | | | | |
| 1 tbsp. ............. | 0 | tr. | tr. | .01 | .10 | n.a. | n.a. | 0 |
| strained or extracted, | | | | | | | | |
| 1 tbsp. ............ | 0 | tr. | 0 | .01 | .03 | .01 | 0 | 0 |
| **Honey loaf[1], pork and** | | | | | | | | |
| beef, 1-oz. slice ...... | n.a. | 6 | .14 | .07 | .89 | .09 | n.a. | .31 |
| **Honey roll sausage[1],** | | | | | | | | |
| beef, 1 oz........... | n.a. | 5 | .02 | .05 | 1.18 | .08 | n.a. | .67 |
| **Honeydew melon:** | | | | | | | | |
| untrimmed, 1 lb. ....... | 83 | 52 | .16 | .04 | 1.25 | .12 | n.a. | 0 |
| 1⁄10 of 7"-diam. melon, | | | | | | | | |
| 2" slice, approx. 8 oz. | 52 | 32 | .10 | .02 | .77 | .08 | n.a. | 0 |
| pulp, cubed, ½ cup ..... | 34 | 21 | .07 | .02 | .51 | .05 | n.a. | 0 |
| **Horseradish-tree,** fresh: | | | | | | | | |
| leafy tips: | | | | | | | | |
| raw, untrimmed, | | | | | | | | |
| 1 lb. ...........| 21,270 | 145 | .72 | 1.86 | 6.24 | 3.37 | n.a. | 0 |
| raw, trimmed, | | | | | | | | |
| chopped, ½ cup .. | 756 | 5 | .03 | .07 | .22 | .12 | n.a. | 0 |
| boiled, drained, | | | | | | | | |
| chopped, ½ cup .. | 1473 | 7 | .05 | .11 | 42 | n.a. | n.a. | 0 |
| pods: | | | | | | | | |
| raw, untrimmed, | | | | | | | | |
| 1 lb. ............ | 175 | n.a. | .13 | .18 | 1.46 | .28 | n.a. | 0 |

---

[1] *With added ascorbic acid or sodium ascorbate; vitamin C value for product without additives would be negliglible.*

| | Vitamin A | Vitamin C | Thiamin | Riboflavin | Niacin | B6 | Folacin | B12 |
|---|---|---|---|---|---|---|---|---|
| | (IU) | (Mg) | (Mg) | (Mg) | (Mg) | (Mg) | (Mcg) | (Mcg) |

**Horseradish-tree, pods,** *continued*
| | | | | | | | | |
|---|---|---|---|---|---|---|---|---|
| raw, trimmed, sliced, ½ cup . . . . . . . . . | 37 | n.a. | .03 | .04 | .32 | .06 | n.a. | 0 |
| boiled, drained, sliced, ½ cup . . . . . | 41 | n.a. | .03 | .04 | .35 | n.a. | n.a. | 0 |
| **Hubbard squash:** | | | | | | | | |
| raw, untrimmed, 1 lb. . . . | 16,676 | 32 | .20 | .12 | 1.45 | .45 | 47.7 | 0 |
| raw, cubed, ½ cup . . . . . | 3132 | 6 | .04 | .02 | .29 | .09 | 9.5 | 0 |
| boiled, drained, cubed, ½ cup . . . . . . . . . . . . . . | 6156 | 10 | .08 | .05 | .57 | .18 | 16.5 | 0 |
| boiled, drained, mashed, ½ cup . . . . . . . . . . . . | 4726 | 8 | .05 | .03 | .39 | .12 | 11.5 | 0 |
| **Hummus[1]:** | | | | | | | | |
| 1 lb. . . . . . . . . . . . . . . . | 112 | 36 | .42 | .24 | 1.86 | 1.81 | 269.3 | 0 |
| 1 cup . . . . . . . . . . . . . . | 61 | 19 | .23 | .13 | 1.01 | .98 | 146.1 | 0 |
| **Hyacinth beans,** fresh: | | | | | | | | |
| raw, untrimmed, 1 lb. . . . | 460 | 55 | .33 | .39 | 2.19 | n.a. | n.a. | 0 |
| raw, ½ cup . . . . . . . . . . | 44 | 5 | .03 | .04 | .21 | n.a. | n.a. | 0 |
| boiled, drained, ½ cup . . . | 62 | 2 | .03 | .04 | .21 | n.a. | n.a. | 0 |
| **Hyacinth beans,** dried: | | | | | | | | |
| uncooked, 1 lb. . . . . . . . . | n.a. | 0 | 5.13 | .62 | 7.30 | n.a. | n.a. | 0 |
| uncooked, ½ cup. . . . . . . | n.a. | 0 | 1.19 | .14 | 1.69 | n.a. | n.a. | 0 |
| boiled, ½ cup . . . . . . . . . | n.a. | 0 | .26 | .04 | .40 | n.a. | n.a. | 0 |

---

[1] *Recipe: chickpeas, lemon juice, tahini, olive oil, and garlic.*

# I

| | Vitamin A | Vitamin C | Thiamin | Riboflavin | Niacin | B6 | Folacin | B12 |
|---|---|---|---|---|---|---|---|---|
| | (IU) | (Mg) | (Mg) | (Mg) | (Mg) | (Mg) | (Mcg) | (Mcg) |
| **Ice, Italian**, lime, ½ cup | 0 | 1 | n.a. | n.a. | n.a. | n.a. | n.a. | 0 |
| **Ice bar:** | | | | | | | | |
| 2-fl.-oz. bar . . . . . . . . . . | 0 | 0 | 0 | 0 | 0 | n.a. | n.a. | 0 |
| fruit, reduced calorie, | | | | | | | | |
|   1.8-oz. bar . . . . . . . . . | 0 | 0 | 0 | 0 | .08 | 0 | 0 | 0 |
| **Ice cream**, ½ cup: | | | | | | | | |
| chocolate. . . . . . . . . . . . | 275 | 1 | .03 | .13 | .15 | .04 | 10.0 | .19 |
| strawberry . . . . . . . . . . . | 211 | 5 | .03 | .17 | .11 | .03 | 8.0 | .20 |
| vanilla: | | | | | | | | |
| hardened, 16% fat . . . . . . | 476 | <1 | .03 | .12 | .06 | .03 | 4.0 | .27 |
| hardened, 10% fat . . . . . . | 270 | <1 | .03 | .16 | .08 | .03 | 3.0 | .26 |
| French, soft serve . . . . . . | 464 | 1 | .04 | .16 | .08 | .04 | 7.0 | .43 |
| **Ice cream cone**, unfilled: | | | | | | | | |
| plain, wafer type, | | | | | | | | |
|   1 piece . . . . . . . . . . . | 0 | 0 | .01 | .01 | .17 | tr. | 0 | 0 |
| sugar type, 1 piece . . . . . | 0 | 0 | .05 | .04 | .51 | .01 | 1.0 | 0 |
| **Ice cream nuggets**, chocolate coated: | | | | | | | | |
| dark chocolate (*Carnation* | | | | | | | | |
|   *Bon Bons*), 5 pieces . . | 160 | <1 | .02 | .08 | .05 | n.a. | n.a. | .16 |
| milk chocolate (*Carnation* | | | | | | | | |
|   *Bon Bons*), 5 pieces . . | 170 | <1 | .02 | **.10** | .07 | n.a. | n.a. | .23 |
| **Ice milk:** | | | | | | | | |
| vanilla, hardened, | | | | | | | | |
|   ½ cup . . . . . . . . . . . . . | 109 | <1 | .04 | .18 | .06 | .04 | 4.0 | .44 |
| vanilla, soft serve, | | | | | | | | |
|   ½ cup . . . . . . . . . . . . . | 90 | 1 | .05 | .17 | .10 | .04 | 6.0 | .44 |
| **Italian sausage**, pork: | | | | | | | | |
| raw, 4-oz. link . . . . . . . . | 0 | 3 | .64 | .19 | 3.67 | .34 | n.a. | 1.03 |
| cooked, 3 oz. | | | | | | | | |
|   (4-oz. raw link) . . . . . . | 0 | 1 | .52 | .19 | 3.46 | .28 | n.a. | 1.08 |
| **Italian seasoning** (*Tone's* | | | | | | | | |
|   *Perc*), ¼ tsp. . . . . . . . . | 7 | <1 | tr. | tr. | .01 | .01 | tr. | 0 |

# J

| | Vitamin A | Vitamin C | Thiamin | Riboflavin | Niacin | B6 | Folacin | B12 |
|---|---|---|---|---|---|---|---|---|
| | (IU) | (Mg) | (Mg) | (Mg) | (Mg) | (Mg) | (Mcg) | (Mcg) |
| **Jackfruit:** | | | | | | | | |
| untrimmed, 1 lb. . . . . . . | 378 | 9 | .04 | n.a. | .51 | .14 | n.a. | 0 |
| trimmed, 1 oz. . . . . . . . . . | 84 | 2 | .01 | n.a. | .11 | .03 | n.a. | 0 |
| **Jam and preserves:** | | | | | | | | |
| all flavors, except cherry and strawberry, 1 tbsp. . . . . . . . . . . . . | tr. | tr. | tr. | .01 | tr. | n.a. | n.a. | 0 |
| cherry, 1 tbsp. . . . . . . . . . | tr. | tr. | tr. | .01 | tr. | n.a. | n.a. | 0 |
| strawberry, 1 tbsp. . . . . . . | 2 | 2 | 0 | n.a. | .01 | .tr. | 7.0 | 0 |
| **Java plum:** | | | | | | | | |
| untrimmed, 1 lb. . . . . . . | 12 | 53 | .02 | .04 | 1.00 | .14 | n.a. | 0 |
| seeded, ½ cup . . . . . . . . | 3 | 10 | <.01 | .01 | .18 | .03 | n.a. | 0 |
| **Jelly:** | | | | | | | | |
| all flavors except apple and guava, 1 tbsp. . . . . | tr. | 1 | tr. | .01 | tr. | n.a. | n.a. | 0 |
| apple, 1 tbsp. . . . . . . . . | 3 | tr. | 0 | n.a. | .01 | tr. | 0 | 0 |
| guava, 1 tbsp. . . . . . . . . | tr. | 7 | tr. | .01 | tr. | n.a. | n.a. | 0 |
| **Jerusalem artichoke:** | | | | | | | | |
| raw, untrimmed, 1 lb. . . . | 63 | 13 | .63 | .19 | 4.07 | n.a. | n.a. | 0 |
| raw, sliced, ½ cup . . . . . . | 15 | 3 | .15 | .05 | .98 | n.a. | n.a. | 0 |
| **Jujube:** | | | | | | | | |
| fresh, untrimmed, 1 lb. . . | 169 | 291 | .08 | .17 | 3.77 | .34 | n.a. | 0 |
| fresh, seeded, 1 oz. . . . . . | 11 | 20 | .01 | .01 | .26 | .02 | n.a. | 0 |
| dried, untrimmed, 1 lb. . . | n.a. | 53 | .85 | 1.45 | 2.02 | n.a. | n.a. | 0 |
| **Jute,** potherb: | | | | | | | | |
| raw, untrimmed, 1 lb. . . . | 15,632 | 104 | .37 | 1.54 | 3.54 | 1.69 | 345.9 | 0 |
| raw, trimmed, ½ cup . . . . | 778 | 5 | .02 | .08 | .18 | .08 | 17.2 | 0 |
| boiled, drained, ½ cup . . . | 2230 | 14 | .04 | .08 | .38 | n.a. | n.a. | 0 |

# K

| | Vitamin A | Vitamin C | Thiamin | Riboflavin | Niacin | B₆ | Folacin | B₁₂ |
|---|---|---|---|---|---|---|---|---|
| | (IU) | (Mg) | (Mg) | (Mg) | (Mg) | (Mg) | (Mcg) | (Mcg) |

**Kale:**
fresh:
raw, untrimmed,

| | Vitamin A | Vitamin C | Thiamin | Riboflavin | Niacin | $B_6$ | Folacin | $B_{12}$ |
|---|---|---|---|---|---|---|---|---|
| 1 lb. . . . . . . . . . | 24,626 | 332 | .30 | .36 | 2.77 | .75 | 81.1 | 0 |
| raw, trimmed, chopped, ½ cup . . | 3026 | 41 | .04 | .04 | .34 | .09 | 10.0 | 0 |
| boiled, drained, chopped, ½ cup . . | 4810 | 27 | .03 | .05 | .33 | .09 | 8.6 | 0 |
| frozen, 10-oz. pkg. . . . . . . | 17,759 | 112 | .16 | .32 | 1.98 | .26 | 47.6 | 0 |
| frozen, boiled, drained, chopped, ½ cup . . . . . | 4130 | 16 | .03 | .07 | .44 | .06 | 9.3 | 0 |
| **Kale, Scotch:** | | | | | | | | |
| raw, untrimmed, 1 lb. . . . | 8578 | 360 | .19 | .17 | 3.60 | .63 | n.a. | 0 |
| raw, trimmed, chopped, ½ cup. . . . . . . . . . . . | 1054 | 44 | .02 | .02 | .44 | .08 | n.a. | 0 |
| boiled, drained, chopped, ½ cup. . . . . . . . . . . . | 1296 | 34 | .03 | .03 | .52 | .09 | 8.6 | 0 |
| **Kanpyo,** dried, 3 strips, approx. .75 oz. . . . . . . | 0 | 0 | 0 | .01 | .55 | n.a. | n.a. | 0 |
| **Kelp,** see "Seaweed" | | | | | | | | |
| **Kidney[1]:** | | | | | | | | |
| beef, simmered, 4 oz. . . . | 1407 | 1 | .22 | 4.60 | 6.83 | .59 | 111.1 | 58.17 |
| lamb, braised, 4 oz. . . . . . | 516 | 14 | .40 | 2.35 | 6.79 | .14 | 91.9 | 89.47 |
| pork, braised, 4 oz. . . . . . | 295 | 12 | .45 | 1.80 | 6.56 | .52 | 46.5 | 8.63 |
| veal, braised, 4 oz. . . . . . | 759 | 9 | .22 | 2.26 | 5.25 | .20 | 23.8 | 41.84 |
| **Kidney beans,** red, dried: | | | | | | | | |
| uncooked, 1 lb. . . . . . . . . | 36 | 20 | 2.76 | .98 | 9.57 | 1.80 | 1787.6 | 0 |
| uncooked, ½ cup. . . . . . . | 7 | 4 | .56 | .20 | 1.94 | .37 | 362.6 | 0 |
| boiled, ½ cup . . . . . . . . . | 0 | 1 | .14 | .05 | .51 | .11 | 114.1 | 0 |
| canned, w/liquid, 8 oz. . . . | 0 | 3 | .24 | .20 | 1.03 | .05 | 114.7 | 0 |

---

[1] *Prepared without added ingredients.*

| | Vitamin A | Vitamin C | Thiamin | Riboflavin | Niacin | B6 | Folacin | B12 |
|---|---|---|---|---|---|---|---|---|
| | (IU) | (Mg) | (Mg) | (Mg) | (Mg) | (Mg) | (Mcg) | (Mcg) |
| Kidney beans, *continued* | | | | | | | | |
| canned, w/liquid, | | | | | | | | |
| ½ cup............. | 0 | 2 | .13 | .11 | .58 | .03 | 64.7 | 0 |
| **Kidney beans, sprouted,** mature seeds: | | | | | | | | |
| raw, 1 lb.............. | 8 | 176 | 1.68 | 1.13 | 13.25 | n.a. | n.a. | 0 |
| raw, 1 cup............ | 3 | 71 | .68 | .46 | 5.37 | n.a. | n.a. | 0 |
| **Kielbasa**[1] (see also "Polish sausage"), | | | | | | | | |
| pork and beef, 1 oz.... | (0) | 6 | .07 | .06 | .82 | .05 | n.a. | .46 |
| **Kiwifruit:** | | | | | | | | |
| untrimmed, 1 lb. ....... | 683 | 382 | .08 | .20 | 1.95 | n.a. | n.a. | 0 |
| 1 medium, approx. | | | | | | | | |
| 3.1 oz............ | 133 | 75 | .02 | .04 | .38 | n.a. | n.a. | 0 |
| **Knockwurst**[1], pork and | | | | | | | | |
| beef, 1 oz........... | (0) | 8 | .10 | .04 | .78 | .05 | n.a. | .33 |
| **Kohlrabi:** | | | | | | | | |
| raw, untrimmed, 1 lb. | 75 | 129 | .10 | .04 | .84 | .31 | n.a. | 0 |
| raw, trimmed, sliced, | | | | | | | | |
| ½ cup............. | 25 | 43 | .04 | .01 | .28 | .11 | n.a. | 0 |
| boiled, drained, sliced, | | | | | | | | |
| ½ cup............. | 29 | 44 | .03 | .02 | .32 | n.a. | n.a. | 0 |
| **Koyadofu,** see "Tofu, dried-frozen" | | | | | | | | |
| **Kumquat,** fresh: | | | | | | | | |
| untrimmed, 1 lb. ....... | 1272 | 158 | .34 | .42 | n.a. | n.a. | n.a. | 0 |
| seeded, 1 oz........... | 86 | 11 | .02 | .03 | n.a. | n.a. | n.a. | 0 |

---

[1] *With added ascorbic acid or sodium ascorbate; vitamin C value for product without additives would be negligible. Nonfat dry milk added.*

# L

| | Vitamin A | Vitamin C | Thiamin | Riboflavin | Niacin | B6 | Folacin | B12 |
|---|---|---|---|---|---|---|---|---|
| | (IU) | (Mg) | (Mg) | (Mg) | (Mg) | (Mg) | (Mcg) | (Mcg) |

**Lamb[1], domestic, meat only, 4 oz.:**
cubed, for stew or kabob, leg and shoulder:

| | Vitamin A | Vitamin C | Thiamin | Riboflavin | Niacin | B6 | Folacin | B12 |
|---|---|---|---|---|---|---|---|---|
| braised, lean only .... | 0 | 0 | .08 | .27 | 6.75 | .14 | 23.8 | 3.10 |
| broiled, lean only .... | 0 | 0 | .12 | .34 | 7.50 | .16 | 26.1 | 3.44 |
| foreshank, braised: | | | | | | | | |
| lean w/fat ......... | 0 | 0 | .06 | .22 | 6.19 | .11 | 19.3 | 2.59 |
| lean only .......... | 0 | 0 | .05 | .22 | 5.75 | .12 | 21.5 | 2.56 |
| ground, broiled ........ | 0 | 0 | .11 | .28 | 7.60 | .16 | 21.5 | 2.96 |
| leg, roasted: | | | | | | | | |
| whole, lean w/fat .... | 0 | 0 | .11 | .31 | 7.47 | .17 | 22.7 | 2.94 |
| whole, lean only..... | 0 | 0 | .12 | .33 | 7.19 | .19 | 26.1 | 2.99 |
| shank half, lean w/fat | 0 | 0 | .11 | .31 | 7.43 | .18 | 24.9 | 3.03 |
| shank half, lean only | 0 | 0 | .12 | .32 | 7.25 | .19 | 27.2 | 3.07 |
| sirloin, lean w/fat.... | 0 | 0 | .12 | .32 | 7.51 | .16 | 19.3 | 2.87 |
| sirloin, lean only .... | 0 | 0 | .14 | .35 | 7.11 | .19 | 23.8 | 2.93 |
| loin: | | | | | | | | |
| broiled, lean w/fat ... | 0 | 0 | .11 | .28 | 8.05 | .15 | 20.4 | 2.80 |
| broiled, lean only.... | 0 | 0 | .12 | .32 | 7.77 | .18 | 27.2 | 2.86 |
| roasted, lean w/fat ... | 0 | 0 | .11 | .27 | 8.05 | .12 | 21.5 | 2.51 |
| roasted, lean only ... | 0 | 0 | .11 | .31 | 7.75 | .18 | 28.4 | 2.45 |
| rib: | | | | | | | | |
| broiled, lean w/fat ... | 0 | 0 | .10 | .25 | 7.94 | .12 | 15.9 | 2.88 |
| broiled, lean only.... | 0 | 0 | .11 | .28 | 7.43 | .17 | 23.8 | 2.99 |
| roasted, lean w/fat ... | 0 | 0 | .10 | .24 | 7.65 | .12 | 17.0 | 2.53 |
| roasted, lean only ... | 0 | 0 | .10 | .26 | 6.99 | .17 | 24.9 | 2.45 |
| shoulder, whole: | | | | | | | | |
| braised, lean w/fat ... | 0 | 0 | .08 | .25 | 7.18 | .11 | 19.3 | 3.18 |
| braised, lean only.... | 0 | 0 | .07 | .26 | 6.76 | .14 | 23.8 | 3.30 |
| broiled, lean w/fat ... | 0 | 0 | .10 | .29 | 7.31 | .14 | 21.5 | 3.37 |
| broiled, lean only.... | 0 | 0 | .11 | .32 | 6.97 | .16 | 26.1 | 3.53 |
| roasted, lean w/fat ... | 0 | 0 | .10 | .27 | 6.97 | .15 | 23.8 | 2.99 |
| roasted, lean only ... | 0 | 0 | .10 | .29 | 6.53 | .17 | 28.4 | 3.06 |

[1] *Prepared without added ingredients.*

| | Vitamin A | Vitamin C | Thiamin | Riboflavin | Niacin | B6 | Folacin | B12 |
|---|---|---|---|---|---|---|---|---|
| | (IU) | (Mg) | (Mg) | (Mg) | (Mg) | (Mg) | (Mcg) | (Mcg) |

**Lamb,** *continued*
shoulder, arm:

| | | | | | | | | |
|---|---|---|---|---|---|---|---|---|
| braised, lean w/fat . . . | 0 | 0 | .08 | .28 | 7.55 | .12 | 20.4 | 2.93 |
| braised, lean only. . . . | 0 | 0 | .08 | .31 | 7.18 | .15 | 24.9 | 3.01 |
| broiled, lean w/ fat. . . | 0 | 0 | .11 | .31 | 7.96 | .14 | 20.4 | 3.24 |
| broiled, lean only. . . . | 0 | 0 | .11 | .33 | 7.72 | .16 | 26.1 | 3.40 |
| roasted, lean w/fat . . . | 0 | 0 | .10 | .28 | 7.55 | .14 | 22.7 | 2.89 |
| roasted, lean only . . . | 0 | 0 | .11 | .31 | 7.19 | .16 | 28.4 | 2.96 |

shoulder, blade:

| | | | | | | | | |
|---|---|---|---|---|---|---|---|---|
| braised, lean w/fat . . . | 0 | 0 | .07 | .24 | 6.85 | .12 | 20.4 | 3.21 |
| braised, lean only. . . . | 0 | 0 | .07 | .25 | 6.38 | .14 | 23.8 | 3.33 |
| broiled, lean w/fat . . . | 0 | 0 | .10 | .28 | 7.23 | .17 | 20.4 | 3.10 |
| broiled, lean only. . . . | 0 | 0 | .11 | .29 | 6.88 | .19 | 23.9 | 3.19 |
| roasted, lean w/fat . . . | 0 | 0 | .10 | .26 | 6.70 | .12 | 23.8 | 3.03 |
| roasted, lean only . . . | 0 | 0 | .10 | .28 | 6.20 | .17 | 28.4 | 3.11 |

**Laver,** see "Seaweed"
**Leek,** fresh:
raw:

| | | | | | | | | |
|---|---|---|---|---|---|---|---|---|
| untrimmed, 1 lb. . . . . | 190 | 24 | .12 | .06 | .80 | n.a. | 127.9 | 0 |
| trimmed, 1 medium, 4.5 oz. . . . . . . . . . | 118 | 15 | .07 | .04 | .50 | n.a. | 79.5 | 0 |
| trimmed, chopped, ½ cup . . . . . . . . . | 50 | 6 | .03 | .02 | .21 | n.a. | 33.4 | 0 |
| boiled, drained, 1 medium . . . . . . . . . | 57 | 5 | .03 | .03 | .25 | n.a. | 30.1 | 0 |
| boiled, drained, chopped, ½ cup . . . . . . . . . . . | 24 | 2 | .01 | .01 | .10 | n.a. | 12.6 | 0 |

**Leek, freeze-dried:**

| | | | | | | | | |
|---|---|---|---|---|---|---|---|---|
| ¼ cup . . . . . . . . . . . . . . | 2 | 1 | .01 | tr. | .03 | n.a. | 2.9 | 0 |
| 1 tbsp. . . . . . . . . . . . . . | 1 | tr. | tr. | tr. | .01 | n.a. | .7 | 0 |

**Lemon,** w/peel, except as noted:

| | | | | | | | | |
|---|---|---|---|---|---|---|---|---|
| untrimmed, 1 lb. . . . . . . . | 70 | 127 | .10 | .05 | .24 | .19 | 25.5 | 0 |
| 2⅛"-diam. fruit, 3.9 oz. . . | 32 | 83 | .05 | .04 | .22 | .12 | n.a. | 0 |
| 1-oz. wedge, ¼ medium . . | 8 | 21 | .01 | .01 | .05 | .03 | n.a. | 0 |

| | Vitamin A | Vitamin C | Thiamin | Riboflavin | Niacin | B6 | Folacin | B12 |
|---|---|---|---|---|---|---|---|---|
| | (IU) | (Mg) | (Mg) | (Mg) | (Mg) | (Mg) | (Mcg) | (Mcg) |
| pulp from 2⅛"-diam. fruit............. | 17 | 31 | .02 | .01 | .06 | .05 | 6.2 | 0 |
| **Lemon extract** (*Virginia Dare*), 1 tsp......... | 0 | 0 | 0 | 0 | 0 | 0 | 0 | 0 |
| **Lemon juice:** | | | | | | | | |
| fresh, 2 tbsp. or 1 fl. oz............. | 6 | 14 | .01 | <.01 | .03 | .02 | 3.9 | 0 |
| canned or bottled, 1 fl. oz............. | 5 | 8 | .01 | <.01 | .06 | .01 | 3.1 | 0 |
| frozen, single strength, 1 fl. oz............. | 4 | 10 | .02 | <.01 | .04 | .02 | 2.9 | 0 |
| **Lemon peel,** fresh, 1 tsp. | 1 | 3 | <.01 | <.01 | .01 | <.01 | n.a. | 0 |
| **Lemon seasoning:** | | | | | | | | |
| and pepper (*Tone's Perc*), ¼ tsp......... | 1 | tr. | tr. | tr. | .01 | 0 | 0 | 0 |
| and spice (*Tone's Perc*), ¼ tsp......... | 7 | <1 | tr. | tr. | tr. | .01 | .08 | 0 |
| **Lemonade:** | | | | | | | | |
| frozen, diluted, 8 fl. oz. ... | 53 | 10 | <.01 | .01 | .01 | .02 | 5.5 | 0 |
| mix, 2 tbsp. or 1 scoop............ | 0 | 9 | <.01 | n.a. | .04 | .01 | 3.5 | 0 |
| **Lemonade flavor drink mix**[1], 2 tbsp. or ½ scoop............ | 0 | 34 | <.01 | <.01 | 0 | 0 | 0 | 0 |
| **Lentils,** dried: | | | | | | | | |
| uncooked, 1 lb......... | 177 | 28 | 2.16 | 1.11 | 11.89 | 2.43 | 1963.2 | 0 |
| uncooked, ½ cup....... | 75 | 12 | .91 | .47 | 5.03 | 1.03 | 831.0 | 0 |
| boiled, ½ cup ......... | 8 | 2 | .17 | .07 | 1.05 | .18 | 178.9 | 0 |
| **Lentils,** sprouted: | | | | | | | | |
| raw, untrimmed, 1 lb. ... | 204 | 75 | 1.03 | .58 | 5.12 | .86 | 453.1 | 0 |
| raw, ½ cup ............ | 17 | 6 | .09 | .05 | .43 | .07 | 38.0 | 0 |
| stir-fried[2], 4 oz......... | 46 | 14 | .25 | .10 | 1.36 | n.a. | n.a. | 0 |

[1] *With added ascorbic acid.*
[2] *No fat added in cooking.*

| | Vitamin A | Vitamin C | Thiamin | Riboflavin | Niacin | B6 | Folacin | B12 |
|---|---|---|---|---|---|---|---|---|
| | (IU) | (Mg) | (Mg) | (Mg) | (Mg) | (Mg) | (Mcg) | (Mcg) |

**Lettuce:**
Bibb, Boston, or butterhead:

| | | | | | | | | |
|---|---|---|---|---|---|---|---|---|
| untrimmed, 1 lb. .... | 3256 | 26.9 | .20 | .20 | 1.01 | n.a. | 246.0 | 0 |
| 5"-diam. head, trimmed, 5.7 oz. ... | 1581 | 13 | .10 | .10 | .49 | n.a. | 118.7 | 0 |
| cos or romaine: | | | | | | | | |
| untrimmed, 1 lb. .....| 11,086 | 102.3 | .43 | .43 | 2.13 | n.a. | 578.7 | 0 |
| shredded, ½ cup, approx. 1 oz...... | 728 | 7 | .03 | .03 | .14 | n.a. | 38.0 | 0 |
| iceberg: | | | | | | | | |
| untrimmed, 1 lb. .... | 1420 | 16.8 | .20 | .13 | .81 | .17 | 241.0 | 0 |
| 6"-diam. head, cored, 1.25 lbs. ........ | 1779 | 21 | .25 | .16 | 1.01 | .22 | 301.8 | 0 |
| 1 leaf, .7 oz. ....... | 66 | 1 | .01 | .01 | .04 | .01 | 11.2 | 0 |
| loose leaf: | | | | | | | | |
| untrimmed, 1 lb. .... | 5516 | 52.3 | .15 | .23 | 1.61 | .16 | n.a. | 0 |
| shredded, 1 oz. or ½ cup.......... | 532 | 5 | .01 | .02 | .11 | .02 | n.a. | 0 |

**Lima beans:**
fresh:
raw, untrimmed (in

| | | | | | | | | |
|---|---|---|---|---|---|---|---|---|
| pods), 1 lb. ...... | 605 | 47 | .43 | .21 | 2.94 | .41 | n.a. | 0 |
| raw, trimmed, ½ cup | 236 | 18 | .17 | .08 | 1.15 | .16 | n.a. | 0 |
| boiled, drained, ½ cup.......... | 315 | 9 | .12 | .08 | .88 | .16 | n.a. | 0 |
| canned, w/liquid, ½ cup............. | 214 | 11 | .04 | .05 | .66 | .12 | n.a. | 0 |
| frozen: | | | | | | | | |
| baby, 10-oz. pkg..... | 537 | 30 | .32 | .21 | 2.91 | .45 | n.a. | 0 |
| baby, boiled, drained, ½ cup.......... | 150 | 5 | .06 | .05 | .16 | .10 | n.a. | 0 |
| Fordhook, 10-oz. pkg............. | 634 | 55 | .26 | .19 | 3.37 | .39 | n.a. | 0 |
| Fordhook, boiled, drained, ½ cup ... | 162 | 11 | .06 | .05 | .91 | .10 | n.a. | 0 |

| | Vitamin A | Vitamin C | Thiamin | Riboflavin | Niacin | B6 | Folacin | B12 |
|---|---|---|---|---|---|---|---|---|
| | (IU) | (Mg) | (Mg) | (Mg) | (Mg) | (Mg) | (Mcg) | (Mcg) |
| **Lima beans, dried:** | | | | | | | | |
| large: | | | | | | | | |
| uncooked, 1 lb...... | 0 | 0 | 2.30 | .92 | 6.97 | 2.32 | 1792.0 | 0 |
| uncooked, ½ cup.... | 0 | 0 | .45 | .18 | 1.37 | .46 | 351.6 | 0 |
| boiled, ½ cup ...... | 0 | 0 | .15 | .05 | .40 | .15 | 78.1 | 0 |
| canned, w/liquid, 8 oz............ | 0 | 0 | .12 | .08 | .59 | .21 | 114.3 | 0 |
| canned, w/liquid, ½ cup.......... | 0 | 0 | .07 | .04 | .31 | .11 | 60.5 | 0 |
| baby: | | | | | | | | |
| uncooked, 1 lb...... | 23 | 0 | 2.60 | .99 | 7.77 | 1.48 | 1815.2 | 0 |
| uncooked, ½ cup.... | 5 | 0 | .58 | .22 | 1.73 | .33 | 404.2 | 0 |
| boiled, ½ cup ...... | 0 | 0 | .15 | .05 | .60 | .07 | 136.4 | 0 |
| **Lime:** | | | | | | | | |
| untrimmed, 1 lb........ | 38 | 111 | .11 | .08 | .76 | n.a. | 31.2 | 0 |
| 2"-diam. fruit, 2.8 oz..... | 7 | 20 | .02 | .01 | .13 | n.a. | 5.5 | 0 |
| **Lime juice:** | | | | | | | | |
| fresh, 2 tbsp. or 1 fl. oz............ | 3 | 9 | .01 | <.01 | .03 | .01 | n.a. | 0 |
| canned or bottled, 1 fl. oz............ | 5 | 2 | .01 | tr. | .05 | .01 | 2.4 | 0 |
| **Ling,** meat only: | | | | | | | | |
| raw, 1 lb............. | 454 | (0) | .50 | .86 | 10.43 | 1.38 | n.a. | 2.54 |
| baked, broiled, or microwaved[1], 4 oz. ... | 130 | (0) | .14 | .26 | 3.18 | .40 | n.a. | .74 |
| **Litchis:** | | | | | | | | |
| fresh, untrimmed, 1 lb. | 0 | 195 | .03 | .18 | 1.64 | n.a. | n.a. | 0 |
| fresh, shelled and seeded, ½ cup............. | 0 | 68 | .01 | .06 | .57 | n.a. | n.a. | 0 |
| dried, untrimmed, 1 lb. | 0 | 448 | .02 | 1.40 | 7.59 | n.a. | n.a. | 0 |
| dried, 1 oz. .......... | 0 | 52 | <.01 | .16 | .88 | n.a. | n.a. | 0 |
| **Liver[2],** 4 oz.: | | | | | | | | |
| beef, braised .......... | 40,460 | 26 | .23 | 4.65 | 12.16 | 1.03 | 246.1 | 80.51 |

[1] *Prepared without added ingredients.*

[2] *Prepared without added ingredients, except as noted.*

| | Vitamin A | Vitamin C | Thiamin | Riboflavin | Niacin | B6 | Folacin | B12 |
|---|---|---|---|---|---|---|---|---|
| | (IU) | (Mg) | (Mg) | (Mg) | (Mg) | (Mg) | (Mcg) | (Mcg) |
| **Liver,** *continued* | | | | | | | | |
| beef, pan-fried in | | | | | | | | |
|   vegetable oil . . . . . . . . | 40,943 | 26 | .24 | 4.69 | 16.37 | 1.62 | 249.5 | 126.78 |
| chicken, simmered . . . . . . | 18,569 | 18 | .17 | 1.98 | 5.05 | .66 | 873.2 | 21.99 |
| lamb, braised . . . . . . . . . | 28,288 | 5 | .26 | 4.57 | 13.78 | .56 | 82.8 | 86.75 |
| lamb, pan-fried in | | | | | | | | |
|   vegetable oil . . . . . . . . | 29,482 | 15 | .40 | 5.21 | 18.92 | 1.08 | 453.6 | 97.18 |
| pork, braised . . . . . . . . . | 20,409 | 27 | .29 | 2.49 | 9.57 | .65 | 184.8 | 21.17 |
| turkey, simmered . . . . . . . | 14,267 | 2 | .06 | 1.61 | 6.74 | .59 | 755.2 | 53.90 |
| veal (calf), braised . . . . . . | 30,485 | 35 | .15 | 2.20 | 9.62 | .56 | 860.7 | 41.39 |
| veal (calf), pan-fried in | | | | | | | | |
|   vegetable oil . . . . . . . . | 21,317 | 25 | .28 | 3.81 | 19.19 | .98 | 362.9 | 72.52 |
| **Liver cheese,** pork, 1 oz. | 4958 | 1 | .06 | .63 | 3.34 | .13 | n.a. | 6.96 |
| **Liver pâté,** see "Pâté" | | | | | | | | |
| **Liverwurst** (see also "Braunschweiger"), | | | | | | | | |
|   pork, 1 oz. . . . . . . . . . . | n.a. | n.a. | .08 | .29 | n.a. | .05 | 9.0 | 3.81 |
| **Lobster,** northern, meat only: | | | | | | | | |
| boiled or steamed[1], | | | | | | | | |
|   4 oz. . . . . . . . . . . . . . | 99 | n.a. | .01 | .07 | 1.21 | .09 | 12.6 | 3.53 |
| boiled or steamed[1], | | | | | | | | |
|   1 cup . . . . . . . . . . . . | 126 | n.a. | .01 | .10 | 1.55 | .11 | 16.1 | 4.51 |
| **Loganberry:** | | | | | | | | |
| fresh, trimmed, 1 cup . . . | 290 | 35 | .04 | .06 | .60 | n.a. | n.a. | 0 |
| frozen, ½ cup . . . . . . . . . | 26 | 11 | .04 | .03 | .62 | .05 | 18.9 | 0 |
| **Longan,** fresh, | | | | | | | | |
|   untrimmed, 1 lb. . . . . . . | n.a. | 202 | .08 | .34 | .72 | n.a. | n.a. | 0 |
| **Loquat:** | | | | | | | | |
| untrimmed, 1 lb. . . . . . . . | 4297 | 3 | .05 | .07 | .51 | n.a. | n.a. | 0 |
| peeled and seeded, | | | | | | | | |
|   1 oz. . . . . . . . . . . . . . | 433 | <1 | .01 | .01 | .05 | n.a. | n.a. | 0 |
| **Lotus root:** | | | | | | | | |
| raw, 10 slices, 2.9 oz. . . . | 0 | 36 | .13 | .18 | .32 | n.a. | n.a. | 0 |
| boiled, drained, | | | | | | | | |
|   10 slices . . . . . . . . . . . | 0 | 24 | .11 | .01 | .27 | n.a. | n.a. | 0 |

[1] *Prepared without added ingredients.*

| | Vitamin A | Vitamin C | Thiamin | Riboflavin | Niacin | B6 | Folacin | B12 |
|---|---|---|---|---|---|---|---|---|
| | (IU) | (Mg) | (Mg) | (Mg) | (Mg) | (Mg) | (Mcg) | (Mcg) |
| **Lotus seeds:** | | | | | | | | |
| raw, 1 oz. . . . . . . . . . . | 4 | 0 | .05 | .01 | .12 | n.a. | n.a. | 0 |
| dried, 1 oz. . . . . . . . . . | 14 | 0 | .18 | .04 | .45 | n.a. | n.a. | 0 |
| **Luncheon meat[2] (see also specific listings):** | | | | | | | | |
| pork and beef, 1-oz. slice | 0 | 4 | .09 | .04 | .80 | .06 | 2.0 | .36 |
| pork and beef, sausage, | | | | | | | | |
| 1 oz. . . . . . . . . . . . . . | 0 | 5 | .06 | .06 | 1.00 | .06 | n.a. | .56 |
| canned, pork, 1 oz. . . . . . | tr. | 0 | .10 | .06 | .89 | .06 | 2.0 | .26 |
| **Lung[1]:** | | | | | | | | |
| beef, braised . . . . . . . . . . | 44 | 37 | .04 | .16 | 2.83 | .02 | 9.1 | 2.94 |
| pork, braised . . . . . . . . . . | 0 | 9 | .09 | .37 | 2.15 | .09 | n.a. | 2.30 |
| **Lupines:** | | | | | | | | |
| raw, 1 lb.. . . . . . . . . . . . | n.a. | n.a. | 2.90 | 1.00 | 9.93 | n.a. | n.a. | 0 |
| raw, ½ cup . . . . . . . . . . | n.a. | n.a. | .57 | .20 | 1.97 | n.a. | n.a. | 0 |
| boiled, ½ cup . . . . . . . . | n.a. | n.a. | .11 | .04 | .41 | n.a. | n.a. | 0 |
| **Luxury loaf[2], pork,** | | | | | | | | |
| 1-oz. slice . . . . . . . . . . | 0 | 6 | .20 | .08 | .99 | .09 | n.a. | .39 |
| **Lychees, see "Litchis"** | | | | | | | | |

[1] Prepared without added ingredients.
[2] With added ascorbic acid or sodium ascorbate; vitamin C value for product without additives would be negligible.

# M

| | Vitamin A (IU) | Vitamin C (Mg) | Thiamin (Mg) | Riboflavin (Mg) | Niacin (Mg) | B6 (Mg) | Folacin (Mcg) | B12 (Mcg) |
|---|---|---|---|---|---|---|---|---|
| **Macadamia nut:** | | | | | | | | |
| dried, in shell, 1 lb...... | 0 | 0 | .49 | .16 | 3.01 | n.a. | n.a. | 0 |
| dried, 1 oz. .......... | 0 | 0 | .10 | .03 | .61 | n.a. | n.a. | 0 |
| oil-roasted, 1 oz. ....... | 3 | 0 | .06 | .03 | .57 | n.a. | n.a. | 0 |
| oil-roasted, wholes or | | | | | | | | |
|   halves, 1 cup ........ | 12 | 0 | .29 | .15 | 2.71 | n.a. | n.a. | 0 |
| **Macaroni** (see also "Pasta"), dry: | | | | | | | | |
| uncooked: | | | | | | | | |
|   enriched, 2 oz...... | 0 | 0 | .59 | .25 | 4.28 | .06 | 10.0 | 0 |
|   protein fortified, 2 oz... | 0 | 0 | .68 | .27 | 4.36 | .10 | 11.0 | 0 |
|   vegetable (tricolor), 2 oz. | 91 | 0 | .59 | .30 | 4.18 | .07 | 10.0 | 0 |
|   whole wheat, 2 oz.... | 0 | 0 | .28 | .08 | 2.92 | .13 | 32.0 | 0 |
| cooked: | | | | | | | | |
|   enriched, 4 oz....... | 0 | 0 | .23 | .11 | 1.90 | .04 | 7.9 | 0 |
|   elbow, enriched, 1 cup | 0 | 0 | .29 | .14 | 2.34 | .05 | 10.0 | 0 |
|   protein fortified, 4 oz. | 0 | 0 | .34 | .18 | 2.08 | .07 | 12.5 | 0 |
|   vegetable (tricolor), | | | | | | | | |
|     4 oz............ | 60 | 0 | .13 | .07 | 1.21 | .03 | 6.8 | 0 |
|   whole wheat, 4 oz. | 0 | 0 | .12 | .05 | .80 | .09 | 5.7 | 0 |
| **Mace,** ground, 1 tsp..... | 14 | n.a. | .01 | .01 | .02 | n.a. | n.a. | 0 |
| **Mackerel,** meat only: | | | | | | | | |
| Atlantic: | | | | | | | | |
|   raw, 1 lb........... | 748 | 2 | .80 | 1.42 | 41.19 | 1.81 | n.a. | 39.51 |
|   baked, broiled, or | | | | | | | | |
|     microwaved[1], 4 oz. | 204 | <1 | .18 | .47 | .78 | .52 | n.a. | 21.54 |
| king: | | | | | | | | |
|   raw, 1 lb........... | 3298 | (0) | .45 | 2.16 | 38.96 | 2.01 | 34.2 | 70.76 |
|   baked, broiled, or | | | | | | | | |
|     microwaved[1], 4 oz. | 951 | (0) | .13 | .66 | 11.86 | .57 | 10.2 | 20.41 |
| Pacific or jack: | | | | | | | | |
|   raw, 1 lb........... | 195 | (0) | .50 | 1.91 | 37.74 | 1.50 | 9.0 | 19.98 |

---

[1] Prepared without added ingredients.

| | Vitamin A | Vitamin C | Thiamin | Riboflavin | Niacin | B6 | Folacin | B12 |
|---|---|---|---|---|---|---|---|---|
| | (IU) | (Mg) | (Mg) | (Mg) | (Mg) | (Mg) | (Mcg) | (Mcg) |
| baked, broiled, or microwaved[1], 4 oz. | 53 | (0) | .15 | .61 | 12.10 | .43 | 2.27 | 4.80 |
| **Mackerel, canned,** jack, drained, 4 oz. . . . . . . . | 492 | 1 | .05 | .24 | 7.01 | .24 | 5.7 | 7.87 |
| **Malted milk:** | | | | | | | | |
| natural flavor: | | | | | | | | |
| powder, ¾ oz. or 2–3 heaping tsp. . . | 68 | 0 | .11 | .14 | 1.07 | .08 | 10.0 | .16 |
| prepared[2] . . . . . . . . . | 376 | 2 | .20 | .54 | 1.28 | .18 | 22.0 | 1.04 |
| chocolate flavor: | | | | | | | | |
| powder, ¾ oz. or 2–3 heaping tsp. . . | 20 | n.a. | .04 | .04 | .43 | .03 | 5.0 | .05 |
| prepared[2] . . . . . . . . . | 326 | 2 | .14 | .43 | .69 | .13 | 17.0 | .92 |
| **Mammy apple:** | | | | | | | | |
| untrimmed, 1 lb. . . . . . . . | 626 | 38 | .05 | .11 | 1.09 | n.a. | n.a. | 0 |
| peeled and seeded, 1 oz. . . . | 65 | 4 | .01 | .01 | .11 | n.a. | n.a | 0 |
| **Mango:** | | | | | | | | |
| untrimmed, 1 lb. . . . . . . . | 12,187 | 87 | .18 | .18 | 1.83 | .42 | n.a. | 0 |
| 1 medium, approx. 10.5 oz. . . . . . . . . . . | 8060 | 57 | .12 | .19 | 1.21 | .28 | n.a. | 0 |
| peeled and seeded, sliced, ½ cup . . . . . . . . . . . . | 3213 | 23 | .05 | .05 | .48 | .11 | n.a. | 0 |
| **Maple syrup** (see also "Syrup, table blends"), 1 tbsp. . . . . . . . . . . . | 0 | 0 | tr. | tr. | .01 | .01 | 0 | 0 |
| **Margarine:** | | | | | | | | |
| regular: | | | | | | | | |
| stick, 4-oz. stick . . . . . | 3750 | tr. | .01 | .04 | .03 | .01 | 1.34 | .11 |
| stick, 1 tsp. . . . . . . . . | 155 | tr. | 0 | tr. | tr. | 0 | .06 | tr. |
| tub, soft, 1 cup . . . . . | 7507 | tr. | .02 | .07 | .05 | .02 | 2.37 | .19 |
| tub, soft, 1 tsp. . . . . . | 155 | tr. | 0 | tr. | tr. | 0 | .05 | tr. |
| liquid, 1 cup . . . . . . . | 7507 | 1 | .05 | .18 | .11 | .04 | 5.96 | .48 |
| liquid, 1 tsp. . . . . . . . | 155 | tr. | tr. | tr. | tr. | tr. | .12 | .01 |

[1] Prepared without added ingredients.
[2] One cup whole milk and ¾ oz. powder.

| | Vitamin A | Vitamin C | Thiamin | Riboflavin | Niacin | B6 | Folacin | B12 |
|---|---|---|---|---|---|---|---|---|
| | (IU) | (Mg) | (Mg) | (Mg) | (Mg) | (Mg) | (Mcg) | (Mcg) |

**Margarine,** *continued*
blend:

| | | | | | | | | |
|---|---|---|---|---|---|---|---|---|
| 40% fat, 1 cup | 7672 | tr. | .01 | .05 | .03 | .01 | 2.64 | .13 |
| 40% fat, 1 tsp. | 159 | tr. | 0 | tr. | tr. | 0 | .03 | tr. |
| 60% corn oil, 40% butter, 4-oz. stick | 3624 | tr. | .01 | .04 | .04 | .01 | 2.00 | .06 |
| 60% corn oil, 40% butter, 1 tsp. | 160 | 0 | 0 | tr. | tr. | tr. | 0 | 0 |
| **Marinara sauce,** see "Tomato sauce" | | | | | | | | |
| **Marjoram,** dried, 1 tsp. | 48 | <1 | <.01 | <.01 | .03 | n.a. | n.a. | 0 |
| **Marmalade:** | | | | | | | | |
| citrus, 1 tbsp. | n.a. | 1 | tr. | tr. | tr. | n.a. | n.a. | 0 |
| orange, 1 tbsp. | 9 | 1.0 | tr. | n.a. | .01 | n.a. | 7.0 | 0 |
| **Marshmallow,** see "Candy" | | | | | | | | |
| **Marshmallow creme topping,** 1 oz. | 0 | n.a. | 0 | 0 | .02 | 0 | 0 | 0 |
| **Mayonnaise dressing,** 1 tbsp. | 32 | 0 | tr. | tr. | tr. | n.a. | n.a. | 0 |
| **Melon,** see specific listings | | | | | | | | |
| **Melon balls** (cantaloupe and honeydew), frozen, ½ cup | 1535 | 5 | .14 | .02 | .55 | .09 | 22.3 | 0 |
| **Mexican seasoning** (*Tone's Perc*), ¼ tsp. | 75 | <1 | tr. | .01 | .08 | .01 | .1 | 0 |
| **Milk,** cow, fluid: | | | | | | | | |
| buttermilk, cultured, 1 cup | 81 | 2 | .08 | .38 | .14 | .08 | n.a. | .54 |
| whole: | | | | | | | | |
| 3.3% fat, 1 cup | 307 | 2 | .09 | .40 | .21 | .10 | 12.0 | .87 |
| 3.7% fat, producer, 1 cup | 337 | 4 | .09 | .39 | .21 | .10 | 12.0 | .87 |
| low sodium, 1 cup | 317 | n.a. | .05 | .26 | .11 | .08 | n.a. | .88 |
| low fat 2%: | | | | | | | | |
| 1 cup | 500 | 2 | .10 | .40 | .21 | .11 | 12.0 | .89 |
| nonfat milk solids added, 1 cup | 500 | 2 | .10 | .42 | .22 | .11 | 13.0 | .94 |

|  | Vitamin A | Vitamin C | Thiamin | Riboflavin | Niacin | B6 | Folacin | B12 |
|---|---|---|---|---|---|---|---|---|
|  | (IU) | (Mg) | (Mg) | (Mg) | (Mg) | (Mg) | (Mcg) | (Mcg) |
| protein fortified, 1 cup | 500 | 3 | .11 | .48 | .25 | .13 | 15.0 | 1.05 |
| low fat 1%: |  |  |  |  |  |  |  |  |
| 1 cup . . . . . . . . . . . . | 500 | 2 | .10 | .41 | .21 | .11 | 12.0 | .90 |
| nonfat milk solids |  |  |  |  |  |  |  |  |
| added, 1 cup . . . . . | 500 | 2 | .10 | .42 | .22 | .11 | 13.0 | .94 |
| protein fortified, 1 cup | 500 | 3 | .11 | .47 | .25 | .12 | 15.0 | 1.05 |
| skim: |  |  |  |  |  |  |  |  |
| 1 cup . . . . . . . . . . . . | 500 | 2 | .09 | .34 | .22 | .10 | 13.0 | .93 |
| nonfat milk solids |  |  |  |  |  |  |  |  |
| added, 1 cup . . . . . | 500 | 2 | .10 | .43 | .22 | .11 | 13.0 | .95 |
| protein fortified, 1 cup | 500 | 3 | .11 | .48 | .25 | .12 | 15.0 | 1.10 |
| **Milk, canned:** |  |  |  |  |  |  |  |  |
| condensed, sweetened, |  |  |  |  |  |  |  |  |
| 1 cup . . . . . . . . . . . . | 1004 | 8 | .28 | 1.27 | .64 | .16 | 34.0 | 1.36 |
| evaporated, whole[1], |  |  |  |  |  |  |  |  |
| 1 cup . . . . . . . . . . . . | 612 | 5 | .12 | .80 | .49 | .13 | 20.0 | .41 |
| evaporated, skim[1], 1 cup. . . | 20 | 3 | .11 | .78 | .44 | .14 | 22.0 | .61 |
| **Milk, dry:** |  |  |  |  |  |  |  |  |
| buttermilk, sweet cream, |  |  |  |  |  |  |  |  |
| 1 oz. . . . . . . . . . . . . . | 62 | 2 | .11 | .45 | .25 | .10 | 13.3 | 1.08 |
| whole, 1 oz. . . . . . . . . . | 261 | 2 | .08 | .34 | .18 | .09 | 10.5 | .92 |
| nonfat: |  |  |  |  |  |  |  |  |
| regular, 1 oz. . . . . . . . | 10 | 2 | .12 | .44 | .27 | .10 | 14.2 | 1.14 |
| calcium reduced, 1 oz. | 2 | n.a. | .05 | .47 | .19 | .08 | n.a. | 1.13 |
| instant[1], 1 oz. . . . . . . | 8 | 2 | .12 | .49 | .25 | .10 | 14.2 | 1.13 |
| **Milk, goat,** fluid, whole, |  |  |  |  |  |  |  |  |
| 1 cup . . . . . . . . . . . . | 451 | 3 | .12 | .34 | .68 | .11 | 1.0 | .16 |
| **Milk, human,** fluid, |  |  |  |  |  |  |  |  |
| whole, 1 cup . . . . . . . . | 593 | 12 | .03 | .09 | .44 | .03 | 13.0 | .11 |
| **Milk, Indian buffalo,** |  |  |  |  |  |  |  |  |
| fluid, whole, 1 cup. . . . | 434 | 5 | .13 | .33 | .22 | .06 | 14.0 | .89 |
| **Milk, sheep,** fluid, whole, |  |  |  |  |  |  |  |  |
| 1 cup . . . . . . . . . . . . | 360 | 10 | .16 | .87 | 1.02 | n.a. | n.a. | 1.74 |

[1] Without added vitamin A.

|  | Vitamin A | Vitamin C | Thiamin | Riboflavin | Niacin | B6 | Folacin | B12 |
|---|---|---|---|---|---|---|---|---|
|  | (IU) | (Mg) | (Mg) | (Mg) | (Mg) | (Mg) | (Mcg) | (Mcg) |
| **Milkfish,** meat only: | | | | | | | | |
| raw, 1 lb.............. | n.a. | (0) | .06 | .25 | 29.21 | 1.92 | n.a. | 15.42 |
| baked, broiled, or | | | | | | | | |
| microwaved[1], 4 oz. .... | n.a. | (0) | .02 | .08 | 9.36 | .55 | n.a. | 3.71 |
| **Millet:** | | | | | | | | |
| uncooked, 1 oz......... | n.a. | 0 | .12 | .08 | 1.34 | .11 | n.a. | 0 |
| uncooked, ½ cup....... | n.a. | 0 | .42 | .29 | 4.72 | .38 | n.a. | 0 |
| cooked, 1 cup ......... | n.a. | 0 | .25 | .20 | 3.19 | .26 | n.a. | 0 |
| **Miso:** | | | | | | | | |
| 1 lb. ................ | 396 | 0 | .44 | 1.13 | 3.90 | .98 | 149.7 | .94 |
| ½ cup ............... | 120 | 0 | .13 | .35 | 1.19 | .30 | 45.5 | .29 |
| **Molasses:** | | | | | | | | |
| 1 tbsp. .............. | 0 | n.a. | .01 | 0 | .19 | .13 | 0 | 0 |
| blackstrap, 1 tbsp....... | 0 | n.a. | .01 | .01 | .22 | .14 | 0 | 0 |
| **Molasses,** cane, | | | | | | | | |
| blackstrap, 1 tbsp..... | 0 | 0 | .02 | .04 | .40 | n.a. | n.a. | 0 |
| **Mortadella[2],** beef and | | | | | | | | |
| pork, 1 oz........... | 0 | 7 | .03 | .04 | .76 | .04 | n.a. | .42 |
| **Moth beans,** dried: | | | | | | | | |
| uncooked, 1 lb......... | 145 | 18 | 2.55 | .41 | 12.70 | n.a. | n.a. | 0 |
| uncooked, ½ cup....... | 31 | 4 | .55 | .09 | 2.74 | n.a. | n.a. | 0 |
| boiled, ½ cup ......... | 9 | 1 | .11 | .02 | .59 | n.a. | n.a. | 0 |
| **Mother's loaf,** pork, 1 oz. | 0 | 0 | .16 | .05 | .89 | .05 | n.a. | .30 |
| **Muffin:** | | | | | | | | |
| blueberry: | | | | | | | | |
| 2-oz. piece......... | n.a. | 1 | .08 | .07 | .63 | .01 | n.a. | 0 |
| toaster type, 1.2-oz. | | | | | | | | |
| piece ........... | 105 | 0 | .08 | .10 | .67 | n.a. | n.a. | 0 |
| toaster type, toasted, | | | | | | | | |
| 1.1-oz. piece ..... | 94 | 0 | .06 | .09 | .6 | n.a. | n.a. | 0 |
| corn: | | | | | | | | |
| 2-oz. piece......... | 118 | n.a. | .16 | .19 | 1.16 | .05 | n.a. | 0 |

[1] *Prepared without added ingredients.*
[2] *With added ascorbic acid or sodium ascorbate; vitamin C value for product without additives would be negligible.*

| | Vitamin A | Vitamin C | Thiamin | Riboflavin | Niacin | B6 | Folacin | B12 |
|---|---|---|---|---|---|---|---|---|
| | (IU) | (Mg) | (Mg) | (Mg) | (Mg) | (Mg) | (Mcg) | (Mcg) |
| toaster type, 1.2-oz. piece . . . . . . . . . . | 32 | 0 | .10 | .12 | .76 | n.a. | n.a. | 0 |
| toaster type, toasted, 1.1-oz. piece . . . . . | 29 | 0 | .08 | .11 | .69 | n.a. | n.a. | 0 |
| English: | | | | | | | | |
| plain, 2-oz. piece . . . . | n.a. | n.a. | .25 | .16 | 2.21 | .03 | n.a. | 0 |
| plain, toasted, 1.8-oz. piece . . . . . . . . . . | n.a. | n.a. | .2 | .14 | 1.98 | .02 | n.a. | 0 |
| mixed grain, 2.3-oz. piece . . . . . . . . . . | n.a. | 0 | .28 | .21 | 2.37 | n.a. | n.a. | 0 |
| mixed grain, toasted, 2.2-oz. piece . . . . . | n.a. | 0 | .23 | .19 | 2.14 | n.a. | n.a. | 0 |
| raisin-cinnamon, 2-oz. piece. . . . . . . | n.a. | n.a. | .22 | .17 | 2.03 | n.a. | n.a. | 0 |
| raisin-cinnamon, toasted, 1.8-oz. piece . . . . . . . . . . | n.a. | n.a. | .17 | .15 | 1.81 | n.a. | n.a. | 0 |
| wheat, 2-oz. piece . . . | n.a. | n.a. | .25 | .17 | 1.91 | n.a. | n.a. | 0 |
| wheat, toasted, 1.8-oz. piece . . . . . | n.a. | n.a. | .20 | .15 | 1.71 | n.a. | n.a. | 0 |
| whole wheat, 2.3-oz. piece . . . . . . . . . . | 0 | 0 | .2 | .09 | 2.25 | .11 | n.a. | 0 |
| whole wheat, toasted, 2.2-oz. piece . . . . . | 0 | 0 | .16 | .08 | 2.04 | .10 | n.a. | 0 |
| (Roman Meal Original), 1 piece. . . | 0 | 0 | .28 | .20 | 2.91 | n.a. | n.a. | n.a. |
| oat bran, 2-oz. piece . . . . | n.a. | n.a. | .15 | .05 | .24 | n.a. | 10.0 | 0 |
| wheat bran, toaster type w/raisins, 1.3-oz. piece | 64 | 0 | .09 | .11 | .87 | n.a. | n.a. | 0 |
| wheat bran, toaster type w/raisins, toasted, 1.2-oz. piece . . . . . . . . | 58 | 0 | .07 | .10 | .79 | n.a. | n.a. | 0 |
| **Muffin mix[1]:** | | | | | | | | |
| blueberry, 1.6-oz. piece | 50 | tr. | .10 | .17 | 1.10 | n.a. | n.a. | 0 |

---

[1] *Prepared according to package directions, with eggs and water.*

| | Vitamin A | Vitamin C | Thiamin | Riboflavin | Niacin | B6 | Folacin | B12 |
|---|---|---|---|---|---|---|---|---|
| | (IU) | (Mg) | (Mg) | (Mg) | (Mg) | (Mg) | (Mcg) | (Mcg) |
| **Muffin mix,** *continued* | | | | | | | | |
| bran, 1.6-oz. piece...... | 100 | 0 | .08 | .12 | 1.90 | n.a. | n.a. | 0 |
| corn, 1.6-oz. piece...... | 90 | tr. | .09 | .09 | .80 | n.a. | n.a. | 0 |
| **Mulberry,** fresh: | | | | | | | | |
| untrimmed, 1 lb. ....... | 113 | 165 | .13 | .46 | 2.81 | n.a. | n.a. | 0 |
| trimmed, ½ cup........ | 18 | 26 | .02 | .07 | .43 | n.a. | n.a. | 0 |
| **Mullet,** striped, meat only: | | | | | | | | |
| raw, 1 lb............. | 553 | 5.4 | n.a. | n.a. | n.a. | 1.93 | 38.6 | n.a. |
| baked, broiled, or | | | | | | | | |
| microwaved[1], 4 oz. ... | 160 | 1 | n.a. | n.a. | n.a. | .56 | 11.1 | n.a. |
| **Mung beans,** dried: | | | | | | | | |
| uncooked, 1 lb......... | 516 | 22 | 2.82 | 1.06 | 10.21 | 1.73 | 2834.4 | 0 |
| uncooked, ½ cup....... | 118 | 5 | .65 | .24 | 2.34 | .40 | 649.9 | 0 |
| boiled, ½ cup ......... | 24 | 1 | .17 | .06 | .58 | .07 | 160.3 | 0 |
| **Mung beans, sprouted,** mature seeds: | | | | | | | | |
| raw: | | | | | | | | |
| 1 lb. ............. | 95 | 60 | .38 | .56 | 3.98 | .40 | 275.8 | 0 |
| 12-oz. pkg. ........ | 71 | 45 | .29 | .42 | 2.56 | .30 | 206.7 | 0 |
| ½ cup............ | 11 | 7 | .04 | .06 | .39 | .05 | 31.6 | 0 |
| boiled, drained, ½ cup... | 8 | 7 | .03 | .06 | .51 | n.a. | n.a. | 0 |
| canned, drained, | | | | | | | | |
| ½ cup............. | 14 | <1 | .02 | .04 | .14 | n.a. | 6.0 | 0 |
| **Mungo beans,** dried: | | | | | | | | |
| uncooked, 1 lb......... | 518 | 22 | 1.61 | 1.27 | 8.17 | 1.25 | 2849.3 | 0 |
| uncooked, ½ cup....... | 119 | 5 | .37 | .29 | 1.87 | .29 | 653.3 | 0 |
| boiled, ½ cup ......... | 28 | 1 | .14 | .07 | 1.35 | .05 | 85.0 | 0 |
| **Mushroom:** | | | | | | | | |
| raw: | | | | | | | | |
| untrimmed, 1 lb. ..... | 0 | 15 | .45 | 1.98 | 18.11 | .43 | 92.8 | 0 |
| 1 medium, .7 oz..... | 0 | 1 | .02 | .08 | .74 | .02 | 3.8 | 0 |
| pieces, ½ cup ...... | 0 | 1 | .04 | .16 | 1.44 | .03 | 7.4 | 0 |
| boiled, drained, pieces, | | | | | | | | |
| ½ cup............. | 0 | 3 | .06 | .23 | 3.48 | .07 | 14.2 | 0 |

[1] *Without added ingredients.*

| | Vitamin A | Vitamin C | Thiamin | Riboflavin | Niacin | B6 | Folacin | B12 |
|---|---|---|---|---|---|---|---|---|
| | (IU) | (Mg) | (Mg) | (Mg) | (Mg) | (Mg) | (Mcg) | (Mcg) |
| canned, drained, pieces, ½ cup . . . . . . . . . . . . | 0 | n.a. | n.a. | n.a. | n.a. | n.a. | 9.6 | 0 |
| **Mushroom, enoki,** raw: | | | | | | | | |
| untrimmed, 1 lb . . . . . . . | 28 | 45 | .33 | .40 | 13.89 | .17 | 114.0 | 0 |
| 1 medium, .1 oz . . . . . . . | 0 | <1 | tr. | tr. | .12 | tr. | 1.0 | 0 |
| **Mushroom, shiitake:** | | | | | | | | |
| dried, 4 oz. . . . . . . . . . . | 0 | 4 | .03 | 1.44 | 15.88 | n.a. | n.a. | 0 |
| dried, 1 medium, .1 oz. . . | 0 | tr. | .01 | .05 | .51 | n.a. | n.a. | 0 |
| cooked, pieces, 1 cup . . . | 0 | tr. | .03 | .12 | 1.08 | n.a. | n.a. | 0 |
| **Mushroom gravy:** | | | | | | | | |
| canned, ¼ cup . . . . . . . . | 0 | 0 | .02 | .04 | .40 | .01 | n.a. | 0 |
| mix, vegetarian (*Loma Linda Gravy Quik*), 1 tbsp., .2 oz. . . . . . . . | 0 | 0 | tr. | .01 | 0 | .01 | n.a. | 0 |
| **Mustard,** prepared, yellow, 1 tsp . . . . . . . . | 0 | tr. | tr. | .01 | tr. | 0 | n.a. | 0 |
| **Mustard greens:** | | | | | | | | |
| fresh: | | | | | | | | |
| raw, untrimmed, 1 lb. . . . . . . . . . . | 22,355 | 295 | .34 | .46 | 3.37 | n.a. | n.a. | 0 |
| raw, trimmed, chopped, ½ cup . . | 1484 | 20 | .02 | .03 | .22 | n.a. | n.a. | 0 |
| boiled, drained, chopped, ½ cup . . | 2122 | 18 | .03 | .04 | .30 | n.a. | n.a. | 0 |
| frozen: | | | | | | | | |
| 10-oz. pkg. . . . . . . . . | 14,639 | 72 | .14 | .17 | .89 | .37 | n.a. | 0 |
| boiled, drained, ⅓ of 10-oz. pkg. . . . . . . | 3158 | 10 | .03 | .04 | .18 | .08 | n.a. | 0 |
| boiled, drained, chopped, ½ cup . . | 3352 | 10 | .03 | .04 | .19 | .08 | n.a. | 0 |
| **Mustard seeds,** yellow, 1 tsp. . . . . . . . . . . . . | 2 | n.a. | .02 | .01 | .26 | n.a. | n.a. | 0 |

# N

| | Vitamin A | Vitamin C | Thiamin | Riboflavin | Niacin | B6 | Folacin | B12 |
|---|---|---|---|---|---|---|---|---|
| | (IU) | (Mg) | (Mg) | (Mg) | (Mg) | (Mg) | (Mcg) | (Mcg) |
| **Natto:** | | | | | | | | |
| 1 lb. . . . . . . . . . . . . . . . | 0 | 59 | .73 | .86 | 0 | n.a. | n.a. | 0 |
| ½ cup . . . . . . . . . . . . . | 0 | 11 | .14 | .17 | 0 | n.a. | n.a. | 0 |
| **Navy beans,** dried: | | | | | | | | |
| uncooked, 1 lb. . . . . . . . . | 20 | 14 | 2.93 | 1.05 | 9.36 | 1.98 | 1677.0 | 0 |
| uncooked, ½ cup. . . . . . . | 5 | 3 | .67 | .24 | 2.15 | .45 | 384.5 | 0 |
| boiled, ½ cup . . . . . . . . . | 2 | 1 | .18 | .06 | .48 | .15 | 127.3 | 0 |
| canned, w/liquid, 8 oz. . . . | 3 | 2 | .32 | .12 | 1.10 | .23 | 141.4 | 0 |
| canned, w/liquid, | | | | | | | | |
| ½ cup . . . . . . . . . . . . . | 2 | 1 | .19 | .07 | .64 | .13 | 81.7 | 0 |
| **Nectarine:** | | | | | | | | |
| untrimmed, 1 lb. . . . . . . . | 3040 | 22 | .07 | .17 | 4.09 | .10 | 15.4 | 0 |
| 1 medium, 2½" diam., | | | | | | | | |
| 5.3 oz. . . . . . . . . . . . | 1001 | 7 | .02 | .06 | 1.35 | .03 | 5.1 | 0 |
| pitted, sliced, ½ cup . . . . | 508 | 4 | .01 | .03 | .68 | .02 | 2.6 | 0 |
| **New England brand** | | | | | | | | |
| **sausage**[1], pork and | | | | | | | | |
| beef, 1 oz. . . . . . . . . . . | n.a. | 6 | .18 | .07 | .99 | .10 | 2.0 | .38 |
| **New Zealand spinach:** | | | | | | | | |
| raw, untrimmed, 1 lb. . . . | 14,370 | 98 | .13 | .43 | 1.63 | n.a. | n.a. | 0 |
| raw, trimmed, chopped, | | | | | | | | |
| ½ cup . . . . . . . . . . . . . | 1232 | 8 | .01 | .04 | .14 | n.a. | n.a. | 0 |
| boiled, drained, chopped, | | | | | | | | |
| ½ cup . . . . . . . . . . . . . | 3260 | 14 | .03 | .10 | .35 | n.a. | n.a. | 0 |
| **Noodle,** egg, enriched, dry: | | | | | | | | |
| uncooked, plain, 2 oz. . . . | 35 | 0 | .61 | .27 | 4.58 | .07 | 17.0 | .23 |
| uncooked, spinach, | | | | | | | | |
| 2 oz. . . . . . . . . . . . . . | 180 | 0 | .62 | .27 | 3.75 | .24 | 50.0 | .23 |
| cooked, plain, 1 cup . . . . | 32 | 0 | .30 | .13 | 2.38 | .06 | 11.0 | .14 |
| cooked, spinach, 1 cup | 165 | 0 | .39 | .20 | 2.36 | .18 | 34.0 | .22 |

---

[1] With added ascorbic acid or sodium ascorbate; vitamin C value for product without additives would be negligible.

| | Vitamin A | Vitamin C | Thiamin | Riboflavin | Niacin | B6 | Folacin | B12 |
|---|---|---|---|---|---|---|---|---|
| | (IU) | (Mg) | (Mg) | (Mg) | (Mg) | (Mg) | (Mcg) | (Mcg) |

**Noodle, Chinese,** dehydrated:

| | | | | | | | | |
|---|---|---|---|---|---|---|---|---|
| chow mein, 1 cup . . . . . . | 38 | 0 | .26 | .19 | 2.68 | .05 | 10.0 | 0 |
| long rice or cellophane, uncooked, 2 oz. . . . . . . | 0 | 0 | .09 | 0 | .10 | n.a. | n.a. | 0 |
| long rice, mung bean, uncooked, ½ cup. . . . . | 0 | 0 | .11 | 0 | .14 | n.a. | n.a. | 0 |
| **Noodle, Japanese,** dry: | | | | | | | | |
| soba, uncooked, 2 oz. . . . | n.a. | 0 | .27 | .07 | 1.83 | .14 | 34.0 | 0 |
| soba, cooked, 1 cup, approx. 4 oz. . . . . . . . . | n.a. | 0 | .11 | .03 | .58 | .05 | 8.0 | 0 |
| somen, uncooked, 2 oz. . . . . . . . . . . . . | n.a. | 0 | .06 | .02 | .50 | .03 | 8.0 | 0 |
| somen, cooked, 1 cup . . . | n.a. | 0 | .03 | .06 | .17 | .02 | 3.0 | 0 |
| **Nopal:** | | | | | | | | |
| raw, untrimmed, 1 lb. . . . | 1806 | 58 | .05 | .18 | 2.28 | .32 | 13.0 | 0 |
| raw, trimmed, sliced, ½ cup. . . . . . . . . . . . | 178 | 6 | .01 | .02 | .23 | .03 | 1.0 | 0 |
| boiled, drained, 1 cup . . . | 685 | 8 | .02 | .06 | .44 | .10 | 4.0 | 0 |
| **Nut topping,** in syrup, 2 tbsp. . . . . . . . . . . | n.a. | n.a. | .07 | .05 | n.a. | n.a. | n.a. | 0 |
| **Nutmeg,** ground, 1 tsp. | 2 | n.a. | .01 | <.01 | .03 | n.a. | n.a. | 0 |
| **Nuts,** see specific listings | | | | | | | | |
| **Nuts, mixed:** | | | | | | | | |
| w/peanuts[1]: | | | | | | | | |
| dry-roasted, 1 oz. . . . | 4 | <1 | .06 | .06 | 1.34 | .08 | 14.3 | 0 |
| dry-roasted, 1 cup . . . | 21 | 1 | .27 | .27 | 6.44 | .41 | 69.0 | 0 |
| oil-roasted, 1 oz. . . . . | 6 | <1 | .14 | .06 | 1.44 | .07 | 23.6 | 0 |
| oil-roasted, 1 cup. . . . | 28 | 1 | .71 | .32 | 7.19 | .34 | 117.9 | 0 |
| w/out peanuts[2], oil-roasted, 1 oz. . . . . . . . | 6 | <1 | .14 | .14 | .56 | .05 | 16.0 | 0 |
| w/out peanuts[2], oil-roasted, 1 cup . . . . . . . | 29 | 1 | .73 | .70 | 2.83 | .26 | 81.2 | 0 |

[1] *Mixture of cashews, peanuts, Brazil nuts, filberts, almonds, and pecans.*
[2] *Mixture of cashews, almonds, Brazil nuts, pecans, and filberts.*

# O

| | Vitamin A | Vitamin C | Thiamin | Riboflavin | Niacin | B6 | Folacin | B12 |
|---|---|---|---|---|---|---|---|---|
| | (IU) | (Mg) | (Mg) | (Mg) | (Mg) | (Mg) | (Mcg) | (Mcg) |
| **Oat** (see also "Cereal"): | | | | | | | | |
| whole grain, 1 cup . . . . . | n.a. | 0 | 1.19 | .22 | 1.50 | .19 | 87.0 | 0 |
| rolled or oatmeal: | | | | | | | | |
|    uncooked, 1 oz. . . . . . | 29 | 0 | .21 | .04 | .22 | .03 | 9.1 | 0 |
|    uncooked, 1 cup . . . . | 82 | 0 | .59 | .11 | .63 | .10 | 26.0 | 0 |
|    cooked, 1 cup . . . . . . | 38 | 0 | .26 | .05 | .30 | .05 | 9.0 | 0 |
| **Oat bran** (see also "Cereal, ready-to-eat"): | | | | | | | | |
| uncooked, 1 oz. . . . . . . . | n.a. | 0 | .33 | .06 | .26 | .05 | 14.7 | 0 |
| uncooked, ½ cup. . . . . . | 0 | 0 | .55 | .10 | .44 | .08 | 24.0 | 0 |
| cooked, 1 cup . . . . . . . . | n.a. | 0 | .35 | .07 | .32 | .06 | 14.0 | 0 |
| **Ocean perch,** Atlantic, meat only: | | | | | | | | |
| raw, 1 lb. . . . . . . . . . . . . | 181 | (0) | n.a. | .50 | 9.07 | n.a. | n.a. | 4.54 |
| baked, broiled, or | | | | | | | | |
|   microwaved[1], 4 oz. . . . | 52 | (0) | n.a. | .15 | 2.76 | n.a. | n.a. | 1.31 |
| **Oheloberry:** | | | | | | | | |
| 1 lb. . . . . . . . . . . . . . . . | 3765 | 27 | .08 | .16 | 1.23 | n.a. | n.a. | 0 |
| ½ cup . . . . . . . . . . . . . | 581 | 4 | .01 | .03 | .19 | n.a. | n.a. | 0 |
| **Oil,** corn, olive, peanut, safflower, soybean (hydrogenated), soybean-cottonseed blend (hydrogenated), or sunflower, | | | | | | | | |
| 1 tbsp. . . . . . . . . . . . | 0 | 0 | 0 | 0 | 0 | n.a. | n.a. | 0 |
| **Okra:** | | | | | | | | |
| fresh: | | | | | | | | |
|    raw, untrimmed, 1 lb. | 2575 | 82 | .78 | .23 | 3.90 | .84 | 342.4 | 0 |
|    raw, trimmed, sliced, | | | | | | | | |
|      ½ cup . . . . . . . . . | 330 | 11 | .10 | .03 | .50 | .11 | 43.9 | 0 |
|    boiled, drained, | | | | | | | | |
|      sliced, ½ cup. . . . . | 460 | 13 | .11 | .04 | .70 | .15 | 36.5 | 0 |
| frozen: | | | | | | | | |
|    10-oz. pkg. . . . . . . . . | 1314 | 35 | .25 | .30 | 2.01 | .12 | 419.3 | 0 |

[1] Prepared without added ingredients.

| | Vitamin A | Vitamin C | Thiamin | Riboflavin | Niacin | B6 | Folacin | B12 |
|---|---|---|---|---|---|---|---|---|
| | (IU) | (Mg) | (Mg) | (Mg) | (Mg) | (Mg) | (Mcg) | (Mcg) |
| boiled, drained, ⅓ of 10-oz. pkg. . . . . . . | 437 | 10 | .08 | .10 | .67 | .04 | 123.8 | 0 |
| frozen, boiled, drained, sliced, ½ cup. . . . . . . | 473 | 11 | .09 | .11 | .72 | .04 | 134.0 | 0 |
| **Olive,** ripe, pitted, canned: | | | | | | | | |
| Mission and Manzanilla: | | | | | | | | |
| all sizes, 1 oz. . . . . . | 114 | <1 | tr. | (0) | .01 | tr. | 0 | 0 |
| 10 small, 1.1 oz. . . . . | 129 | <1 | tr. | (0) | .01 | tr. | 0 | 0 |
| 10 large, 1.6 oz. . . . . | 177 | <1 | tr. | (0) | .02 | tr. | 0 | 0 |
| Sevillano and Ascolano: | | | | | | | | |
| all sizes, 1 oz. . . . . . . | 98 | <1 | (0) | (0) | <.01 | <.01 | 0 | 0 |
| 10 jumbo, 2.9 oz. . . . | 287 | 1 | (0) | (0) | .02 | .01 | 0 | 0 |
| 10 supercolossal, 5.4 oz. . . . . . . . . . | 526 | 2 | (0) | (0) | .03 | .02 | 0 | 0 |
| **Olive loaf**[1], pork, 1-oz. slice . . . . . . . . . . | n.a. | 2 | .08 | .07 | .52 | .07 | n.a. | .36 |
| **Onion,** mature: | | | | | | | | |
| fresh: | | | | | | | | |
| raw, untrimmed, 1 lb. | 0 | 26 | .17 | .08 | .60 | .47 | 76.0 | 0 |
| raw, trimmed, chopped, ½ cup . . | 0 | 5 | .03 | .02 | .12 | .09 | 15.0 | 0 |
| boiled, drained, chopped, ½ cup . . | 0 | 6 | .05 | .02 | .17 | .14 | 16.0 | 0 |
| frozen: | | | | | | | | |
| whole, 10-oz. pkg. . . . | 74 | 23 | .07 | .07 | .50 | .26 | 60.1 | 0 |
| chopped, 10-oz. pkg. | 99 | 10 | .09 | .08 | .43 | .21 | 49.2 | 0 |
| boiled, drained, chopped, ½ cup . . | 36 | 3 | .02 | .03 | .15 | .07 | 14.1 | 0 |
| **Onion, green** (scallion), w/top[2], raw: | | | | | | | | |
| untrimmed, 1 lb. . . . . . . . | 1677 | 82 | .24 | .35 | 2.29 | n.a. | 279.0 | 0 |
| chopped, ½ cup . . . . . . . | 193 | 9 | .03 | .04 | .26 | n.a. | 32.0 | 0 |

[1] *With added ascorbic acid or sodium ascorbate; vitamin C value for product without additives would be negligible.*
[2] *Vitamin A value varies depending on proportion of bulb and top (leaves).*

| | Vitamin A | Vitamin C | Thiamin | Riboflavin | Niacin | B6 | Folacin | B12 |
|---|---|---|---|---|---|---|---|---|
| | (IU) | (Mg) | (Mg) | (Mg) | (Mg) | (Mg) | (Mcg) | (Mcg) |
| **Onion, green,** *continued* | | | | | | | | |
| chopped, 1 tbsp........ | 23 | 1 | <.01 | .01 | <.01 | n.a. | 4.0 | 0 |
| **Onion flakes,** dehydrated, | | | | | | | | |
| 1 tbsp. ............ | 0 | 4 | .03 | .01 | .05 | .08 | 8.3 | 0 |
| **Onion gravy mix** (*Loma* | | | | | | | | |
| *Linda Gravy Quik*), | | | | | | | | |
| 1 tbsp., .2 oz. ....... | 0 | 0 | .03 | .02 | 0 | .02 | n.a. | 0 |
| **Onion powder,** 1 tsp. .... | tr. | <1 | .01 | <.01 | .01 | n.a. | n.a. | 0 |
| **Onion rings**[1], frozen: | | | | | | | | |
| 9-oz. pkg. ........... | 449 | 12 | .23 | .20 | 1.77 | n.a. | n.a. | 0 |
| oven heated, 2 rings, | | | | | | | | |
| .75 oz.............. | 45 | <1 | .06 | .03 | .72 | .02 | 2.6 | 0 |
| **Orange,** fresh: | | | | | | | | |
| all varieties: | | | | | | | | |
| untrimmed, 1 lb. ..... | 679 | 176 | .29 | .13 | .93 | .20 | 100.3 | 0 |
| 1 medium, 2⅝" | | | | | | | | |
| diam., 6.3 oz. ..... | 269 | 70 | .11 | .05 | .37 | .08 | 39.7 | 0 |
| sections, w/out | | | | | | | | |
| membrane, ½ cup | 369 | 96 | .16 | .07 | .51 | .11 | 54.5 | 0 |
| California navel: | | | | | | | | |
| untrimmed, 1 lb. ..... | 565 | 177 | .27 | .12 | .89 | .21 | 104.0 | 0 |
| 1 medium, 2⅞" | | | | | | | | |
| diam., 7.3 oz. ..... | 256 | 80 | .12 | .06 | .41 | .10 | 47.2 | 0 |
| sections, w/out | | | | | | | | |
| membrane, ½ cup | 151 | 47 | .07 | .03 | .24 | .06 | 27.8 | 0 |
| California Valencia: | | | | | | | | |
| untrimmed, 1 lb. ..... | 782 | 165 | .30 | .14 | .93 | .21 | 131.3 | 0 |
| 1 medium, 2⅝" | | | | | | | | |
| diam., 5.7 oz. ..... | 278 | 59 | .11 | .05 | .33 | .08 | 46.7 | 0 |
| sections, w/out | | | | | | | | |
| membrane, ½ cup | 207 | 44 | .08 | .04 | .25 | .06 | 34.8 | 0 |
| Florida: | | | | | | | | |
| untrimmed, 1 lb. ..... | 671 | 151 | .34 | .13 | 1.34 | .17 | 58.1 | 0 |

---

[1] *Breaded and par-fried in vegetable oil.*

| | Vitamin A | Vitamin C | Thiamin | Riboflavin | Niacin | B6 | Folacin | B12 |
|---|---|---|---|---|---|---|---|---|
| | (IU) | (Mg) | (Mg) | (Mg) | (Mg) | (Mg) | (Mcg) | (Mcg) |
| 1 medium, 2¹¹⁄₁₆" diam., 7.2 oz. .... | 302 | 68 | .15 | .06 | .60 | .08 | 26.1 | 0 |
| sections, w/out membrane, ½ cup | 185 | 42 | .09 | .04 | .37 | .05 | 16.0 | 0 |
| **Orange, canned,** see "Tangerine" | | | | | | | | |
| **Orange drink¹,** canned, 8 fl. oz. . . . . . . . . . . . | 45 | 85 | .01 | .01 | .08 | .02 | n.a. | 0 |
| **Orange extract** (*Virginia Dare*), 1 tsp. . . . . . . . . | 0 | 0 | 0 | 0 | 0 | 0 | 0 | 0 |
| **Orange flavor drink¹,** breakfast: | | | | | | | | |
| frozen, w/orange pulp, diluted, 1 fl. oz. . . . . . . | 0 | 22 | .04 | .01 | 0 | 0 | n.a. | 0 |
| frozen, w/orange juice and pulp, diluted, 1 fl. oz. . . . | 2 | 17 | .03 | .33 | .08 | .02 | 10.1 | 0 |
| mix, 3 rounded tsp. . . . . . | 0 | 22 | .04 | .01 | 0 | 0 | n.a. | 0 |
| **Orange juice:** | | | | | | | | |
| fresh, juice from 1 average fruit . . . . . . . | 172 | 43 | .08 | .03 | .34 | .03 | n.a. | 0 |
| fresh, 6 fl oz . . . . . . . . . | 372 | 93 | .17 | .06 | .74 | .07 | n.a. | 0 |
| canned, 6 fl. oz. . . . . . . . | 330 | 64 | .11 | .05 | .59 | .16 | n.a. | 0 |
| chilled, 6 fl. oz. . . . . . . . | 144 | 61 | .21 | .04 | .52 | .10 | 33.6 | 0 |
| frozen, diluted, 6 fl. oz. . . . | 144 | 73 | .15 | .04 | .38 | .08 | 81.6 | 0 |
| **Orange peel,** fresh, 1 tsp. . . . | 8 | 3 | <.01 | <.01 | .02 | <.01 | n.a. | 0 |
| **Orange-apricot juice drink,** canned, 8 fl. oz. | 1450 | 50 | .05 | .03 | .50 | n.a. | n.a. | 0 |
| **Orange-grapefruit juice,** canned, 6 fl. oz. . . . . . . | 222 | 54 | .10 | .05 | .62 | .04 | n.a. | 0 |
| **Oregano,** ground, 1 tsp. | 104 | n.a. | .01 | n.a. | .09 | n.a. | n.a. | 0 |
| **Oriental seasoning** (*Tone's Perc*), ¼ tsp. | 38 | 6 | tr. | tr. | .02 | .03 | .3 | 0 |
| **Oyster, Eastern,** meat only: | | | | | | | | |
| wild: raw, 1 lb. . . . . . . . . | 454 | 17 | .45 | .43 | 6.26 | .28 | 43.0 | 88.26 |

¹ *With added nutrients.*

| | Vitamin A | Vitamin C | Thiamin | Riboflavin | Niacin | B6 | Folacin | B12 |
|---|---|---|---|---|---|---|---|---|
| | (IU) | (Mg) | (Mg) | (Mg) | (Mg) | (Mg) | (Mcg) | (Mcg) |
| **Oyster, Eastern, wild**, *continued* | | | | | | | | |
| raw, 6 medium, approx. 3 oz...... | 84 | 3 | .08 | .08 | 1.16 | .05 | 8.0 | 16.34 |
| raw, 1 cup......... | 248 | 9 | .25 | .24 | 3.42 | .46 | 24.0 | 48.25 |
| baked, broiled, or microwaved[1], 4 oz. | n.a. | 5 | .10 | .09 | 1.90 | .11 | 20.4 | 31.53 |
| baked, broiled, or microwaved[1], 6 medium ....... | n.a. | 2 | .05 | .05 | .99 | .06 | 11.0 | 16.40 |
| boiled or steamed[1], 4 oz............ | 204 | 7 | .21 | .21 | 2.82 | .14 | 15.8 | 39.71 |
| boiled or steamed[1], 6 medium ....... | 76 | 3 | .08 | .08 | 1.04 | .05 | 6.0 | 14.71 |
| farmed: | | | | | | | | |
| raw, 1 lb........... | 113 | 21.5 | .48 | .30 | 5.75 | .27 | 84.0 | 73.48 |
| raw, 6 medium, approx. 3 oz...... | 21 | 4 | .09 | .06 | 1.07 | .05 | 16.0 | 13.61 |
| baked, broiled, or microwaved[1], 4 oz. | 71 | 7 | .15 | .06 | 2.03 | .09 | 27.2 | 27.56 |
| baked, broiled, or microwaved[1], 6 medium | 37 | 4 | .08 | .32 | 1.06 | .05 | 14.0 | 14.34 |
| **Oyster, Eastern, canned:** | | | | | | | | |
| w/liquid, 4 oz.......... | n.a. | n.a. | n.a. | .19 | 1.41 | .11 | 10.1 | 21.70 |
| w/liquid, 1 cup......... | n.a. | n.a. | n.a. | .41 | 3.09 | .24 | 22.1 | 47.45 |
| **Oyster, Pacific**, meat only: | | | | | | | | |
| raw, 1 lb.............. | n.a. | n.a. | .30 | 1.06 | 9.12 | n.a. | n.a. | n.a. |
| raw, 1 medium, approx. 1.75 oz............ | n.a. | n.a. | .03 | .12 | 1.01 | n.a. | n.a. | n.a. |
| boiled or steamed[1], 4 oz... | n.a. | n.a. | .14 | .50 | 4.10 | n.a. | n.a. | n.a. |

**Oyster plant,** see "Salsify"
**Oyster stew,** see "Soup, canned, condensed"

---

[1] *Prepared without added ingredients.*

# P

| | Vitamin A | Vitamin C | Thiamin | Riboflavin | Niacin | B6 | Folacin | B12 |
|---|---|---|---|---|---|---|---|---|
| | (IU) | (Mg) | (Mg) | (Mg) | (Mg) | (Mg) | (Mcg) | (Mcg) |
| **Palm, hearts of,** canned: | | | | | | | | |
| 1 cup . . . . . . . . . . . . . . . | 0 | 12 | .02 | .08 | .64 | .03 | 57.0 | 0 |
| 1 heart, 1.1 oz. . . . . . . . . | 0 | 3 | tr. | .02 | .14 | .01 | 13.0 | 0 |
| **Pancake,** frozen, microwaved, 4" cake, 1.3 oz. . . . . . . . . . . . . | 36 | n.a. | .14 | .17 | 1.44 | n.a. | n.a. | n.a. |
| **Pancake mix,** prepared, 4"-diam. cake, 1.3 oz. | 12 | 0 | .08 | .08 | .65 | .04 | n.a. | .07 |
| **Pancake syrup,** see "Syrup, table blends" | | | | | | | | |
| **Pancreas,** braised[1]: | | | | | | | | |
| beef, 4 oz. . . . . . . . . . . . | 0 | 23 | .20 | .55 | 4.50 | j.20 | n.a. | 18.82 |
| lamb, 4 oz. . . . . . . . . . . | 0 | 23 | .02 | .24 | 2.90 | .06 | 14.7 | 6.28 |
| pork, 4 oz.. . . . . . . . . . . | 0 | 6 | .10 | .75 | 3.64 | n.a. | n.a. | 19.36 |
| **Papaya:** | | | | | | | | |
| untrimmed, 1-lb. fruit, 3½" × 5⅛" . . . . . . . . . | 6122 | 188 | .08 | .10 | 1.03 | .06 | n.a. | 0 |
| peeled and seeded, cubed, ½ cup . . . . . . . | 1410 | 43 | .02 | .02 | .24 | .01 | n.a. | 0 |
| **Papaya nectar,** canned, 6 fl. oz.. . . . . . . . . . . . | 210 | 5 | .01 | .01 | .28 | .02 | 3.6 | 0 |
| **Paprika,** 1 tsp. . . . . . . . . | 1273 | 1 | .01 | .04 | .32 | n.a. | n.a. | 0 |
| **Parsley,** fresh, raw: | | | | | | | | |
| untrimmed, 1 lb. . . . . . . | 22,407 | 573 | .37 | .42 | 5.66 | .39 | 656.0 | 0 |
| trimmed, chopped, 10 sprigs. . . . . . . . . . | 520 | 13 | .01 | .01 | .13 | .01 | 15.0 | 0 |
| trimmed, chopped, ½ cup. . . . . . . . . . . . | 1560 | 40 | .03 | .03 | .39 | .03 | 46.0 | 0 |
| **Parsley, Chinese,** see "Coriander" | | | | | | | | |
| **Parsley, dried:** | | | | | | | | |
| dried, 1 tsp. . . . . . . . . . . | 70 | <1 | .01 | .01 | .02 | <.01 | n.a. | 0 |
| freeze-dried, ¼ cup . . . . . | 885 | 2 | .02 | .03 | .15 | .02 | 21.5 | 0 |
| freeze-dried, 1 tbsp. . . . . . | 253 | 1 | tr. | .01 | .04 | .01 | 6.1 | 0 |

[1] *Prepared without added ingredients.*

| | Vitamin A | Vitamin C | Thiamin | Riboflavin | Niacin | B6 | Folacin | B12 |
|---|---|---|---|---|---|---|---|---|
| | (IU) | (Mg) | (Mg) | (Mg) | (Mg) | (Mg) | (Mcg) | (Mcg) |
| **Parsnip:** | | | | | | | | |
| raw, untrimmed, 1 lb. .... | 0 | 66 | .35 | .19 | 2.70 | .35 | 257.6 | 0 |
| raw, trimmed, sliced, | | | | | | | | |
| ½ cup.............. | 0 | 11 | .06 | .03 | .47 | .06 | 44.8 | 0 |
| boiled, drained, sliced, | | | | | | | | |
| ½ cup.............. | 0 | 10 | .07 | .04 | .57 | .07 | 45.4 | 0 |
| **Passion fruit,** purple: | | | | | | | | |
| untrimmed, 1 lb. ....... | 1651 | 71 | n.a. | .31 | 3.54 | n.a. | n.a. | 0 |
| trimmed, 1 oz.......... | 198 | 9 | n.a. | .04 | .43 | n.a. | n.a. | 0 |
| **Passion fruit juice,** fresh: | | | | | | | | |
| purple, 6 fl. oz. ........ | 1332 | 55 | n.a. | .24 | 2.71 | n.a. | n.a. | 0 |
| yellow, 6 fl. oz. ........ | 4470 | 34 | n.a. | .19 | 4.15 | n.a. | n.a. | 0 |
| **Pasta** (see also "Macaroni"), dry: | | | | | | | | |
| uncooked: | | | | | | | | |
| plain, spaghetti, 2 oz. | 0 | 0 | .59 | .25 | 4.28 | .06 | 10.0 | 0 |
| plain, spaghetti, pro- | | | | | | | | |
| tein fortified, 2 oz. | n.a. | 0 | .68 | .27 | 4.36 | .10 | 11.0 | 0 |
| corn, 2 oz.......... | 97 | 0 | .13 | .05 | 1.39 | .12 | 14.0 | 0 |
| spinach, 2 oz. ...... | n.a. | 0 | .21 | .11 | 2.59 | .18 | 27.0 | 0 |
| whole wheat, 2 oz. | n.a. | 0 | .28 | .08 | 2.92 | .13 | 32.0 | 0 |
| cooked: | | | | | | | | |
| plain, spaghetti, | | | | | | | | |
| 1 cup ........... | 0 | 0 | .29 | .14 | 2.34 | .05 | 10.0 | 0 |
| plain, spaghetti, pro- | | | | | | | | |
| tein fortified, 1 cup | n.a. | 0 | .42 | .23 | 2.57 | .09 | 15.0 | 0 |
| corn, 1 cup ........ | 80 | 0 | .07 | .03 | .78 | .08 | 9.0 | 0 |
| spinach, 1 cup...... | n.a. | 0 | .14 | .14 | 2.14 | .13 | 16.0 | 0 |
| whole wheat, 1 cup | n.a. | 0 | .15 | .06 | .99 | .11 | 7.0 | 0 |
| **Pasta, refrigerated, fresh,** w/egg: | | | | | | | | |
| uncooked, 4.5 oz. ...... | n.a. | 0 | .90 | .56 | 4.29 | .12 | n.a. | .40 |
| uncooked, spinach, | | | | | | | | |
| 4.5 oz............... | n.a. | 0 | .78 | .51 | 4.43 | .40 | n.a. | .40 |
| cooked, 4 oz.......... | n.a. | 0 | .24 | .17 | 1.12 | .04 | n.a. | .16 |
| cooked, spinach, 4 oz. | n.a. | 0 | .20 | .15 | 1.15 | .13 | n.a. | .16 |

| | Vitamin A | Vitamin C | Thiamin | Riboflavin | Niacin | B6 | Folacin | B12 |
|---|---|---|---|---|---|---|---|---|
| | (IU) | (Mg) | (Mg) | (Mg) | (Mg) | (Mg) | (Mcg) | (Mcg) |

**Pasta sauce,** see "Tomato sauce"
**Pâté,** canned:

| | | | | | | | | |
|---|---|---|---|---|---|---|---|---|
| chicken liver, 1 tbsp. | 94 | 1 | .01 | .18 | .98 | n.a. | n.a. | n.a. |
| liver, 1 tbsp. . . . . . . . . . | 429 | 0 | <.01 | .08 | .43 | .01 | 8.0 | .42 |

**Peach:**
fresh:

| | | | | | | | | |
|---|---|---|---|---|---|---|---|---|
| untrimmed, 1 lb. . . . . | 1844 | 23 | .06 | .14 | 3.41 | .06 | 11.7 | 0 |
| 1 medium, 2½" diam., approx. 4 per lb. . . . | 465 | 6 | .02 | .04 | .86 | .02 | 3.0 | 0 |
| pulp, sliced, ½ cup | 455 | 6 | .01 | .04 | .84 | .02 | 2.9 | 0 |
| canned, halves or slices: | | | | | | | | |
| in water, clingstone, ½ cup . . . . . . . . . | 649 | 4 | .01 | .02 | .64 | .02 | 4.1 | 0 |
| in juice, clingstone or freestone, ½ cup | 473 | 4 | .01 | .02 | .72 | n.a. | n.a. | 0 |
| in light syrup, clingstone, ½ cup . . . . . | 444 | 3 | .01 | .03 | .74 | .02 | 4.1 | 0 |
| in heavy syrup, clingstone or freestone, ½ cup . . . . . . . . . | 425 | 4 | .01 | .03 | .79 | .02 | 4.1 | 0 |
| canned, spiced, whole, in heavy syrup, ½ cup | 384 | 6 | .01 | .04 | .65 | n.a. | n.a. | 0 |
| dehydrated, sulfured: | | | | | | | | |
| uncooked, 1 lb. . . . . . | 6428 | 48 | .18 | .50 | 21.89 | .72 | 29.9 | 0 |
| uncooked, ½ cup. . . . | 822 | 6 | .02 | .06 | 2.80 | .09 | 3.8 | 0 |
| cooked, ½ cup . . . . . | 479 | 8 | .01 | .07 | 2.46 | .07 | 3.4 | 0 |
| dried, sulfured, halves: | | | | | | | | |
| uncooked, 1 lb. . . . . . | 9813 | 22 | .01 | .96 | 19.85 | .30 | n.a. | 0 |
| uncooked, 10 halves, 4.5 oz. . . . . . . . | 2812 | 6 | <.01 | .28 | 5.69 | .09 | n.a. | 0 |
| uncooked, ½ cup. . . . | 1731 | 4 | <.01 | .17 | 3.50 | .05 | n.a. | 0 |
| cooked, unsweetened, ½ cup . . . . . . . . . . | 254 | 5 | .01 | .03 | 1.96 | .05 | .1 | 0 |
| cooked, sweetened, ½ cup . . . . . . . . . | 243 | 5 | .01 | .03 | 1.87 | .22 | .1 | 0 |

| | Vitamin A | Vitamin C | Thiamin | Riboflavin | Niacin | B6 | Folacin | B12 |
|---|---|---|---|---|---|---|---|---|
| | (IU) | (Mg) | (Mg) | (Mg) | (Mg) | (Mg) | (Mcg) | (Mcg) |
| **Peach,** *continued* | | | | | | | | |
| frozen[1], sweetened, | | | | | | | | |
| sliced, 10-oz. pkg. . . . . | 806 | 267 | .04 | .10 | 1.86 | .05 | n.a. | 0 |
| frozen[1], sweetened, | | | | | | | | |
| sliced, ½ cup. . . . . . . | 355 | 118 | .02 | .04 | .82 | .02 | n.a. | 0 |
| **Peach nectar,** canned[2], | | | | | | | | |
| 6 fl. oz. . . . . . . . . . . . | 480 | 10 | .01 | .02 | .54 | n.a. | n.a. | 0 |
| **Peanut,** shelled, except as noted: | | | | | | | | |
| all types: | | | | | | | | |
| raw, in shell, 1 lb. . . . | 0 | 0 | 2.12 | .44 | 39.95 | 1.15 | 793.88 | 0 |
| raw, 1 oz. . . . . . . . . | 0 | 0 | .18 | .04 | 3.38 | .10 | 67.1 | 0 |
| raw, 1 cup. . . . . . . . | 0 | 0 | .93 | .20 | 17.62 | .51 | 350.0 | 0 |
| boiled, 1 oz. . . . . . . . | 0 | 0 | .08 | .02 | 1.68 | .05 | 23.9 | 0 |
| dry-roasted, 1 oz. . . . | 0 | 0 | .12 | .03 | 3.79 | .07 | 40.7 | 0 |
| dry-roasted, 1 cup . . . | 0 | 0 | .64 | .14 | 19.75 | .37 | 212.2 | 0 |
| oil-roasted, 1 oz. . . . . | 0 | 0 | .07 | .03 | 4.00 | .07 | 35.2 | 0 |
| oil-roasted, 1 cup. . . . | 0 | 0 | .36 | .16 | 20.56 | .37 | 181.0 | 0 |
| Spanish: | | | | | | | | |
| raw, 1 oz. . . . . . . . . | 0 | 0 | .19 | .04 | 4.46 | .10 | 67.2 | 0 |
| raw, 1 cup. . . . . . . . | 0 | 0 | .99 | .20 | 23.24 | .51 | 350.4 | 0 |
| oil-roasted, 1 oz. . . . . | 0 | 0 | .09 | .02 | 4.18 | .07 | 35.3 | 0 |
| oil-roasted, 1 cup. . . . | 0 | 0 | .47 | .13 | 21.95 | .38 | 185.1 | 0 |
| Valencia: | | | | | | | | |
| raw, 1 oz. . . . . . . . . | 0 | 0 | .18 | .08 | 3.61 | .10 | 68.7 | 0 |
| raw, 1 cup. . . . . . . . | 0 | 0 | .93 | .44 | 18.80 | .50 | 358.4 | 0 |
| oil-roasted, 1 oz. . . . . | 0 | 0 | .03 | .04 | 4.02 | .07 | 35.1 | 0 |
| oil-roasted, 1 cup. . . . | 0 | 0 | .13 | .22 | 20.65 | .35 | 180.7 | 0 |
| Virginia: | | | | | | | | |
| raw, 1 oz. . . . . . . . . | 0 | 0 | .18 | .04 | 3.47 | .10 | 66.8 | 0 |
| raw, 1 cup. . . . . . . . | 0 | 0 | .95 | .19 | 18.07 | .51 | 348.5 | 0 |
| oil-roasted, 1 oz. . . . . | 0 | 0 | .08 | .03 | 4.12 | .07 | 35.1 | 0 |
| oil-roasted, 1 cup. . . . | 0 | 0 | .40 | .16 | 21.20 | .36 | 179.4 | 0 |

[1] *With added ascorbic acid.*
[2] *Without added ascorbic acid.*

| | Vitamin A | Vitamin C | Thiamin | Riboflavin | Niacin | B6 | Folacin | B12 |
|---|---|---|---|---|---|---|---|---|
| | (IU) | (Mg) | (Mg) | (Mg) | (Mg) | (Mg) | (Mcg) | (Mcg) |
| **Peanut butter:** | | | | | | | | |
| chunk style, 2 tbsp...... | 0 | 0 | .04 | .04 | 4.38 | .14 | 29.4 | 0 |
| smooth style, 2 tbsp..... | 0 | 0 | .03 | .03 | 4.29 | .15 | 24.0 | 0 |
| **Peanut flour,** defatted: | | | | | | | | |
| 1 oz................. | 0 | 0 | .20 | .13 | 7.56 | .14 | 69.5 | 0 |
| 1 cup .............. | 0 | 0 | .42 | .29 | 16.20 | .30 | 148.9 | 0 |
| **Pear:** | | | | | | | | |
| fresh: | | | | | | | | |
| untrimmed, 1 lb..... | 83 | 17 | .08 | .17 | .42 | .08 | 30.4 | 0 |
| Bartlett, 2½" diam. × 3½", approx. 2½ per lb......... | 33 | 7 | .03 | .07 | .17 | .03 | 12.1 | 0 |
| trimmed, w/skin, sliced, ½ cup..... | 17 | 3 | .02 | .03 | .08 | .02 | 6.0 | 0 |
| canned, halves: | | | | | | | | |
| in water, ½ cup..... | 0 | 1 | .01 | .01 | .07 | .02 | 1.5 | 0 |
| in juice, ½ cup ..... | 7 | 2 | .01 | .01 | .25 | n.a. | n.a. | 0 |
| in light syrup, ½ cup.......... | 0 | 1 | .01 | .02 | .19 | .02 | 1.5 | 0 |
| in heavy or extra heavy syrup, ½ cup.......... | 0 | 2 | .01 | .03 | .31 | .02 | 1.5 | 0 |
| dried, sulfured, halves: | | | | | | | | |
| uncooked, 1 lb...... | 15 | 32 | .04 | .66 | 6.22 | n.a. | n.a. | 0 |
| uncooked, 10 halves, 6.2 oz.......... | 6 | 12 | .01 | .25 | 2.4 | n.a. | n.a. | 0 |
| uncooked, ½ cup.... | 3 | 6 | .01 | .13 | 1.24 | n.a. | n.a. | 0 |
| cooked, unsweetened, ½ cup.......... | 54 | 5 | .01 | .03 | .45 | .04 | 0 | 0 |
| cooked, sweetened, ½ cup.......... | 56 | 5 | .01 | .03 | .47 | .05 | 0 | 0 |
| **Pear, Asian,** fresh: | | | | | | | | |
| untrimmed, 1 lb........ | 0 | 5 | .04 | .04 | .91 | .09 | 34.0 | 0 |
| 1 fruit, 2½" diam., 4.3 oz.............. | 0 | 2 | .01 | .01 | .27 | .03 | 10.0 | 0 |

| | Vitamin A | Vitamin C | Thiamin | Riboflavin | Niacin | B6 | Folacin | B12 |
|---|---|---|---|---|---|---|---|---|
| | (IU) | (Mg) | (Mg) | (Mg) | (Mg) | (Mg) | (Mcg) | (Mcg) |
| **Pear nectar,** canned[1], | | | | | | | | |
| 6 fl. oz. . . . . . . . . . . . | 2 | 2 | .01 | .02 | .24 | n.a. | n.a. | 0 |
| **Peas, edible-podded:** | | | | | | | | |
| fresh: | | | | | | | | |
| raw, untrimmed, | | | | | | | | |
| 1 lb. . . . . . . . . . . | 620 | 256 | .64 | .34 | 2.56 | .68 | n.a. | 0 |
| raw, trimmed, | | | | | | | | |
| ½ cup . . . . . . . . . | 105 | 43 | .11 | .06 | .43 | .12 | n.a. | 0 |
| boiled, drained, | | | | | | | | |
| ½ cup . . . . . . . . . | 104 | 38 | .10 | .06 | .43 | .12 | n.a. | 0 |
| frozen: | | | | | | | | |
| 10-oz. pkg. . . . . . . . | 398 | 63 | .17 | .28 | 1.42 | .44 | n.a. | 0 |
| boiled, drained, ⅓ of | | | | | | | | |
| 10-oz. pkg. . . . . . . | 140 | 19 | .05 | .10 | .47 | .15 | n.a. | 0 |
| boiled, drained, | | | | | | | | |
| ½ cup . . . . . . . . . | 133 | 18 | .05 | .10 | .45 | .14 | n.a. | 0 |
| **Peas, green** (sweet): | | | | | | | | |
| fresh: | | | | | | | | |
| raw, in pods, 1 lb. . . . | 1103 | 69 | .46 | .23 | 3.60 | .29 | 112.0 | 0 |
| raw, shelled, ½ cup | 461 | 29 | .19 | .10 | 1.51 | .12 | 47.0 | 0 |
| boiled, drained, | | | | | | | | |
| ½ cup . . . . . . . . . | 478 | 11 | .21 | .12 | 1.62 | .17 | 50.7 | 0 |
| canned: | | | | | | | | |
| w/liquid, ½ cup . . . . . | 470 | 14 | .14 | .09 | 1.04 | .08 | 35.4 | 0 |
| drained, ½ cup . . . . . | 653 | 8 | .10 | .07 | .62 | .05 | 37.7 | 0 |
| seasoned, w/liquid, | | | | | | | | |
| ½ cup . . . . . . . . . | 494 | 13 | .11 | .08 | .79 | n.a. | n.a. | 0 |
| frozen: | | | | | | | | |
| 10-oz. pkg. . . . . . . . | 2064 | 51 | .73 | .28 | 4.85 | .35 | 150.9 | 0 |
| boiled, drained, ⅓ of | | | | | | | | |
| 10-oz. pkg. . . . . . . | 563 | 8 | .24 | .08 | 1.25 | .10 | 49.4 | 0 |
| boiled, drained, | | | | | | | | |
| ½ cup . . . . . . . . . | 534 | 8 | .23 | .08 | 1.18 | .09 | 46.9 | 0 |
| **Peas, pigeon,** see "Pigeon peas" | | | | | | | | |

[1] *Without added ascorbic acid.*

| | Vitamin A | Vitamin C | Thiamin | Riboflavin | Niacin | B6 | Folacin | B12 |
|---|---|---|---|---|---|---|---|---|
| | (IU) | (Mg) | (Mg) | (Mg) | (Mg) | (Mg) | (Mcg) | (Mcg) |

**Peas, snow or Chinese,** see "Peas, edible-podded"

**Peas, split,** dried:

| | | | | | | | | |
|---|---|---|---|---|---|---|---|---|
| uncooked, 1 lb. . . . . . . . | 675 | 8 | 3.29 | .98 | 13.11 | .79 | 1242.0 | 0 |
| uncooked, ½ cup . . . . . . . | 146 | 2 | .71 | .21 | 2.83 | .17 | 268.3 | 0 |
| boiled, ½ cup . . . . . . . . . | 7 | <1 | .19 | .06 | .87 | .05 | 63.6 | 0 |

**Peas, sprouted,** mature seeds:

| | | | | | | | | |
|---|---|---|---|---|---|---|---|---|
| raw, untrimmed, 1 lb. . . . | 753 | 47 | 1.02 | .70 | 14.01 | 1.20 | 653.2 | 0 |
| raw, ½ cup . . . . . . . . . . . | 100 | 6 | .14 | .09 | 1.85 | .16 | 86.4 | 0 |

**Peas, sugar snap,** see "Peas, edible-podded"

**Peas, sweet,** see "Peas, green"

**Peas and carrots:**

canned, w/liquid,

| | | | | | | | | |
|---|---|---|---|---|---|---|---|---|
| ½ cup . . . . . . . . . . . . | 7386 | 8 | .10 | .07 | .74 | .11 | 23.5 | 0 |
| frozen, 10-oz. pkg. . . . . . . | 26,972 | 32 | .54 | .23 | 4.01 | .29 | 101.5 | 0 |

frozen, boiled, drained,

| | | | | | | | | |
|---|---|---|---|---|---|---|---|---|
| ½ cup . . . . . . . . . . . . | 6209 | 7 | .18 | .05 | .92 | .07 | 20.8 | 0 |

**Peas and onions:**

canned, w/liquid,

| | | | | | | | | |
|---|---|---|---|---|---|---|---|---|
| ½ cup . . . . . . . . . . . | 96 | 2 | .06 | .04 | .77 | n.a. | n.a. | 0 |
| frozen, 10-oz. pkg. . . . . . . | 1544 | 40 | .84 | .32 | 4.89 | n.a. | n.a. | 0 |

frozen, boiled, drained,

| | | | | | | | | |
|---|---|---|---|---|---|---|---|---|
| ½ cup . . . . . . . . . . . . | 313 | 6 | .14 | .06 | .94 | n.a. | n.a. | 0 |

**Pecan,** shelled, except as noted:

dried:

| | | | | | | | | |
|---|---|---|---|---|---|---|---|---|
| in shell, 1 lb. . . . . . . . | 308 | 5 | 2.04 | .31 | 2.13 | .45 | 94.1 | 0 |
| 1 oz. . . . . . . . . . . . . | 36 | 1 | .24 | .04 | .25 | .05 | 11.1 | 0 |
| halves, 1 cup . . . . . . . | 138 | 2 | .92 | .14 | .96 | .20 | 42.3 | 0 |
| dry-roasted, 1 oz. . . . | n.a. | n.a. | .09 | .03 | n.a. | n.a. | 11.6 | 0 |

**Pectin,** unsweetened,

powdered,

| | | | | | | | | |
|---|---|---|---|---|---|---|---|---|
| 1.75-oz. pkg. . . . . . . . . | 1 | n.a. | tr. | .03 | tr. | .01 | 0 | 0 |

**Pepper, chili, hot:**

green, 1 medium,

| | | | | | | | | |
|---|---|---|---|---|---|---|---|---|
| 1.6 oz. . . . . . . . . . . . . | 346 | 109 | .04 | .04 | .43 | .13 | 10.5 | 0 |
| green, chopped, ½ cup | 578 | 182 | .07 | .07 | .71 | .21 | 17.5 | 0 |

| | Vitamin A | Vitamin C | Thiamin | Riboflavin | Niacin | B6 | Folacin | B12 |
|---|---|---|---|---|---|---|---|---|
| | (IU) | (Mg) | (Mg) | (Mg) | (Mg) | (Mg) | (Mcg) | (Mcg) |

**Pepper, chili, hot,** *continued*
red:

| | | | | | | | | |
|---|---|---|---|---|---|---|---|---|
| 1 medium, 1.6 oz.... | 4838 | 109 | .04 | .04 | .43 | .13 | 10.5 | 0 |
| chopped, ½ cup .... | 8063 | 182 | .07 | .07 | .71 | .21 | 17.5 | 0 |
| sun-dried, 1 cup, | | | | | | | | |
| 1.3 oz.......... | 9801 | 11.6 | .03 | .45 | 3.21 | .30 | 19.0 | 0 |
| canned, chopped, | | | | | | | | |
| ½ cup............ | 415 | 46.2 | .01 | .03 | .54 | n.a. | n.a. | 0 |
| **Pepper, ground:** | | | | | | | | |
| black, 1 tsp. ......... | 4 | tr. | <.01 | .01 | .02 | n.a. | n.a. | 0 |
| red or cayenne, 1 tsp. .... | 749 | 1 | .01 | .02 | .16 | n.a. | n.a. | 0 |
| **Pepper, jalapeño,** | | | | | | | | |
| canned, w/liquid, | | | | | | | | |
| chopped, ½ cup ..... | 1156 | 9 | .02 | .03 | .34 | n.a. | n.a. | 0 |

**Pepper, sweet** (bell), **fresh:**
green:

| | | | | | | | | |
|---|---|---|---|---|---|---|---|---|
| raw, untrimmed, | | | | | | | | |
| 1 lb. ........... | 2351 | 332.1 | .25 | .11 | 1.89 | .92 | 80.0 | 0 |
| raw, 1 medium, | | | | | | | | |
| 3.2 oz.......... | 468 | 66 | .05 | .02 | .38 | .18 | 16.0 | 0 |
| raw, chopped, ½ cup | 316 | 45 | .03 | .02 | .26 | .12 | 11.0 | 0 |
| boiled, drained, | | | | | | | | |
| chopped, ½ cup .. | 403 | 51 | .04 | .02 | .33 | .16 | 11.0 | 0 |

red:

| | | | | | | | | |
|---|---|---|---|---|---|---|---|---|
| raw, untrimmed, | | | | | | | | |
| 1 lb. ...........| 25,855 | 862.6 | .25 | .11 | 1.89 | .92 | 80.0 | 0 |
| raw, 1 medium, | | | | | | | | |
| 3.2 oz.......... | 4218 | 141 | .05 | .02 | .38 | .18 | 16.0 | 0 |
| raw, chopped, ½ cup | 2850 | 95 | .03 | .02 | .26 | .12 | 11.0 | 0 |
| boiled, drained, | | | | | | | | |
| chopped, ½ cup .. | 2557 | 116 | .04 | .02 | .33 | .16 | 11.0 | 0 |

yellow, raw:

| | | | | | | | | |
|---|---|---|---|---|---|---|---|---|
| untrimmed, 1 lb. ..... | 884 | 683 | .10 | .10 | 3.31 | .63 | 97.0 | 0 |
| 1 large, 6.6 oz. ...... | 442 | 341 | .05 | .05 | 1.66 | .31 | 48.0 | 0 |
| 10 strips, 1.8 oz..... | 124 | 95 | .02 | .01 | .46 | .09 | 14.0 | 0 |

| | Vitamin A | Vitamin C | Thiamin | Riboflavin | Niacin | B6 | Folacin | B12 |
|---|---|---|---|---|---|---|---|---|
| | (IU) | (Mg) | (Mg) | (Mg) | (Mg) | (Mg) | (Mcg) | (Mcg) |
| **Pepper, sweet, canned,** w/liquid: | | | | | | | | |
| green, halves, ½ cup . . . . | 109 | 33 | .02 | .02 | .39 | n.a. | n.a. | 0 |
| red, halves, ½ cup . . . . . . | 364 | 33 | .02 | .02 | .39 | n.a. | n.a. | 0 |
| **Pepper, sweet, frozen:** | | | | | | | | |
| green, chopped, | | | | | | | | |
| 10-oz. pkg. . . . . . . . . | 1041 | 167 | .20 | .11 | 3.89 | .39 | 40.0 | 0 |
| red, chopped, | | | | | | | | |
| 10-oz. pkg. . . . . . . . .13,524 | | 167 | .20 | .11 | 3.89 | .39 | 40.0 | 0 |
| **Pepper, sweet, freeze-dried:** | | | | | | | | |
| green, ¼ cup . . . . . . . . . | 100 | 30 | .02 | .02 | .12 | .04 | 3.7 | 0 |
| green, 1 tbsp. . . . . . . . . | 25 | 8 | .01 | .01 | .03 | .01 | .9 | 0 |
| red, ¼ cup . . . . . . . . . . | 1236 | 30 | .02 | .02 | .12 | .04 | 3.7 | 0 |
| red, 1 tbsp. . . . . . . . . . | 309 | 8 | .01 | .01 | .03 | .01 | .9 | 0 |
| **Pepper sauce, hot:** | | | | | | | | |
| 1 tsp. . . . . . . . . . . . . . . | 14 | 3.5 | tr. | tr. | .01 | .01 | 0 | 0 |
| (*Tabasco*), 1 tsp. . . . . . . . | 77 | .2 | tr. | tr. | .01 | .01 | 0 | 0 |
| **Peppered loaf**[1], pork and | | | | | | | | |
| beef, 1-oz. slice . . . . . . . . | 0 | 7 | .11 | .09 | .87 | .08 | n.a. | .56 |
| **Pepperoni,** pork and | | | | | | | | |
| beef, 1 oz. . . . . . . . . . . | 0 | n.a. | .09 | .07 | 1.41 | .07 | n.a. | .71 |
| **Persimmon,** Japanese: | | | | | | | | |
| fresh, untrimmed, 1 lb. | 8255 | 29 | .11 | .08 | .48 | n.a. | 28.6 | 0 |
| fresh, 1 medium, 2½" × | | | | | | | | |
| 3½", 1.1 oz. . . . . . . . | 3640 | 13 | .05 | .03 | .17 | n.a. | 12.6 | 0 |
| dried, untrimmed, 1 lb. | 2329 | 0 | n.a. | .12 | .75 | n.a. | n.a. | 0 |
| dried, 1 oz. . . . . . . . . . . | 158 | 0 | n.a. | .01 | .05 | n.a. | n.a. | 0 |
| **Pheasant,** raw, | | | | | | | | |
| meat w/skin, 1 oz. . . . . | 50 | 2 | .02 | .04 | 1.82 | .19 | n.a. | .22 |
| **Phyllo dough,** .7-oz. | | | | | | | | |
| sheet . . . . . . . . . . . . . | 0 | 0 | .10 | .07 | .77 | .01 | 3.0 | 0 |
| **Picante sauce** (see also "Salsa") | | | | | | | | |
| (*Pace*), 2 tbsp. . . . . . . . | 64 | 2 | .02 | .01 | .25 | n.a. | n.a. | n.a. |

[1] *With added ascorbic acid or sodium ascorbate; vitamin C value for product without additives would be negligible.*

|  | Vitamin A | Vitamin C | Thiamin | Riboflavin | Niacin | B6 | Folacin | B12 |
|---|---|---|---|---|---|---|---|---|
|  | (IU) | (Mg) | (Mg) | (Mg) | (Mg) | (Mg) | (Mcg) | (Mcg) |

**Pickle**, cucumber:

dill, 1 large, 3¾" long,

2.3 oz. . . . . . . . . . . . | 214 | 1 | .01 | .02 | .04 | .01 | 1.0 | 0

dill, 1 slice, .2 oz. . . . . . . | 20 | <1 | tr. | <.01 | <.01 | <.01 | 0 | 0

sour, 1 medium, 3¾"

long, 1.2 oz. . . . . . . | 51 | <1 | 0 | <.01 | 0 | n.a. | n.a. | 0

sour, 1 slice, .25 oz. . . . . | 10 | <1 | 0 | tr. | 0 | n.a. | n.a. | 0

sweet, 1 large, 3" long,

1.2 oz. . . . . . . . . . . . . | 44 | <1 | <.01 | .01 | .06 | .01 | 0 | 0

sweet, 1 slice, .2 oz. . . . . | 8 | <1 | tr. | <.01 | .01 | tr. | 0 | 0

**Pickle and pimiento loaf**[1],

pork, 1-oz. slice . . . . . . | n.a. | 4 | .08 | .07 | .58 | .05 | n.a. | .33

**Pickle relish**, see "Relish"

**Picnic loaf**[1], pork and

beef, 1-oz. slice . . . . . . | 0 | 5 | .11 | .07 | .65 | .09 | n.a. | .42

**Pie**, ready-to-serve:

apple, ⅛ of 9" pie . . . . . . | 154 | 4 | .04 | .03 | .33 | .05 | 5.0 | 0

blueberry, ⅛ of 9" pie . . . | 175 | n.a. | .01 | .04 | .38 | .05 | n.a. | 0

cherry, ⅛ of 9" pie . . . . . | n.a. | n.a. | .03 | .04 | .25 | .05 | 10.0 | 0

chocolate cream, ⅙ of

8" pie . . . . . . . . . . . . | n.a. | n.a. | .04 | .12 | .77 | .02 | 8.0 | n.a.

coconut creme, ⅙ of

7" pie . . . . . . . . . . . . | 58 | 0 | .03 | .05 | .13 | n.a. | n.a. | 0

coconut custard, ⅙ of

8" pie . . . . . . . . . . . . | 114 | n.a. | .09 | .15 | .42 | .01 | n.a. | n.a.

custard . . . . . . . . . . . . | 350 | 0 | .14 | .32 | .90 | n.a. | n.a. | n.a.

egg custard, ⅙ of

8" pie . . . . . . . . . . . . | n.a. | n.a. | .04 | .22 | .31 | .05 | 21.0 | .45

lemon meringue, ⅙ of

8" pie . . . . . . . . . . . . | 198 | 4 | .07 | .24 | .73 | .03 | 10.0 | n.a.

peach, ⅙ of 8" pie . . . . . . | 123 | n.a. | .07 | .04 | .23 | .03 | n.a. | 0

pecan, ⅙ of 8" pie . . . . . . | 198 | 1 | .10 | .14 | .28 | .02 | 7.0 | n.a.

---

[1] *With added ascorbic acid or sodium ascorbate; vitamin C value for product without additives would be negligible.*

| | Vitamin A | Vitamin C | Thiamin | Riboflavin | Niacin | B₆ | Folacin | B₁₂ |
|---|---|---|---|---|---|---|---|---|
| | (IU) | (Mg) | (Mg) | (Mg) | (Mg) | (Mg) | (Mcg) | (Mcg) |
| pumpkin, ⅙ of 8" pie . . . . | n.a. | n.a. | .06 | .17 | .20 | .06 | 17.0 | n.a. |
| **Pie, frozen, baked:** | | | | | | | | |
| apple, ⅙ of 8" pie . . . . . . | 10 | 1 | .01 | .01 | .20 | n.a. | n.a. | n.a. |
| cherry, ⅙ of 8" pie . . . . . | 280 | 2 | .02 | .02 | .20 | n.a. | n.a. | n.a. |
| coconut custard, ⅙ of | | | | | | | | |
| 8" pie . . . . . . . . . . . . | 160 | tr. | .04 | .16 | .20 | n.a. | n.a. | n.a. |
| **Pie crust, frozen,** | | | | | | | | |
| 9" crust . . . . . . . . . . . | n.a. | n.a. | .44 | .54 | 3.4 | .10 | n.a. | n.a. |
| **Pie crust mix¹, 9" crust** | 0 | 0 | .49 | .30 | 3.8 | .09 | n.a. | 0 |
| **Pie filling, canned:** | | | | | | | | |
| apple, 21-oz. can . . . . . . . | n.a. | n.a. | .07 | .07 | .21 | .10· | 0 | 0 |
| cherry, 21-oz. can . . . . . . | 1220 | n.a. | .15 | .10 | .83 | .22 | 24.0 | 0 |
| **Pigeon peas, fresh:** | | | | | | | | |
| raw, untrimmed (in | | | | | | | | |
| pods), 1 lb. . . . . . . . . | 305 | 85 | .87 | .37 | 4.79 | n.a. | n.a. | 0 |
| raw, trimmed, ½ cup . . . . | 108 | 30 | .31 | .13 | 1.69 | n.a. | n.a. | 0 |
| boiled, drained, ½ cup . . . | 100 | 22 | .27 | .13 | 1.66 | n.a. | n.a. | 0 |
| **Pigeon peas, dried:** | | | | | | | | |
| raw, 1 lb. . . . . . . . . . . . . | 125 | 0 | 2.92 | .85 | 13.45 | 1.28 | 2068.4 | 0 |
| raw, ½ cup . . . . . . . . . . | 28 | 0 | .66 | .19 | 3.02 | .29 | 465.1 | 0 |
| boiled, ½ cup . . . . . . . . . | 2 | 0 | .12 | .05 | .66 | .04 | 93.0 | 0 |
| **Pignoli nut, see "Pine nut"** | | | | | | | | |
| **Pike, northern, meat only:** | | | | | | | | |
| raw, 1 lb. . . . . . . . . . . . | 318 | 17 | .26 | .29 | n.a. | .53 | n.a. | n.a. |
| baked, broiled, or | | | | | | | | |
| microwaved², 4 oz. . . . | 92 | 4 | .08 | .09 | n.a. | .15 | n.a. | n.a. |
| **Pimiento, canned:** | | | | | | | | |
| 1 oz. . . . . . . . . . . . . . . . | 753 | 24 | <.01 | .02 | .17 | .06 | 1.7 | 0 |
| 1 tbsp. . . . . . . . . . . . . . | 319 | 10 | <.01 | .01 | .07 | .03 | 1.0 | 0 |
| **Pine nut, shelled, except as noted:** | | | | | | | | |
| pignoli, dried: | | | | | | | | |
| in shell, 1 lb. . . . . . . . | n.a. | n.a. | 2.83 | .66 | 12.47 | n.a. | n.a. | 0 |

¹ *Prepared according to package directions, with enriched flour and vegetable shortening.*
² *Prepared without added ingredients.*

| | Vitamin A | Vitamin C | Thiamin | Riboflavin | Niacin | B6 | Folacin | B12 |
|---|---|---|---|---|---|---|---|---|
| | (IU) | (Mg) | (Mg) | (Mg) | (Mg) | (Mg) | (Mcg) | (Mcg) |
| **Pine nut, pignoli, dried,** *continued* | | | | | | | | |
| 1 oz. . . . . . . . . . . . . | n.a. | n.a. | .23 | .05 | 1.01 | n.a. | n.a. | 0 |
| 1 tbsp. . . . . . . . . . . | n.a. | n.a. | .08 | .02 | .36 | n.a. | n.a. | 0 |
| **piñon, dried:** | | | | | | | | |
| in shell, 1 lb. . . . . . . . | 75 | 5 | 3.21 | .58 | 11.30 | n.a. | n.a. | 0 |
| 1 oz. . . . . . . . . . . | 0 | 1 | .35 | .06 | 1.24 | n.a. | n.a. | 0 |
| 10 kernels . . . . . . . . | 0 | 0 | .01 | tr. | .04 | n.a. | n.a. | 0 |
| **Pineapple:** | | | | | | | | |
| fresh: | | | | | | | | |
| untrimmed, 1 lb. . . . . | 54 | 36 | .22 | .09 | .99 | .21 | 25.0 | 0 |
| trimmed, 1 slice, 3½" | | | | | | | | |
| diam. × ¾". . . . . . | 19 | 13 | .08 | .03 | .35 | .07 | 8.9 | 0 |
| trimmed, diced, | | | | | | | | |
| ½ cup . . . . . . . . . | 18 | 12 | .07 | .03 | .33 | .07 | 8.2 | 0 |
| canned: | | | | | | | | |
| in water, tidbits, | | | | | | | | |
| ½ cup . . . . . . . . . | 19 | 10 | .11 | .03 | .37 | .09 | 6.0 | 0 |
| in juice, chunks or | | | | | | | | |
| tidbits, ½ cup . . . . | 48 | 12 | .12 | .02 | .36 | n.a. | n.a. | 0 |
| in light syrup, ½ cup | 19 | 10 | .11 | .03 | .37 | .09 | 6.0 | 0 |
| in heavy syrup, | | | | | | | | |
| chunks, tidbits or | | | | | | | | |
| crushed, ½ cup . . . | 19 | 10 | .12 | .03 | .37 | .09 | 5.9 | 0 |
| frozen, sweetened, | | | | | | | | |
| chunks, ½ cup . . . . . . | 37 | 10 | .12 | .04 | .37 | .09 | n.a. | 0 |
| **Pineapple juice:** | | | | | | | | |
| canned[1], 6 fl. oz. . . . . . . . | 6 | 20 | .10 | .04 | .48 | .18 | 43.2 | 0 |
| frozen, diluted, 6 fl. oz. . . | 18 | 22 | .13 | .04 | .37 | .14 | n.a. | 0 |
| **Pineapple topping,** | | | | | | | | |
| 2 tbsp. . . . . . . . . . . . | 9 | 25 | .01 | tr. | .04 | .01 | 1.0 | 0 |
| **Pineapple-grapefruit** | | | | | | | | |
| **juice drink[2], canned,** | | | | | | | | |
| 8 fl. oz. . . . . . . . . . . . | 88 | 115 | .08 | .04 | .67 | .11 | 26.2 | 0 |

[1] *Without added ascorbic acid.*
[2] *With added ascorbic acid.*

| | Vitamin A | Vitamin C | Thiamin | Riboflavin | Niacin | B₆ | Folacin | B₁₂ |
|---|---|---|---|---|---|---|---|---|
| | (IU) | (Mg) | (Mg) | (Mg) | (Mg) | (Mg) | (Mcg) | (Mcg) |
| **Pineapple-orange juice** | | | | | | | | |
| **drink**[1], canned, 8 fl. oz. | 1328 | 56 | .08 | .05 | .52 | .12 | 27.2 | 0 |
| **Pink beans,** dried: | | | | | | | | |
| uncooked, 1 lb. . . . . . . . | 0 | 0 | 3.50 | .87 | 8.58 | 2.39 | 2199.9 | 0 |
| uncooked, ½ cup. . . . . . | 0 | 0 | .81 | .20 | 1.99 | .55 | 486.3 | 0 |
| boiled, ½ cup . . . . . . . . | 0 | 0 | .22 | .05 | .48 | .15 | 141.3 | 0 |
| **Pinto beans,** dried: | | | | | | | | |
| uncooked, 1 lb. . . . . . . . | 24 | 33 | 2.52 | 1.08 | 6.56 | 2.01 | 2296.6 | 0 |
| uncooked, ½ cup. . . . . . | 5 | 7 | .53 | .23 | 1.39 | .43 | 486.1 | 0 |
| boiled, ½ cup . . . . . . . . | 2 | 2 | .16 | .08 | .34 | .13 | 146.2 | 0 |
| canned, w/liquid, 8 oz. . . . | 3 | 2 | .23 | .14 | .66 | .17 | 136.7 | 0 |
| canned, w/liquid, | | | | | | | | |
| ½ cup . . . . . . . . . . . | 1 | 1 | .12 | .08 | .35 | .09 | 72.3 | 0 |
| **Pistachio nut,** shelled, except as noted: | | | | | | | | |
| dried: | | | | | | | | |
| in shell, 1 lb. . . . . . . . | 530 | n.a. | 1.86 | .40 | 2.45 | n.a. | n.a. | 0 |
| 1 oz. . . . . . . . . . . . . | 66 | n.a. | .23 | .05 | .31 | n.a. | n.a. | 0 |
| 1 cup . . . . . . . . . . . . | 299 | n.a. | 1.05 | .22 | 1.38 | n.a. | n.a. | 0 |
| dry-roasted, 1 oz. . . . . . . | n.a. | n.a. | .12 | .07 | .40 | n.a. | n.a. | 0 |
| **Pitanga:** | | | | | | | | |
| untrimmed, 1 lb. . . . . . . | 5988 | 105 | .12 | .16 | 1.20 | n.a. | n.a. | 0 |
| trimmed, ½ cup. . . . . . . | 1298 | 23 | .03 | .03 | .26 | n.a. | n.a. | 0 |
| **Pizza,** see "Fast foods" | | | | | | | | |
| **Plantain,** fresh: | | | | | | | | |
| raw: | | | | | | | | |
| untrimmed, 1 lb. . . . . | 3322 | 54 | .15 | .16 | 2.02 | .88 | 64.9 | 0 |
| 1 medium, 9.7 oz. . . . | 2017 | 33 | .09 | .10 | 1.23 | .54 | 39.4 | 0 |
| trimmed, sliced, | | | | | | | | |
| ½ cup . . . . . . . . . | 834 | 14 | .04 | .04 | .51 | .22 | 16.3 | 0 |
| cooked, sliced, ½ cup . . . | 700 | 8 | .04 | .04 | .58 | .19 | 20.0 | 0 |
| **Plum:** | | | | | | | | |
| fresh: | | | | | | | | |
| untrimmed, 1 lb. . . . . | 1377 | 41 | .18 | .41 | 2.13 | .25 | 9.2 | 0 |

[1] With added ascorbic acid.

| | Vitamin A | Vitamin C | Thiamin | Riboflavin | Niacin | B6 | Folacin | B12 |
|---|---|---|---|---|---|---|---|---|
| | (IU) | (Mg) | (Mg) | (Mg) | (Mg) | (Mg) | (Mcg) | (Mcg) |
| **Plum, fresh,** *continued* | | | | | | | | |
| Japanese or hybrid, | | | | | | | | |
| 1 medium, 2⅛" | | | | | | | | |
| diam., 2.3 oz. . . . . | 213 | 6 | .03 | .06 | .33 | .05 | 1.4 | 0 |
| pitted, sliced, ½ cup | 267 | 8 | .04 | .08 | .41 | .07 | 1.8 | 0 |
| canned, purple: | | | | | | | | |
| in water, ½ cup. . . . . | 1138 | 3 | .03 | .05 | .46 | .03 | 3.3 | 0 |
| in juice, ½ cup . . . . . | 1271 | 4 | .03 | .07 | .60 | n.a. | n.a. | 0 |
| in light syrup, ½ cup | 333 | 1 | .02 | .05 | .37 | .03 | n.a. | 0 |
| in heavy syrup, | | | | | | | | |
| ½ cup, . . . . . . . . | 334 | 1 | .02 | .05 | .38 | .04 | 3.3 | 0 |
| **Poi,** ½ cup . . . . . . . . . . | 24 | 5 | .16 | .05 | 1.32 | n.a. | n.a. | 0 |
| **Pokeberry shoots:** | | | | | | | | |
| raw, ½ cup . . . . . . . . . . | 6960 | 109 | .06 | .26 | .96 | n.a. | n.a. | 0 |
| boiled, drained, ½ cup. . . | 7134 | 67 | .06 | .21 | .91 | n.a. | n.a. | 0 |
| **Polish sausage** (see also | | | | | | | | |
| "Kielbasa"), pork, 1 oz. | 0 | 0 | .14 | .04 | .98 | .05 | n.a. | .28 |
| **Pollock,** meat only: | | | | | | | | |
| Atlantic: | | | | | | | | |
| raw, 1 lb. . . . . . . . . . | 159 | (0) | .21 | .84 | 14.83 | 1.62 | n.a. | 14.47 |
| baked, broiled, or | | | | | | | | |
| microwaved[1], 4 oz. | 45 | (0) | .06 | .26 | 4.51 | .38 | n.a. | 4.17 |
| walleye: | | | | | | | | |
| raw, 1 lb. . . . . . . . . . | 299 | (0) | .30 | .26 | 5.85 | .27 | 14.1 | 14.06 |
| baked, broiled, or | | | | | | | | |
| microwaved[1], 4 oz. | 86 | (0) | .08 | .09 | 1.87 | .08 | 4.1 | 4.76 |
| **Pomegranate,** fresh: | | | | | | | | |
| untrimmed, 1 lb. . . . . . . | n.a. | 16 | .08 | .08 | .76 | .27 | n.a. | 0 |
| 1 medium, 3⅜" × 3¾", | | | | | | | | |
| 9.7 oz. . . . . . . . . . . | n.a. | 9 | .05 | .05 | .46 | .16 | n.a. | 0 |
| **Popcorn,** popped: | | | | | | | | |
| air-popped, unsalted, | | | | | | | | |
| 1 cup . . . . . . . . . . . | 16 | 0 | .02 | .02 | .16 | .02 | 2.0 | 0 |
| cheese flavor, 1 cup. . . . . | 27 | .1 | .01 | .03 | .16 | .03 | n.a. | n.a. |

[1] *Prepared without added ingredients.*

| | Vitamin A | Vitamin C | Thiamin | Riboflavin | Niacin | B₆ | Folacin | B₁₂ |
|---|---|---|---|---|---|---|---|---|
| | (IU) | (Mg) | (Mg) | (Mg) | (Mg) | (Mg) | (Mcg) | (Mcg) |
| oil-popped, unsalted, 1 cup | 17 | 0 | .02 | .02 | .17 | .02 | 2.0 | 0 |
| oil-popped, salted, 1 cup | 20 | 0 | .01 | .02 | .10 | n.a. | n.a. | 0 |
| w/caramel coating, 1 cup | 18 | 0 | .02 | .03 | .77 | n.a. | n.a. | n.a. |
| w/caramel coating and peanuts, ⅔ cup | 18 | 0 | .01 | .04 | .56 | .05 | n.a. | 0 |
| **Poppy seeds,** 1 tsp. | tr. | tr. | .02 | .01 | .03 | .01 | n.a. | 0 |
| **Pork**[1]**,** fresh, 4 oz., except as noted (see also "Ham"): | | | | | | | | |
| loin, whole: | | | | | | | | |
| braised, lean and fat | 10 | <1 | .69 | .34 | 6.77 | .41 | 4.5 | .90 |
| braised, lean only | 9 | <1 | .78 | .40 | 7.87 | .51 | 5.7 | .95 |
| broiled, lean and fat | 10 | <1 | .95 | .41 | 5.97 | .43 | 5.7 | 1.11 |
| broiled, lean only | 9 | <1 | 1.10 | .48 | 6.75 | .52 | 5.7 | 1.22 |
| roasted, lean and fat | 9 | <1 | .82 | .36 | 6.11 | .43 | 5.7 | .99 |
| roasted, lean only | 8 | <1 | .91 | .41 | 6.77 | .51 | 6.8 | 1.05 |
| loin, blade: | | | | | | | | |
| braised, lean and fat | 8 | <1 | .56 | .31 | 5.44 | .36 | 4.5 | .86 |
| braised, lean only | 6 | <1 | .62 | .37 | 6.29 | .46 | 5.7 | .93 |
| broiled, lean and fat | 10 | <1 | .75 | .36 | 4.73 | .39 | 4.5 | 1.07 |
| broiled, lean only | 9 | <1 | .86 | .43 | 5.30 | .49 | 5.7 | 1.18 |
| pan-fried[2], lean and fat | 11 | <1 | .69 | .33 | 4.43 | .33 | 1.1 | .99 |
| pan-fried[2], lean only | 9 | <1 | .84 | .42 | 5.13 | .45 | tr. | 1.13 |
| roasted, lean and fat | 10 | <1 | .59 | .33 | 4.80 | .41 | 4.5 | .86 |
| roasted, lean only | 9 | <1 | .65 | .39 | 5.29 | .50 | 5.7 | .91 |
| loin, center: | | | | | | | | |
| braised, lean and fat | 10 | <1 | .88 | .27 | 6.79 | .43 | 4.5 | .69 |
| braised, lean only | 10 | <1 | 1.00 | .31 | 7.71 | .51 | 5.7 | .69 |
| broiled, lean and fat | 10 | <1 | 1.13 | .31 | 5.67 | .45 | 5.7 | .81 |
| broiled, lean only | 9 | <1 | 1.30 | .35 | 6.28 | .53 | 6.8 | .84 |

[1] *Prepared without added ingredients, except as noted.*
[2] *In hydrogenated soybean and cottonseed oils.*

|  | Vitamin A | Vitamin C | Thiamin | Riboflavin | Niacin | B6 | Folacin | B12 |
|---|---|---|---|---|---|---|---|---|
|  | (IU) | (Mg) | (Mg) | (Mg) | (Mg) | (Mg) | (Mcg) | (Mcg) |

Pork, loin, center, *continued*

pan-fried[1], lean and

| fat | 10 | <1 | 1.16 | .31 | 5.84 | .44 | 5.7 | .87 |
| pan-fried[1], lean only | 9 | <1 | 1.42 | .37 | 6.82 | .57 | 6.8 | .83 |
| roasted, lean and fat | 9 | <1 | .94 | .27 | 5.72 | .45 | 1.1 | .68 |
| roasted, lean only ... | 9 | <1 | 1.03 | .30 | 6.19 | .51 | 1.1 | .68 |

loin, center rib:

| braised, lean and fat | 11 | <1 | .60 | .31 | 6.40 | .36 | 6.8 | .61 |
| braised, lean only.... | 10 | <1 | .66 | .36 | 7.34 | .44 | 9.1 | .59 |
| broiled, lean and fat | 8 | <1 | .89 | .32 | 5.35 | .39 | 7.9 | .77 |
| broiled, lean only.... | 7 | <1 | 1.01 | .37 | 5.93 | .45 | 10.2 | .79 |

pan-fried[1], lean and

| fat | 10 | <1 | .72 | .32 | 4.97 | .37 | 6.8 | .70 |
| pan-fried[1], lean only | 9 | <1 | .87 | .40 | 5.85 | .50 | 9.1 | .70 |
| roasted, lean and fat | 9 | <1 | .67 | .32 | 5.56 | .40 | 9.1 | .64 |
| roasted, lean only ... | 9 | <1 | .72 | .35 | 6.07 | .45 | 10.2 | .62 |

loin, sirloin:

| braised, lean and fat | 10 | <1 | .74 | .34 | 5.69 | .41 | 4.5 | .75 |
| braised, lean only.... | 9 | <1 | .84 | .39 | 6.42 | .60 | 5.7 | .76 |
| broiled, lean and fat | 10 | <1 | 1.02 | .39 | 4.92 | .50 | 5.7 | .91 |
| broiled, lean only.... | 9 | <1 | 1.17 | .46 | 5.40 | .61 | 6.8 | .95 |
| roasted, lean and fat | 9 | <1 | .84 | .35 | 5.89 | .43 | 5.7 | .86 |
| roasted, lean only ... | 8 | <1 | .90 | .38 | 6.30 | .48 | 6.8 | .88 |

loin, top:

| braised, lean and fat | 11 | <1 | .59 | .30 | 6.25 | .35 | 6.8 | .61 |
| braised, lean only.... | 10 | <1 | .66 | .36 | 7.34 | .44 | 9.1 | .59 |
| broiled, lean and fat | 9 | <1 | .87 | .31 | 5.23 | .39 | 7.9 | .76 |
| broiled, lean only.... | 7 | <1 | 1.01 | .37 | 5.93 | .45 | 10.2 | .79 |

pan-fried[1], lean and

| fat | 10 | <1 | .72 | .32 | 4.96 | .37 | 6.8 | .69 |
| pan-fried[1], lean only | 9 | <1 | .87 | .40 | 5.85 | .50 | 9.1 | .70 |
| roasted, lean and fat | 9 | <1 | .66 | .31 | 5.48 | .39 | 7.9 | .64 |
| roasted, lean only ... | 9 | <1 | .72 | .35 | 6.07 | .45 | 10.2 | .62 |

[1] *In hydrogenated soybean and cottonseed oils.*

|  | Vitamin A (IU) | Vitamin C (Mg) | Thiamin (Mg) | Riboflavin (Mg) | Niacin (Mg) | B6 (Mg) | Folacin (Mcg) | B12 (Mcg) |
|---|---|---|---|---|---|---|---|---|
| shoulder, whole: | | | | | | | | |
| roasted, lean and fat | 9 | <1 | .61 | .36 | 4.52 | .37 | 4.5 | .94 |
| roasted, lean only ... | 8 | <1 | .66 | .41 | 4.88 | .45 | 5.7 | 1.00 |
| shoulder, arm (picnic): | | | | | | | | |
| braised, lean and fat | 10 | <1 | .61 | .35 | 5.92 | .31 | 4.5 | .78 |
| braised, lean only.... | 9 | <1 | .68 | .41 | 6.74 | .46 | 5.7 | .81 |
| roasted, lean and fat | 9 | <1 | .59 | .34 | 4.45 | .32 | 4.5 | .84 |
| roasted, lean only ... | 8 | <1 | .66 | .40 | 4.89 | .46 | 5.7 | .88 |
| shoulder, Boston blade: | | | | | | | | |
| braised, lean and fat | 11 | <1 | .57 | .38 | 4.53 | .26 | 1.1 | .95 |
| braised, lean only.... | 10 | <1 | .63 | .44 | 4.92 | .31 | 5.7 | 1.02 |
| broiled, lean and fat | 10 | <1 | .76 | .43 | 4.52 | .31 | 4.5 | 1.18 |
| broiled, lean only.... | 9 | <1 | .85 | .50 | 4.88 | .35 | 5.7 | 1.28 |
| roasted, lean and fat | 9 | <1 | .62 | .38 | 4.58 | .31 | 4.5 | 1.03 |
| roasted, lean only ... | 8 | <1 | .67 | .42 | 4.88 | .34 | 5.7 | 1.09 |
| spareribs, lean and fat, braised, 6.3 oz. (1 lb. raw w/bone) ........ | 18 | n.a. | .72 | .68 | 9.69 | .62 | 7.0 | 1.91 |
| tenderloin, lean only, roasted ............ | 8 | <1 | 1.07 | .44 | 5.34 | .48 | 6.8 | .62 |
| **Pork ear,** frozen, simmered[1], 4 oz. ..... | 0 | 0 | .02 | .08 | .64 | n.a. | n.a. | n.a. |
| **Pork jowl,** raw, 1 oz..... | 3 | n.a. | .11 | .07 | 1.29 | .03 | 0 | .23 |
| **Potato,** fresh or stored: | | | | | | | | |
| raw: | | | | | | | | |
| pulp, untrimmed, 1 lb. ........... | (0) | 67 | .30 | .12 | 5.05 | .89 | 43.3 | 0 |
| pulp from 1 medium, 2½" diam., 5.3 oz. w/skin ......... | (0) | 22 | .10 | .04 | 1.66 | .29 | 14.3 | 0 |
| pulp, diced, ½ cup... | (0) | 15 | .07 | .03 | 1.11 | .20 | 9.6 | 0 |
| skin from 2½"-diam. potato ......... | (0) | 4 | .01 | .01 | .39 | .09 | 6.6 | 0 |

[1] *Prepared without added ingredients.*

| | Vitamin A | Vitamin C | Thiamin | Riboflavin | Niacin | B6 | Folacin | B12 |
|---|---|---|---|---|---|---|---|---|
| | (IU) | (Mg) | (Mg) | (Mg) | (Mg) | (Mg) | (Mcg) | (Mcg) |

**Potato,** *continued*
**baked in skin:**

| | | | | | | | | |
|---|---|---|---|---|---|---|---|---|
| whole, 1 medium, 4¾" × 2⅓" diam., 7.1 oz. | (0) | 26 | .22 | .07 | 3.32 | .70 | 22.2 | 0 |
| pulp from 4¾"-diam. potato | (0) | 20 | .16 | .03 | 2.18 | .47 | 14.2 | 0 |
| pulp, ½ cup | (0) | 8 | .06 | .01 | .85 | .18 | 5.6 | 0 |
| skin, 2 oz. | (0) | 8 | .07 | .06 | 1.72 | .34 | 12.1 | 0 |
| **boiled:** | | | | | | | | |
| in skin, peeled, 1 medium, 2½" diam., 5.3 oz. w/skin | (0) | 18 | .14 | .03 | 1.96 | .41 | 13.6 | 0 |
| in skin, pulp, ½ cup | (0) | 10 | .08 | .02 | 1.12 | .23 | 7.8 | 0 |
| w/out skin, 2½"-diam. potato | (0) | 10 | .13 | .03 | 1.77 | .36 | 11.9 | 0 |
| w/out skin, pulp, ½ cup | (0) | 6 | .08 | .02 | 1.02 | .21 | 6.9 | 0 |
| **microwaved in skin:** | | | | | | | | |
| whole, 1 medium, 4¾" × 2⅓" diam., 7.1 oz. | (0) | 31 | .24 | .07 | 3.46 | .70 | 24.2 | 0 |
| pulp from 4¾"-diam. potato | (0) | 24 | .20 | .04 | 2.54 | .50 | 19.3 | 0 |
| pulp, ½ cup | (0) | 12 | .10 | .02 | 1.27 | .25 | 9.7 | 0 |
| skin, 2 oz. | (0) | 9 | .04 | .04 | 1.24 | .28 | 9.3 | 0 |
| mashed, w/whole milk, ½ cup | 20 | 7 | .09 | .04 | 1.17 | .25 | 8.6 | .06 |
| mashed, w/whole milk and margarine, ½ cup | 177 | 6 | .09 | .04 | 1.13 | .24 | 8.3 | .05 |
| **Potato, canned, whole:** | | | | | | | | |
| w/liquid, 1-lb. can | (0) | 56.2 | .15 | .09 | 4.03 | .62 | 20.5 | 0 |
| 1"-diam. potato, 1.2 oz. | (0) | 2 | .02 | .01 | .32 | .07 | 2.2 | 0 |
| drained, ½ cup | (0) | 5 | .06 | .01 | .82 | .17 | 5.6 | 0 |

| | Vitamin A | Vitamin C | Thiamin | Riboflavin | Niacin | B6 | Folacin | B12 |
|---|---|---|---|---|---|---|---|---|
| | (IU) | (Mg) | (Mg) | (Mg) | (Mg) | (Mg) | (Mcg) | (Mcg) |
| **Potato, frozen:** | | | | | | | | |
| french-fried[1], heated: | | | | | | | | |
| 9-oz. pkg. . . . . . . . . | 0 | 25 | .27 | .06 | 4.37 | .64 | 30.0 | 0 |
| 10 strips, 1.75 oz. . . . | 0 | 6 | .07 | .02 | 1.15 | .16 | 8.0 | 0 |
| cottage cut, | | | | | | | | |
| 9-oz. pkg. . . . . . . . | 0 | 19 | .24 | .06 | 4.78 | .48 | 32.7 | 0 |
| cottage cut, 10 strips, | | | | | | | | |
| 1.75 oz. . . . . . . . . | 0 | 5 | .06 | .02 | 1.21 | .12 | 8.3 | 0 |
| hash brown: | | | | | | | | |
| 12-oz. pkg. . . . . . . . | n.a. | 28 | .33 | .05 | 5.66 | .30 | n.a. | 0 |
| heated[2], 12-oz. pkg. | n.a. | 13 | .23 | .04 | 4.96 | .26 | n.a. | 0 |
| heated[2], ½ cup . . . . . | n.a. | 5 | .09 | .02 | 1.89 | .10 | n.a. | 0 |
| puffs[1], 1 piece, .25 oz. . . . | 1 | <1 | .01 | .01 | .15 | .02 | 1.2 | 0 |
| **Potato chips[3]:** | | | | | | | | |
| plain, 1 oz. . . . . . . . | 0 | 9 | .05 | .06 | 1.09 | .19 | 13.0 | 0 |
| plain, light, 1 oz. . . . . . . . | 0 | 7 | .06 | .08 | 1.98 | .19 | n.a. | 0 |
| barbecue flavor, 1 oz. . . . | 62 | 10 | .06 | .06 | 1.3 | .18 | 24.0 | 0 |
| cheese flavor, 1 oz. . . . . . | n.a. | 15 | .04 | .05 | 1.42 | .10 | 0 | n.a. |
| sour cream and onion | | | | | | | | |
| flavors, 1 oz. . . . . . . . | 48 | 11 | .05 | .06 | 1.14 | .19 | 18.0 | n.a. |
| **Potato flour,** ½ cup . . . . . | 0 | 17 | .38 | .13 | 3.06 | n.a. | n.a. | 0 |
| **Potato mix[4]:** | | | | | | | | |
| mashed[5], flakes, ½ cup . . | 189 | 10 | .12 | .05 | .70 | .01 | 7.8 | .08 |
| mashed[5], granules, | | | | | | | | |
| ½ cup . . . . . . . . . . . | 195 | 6 | .08 | .08 | .80 | .14 | 8.0 | 0 |
| **Potato sticks,** 1-oz. pkg. . . . | 0 | 13 | .03 | .03 | 1.36 | .09 | 11.0 | 0 |
| **Poultry,** see specific listings | | | | | | | | |
| **Poultry salad sandwich** | | | | | | | | |
| **spread** (chicken and | | | | | | | | |
| turkey), 1 tbsp. . . . . . . | 18 | 0 | <.01 | .01 | .22 | .01 | 1.0 | .05 |

[1] Par-fried in vegetable oil.
[2] Prepared in vegetable oil.
[3] Includes rippled, salt and vinegar, and kettle-cooked varieties.
[4] Flakes and granules without milk.
[5] Prepared according to package directions, with whole milk and butter.

|  | Vitamin A | Vitamin C | Thiamin | Riboflavin | Niacin | B6 | Folacin | B12 |
|---|---|---|---|---|---|---|---|---|
|  | (IU) | (Mg) | (Mg) | (Mg) | (Mg) | (Mg) | (Mcg) | (Mcg) |
| **Poultry seasoning**, 1 tsp. | 39 | <1 | <.01 | <.01 | .05 | n.a. | n.a. | 0 |
| **Pretzels:** | | | | | | | | |
| plain, 1 oz. . . . . . . . . . . | 0 | 0 | .13 | .18 | 1.49 | .03 | n.a. | 0 |
| whole wheat, 1 oz. . . . . . . | n.a. | n.a. | .13 | .08 | 1.9 | n.a. | n.a. | 0 |
| **Prickly pear:** | | | | | | | | |
| untrimmed, 1 lb. . . . . . . . | 174 | 48 | .05 | .20 | 1.57 | n.a. | n.a. | 0 |
| 1 medium, approx. | | | | | | | | |
| 4.8 oz. . . . . . . . . . . . . | 53 | 14 | .01 | .06 | .47 | n.a. | n.a. | 0 |
| **Prune:** | | | | | | | | |
| canned, in heavy syrup, | | | | | | | | |
| ½ cup . . . . . . . . . . . . . | 933 | 3 | .04 | .14 | 1.01 | n.a. | n.a. | 0 |
| dehydrated, pitted: | | | | | | | | |
| uncooked, 1 lb. . . . . . . | 7992 | 0 | .54 | .75 | 13.59 | 3.38 | 8.6 | 0 |
| uncooked, ½ cup. . . . | 1163 | 0 | .08 | .25 | 1.98 | .49 | 1.3 | 0 |
| cooked, ½ cup . . . . . | 732 | 0 | .06 | .04 | 1.38 | .27 | .2 | 0 |
| dried, w/pits: | | | | | | | | |
| uncooked, 1 lb. . . . . . . | 7840 | 13 | .32 | .64 | 7.74 | 1.04 | 14.4 | 0 |
| uncooked, 10 fruits, | | | | | | | | |
| approx. 3.5 oz. . . . | 1669 | 3 | .07 | .14 | 1.65 | .22 | 3.1 | 0 |
| uncooked, ½ cup. . . . | 1600 | 3 | .07 | .13 | 1.58 | .21 | 3.0 | 0 |
| cooked, stewed, | | | | | | | | |
| unsweetened, | | | | | | | | |
| ½ cup . . . . . . . . . | 324 | 3 | .03 | .11 | .77 | .23 | .1 | 0 |
| cooked, stewed, | | | | | | | | |
| sweetened, ½ cup | 340 | 3 | .03 | .11 | .80 | .24 | .1 | 0 |
| dried, pitted: | | | | | | | | |
| uncooked, 4 oz. . . . . . | 2253 | 4 | .09 | .18 | 2.22 | .30 | 4.2 | 0 |
| cooked, stewed, | | | | | | | | |
| unsweetened, 4 oz. | 347 | 3 | .03 | .11 | .82 | .25 | .1 | 0 |
| cooked, stewed, | | | | | | | | |
| sweetened, 4 oz. . . | 323 | 3 | .02 | .11 | .77 | .23 | .1 | 0 |
| **Prune juice,** canned, | | | | | | | | |
| 6 fl. oz. . . . . . . . . . . . . | 6 | 8 | .03 | .13 | 1.51 | n.a. | .6 | 0 |
| **Pudding,** ready-to-serve: | | | | | | | | |
| banana, 5-oz. can . . . . . . | n.a. | tr. | .21 | .23 | n.a. | n.a. | n.a. | n.a. |
| chocolate, 5-oz. can. . . . . | 51 | 3 | .04 | .22 | .49 | .04 | 4.0 | 0 |

| | Vitamin A | Vitamin C | Thiamin | Riboflavin | Niacin | B6 | Folacin | B12 |
|---|---|---|---|---|---|---|---|---|
| | (IU) | (Mg) | (Mg) | (Mg) | (Mg) | (Mg) | (Mcg) | (Mcg) |
| lemon, 5-oz. can . . . . . . . | n.a. | n.a. | n.a. | n.a. | n.a. | n.a. | n.a. | 0 |
| rice, 5-oz. can . . . . . . . . . | n.a. | n.a. | .03 | .10 | .23 | n.a. | n.a. | n.a. |
| tapioca, 5-oz. can . . . . . . | 0 | n.a. | .03 | .14 | .44 | n.a. | n.a. | n.a. |
| vanilla, 5-oz. can . . . . . . . | 23 | 0 | .03 | .16 | .29 | .01 | 0 | .11 |
| **Pudding, frozen:** | | | | | | | | |
| butterscotch (*Rich's*), | | | | | | | | |
|    3.5 oz. . . . . . . . . . . . . | 2 | <1 | .02 | .08 | .05 | .02 | 0 | .20 |
| chocolate (*Rich's*), | | | | | | | | |
|    3.5 oz. . . . . . . . . . . . . | 2 | <1 | .02 | .08 | .09 | .02 | 0 | .18 |
| vanilla (*Rich's*), 3.5 oz. . . | 2 | <1 | .02 | .08 | .05 | .02 | 0 | .20 |
| **Pudding bar:** | | | | | | | | |
| chocolate, 1.7-oz. bar. . . . | 52 | tr. | .02 | .08 | .06 | .02 | 1.0 | .25 |
| vanilla, 1.7-oz. bar . . . . . . | 81 | tr. | .02 | .09 | .02 | .02 | 2.0 | .17 |
| **Pudding mix[1]:** | | | | | | | | |
| chocolate, ½ cup . . . . . . . | 140 | 1 | .05 | .20 | .10 | n.a. | n.a. | n.a. |
| chocolate, instant, | | | | | | | | |
|    ½ cup . . . . . . . . . . . . . | 130 | 1 | .04 | .18 | .10 | n.a. | n.a. | n.a. |
| rennet custard: | | | | | | | | |
|    caramel, fruit | | | | | | | | |
|      flavored, or vanilla, | | | | | | | | |
|      ½ cup . . . . . . . . . | 190 | 2 | .04 | .20 | .15 | n.a. | n.a. | n.a. |
|      chocolate, ½ cup. . . . | 180 | 2 | .04 | .19 | .15 | n.a. | n.a. | n.a. |
| rice, ½ cup . . . . . . . . . . . | 140 | 1 | .10 | .18 | .60 | n.a. | n.a. | n.a. |
| vanilla, ½ cup . . . . . . . . . | 140 | 1 | .04 | .18 | .10 | n.a. | n.a. | n.a. |
| vanilla, instant, ½ cup . . . | 140 | 1 | .04 | .17 | .10 | n.a. | n.a. | n.a. |
| **Puff pastry,** frozen, | | | | | | | | |
|    1.7-oz. shell. . . . . . . . | 0 | 0 | .19 | .13 | 1.96 | .01 | 6.0 | 0 |
| **Pummelo:** | | | | | | | | |
| untrimmed, 1 lb. . . . . . . . | 0 | 155 | .09 | .07 | .56 | .10 | n.a. | 0 |
| trimmed, sections, | | | | | | | | |
|    ½ cup. . . . . . . . . . . . . | 0 | 58 | .03 | .03 | .21 | .03 | n.a. | 0 |
| **Pumpkin:** | | | | | | | | |
| fresh: | | | | | | | | |
|    untrimmed, 1 lb. . . . . | 5080 | 29 | .16 | .35 | 1.91 | n.a. | n.a. | 0 |

[1] *Prepared according to package directions, with whole milk.*

| | Vitamin A | Vitamin C | Thiamin | Riboflavin | Niacin | B6 | Folacin | B12 |
|---|---|---|---|---|---|---|---|---|
| | (IU) | (Mg) | (Mg) | (Mg) | (Mg) | (Mg) | (Mcg) | (Mcg) |

**Pumpkin, fresh,** *continued*
| trimmed, cubed, | | | | | | | | |
| ½ cup . . . . . . . . . | 928 | 5 | .03 | .06 | .35 | n.a. | n.a. | 0 |
| boiled, drained, | | | | | | | | |
| mashed, ½ cup . . . | 1320 | 6 | .04 | .10 | .50 | n.a. | n.a. | 0 |
| canned, ½ cup . . . . . . . | 26,908 | 5 | .03 | .07 | .45 | .07 | 15.0 | 0 |
| **Pumpkin pie mix,** | | | | | | | | |
| canned, ½ cup . . . . . . | 11,203 | 5 | .02 | .16 | .51 | n.a. | n.a. | 0 |
| **Pumpkin pie spice,** | | | | | | | | |
| 1 tsp. . . . . . . . . . . . . | 4 | <1 | <.01 | <.01 | .04 | n.a. | n.a. | 0 |
| **Pumpkin seeds,** kernels: | | | | | | | | |
| dried, 1 oz. . . . . . . . . . . | 108 | n.a. | .06 | .09 | .50 | n.a. | n.a. | 0 |
| dried, 1 cup. . . . . . . . . . | 525 | n.a. | .29 | .44 | 2.41 | n.a. | n.a. | 0 |
| **Purslane:** | | | | | | | | |
| raw, untrimmed, 1 lb. . . . | 4550 | 72 | .16 | .39 | 1.66 | n.a. | n.a. | 0 |
| raw, trimmed, ½ cup . . . . | 284 | 5 | .01 | .02 | .10 | n.a. | n.a. | 0 |
| boiled, drained, ½ cup . . . | 1074 | 6 | .02 | .05 | .27 | n.a. | n.a. | 0 |

# Q

| | Vitamin A | Vitamin C | Thiamin | Riboflavin | Niacin | B6 | Folacin | B12 |
|---|---|---|---|---|---|---|---|---|
| | (IU) | (Mg) | (Mg) | (Mg) | (Mg) | (Mg) | (Mcg) | (Mcg) |
| **Quail,** raw, meat w/skin, 1 oz. . . . . . . . . . . . . . | 69 | 2 | .07 | .07 | 2.14 | .17 | 2.3 | n.a. |
| **Quince:** | | | | | | | | |
| untrimmed, 1 lb. . . . . . . . | 111 | 42 | .06 | .08 | .55 | .11 | n.a. | 0 |
| 1 medium, 5.3 oz. . . . . . . | 37 | 14 | .02 | .03 | .18 | .04 | n.a. | 0 |
| **Quinoa,** uncooked, 1 cup | n.a. | 0 | .34 | .67 | 4.98 | n.a. | n.a. | 0 |

# R

| | Vitamin A | Vitamin C | Thiamin | Riboflavin | Niacin | B6 | Folacin | B12 |
|---|---|---|---|---|---|---|---|---|
| | (IU) | (Mg) | (Mg) | (Mg) | (Mg) | (Mg) | (Mcg) | (Mcg) |
| **Rabbit[1]**, domesticated, meat only: | | | | | | | | |
| roasted, 4 oz. . . . . . . . . | 0 | 0 | .08 | .18 | 7.50 | .42 | 10.2 | 7.38 |
| stewed, 4 oz. . . . . . . . . . | 0 | 0 | .07 | .19 | 8.12 | .39 | 10.2 | 7.38 |
| **Radicchio**, fresh: | | | | | | | | |
| untrimmed, 1 lb. . . . . . . . | 113 | 33 | .07 | .12 | 1.05 | .24 | 249.0 | 0 |
| trimmed, 1 leaf, approx. | | | | | | | | |
| .25 oz. . . . . . . . . . . . . | 2 | 1 | tr. | tr. | .02 | .01 | 5.0 | 0 |
| trimmed, shredded, | | | | | | | | |
| ½ cup . . . . . . . . . . . . | 5 | 2 | tr. | .01 | .05 | .01 | 12.0 | 0 |
| **Radish**, fresh: | | | | | | | | |
| untrimmed, 1 lb. . . . . . . . | 31 | 93 | .02 | .18 | 1.23 | .29 | 110.2 | 0 |
| 10 medium, 1.75 oz. . . . . | 3 | 10 | <.01 | .02 | .14 | .03 | 12.2 | 0 |
| trimmed, sliced, ½ cup . . | 4 | 13 | <.01 | .03 | .17 | .04 | 15.7 | 0 |
| **Radish, Oriental:** | | | | | | | | |
| fresh: | | | | | | | | |
| raw, untrimmed, | | | | | | | | |
| 1 lb. . . . . . . . . . . . | 0 | 79 | .07 | .07 | .72 | n.a. | n.a. | 0 |
| raw, trimmed, | | | | | | | | |
| 1 medium, approx. | | | | | | | | |
| 12 oz. . . . . . . . . . | 0 | 74 | .07 | .07 | .68 | n.a. | n.a. | 0 |
| raw, trimmed, sliced, | | | | | | | | |
| ½ cup . . . . . . . . . | 0 | 10 | .01 | .01 | .09 | n.a. | n.a. | 0 |
| boiled, drained, | | | | | | | | |
| sliced, ½ cup. . . . . | 0 | 11 | 0 | .02 | .11 | n.a. | n.a. | 0 |
| dried, ½ cup . . . . . . . . . | 0 | 0 | .16 | .39 | 1.97 | n.a. | n.a. | 0 |
| **Radish, white icicle:** | | | | | | | | |
| untrimmed, 1 lb. . . . . . . . | 0 | 86 | .09 | .06 | .88 | .22 | 42.0 | 0 |
| trimmed, 1 medium, | | | | | | | | |
| .6 oz. . . . . . . . . . . . . . | 0 | 5 | .01 | <.01 | .05 | .01 | 2.0 | 0 |
| trimmed, sliced, ½ cup | 0 | 15 | .02 | .01 | .15 | .04 | 7.0 | 0 |
| **Radish seeds, sprouted:** | | | | | | | | |
| raw, 1 lb. . . . . . . . . . . . | 1774 | 131 | .46 | .47 | 12.94 | 1.29 | 429.6 | 0 |
| raw, ½ cup . . . . . . . . . . | 74 | 6 | .02 | .02 | .54 | .05 | 18.0 | 0 |

[1] *Prepared without added ingredients.*

| | Vitamin A | Vitamin C | Thiamin | Riboflavin | Niacin | B6 | Folacin | B12 |
|---|---|---|---|---|---|---|---|---|
| | (IU) | (Mg) | (Mg) | (Mg) | (Mg) | (Mg) | (Mcg) | (Mcg) |

**Raisins:**
seeded:

| | | | | | | | | |
|---|---|---|---|---|---|---|---|---|
| 1 lb. . . . . . . . . . . . . | 0 | 25 | .51 | .83 | 5.05 | .85 | 15.2 | 0 |
| 1 oz. . . . . . . . . . . . . | 0 | 2 | .03 | .05 | .32 | .05 | .09 | 0 |
| ½ cup not packed . . . | 0 | 4 | .08 | .13 | .81 | .14 | 2.4 | 0 |
| seedless: | | | | | | | | |
| 1 lb. . . . . . . . . . . . . | 35 | 15 | .71 | .40 | 3.71 | 1.13 | 15.2 | 0 |
| 1 oz. . . . . . . . . . . . . | 2 | 1 | .04 | .02 | .23 | .07 | .9 | 0 |
| ½ cup not packed . . . | 6 | 2 | .11 | .06 | .59 | .18 | 2.4 | 0 |
| seedless, golden: | | | | | | | | |
| 1 lb. . . . . . . . . . . . . | 200 | 14 | .04 | .87 | 5.18 | 1.47 | 15.2 | 0 |
| 1 oz. . . . . . . . . . . . . | 12 | 1 | <.01 | .05 | .32 | .09 | .9 | 0 |
| ½ cup not packed . . . | 32 | 2 | .01 | .14 | .83 | .23 | 2.4 | 0 |

**Raspberry:**
fresh:

| | | | | | | | | |
|---|---|---|---|---|---|---|---|---|
| untrimmed, 1 lb. . . . . | 566 | 109 | .13 | .39 | 3.92 | .25 | n.a. | 0 |
| 1 pint, 11.5 oz. . . . . . | 406 | 78 | .09 | .28 | 2.81 | .18 | n.a. | 0 |
| trimmed, ½ cup. . . . . | 80 | 15 | .02 | .06 | .55 | .04 | n.a. | 0 |
| canned, red, in heavy syrup, ½ cup. . . . . . . . | 43 | 11 | .03 | .04 | .57 | .05 | 13.4 | 0 |
| frozen, red, sweetened, 10-oz. pkg. . . . . . . . . . | 169 | 47 | .05 | .13 | .65 | .10 | 73.8 | 0 |
| frozen, red, sweetened, ½ cup. . . . . . . . . . . . | 75 | 21 | .02 | .06 | .29 | .04 | 32.5 | 0 |

**Redfish,** see "Ocean perch"

**Refried beans,** canned:

| | | | | | | | | |
|---|---|---|---|---|---|---|---|---|
| 8 oz. . . . . . . . . . . . . . | 0 | 14 | .06 | .04 | .71 | .33 | 25.0 | 0 |
| ½ cup. . . . . . . . . . . . . | 0 | 8 | .03 | .02 | .40 | .18 | 14.0 | 0 |

**Relish, pickle:**

| | | | | | | | | |
|---|---|---|---|---|---|---|---|---|
| hamburger, ½ cup. . . . . | 325 | 3 | .02 | .05 | .75 | n.a. | n.a. | 0 |
| hamburger, 1 tbsp. . . . . | 40 | <1 | tr. | .01 | .09 | n.a. | n.a. | 0 |
| hot dog, ½ cup. . . . . . . | 203 | 1 | .05 | .05 | .61 | n.a. | n.a. | 0 |
| hot dog, 1 tbsp.. . . . . . . | 25 | <1 | .01 | .01 | .08 | n.a. | n.a. | 0 |
| sweet, ½ cup . . . . . . . . | 189 | 1 | 0 | .04 | .28 | n.a. | n.a. | 0 |
| sweet, 1 tbsp. . . . . . . . . | 23 | <1 | 0 | .01 | .04 | n.a. | n.a. | 0 |

| | Vitamin A | Vitamin C | Thiamin | Riboflavin | Niacin | B₆ | Folacin | B₁₂ |
|---|---|---|---|---|---|---|---|---|
| | (IU) | (Mg) | (Mg) | (Mg) | (Mg) | (Mg) | (Mcg) | (Mcg) |
| **Rhubarb:** | | | | | | | | |
| fresh, untrimmed, 1 lb. | 340 | 27 | .07 | .10 | 1.10 | .08 | 24.2 | 0 |
| fresh, trimmed, diced, | | | | | | | | |
| ½ cup . . . . . . . . . . . . | 61 | 5 | .01 | .02 | .18 | .02 | 4.3 | 0 |
| frozen, ½ cup . . . . . . . . | 73 | 3 | .02 | .02 | .14 | .02 | 5.6 | 0 |
| frozen, cooked, | | | | | | | | |
| sweetened, ½ cup . . . . | 83 | 4 | .02 | .03 | .24 | .02 | 6.4 | 0 |
| **Rice[1]:** | | | | | | | | |
| uncooked, ½ cup: | | | | | | | | |
| brown long grain . . . . | 0 | 0 | .37 | .09 | 4.68 | .47 | 18.0 | 0 |
| brown medium grain | 0 | 0 | .39 | .04 | 4.09 | .48 | 19.0 | 0 |
| white long grain, | | | | | | | | |
| regular. . . . . . . . . | 0 | 0 | .53 | .05 | 3.86 | .15 | 8.0 | 0 |
| white long grain, | | | | | | | | |
| parboiled . . . . . . . . | 0 | 0 | .55 | .06 | 3.34 | .32 | 15.0 | 0 |
| white long grain, | | | | | | | | |
| precooked or | | | | | | | | |
| instant . . . . . . . . . | 0 | 0 | .30 | .03 | 2.63 | .02 | .03 | 0 |
| white medium grain | 0 | 0 | .57 | .05 | 4.99 | .14 | 9.0 | 0 |
| white short grain . . . . | 0 | 0 | .57 | .05 | 4.11 | .17 | 6.0 | 0 |
| cooked, ½ cup: | | | | | | | | |
| brown long grain . . . . | 0 | 0 | .09 | .02 | 1.50 | .14 | 4.0 | 0 |
| brown medium grain | 0 | 0 | .10 | .01 | 1.30 | .15 | 4.0 | 0 |
| white long grain, | | | | | | | | |
| regular. . . . . . . . . | 0 | 0 | .13 | .01 | 1.12 | .07 | 3.0 | 0 |
| white long grain, | | | | | | | | |
| parboiled . . . . . . . . | 0 | 0 | .22 | .02 | 1.23 | .02 | 3.0 | 0 |
| white long grain, | | | | | | | | |
| precooked or | | | | | | | | |
| instant | 0 | 0 | .06 | .04 | .72 | .01 | 3.0 | 0 |
| white medium grain | 0 | 0 | .16 | .01 | 1.71 | .05 | 2.0 | 0 |
| white short grain . . . . | 0 | 0 | .15 | .02 | 1.39 | .06 | 2.0 | 0 |
| **Rice, glutinous:** | | | | | | | | |
| uncooked, ½ cup. . . . . . | 0 | 0 | .17 | .05 | 1.97 | .10 | 6.0 | 0 |
| cooked, 1 cup . . . . . . . . | 0 | 0 | .05 | .03 | .70 | .06 | 3.0 | 0 |

[1] *White rice is enriched.*

| | Vitamin A | Vitamin C | Thiamin | Riboflavin | Niacin | B6 | Folacin | B12 |
|---|---|---|---|---|---|---|---|---|
| | (IU) | (Mg) | (Mg) | (Mg) | (Mg) | (Mg) | (Mcg) | (Mcg) |

**Rice, wild,** see "Wild rice"

| | | | | | | | | |
|---|---|---|---|---|---|---|---|---|
| **Rice bran,** crude, 1 cup | 0 | 0 | 2.29 | .24 | 28.22 | 3.38 | 52.0 | 0 |
| **Rice cakes,** brown rice: | | | | | | | | |
| plain, 1 piece.......... | 0 | 0 | .01 | .02 | .70 | .01 | 2.0 | 0 |
| buckwheat, 1 piece ..... | 0 | 0 | .01 | .01 | .73 | .01 | 2.0 | 0 |
| corn, 1 piece.......... | 0 | 0 | .01 | .02 | .58 | .01 | 2.0 | 0 |
| multigrain, 1 piece...... | 0 | 0 | .01 | .02 | .59 | .01 | 2.0 | 0 |
| rye, 1 piece.......... | 0 | 0 | .01 | .01 | .63 | .01 | 0 | 0 |
| sesame seed, 1 piece.... | 0 | 0 | tr. | .01 | .65 | .01 | 2.0 | 0 |
| **Rice flour:** | | | | | | | | |
| brown, 1 cup.......... | 0 | 0 | .70 | .13 | 10.02 | 1.16 | 25.0 | 0 |
| white, 1 cup .......... | 0 | 0 | .22 | .03 | 4.09 | .69 | 6.0 | 0 |
| **Rice pudding,** see "Pudding" and "Pudding mix" | | | | | | | | |
| **Rockfish,** Pacific, mixed species, meat only: | | | | | | | | |
| raw, 1 lb............... | 862 | (0) | .17 | .31 | 14.60 | n.a. | n.a. | n.a. |
| baked, broiled, or | | | | | | | | |
| microwaved[1], 4 oz. .... | 248 | (0) | .05 | .10 | 4.44 | n.a. | n.a. | n.a. |
| **Roll:** | | | | | | | | |
| brown and serve: | | | | | | | | |
| dinner or pan, 1-oz. | | | | | | | | |
| piece............ | tr. | tr. | .07 | .06 | .60 | n.a. | n.a. | n.a. |
| Parkerhouse, 1-oz. | | | | | | | | |
| piece............ | tr. | tr. | .06 | .06 | .60 | n.a. | n.a. | n.a. |
| (*Roman Meal*), | | | | | | | | |
| 2 rolls.......... | 0 | 0 | .27 | .19 | 2.79 | n.a. | n.a. | n.a. |
| dinner: | | | | | | | | |
| 1-oz. roll.......... | tr. | tr. | .14 | .09 | 1.14 | .02 | 8.0 | n.a. |
| egg, 1-oz. roll ...... | n.a. | 0 | .18 | .18 | 1.15 | n.a. | n.a. | .08 |
| oat bran, 1-oz. roll... | n.a. | 0 | .15 | .10 | 1.63 | n.a. | n.a. | 0 |
| rye, 1-oz. roll....... | n.a. | 0 | .11 | .08 | 1.11 | n.a. | n.a. | 0 |
| wheat, 1-oz. roll..... | 0 | 0 | .12 | .08 | 1.16 | n.a. | n.a. | 0 |
| whole-wheat, 1-oz. | | | | | | | | |
| roll ............ | 0 | 0 | .07 | .04 | 1.04 | .06 | 8.0 | 0 |
| (*Roman Meal*), | | | | | | | | |
| 2 rolls .......... | 0 | 0 | .26 | .18 | 2.69 | n.a. | n.a. | n.a. |

[2] *Prepared without added ingredients.*

| | Vitamin A (IU) | Vitamin C (Mg) | Thiamin (Mg) | Riboflavin (Mg) | Niacin (Mg) | B6 (Mg) | Folacin (Mcg) | B12 (Mcg) |
|---|---|---|---|---|---|---|---|---|
| Roll, *continued* | | | | | | | | |
| French, 1.3-oz. roll . . . . . | n.a. | 0 | .2 | .11 | 1.65 | n.a. | n.a. | 0 |
| hard, 2-oz. roll . . . . . . . . | 0 | 0 | .27 | .19 | 2.42 | n.a. | 8.0 | 0 |
| hoagie or submarine, | | | | | | | | |
| 11½" long, 4.8-oz. roll | 0 | 0 | .54 | .33 | 4.50 | n.a. | n.a. | n.a. |
| hot dog or hamburger: | | | | | | | | |
| plain, 1.5-oz. roll . . . . | n.a. | n.a. | .21 | .13 | 1.69 | n.a. | n.a. | n.a. |
| plain (*Roman Meal* Hamburger), 1 roll | 0 | 0 | .21 | .15 | 2.18 | n.a. | n.a. | n.a. |
| plain (*Roman Meal* Hot Dog), 1 roll . . . | 0 | 0 | .20 | .14 | 2.04 | n.a. | n.a. | n.a. |
| light, 1.5-oz. roll . . . . | n.a. | n.a. | .17 | .08 | 2.12 | n.a. | n.a. | n.a. |
| mixed grain, 1.5-oz. roll . . . . . . . . . . . | n.a. | 0 | .2 | .13 | 1.9 | .04 | n.a. | 0 |
| sandwich (*Roman Meal*), 1 roll . . . . . . . . . . . . . | 0 | 0 | .36 | .25 | 3.73 | n.a. | n.a. | n.a. |
| **Roll, sweet:** | | | | | | | | |
| cheese, 2.3-oz. roll . . . . . | n.a. | n.a. | .10 | .09 | .55 | n.a. | n.a. | n.a. |
| cinnamon w/raisin, 2.1-oz. roll . . . . . . . . . | 129 | 1 | .20 | .16 | 1.43 | .06 | 14.0 | n.a. |
| **Roll, sweet, refrigerated dough,** cinnamon, w/frosting, 1.1-oz. roll | n.a. | n.a. | .14 | .08 | 1.11 | n.a. | n.a. | n.a. |
| **Roll mix[1],** cloverleaf, 1.2-oz. roll . . . . . . . . . | tr. | tr. | .02 | .04 | .20 | n.a. | n.a. | n.a. |
| **Rose apple:** | | | | | | | | |
| untrimmed, 1 lb. . . . . . . . | 1029 | 68 | .06 | .09 | 2.41 | n.a. | n.a. | 0 |
| trimmed, 1 oz. . . . . . . . . . | 96 | 6 | .01 | .01 | .23 | n.a. | n.a. | 0 |
| **Roselle:** | | | | | | | | |
| untrimmed, 1 lb. . . . . . . . | 793 | 33 | .03 | .08 | .86 | n.a. | n.a. | 0 |
| trimmed, 1 oz. or ½ cup | 81 | 3 | <.01 | .01 | .09 | n.a. | n.a. | 0 |
| **Rosemary,** dried, 1 tsp. | 38 | 1 | .01 | n.a. | .01 | n.a. | n.a. | 0 |

[1] *Prepared according to package directions, with water.*

| | Vitamin A | Vitamin C | Thiamin | Riboflavin | Niacin | B₆ | Folacin | B₁₂ |
|---|---|---|---|---|---|---|---|---|
| | (IU) | (Mg) | (Mg) | (Mg) | (Mg) | (Mg) | (Mcg) | (Mcg) |
| **Rum extract,** artificial (*Virginia Dare*), 1 tsp. | 0 | 0 | tr. | tr. | tr. | tr. | tr. | 0 |
| **Rutabaga:** | | | | | | | | |
| raw, untrimmed, 1 lb. | 2236 | 96 | .35 | .15 | 2.70 | .39 | 79.0 | 0 |
| raw, trimmed, cubed, ½ cup | 406 | 18 | .06 | .03 | .49 | .07 | 14.0 | 0 |
| boiled, drained, cubed, ½ cup | 477 | 16 | .07 | .04 | .61 | .09 | 13.0 | 0 |
| boiled, drained, mashed, ½ cup | 674 | 23 | .10 | .05 | .86 | .12 | 19.0 | 0 |
| **Rye flour:** | | | | | | | | |
| dark, 1 cup | 0 | 0 | .40 | .32 | 5.47 | .57 | 77.0 | 0 |
| light, 1 cup | 0 | 0 | .34 | .09 | .82 | .24 | 23.0 | 0 |
| medium, 1 cup | 0 | 0 | .29 | .12 | 1.76 | .27 | 20.0 | 0 |

# S

| | Vitamin A | Vitamin C | Thiamin | Riboflavin | Niacin | B₆ | Folacin | B₁₂ |
|---|---|---|---|---|---|---|---|---|
| | (IU) | (Mg) | (Mg) | (Mg) | (Mg) | (Mg) | (Mcg) | (Mcg) |
| **Safflower seed kernels,** dried, 1 oz. . . . . . . . . | n.a. | 0 | 2.69 | .96 | 5.23 | n.a. | n.a. | 0 |
| **Safflower seed meal,** partially defatted, 1 oz. . . . . . . . . . . . . . . | n.a. | 0 | .33 | .12 | .64 | n.a. | n.a. | 0 |
| **Sage,** ground, 1 tsp. . . . . | 41 | <1 | .01 | <.01 | .04 | n.a. | n.a. | 0 |
| **Salad dressing,** 1 tbsp.: | | | | | | | | |
| blue cheese . . . . . . . . . . | 32 | <1 | tr. | .02 | tr. | n.a. | n.a. | 0 |
| French, regular or low calorie . . . . . . . . . . . . | tr. | tr. | tr. | tr. | tr. | n.a. | n.a. | 0 |
| Italian . . . . . . . . . . . . . | 30 | tr. | tr. | tr. | tr. | n.a. | n.a. | 0 |
| Italian, low calorie . . . . . . | tr. | tr. | tr. | tr. | tr. | n.a. | n.a. | 0 |
| mayonnaise type. . . . . . . . | 32 | 0 | tr. | tr. | tr. | n.a. | n.a. | 0 |
| Thousand Island, regular or low calorie . . . . . . . | 50 | 0 | tr. | tr. | tr. | n.a. | n.a. | 0 |
| vinegar and oil. . . . . . . . | 0 | 0 | 0 | 0 | 0 | n.a. | n.a. | 0 |
| **Salami¹:** | | | | | | | | |
| beef, cooked, 1-oz. slice . . . . . . . . . | n.a. | 4 | .04 | .07 | .97 | .06 | 1.0 | 1.37 |
| beef and pork, cooked, 1-oz. slice . . . . . . . . . | n.a. | 3 | .07 | .11 | 1.01 | .06 | 1.0 | 1.04 |
| beer, beef, .8-oz. slice . . . | n.a. | 4 | .02 | .03 | .78 | .04 | 1.0 | .45 |
| beer, pork, 1-oz. slice . . . | n.a. | 8 | .16 | .05 | .92 | .10 | .9 | .25 |
| dry or hard, pork, 1-oz. slice . . . . . . . . . | n.a. | n.a. | .26 | .09 | 1.59 | .16 | n.a. | .79 |
| dry or hard, pork and beef, 1-oz. slice . . . . . . | n.a. | 7 | .17 | .08 | 1.38 | .14 | n.a. | .54 |
| **"Salami," vegetarian** (*Worthington*), 3 slices, 2 oz. . . . . . . . . . . . . . . | 0 | 0 | .76 | .15 | 1.13 | .27 | n.a. | .65 |

¹ With added sodium ascorbate; vitamin C value for product without additives would be negligible.

| | Vitamin A | Vitamin C | Thiamin | Riboflavin | Niacin | B6 | Folacin | B12 |
|---|---|---|---|---|---|---|---|---|
| | (IU) | (Mg) | (Mg) | (Mg) | (Mg) | (Mg) | (Mcg) | (Mcg) |

**Salmon,** meat only:
Atlantic:

| | Vitamin A | Vitamin C | Thiamin | Riboflavin | Niacin | B6 | Folacin | B12 |
|---|---|---|---|---|---|---|---|---|
| wild, raw, 1 lb. . . . . . | 181 | n.a. | 1.03 | 1.72 | 35.65 | 3.71 | n.a. | 14.41 |
| wild, baked, broiled, or microwaved[1], 4 oz. . . . . . . . . . . . | 50 | n.a. | .31 | .55 | 11.42 | 1.07 | n.a. | 3.46 |
| farmed, raw, 1 lb. . . . | 227 | 18 | 1.54 | .54 | 34.04 | 2.87 | 118.0 | 12.70 |
| farmed, baked, broiled, or microwaved[1], 4 oz. . . . . . . | 57 | 4 | .39 | .15 | 9.12 | .73 | 38.6 | 3.18 |
| chinook: | | | | | | | | |
| raw, 1 lb. . . . . . . . . . | n.a. | 18 | .16 | .54 | 35.54 | n.a. | n.a. | n.a. |
| baked, broiled, or microwaved[1], 4 oz. | n.a. | 5 | .05 | .17 | 11.39 | n.a. | n.a. | n.a. |
| smoked, 4 oz. . . . . . . | 100 | n.a. | .03 | .11 | 5.35 | .32 | 2.2 | 3.70 |
| chum, raw, 1 lb. . . . . . . . | 449 | n.a. | .36 | .82 | n.a. | n.a. | n.a. | n.a. |
| chum, baked, broiled, or microwaved[1], 4 oz. . . . | 129 | n.a. | .10 | .25 | n.a. | n.a. | n.a. | n.a. |
| coho: | | | | | | | | |
| wild, raw, 1 lb. . . . . . | 454 | 5 | .51 | .64 | 32.80 | 2.49 | 41.0 | 18.90 |
| wild, baked, broiled, or microwaved[1], 4 oz. . . . . . . . . . . . | 147 | 2 | .09 | .16 | 9.02 | .64 | 14.7 | 5.67 |
| wild, poached or steamed[1], 4 oz. . . . | 122 | 1 | .13 | .18 | 8.82 | .63 | 10.2 | 5.08 |
| farmed, raw, 1 lb. . . . | 854 | 5 | .41 | .50 | 30.91 | 2.99 | 57.0 | 12.10 |
| farmed, baked, broiled, or microwaved[1], 4 oz. | 223 | 2 | .11 | .13 | 8.38 | .64 | 15.9 | 3.59 |
| sockeye (red), raw, 1 lb. | 871 | n.a. | .92 | .68 | 26.22 | .86 | n.a. | 22.68 |
| sockeye (red), baked, broiled, or microwaved[1], 4 oz. . . . . . . . . | 237 | n.a. | .24 | .19 | 7.56 | .25 | n.a. | 6.58 |

---

[1] *Prepared without added ingredients.*

| | Vitamin A | Vitamin C | Thiamin | Riboflavin | Niacin | B6 | Folacin | B12 |
|---|---|---|---|---|---|---|---|---|
| | (IU) | (Mg) | (Mg) | (Mg) | (Mg) | (Mg) | (Mcg) | (Mcg) |
| **Salmon, canned:** | | | | | | | | |
| pink, w/bone and liquid, 16-oz. can.......... | 250 | 0 | .10 | .84 | 29.67 | n.a. | 69.8 | n.a. |
| pink, w/bone and liquid, 4 oz............... | 62 | 0 | .03 | .21 | 7.41 | n.a. | 17.5 | n.a. |
| sockeye (red), w/bone, drained, 13 oz. (16-oz. can w/liquid) .. | 648 | 0 | .06 | .71 | 20.22 | n.a. | 36.2 | n.a. |
| sockeye (red), w/bone, drained, 4 oz. ....... | 200 | 0 | .02 | .22 | 6.21 | n.a. | 11.1 | n.a. |
| **Salsa:** | | | | | | | | |
| ½ cup............... | 861 | 26 | .05 | .04 | .91 | .15 | 19.0 | 0 |
| (*Pace* Thick & Chunky), 2 tbsp. ............ | 85 | 2 | .02 | .01 | .26 | n.a. | n.a. | 0 |
| green chili (*Pace*), 2 tbsp. ............ | 85 | 3 | .02 | .01 | .26 | n.a. | n.a. | 0 |
| **Salsify,** fresh: | | | | | | | | |
| raw, untrimmed, 1 lb. .... | 0 | 32 | .32 | .87 | 1.97 | n.a. | n.a. | 0 |
| raw, trimmed, sliced, ½ cup............. | 0 | 5 | .05 | .15 | .34 | n.a. | n.a. | 0 |
| boiled, drained, sliced, ½ cup............. | 0 | 3 | .04 | .12 | .27 | n.a. | n.a. | 0 |
| **Salt,** 1 tsp. ........... | 0 | 0 | 0 | 0 | 0 | n.a. | n.a. | 0 |
| **Salt, substitute or imitation** (*Instead of Salt*), 1 tsp.......... | 186 | 0 | .01 | 0 | .10 | 0 | <.1 | 0 |
| **Salt pork,** raw, 1 oz. ..... | 0 | 0 | .06 | .02 | .46 | .02 | 0 | .08 |
| **Sandwich spread:** | | | | | | | | |
| pork and beef, 1 tsp..... | n.a. | 0 | .03 | .02 | .26 | .02 | n.a. | .17 |
| vegetarian (*Loma Linda*), ¼ cup, 1.9 oz........ | 104 | 0 | .28 | .32 | 1.78 | .46 | n.a. | 3.61 |
| **Sapodilla:** | | | | | | | | |
| untrimmed, 1 lb. ....... | 218 | 53 | n.a. | .07 | .73 | .13 | n.a. | 0 |
| 1 medium, 3" × 2½", approx. 7.5 oz. ...... | 102 | 25 | n.a. | .03 | .34 | .06 | n.a. | 0 |
| trimmed, ½ cup........ | 73 | 18 | n.a. | .02 | .24 | .04 | n.a. | 0 |

| | Vitamin A | Vitamin C | Thiamin | Riboflavin | Niacin | B6 | Folacin | B12 |
|---|---|---|---|---|---|---|---|---|
| | (IU) | (Mg) | (Mg) | (Mg) | (Mg) | (Mg) | (Mcg) | (Mcg) |
| **Sapote:** | | | | | | | | |
| untrimmed, 1 lb. . . . . . . . | 1321 | 64 | .03 | .06 | 5.80 | n.a. | n.a. | 0 |
| 1 medium, 11.2 oz. . . . . . | 923 | 45 | .02 | .05 | 4.05 | n.a. | n.a. | 0 |
| **Sardines,** canned: | | | | | | | | |
| Atlantic, in soybean oil: | | | | | | | | |
| w/bone, drained, 4 oz. | 254 | (0) | .09 | .26 | 5.95 | .19 | 13.4 | 10.14 |
| w/bone, 2 medium, | | | | | | | | |
| 3" long, .8 oz. . . . . | 54 | (0) | .02 | .05 | 1.26 | .04 | 2.8 | 2.15 |
| Pacific, in tomato sauce: | | | | | | | | |
| drained, 4 oz. . . . . . . | 414 | 1 | .05 | .26 | 4.76 | .14 | 27.6 | 10.20 |
| 1 medium, 4¾" long, | | | | | | | | |
| 1.3 oz. . . . . . . . . | 139 | <1 | .02 | .09 | 1.60 | .05 | 9.2 | 3.42 |
| **Sauce,** see specific listings | | | | | | | | |
| **Sauerkraut,** canned: | | | | | | | | |
| w/liquid, 8 oz. . . . . . . . . | 41 | 33 | .05 | .05 | .32 | .30 | n.a. | 0 |
| w/ liquid, ½ cup . . . . . . . | 21 | 17 | .03 | .03 | .17 | .15 | n.a. | 0 |
| **Sausage** (see also specific listings): | | | | | | | | |
| pork, fresh: | | | | | | | | |
| raw, 1-oz. link . . . . . . | 0 | <1 | .16 | .05 | .80 | .07 | 1.0 | .32 |
| raw, 1 patty, approx. | | | | | | | | |
| 2 oz. . . . . . . . . . . | 0 | <1 | .31 | .09 | 1.62 | .14 | 2.0 | .64 |
| cooked, 1 link, .5 oz. | | | | | | | | |
| (1-oz. raw link) . . . . . . | 0 | 0 | .10 | .03 | .59 | .04 | n.a. | .22 |
| cooked, 1 patty, | | | | | | | | |
| approx. 1 oz. | | | | | | | | |
| (2 oz. raw patty) . . . . . | 0 | 0 | .20 | .07 | 1.22 | .09 | n.a. | .47 |
| pork and beef, fresh: | | | | | | | | |
| cooked, .5 oz. (1-oz. | | | | | | | | |
| raw link) . . . . . . . . | 0 | n.a. | .05 | .02 | .44 | .01 | n.a. | .06 |
| cooked, 1 oz. (2-oz. | | | | | | | | |
| raw patty) . . . . . . . . | 0 | n.a. | .10 | .04 | .91 | .01 | n.a. | .12 |
| smoked, pork, 1 link, | | | | | | | | |
| 4' long × 1⅛". . . . . . . | 0 | 1 | .48 | .18 | 3.08 | .24 | n.a. | 1.11 |

[1] With added sodium ascorbate; vitamin C value for product without additives would be negligible.

| | Vitamin A | Vitamin C | Thiamin | Riboflavin | Niacin | B₆ | Folacin | B₁₂ |
|---|---|---|---|---|---|---|---|---|
| | (IU) | (Mg) | (Mg) | (Mg) | (Mg) | (Mg) | (Mcg) | (Mcg) |
| smoked, pork and beef[1], 1 link, 4" long × 1⅛" | 0 | 13 | .18 | .12 | 2.19 | .12 | n.a. | 1.03 |
| **"Sausage," vegetarian:** | | | | | | | | |
| canned: | | | | | | | | |
| (*Loma Linda Little Links*), 2 links, 1.6 oz. | 0 | 0 | .34 | .43 | 1.32 | .46 | n.a. | 1.71 |
| (*Worthington Saucettes*), 1.3-oz. link | 0 | 0 | .59 | .08 | .10 | .13 | n.a. | .35 |
| frozen: | | | | | | | | |
| (*Morningstar Farms Breakfast Links*), 2 links, 1.6 oz. . . . . | 0 | 0 | 6.95 | .22 | 5.19 | .33 | n.a. | 3.41 |
| (*Morningstar Farms Breakfast Patties*), 1.3-oz. patty . . . . . | 0 | 0 | 5.38 | .13 | 1.84 | .19 | n.a. | 1.49 |
| (*Worthington Prosage Links*), 2 links, 1.6 oz. . . . . . . . . | 0 | 0 | 6.95 | .22 | 5.19 | .33 | n.a. | 3.41 |
| (*Worthington Prosage Patties*), 1.3-oz. patty . . . . . . . . . . | 0 | 0 | .48 | .09 | .52 | .27 | n.a. | 1.51 |
| roll (*Worthington Prosage*), ⅝" slice, 1.9 oz. . . . . . . . . . | 0 | 0 | 1.08 | .19 | 1.55 | .24 | n.a. | .75 |
| **Scallion**, see "Onion, green" | | | | | | | | |
| **Scallop**, mixed species, meat only: | | | | | | | | |
| raw, 1 lb. . . . . . . . . . . . . | n.a. | n.a. | .05 | .30 | 5.22 | n.a. | n.a. | 6.94 |
| raw, 2 large or 5 small, 1.1 oz. . . . . . . . . . . . . | n.a. | n.a. | <.01 | .02 | .35 | n.a. | n.a. | .46 |
| **"Scallop," vegetarian,** canned (*Worthington Skallops*), 3 oz. . . . . . . | 0 | 0 | .03 | .03 | 0 | .01 | n.a. | 0 |
| **Scallop squash:** | | | | | | | | |
| raw, untrimmed, 1 lb. . . . | 484 | 80 | .31 | .13 | 2.67 | .49 | 134.0 | 0 |
| raw, trimmed, sliced, ½ cup . . . . . . . . . . . . | 72 | 12 | .05 | .02 | .39 | .07 | 19.6 | 0 |

| | Vitamin A | Vitamin C | Thiamin | Riboflavin | Niacin | B6 | Folacin | B12 |
|---|---|---|---|---|---|---|---|---|
| | (IU) | (Mg) | (Mg) | (Mg) | (Mg) | (Mg) | (Mcg) | (Mcg) |
| boiled, drained, sliced, ½ cup............ | 77 | 10 | .05 | .02 | .42 | .08 | 18.6 | 0 |
| **Scrod,** see "Cod" | | | | | | | | |
| **Seasoning mix** (see also specific listings): | | | | | | | | |
| all purpose (*Tone's Perc*), ¼ tsp............. | 33 | <1 | tr. | tr. | .02 | .01 | .8 | 0 |
| all purpose, w/herbs (*Tone's Perc*), ¼ tsp. | 21 | 1 | tr. | tr. | .01 | .03 | .7 | 0 |
| garden (*Tone's Perc*), ¼ tsp............. | 15 | 1 | tr. | tr. | .01 | .04 | .6 | 0 |
| garden, extra spicy (*Tone's Perc*), ¼ tsp. | 54 | 4 | tr. | tr. | .02 | .02 | .2 | 0 |
| spice and herb (*Tone's Perc*), ¼ tsp........ | 12 | <1 | tr. | tr. | .02 | .03 | .5 | 0 |
| vegetable (*Tone's Perc*), ¼ tsp............. | 1 | <1 | tr. | tr. | .01 | .02 | 1.0 | 0 |
| zesty country (*Tone's Perc*), ¼ tsp........ | 81 | 3 | tr. | tr. | .02 | .06 | 1.2 | 0 |
| **Seaweed:** | | | | | | | | |
| agar, dried, 1 oz........ | 0 | 0 | <.01 | .01 | <.01 | n.a. | n.a. | 0 |
| kelp, raw, 1 oz......... | 33 | n.a. | <.01 | .04 | .13 | n.a. | 51.0 | 0 |
| laver, raw, 1 oz........ | 1474 | 11 | .03 | .13 | .42 | .05 | n.a. | 0 |
| wakame, raw, 1 oz...... | 102 | 1 | .02 | .06 | .45 | n.a. | n.a. | 0 |
| **Semolina,** whole grain, enriched, 1 cup ...... | n.a. | 0 | 1.35 | .95 | 10.00 | .17 | 120.0 | 0 |
| **Sesame butter:** | | | | | | | | |
| paste, from whole seeds, 1 oz............... | 14 | 0 | .07 | .06 | 1.90 | n.a. | n.a. | 0 |
| paste, from whole seeds, 1 tbsp. ............ | 8 | 0 | .04 | .03 | 1.07 | n.a. | n.a. | 0 |
| tahini: | | | | | | | | |
| from raw and stone-ground kernels, 1 tbsp., .5 oz. .... | n.a. | 0 | .19 | .08 | .89 | n.a. | n.a. | 0 |
| from unroasted kernels, 1 tbsp., .5 oz............. | n.a. | 0 | .22 | .02 | .79 | n.a. | n.a. | 0 |

| | Vitamin A | Vitamin C | Thiamin | Riboflavin | Niacin | B6 | Folacin | B12 |
|---|---|---|---|---|---|---|---|---|
| | (IU) | (Mg) | (Mg) | (Mg) | (Mg) | (Mg) | (Mcg) | (Mcg) |

**Sesame butter, tahini,** *continued*
from roasted and
toasted kernels,

| | | | | | | | | |
|---|---|---|---|---|---|---|---|---|
| 1 tbsp., .5 oz. . . . . | n.a. | 0 | .18 | .07 | .82 | n.a. | n.a. | 0 |
| **Sesame flour:** | | | | | | | | |
| high fat, 1 oz. . . . . . . . . | 20 | 0 | .76 | .08 | 3.80 | .04 | 8.7 | 0 |
| partially defatted, 1 oz.. . . | 20 | 0 | .72 | .08 | 3.58 | .04 | 8.2 | 0 |
| low fat, 1 oz. . . . . . . . . . . | 18 | 0 | .72 | .08 | 3.56 | .04 | 8.2 | 0 |
| **Sesame meal,** partially | | | | | | | | |
| defatted, 1 oz. . . . . . . . | 19 | 0 | .73 | .08 | 3.64 | .04 | 8.4 | 0 |
| **Sesame seeds:** | | | | | | | | |
| whole, dried, 1 cup . . . . . | 13 | 0 | 1.14 | .36 | 6.50 | 1.14 | 139.3 | 0 |
| whole, dried, 1 tbsp. . . . . | 1 | 0 | .07 | .02 | .41 | .07 | 8.7 | 0 |
| kernels, dried, 1 cup . . . . | 99 | 0 | 1.08 | .13 | 7.02 | n.a. | n.a. | 0 |
| kernels, dried, 1 tbsp. . . . | 5 | 0 | .06 | .01 | .38 | n.a. | n.a. | 0 |
| **Sesame sticks,** wheat | | | | | | | | |
| based, 1 oz. . . . . . . . . . | 25 | 0 | .04 | .02 | .44 | n.a. | n.a. | 0 |
| **Sesbania flower,** raw, | | | | | | | | |
| trimmed, 1 cup . . . . . . | 0 | 2 | .02 | .02 | .09 | n.a. | n.a. | 0 |
| **Shallot:** | | | | | | | | |
| raw, chopped, 1 tbsp. . . . | n.a. | 1 | .01 | <.01 | .02 | n.a. | n..a. | 0 |
| freeze-dried, ¼ cup . . . . . | n.a. | 1 | .01 | <.01 | .04 | .06 | 4.2 | 0 |
| freeze-dried, 1 tbsp. . . . . . | n.a. | <1 | <.01 | <.01 | .01 | .02 | 1.0 | 0 |
| **Shark,** mixed species, meat only: | | | | | | | | |
| raw, 1 lb.. . . . . . . . . . . . . | 1058 | (0) | .19 | .28 | 13.38 | n.a. | n.a. | 6.75 |
| batter-dipped, fried, | | | | | | | | |
| 4 oz. . . . . . . . . . . . . . . | 204 | n.a. | .08 | .11 | 3.15 | n.a. | n.a. | 1.37 |
| **Sherbet,** orange, ½ cup | 73 | 4 | .02 | .07 | .09 | .03 | 4.0 | .12 |
| **Shortening,** vegetable, | | | | | | | | |
| 1 tbsp. . . . . . . . . . . . . | 0 | 0 | 0 | 0 | 0 | n.a. | n.a. | 0 |
| **Shrimp,** mixed species, meat only: | | | | | | | | |
| raw, 1 lb.. . . . . . . . . . . . | n.a. | (0) | .13 | .15 | 11.58 | .47 | 13.6 | 5.27 |
| raw, 4 large (32 per lb.), | | | | | | | | |
| 1 oz. . . . . . . . . . . . . . . | n.a. | (0) | .01 | .01 | .72 | .03 | .8 | .33 |

| | Vitamin A | Vitamin C | Thiamin | Riboflavin | Niacin | B6 | Folacin | B12 |
|---|---|---|---|---|---|---|---|---|
| | (IU) | (Mg) | (Mg) | (Mg) | (Mg) | (Mg) | (Mcg) | (Mcg) |
| boiled, poached, or steamed[1], 4 oz. . . . . . | n.a. | (0) | .04 | .04 | 2.94 | .14 | 4.0 | 1.69 |
| boiled, poached, or steamed[1], 4 large. . . . . | n.a. | (0) | .01 | .01 | .57 | .03 | .8 | .33 |
| breaded, fried, 4 oz. . . . . . | n.a. | n.a. | .15 | .15 | 3.48 | .11 | 9.2 | 2.12 |
| breaded, fried, 4 large . . . | n.a. | n.a. | .04 | .04 | .92 | .03 | 2.4 | .56 |
| **Shrimp, canned,** drained: | | | | | | | | |
| 4 oz. . . . . . . . . . . . . . . . . | n.a. | (0) | .03 | .04 | 3.12 | .13 | 2.0 | 1.37 |
| 1 cup . . . . . . . . . . . . . . | n.a. | (0) | .04 | .05 | 3.53 | .14 | 2.3 | 1.44 |
| **Smelt,** rainbow, meat only, raw, 1 lb. . . . . . . | n.a. | (0) | n.a. | .54 | 6.58 | n.a. | n.a. | 15.6 |
| **Snack mix:** | | | | | | | | |
| (*Chex*), ⅔ cup, 1 oz. . . . . | n.a. | 14 | .44 | .14 | 4.77 | .44 | 0 | 3.52 |
| (*Doo Dads*), 1 cup, 2 oz. . . . . . . . . . . . . . | 86 | tr. | .20 | .15 | 3.05 | .12 | 22.0 | .01 |
| **Snail, sea,** see "Whelk" | | | | | | | | |
| **Snap beans,** see "Green beans" | | | | | | | | |
| **Soft drinks and mixers:** | | | | | | | | |
| all flavors, except grape, lemon-lime, orange, and low-calorie cola, 12 fl. oz. . . . . . . . . . . | 0 | 0 | 0 | 0 | 0 | 0 | 0 | 0 |
| cola, low-calorie[2], 12 fl. oz. . . . . . . . . . . | 0 | 0 | .02 | .08 | 0 | 0 | 0 | 0 |
| grape or orange, 12 fl. oz. . . . . . . . . . . | 0 | 0 | 0 | 0 | n.a. | 0 | 0 | 0 |
| lemon-lime, 12 fl. oz. . . . . | 0 | 0 | 0 | 0 | .06 | 0 | 0 | 0 |
| **Sole,** see "Flatfish" | | | | | | | | |
| **Sorghum,** whole grain, 1 cup . . . . . . . . . . . . . | n.a. | 0 | .23 | .14 | 2.81 | n.a. | n.a. | 0 |
| **Sorghum syrup,** 1 tbsp. | n.a. | n.a. | .02 | .03 | .02 | n.a. | n.a. | 0 |

[1] *Prepared without added ingredients.*
[2] *Aspartame sweetened.*

| | Vitamin A (IU) | Vitamin C (Mg) | Thiamin (Mg) | Riboflavin (Mg) | Niacin (Mg) | B6 (Mg) | Folacin (Mcg) | B12 (Mcg) |
|---|---|---|---|---|---|---|---|---|
| **Soup, canned,** ready-to-serve, 1 cup: | | | | | | | | |
| bean (*Grandma Brown's*) .. | <10 | 1 | .11 | .06 | .60 | n.a. | n.a. | n.a. |
| beef, chunky . . . . . . . . . | 2611 | 7 | .06 | .15 | 2.71 | .13 | 13.4 | .61 |
| chicken, chunky. . . . . . . . | 1299 | 1 | .09 | .17 | 4.42 | .05 | 4.6 | .25 |
| chicken rice, chunky . . . . | 5858 | 4 | .02 | .10 | 4.10 | n.a. | 3.8 | n.a. |
| clam chowder, Manhattan . . . . . . . . . | 3292 | 12 | .06 | .06 | 1.85 | .26 | 9.3 | 7.92 |
| crab . . . . . . . . . . . . . | 505 | 0 | .20 | .07 | 1.34 | .12 | n.a. | .20 |
| gazpacho. . . . . . . . . . . . | 200 | 3 | .05 | .02 | .93 | .15 | n.a. | 0 |
| lentil, w/ham . . . . . . . . . | 360 | 4 | .17 | .11 | 1.35 | .22 | 49.6 | .30 |
| pea (*Grandma Brown's*) . . . . . . . . . . | <10 | 1 | .08 | .11 | .98 | n.a. | n.a. | n.a. |
| pea, split, w/ham, chunky . . . . . . . . . . | 4871 | 7 | .12 | .09 | 2.52 | n.a. | 4.7 | n.a. |
| turkey, chunky. . . . . . . . | 7156 | 6 | .04 | .11 | 3.59 | .31 | 11.1 | 2.12 |
| vegetable, chunky . . . . . . | 5877 | 6 | .07 | .07 | 1.20 | .19 | 16.5 | 0 |
| **Soup, canned, condensed**[1], 1 cup: | | | | | | | | |
| asparagus, cream of . . . . | 445 | 3 | .05 | .08 | .78 | .01 | n.a. | n.a. |
| asparagus, cream of[2] . . . . | 599 | 2 | .10 | .28 | .88 | .06 | n.a. | n.a. |
| bean, black . . . . . . . . . . | 506 | 1 | .08 | .05 | .53 | .09 | 24.7 | .02 |
| bean w/bacon . . . . . . . . . | 889 | 2 | .09 | .03 | .57 | .04 | 31.9 | n.a. |
| beef noodle . . . . . . . . . . . | 629 | <1 | .07 | .06 | 1.07 | .04 | 4.4 | .20 |
| celery, cream of. . . . . . . . | 306 | <1 | .03 | .05 | .33 | .01 | 2.4 | n.a. |
| celery, cream of[2] . . . . . . . | 461 | 1 | .07 | .25 | .44 | .06 | 8.5 | n.a. |
| cheese. . . . . . . . . . . . . . | 1088 | 0 | .02 | .14 | .40 | .03 | n.a. | 0 |
| cheese[1] . . . . . . . . . . . . . | 1243 | 1 | .06 | .33 | .50 | .08 | n.a. | .44 |
| chicken: | | | | | | | | |
| broth. . . . . . . . . . . . | 0 | 0 | .01 | .07 | 3.35 | .02 | n.a. | .24 |
| cream of . . . . . . . . . | 560 | <1 | .03 | .06 | .82 | .02 | 1.6 | n.a. |
| cream of[2] . . . . . . . . | 715 | 1 | .07 | .26 | .92 | .07 | 7.7 | n.a. |
| and dumplings. . . . . . | 518 | 0 | .02 | .07 | 1.75 | .04 | n.a. | .16 |

---

[1] *Prepared according to package directions, with water, except as noted.*
[2] *Prepared with whole milk.*

| | Vitamin A | Vitamin C | Thiamin | Riboflavin | Niacin | B6 | Folacin | B12 |
|---|---|---|---|---|---|---|---|---|
| | (IU) | (Mg) | (Mg) | (Mg) | (Mg) | (Mg) | (Mcg) | (Mcg) |
| gumbo. . . . . . . . . . . | 136 | 5 | .02 | .05 | .66 | .06 | n.a. | n.a. |
| noodle. . . . . . . . . . . | 711 | <1 | .05 | .06 | 1.39 | .03 | 2.2 | n.a. |
| rice . . . . . . . . . . . . | 660 | <1 | .02 | .02 | 1.13 | .02 | 1.1 | n.a. |
| vegetable. . . . . . . . . | 2656 | 1 | .04 | .06 | 1.23 | .05 | n.a. | n.a. |
| chili beef . . . . . . . . . . . | 1510 | 4 | .06 | .08 | 1.07 | .16 | n.a. | .32 |
| clam chowder: | | | | | | | | |
| Manhattan . . . . . . . . | 963 | 4 | .03 | .04 | .82 | .10 | 10.0 | 4.06 |
| New England . . . . . . . | 8 | 2 | .02 | .04 | .96 | .08 | 3.7 | 8.01 |
| New England[1] . . . . . . | 164 | 4 | .07 | .24 | 1.03 | .13 | 9.7 | 10.25 |
| consommé, w/gelatin . . . . | 0 | 1 | .02 | .03 | .71 | .02 | 3.0 | 0 |
| minestrone . . . . . . . . . | 2337 | 1 | .05 | .04 | .94 | .10 | 16.1 | 0 |
| mushroom: | | | | | | | | |
| barley . . . . . . . . . . . | 198 | 0 | .02 | .09 | .88 | n.a. | n.a. | 0 |
| w/beef stock . . . . . . . | 1255 | 1 | .03 | .10 | 1.21 | .04 | 9.2 | 0 |
| cream of . . . . . . . . . . | 0 | 1 | .05 | .09 | .73 | .02 | n.a. | .05 |
| cream of[1] . . . . . . . . . | 154 | 2 | .08 | .28 | .91 | .06 | n.a. | n.a. |
| onion. . . . . . . . . . . . . . | 0 | 1 | .03 | .02 | .60 | .05 | 15.2 | 0 |
| oyster stew . . . . . . . . . | 71 | 3 | .02 | .04 | .23 | .01 | n.a. | 2.19 |
| oyster stew[1]. . . . . . . . . | 225 | 4 | .07 | .23 | .34 | .06 | n.a. | 2.63 |
| pea: | | | | | | | | |
| green. . . . . . . . . . . . | 202 | 2 | .11 | .07 | 1.24 | .05 | 1.8 | 0 |
| green[1] . . . . . . . . . . . | 356 | 3 | .16 | .27 | 1.34 | .10 | 7.9 | .44 |
| split, w/ or w/out | | | | | | | | |
| ham . . . . . . . . . . . | 444 | 1 | .15 | .08 | 1.48 | .07 | 2.5 | n.a. |
| pepper pot. . . . . . . . . . | 865 | 1 | .05 | .05 | 1.22 | .06 | n.a. | .17 |
| potato, cream of . . . . . . . | 288 | 0 | .03 | .04 | .54 | .04 | 3.0 | n.a. |
| potato, cream of[1]. . . . . . . | 443 | 1 | .08 | .24 | .64 | .09 | 9.2 | n.a. |
| Scotch broth . . . . . . . . . | 2180 | 1 | .02 | .05 | 1.16 | .07 | n.a. | .27 |
| stockpot . . . . . . . . . . . . | 3980 | 2 | .04 | .05 | 1.22 | .09 | n.a. | 0 |
| tomato: | | | | | | | | |
| plain . . . . . . . . . . . . | 688 | 67 | .09 | .05 | 1.42 | .11 | 14.7 | 0 |
| plain[1]. . . . . . . . . . . . | 849 | 68 | .13 | .25 | 1.52 | .16 | 20.9 | .44 |
| beef w/noodle . . . . . . | 533 | 0 | .08 | .09 | 1.87 | .09 | n.a. | .19 |
| bisque. . . . . . . . . . . | 721 | 6 | .07 | .07 | 1.15 | .09 | n.a. | 0 |

[1] *Prepared with whole milk.*

| | Vitamin A | Vitamin C | Thiamin | Riboflavin | Niacin | B6 | Folacin | B12 |
|---|---|---|---|---|---|---|---|---|
| | (IU) | (Mg) | (Mg) | (Mg) | (Mg) | (Mg) | (Mcg) | (Mcg) |

**Soup, canned, condensed, tomato,** *continued*

| | | | | | | | | |
|---|---|---|---|---|---|---|---|---|
| bisque[1] . . . . . . . . . . | 879 | 7 | .11 | .27 | 1.25 | .14 | n.a. | .44 |
| rice . . . . . . . . . . . . . | 755 | 15 | .06 | .05 | 1.06 | .08 | n.a. | 0 |
| turkey noodle. . . . . . . . . | 292 | <1 | .07 | .06 | 1.40 | .04 | n.a. | n.a. |
| vegetable: | | | | | | | | |
| w/beef . . . . . . . . . . . | 1891 | 2 | .04 | .05 | 1.03 | .08 | 10.6 | .31 |
| w/beef broth . . . . . . . | 2091 | 2 | .05 | .05 | 1.00 | .06 | n.a. | 0 |
| vegetarian . . . . . . . . . | 3005 | 1 | .05 | .05 | .92 | .06 | 10.6 | 0 |
| **Soup mix[2], 1 cup:** | | | | | | | | |
| beef noodle . . . . . . . . . . . | 9 | 1 | .12 | .06 | .69 | .04 | 1.6 | n.a. |
| chicken noodle. . . . . . . . . | 63 | <1 | .07 | .06 | .88 | .01 | 1.4 | n.a. |
| chicken vegetable. . . . . . . | 14 | 1 | .07 | .05 | .69 | .09 | n.a. | n.a. |
| onion. . . . . . . . . . . . . . . | 2 | <1 | .03 | .06 | .48 | n.a. | 1.5 | n.a. |
| pea, green, split or | | | | | | | | |
| w/ham . . . . . . . . . . . . | 49 | tr. | .22 | .15 | 1.34 | .05 | 15.0 | n.a. |
| tomato, regular or | | | | | | | | |
| cream of . . . . . . . . . . . | 832 | 5 | .06 | .05 | .78 | .10 | 6.7 | n.a. |
| tomato, vegetable. . . . . . . | 190 | 6 | .06 | .05 | .79 | n.a. | n.a. | n.a. |
| vegetable beef . . . . . . . . . | 238 | n.a. | .03 | .04 | .46 | .05 | n.a. | n.a. |
| **Soursop:** | | | | | | | | |
| untrimmed, 1 lb. . . . . . . . . | 7 | 63 | .21 | .15 | 2.74 | .18 | n.a. | 0 |
| pulp, ½ cup. . . . . . . . . . . | 3 | 23 | .08 | .06 | 1.01 | .07 | n.a. | 0 |
| **Soy beverage** (see also "Soy milk"), 8 fl. oz.: | | | | | | | | |
| (*EdenSoy* Original) . . . . . . | n.a. | n.a. | .15 | .07 | .86 | .15 | n.a. | 0 |
| (*EdenSoy* Extra Original) | 1176 | n.a. | .12 | .07 | 1.05 | .15 | n.a. | 0 |
| carob (*EdenSoy*) . . . . . . . | n.a. | n.a. | .10 | .07 | 1.10 | .13 | n.a. | 0 |
| vanilla (*EdenSoy*) . . . . . . . | n.a. | n.a. | .12 | .07 | 1.15 | .14 | n.a. | 0 |
| vanilla (*EdenSoy* Extra) . . | 1176 | n.a. | .12 | .07 | 1.27 | .13 | n.a. | 0 |
| **Soy flour,** stirred: | | | | | | | | |
| full fat, 1 cup. . . . . . . . . . | 102 | 0 | .49 | .99 | 3.67 | .39 | 293.3 | 0 |
| full fat, roasted, 1 cup . . . | 93 | 0 | .35 | .80 | 2.79 | .30 | 193.3 | 0 |

[1] *Prepared with whole milk.*
[2] *Prepared according to package directions, with water.*

| | Vitamin A | Vitamin C | Thiamin | Riboflavin | Niacin | B6 | Folacin | B12 |
|---|---|---|---|---|---|---|---|---|
| | (IU) | (Mg) | (Mg) | (Mg) | (Mg) | (Mg) | (Mcg) | (Mcg) |
| defatted, 1 cup ........ | 40 | 0 | .70 | .25 | 2.61 | .57 | 305.4 | 0 |
| low fat, 1 cup ......... | 35 | 0 | .33 | .25 | 1.90 | .46 | 360.8 | 0 |
| **Soy meal,** defatted, 1 cup ............. | 48 | 0 | .84 | .31 | 3.16 | .69 | 361.1 | 0 |
| **Soy milk** (see also "Soy beverage"), fluid, 1 cup ............. | 77 | 0 | .39 | .17 | .35 | .10 | 3.6 | 0 |
| **Soy sauce:** | | | | | | | | |
| from soy (tamari), ¼ cup............. | 0 | 0 | .03 | .09 | 2.29 | .12 | 10.6 | 0 |
| from soy (tamari), 1 tbsp. ............ | 0 | 0 | .01 | .03 | .71 | .04 | 3.3 | 0 |
| from soy and wheat (shoyu), ¼ cup ...... | 0 | 0 | .03 | .08 | 1.95 | .10 | 9.0 | 0 |
| from soy and wheat (shoyu), 1 tbsp....... | 0 | 0 | .01 | .02 | .61 | .03 | 2.8 | 0 |
| **Soybean,** green: | | | | | | | | |
| raw, untrimmed, 1 lb. ... | 433 | 70 | 1.05 | .42 | 3.97 | n.a. | n.a. | 0 |
| raw, trimmed, ½ cup.... | 230 | 37 | .56 | .22 | 2.11 | n.a. | n.a. | 0 |
| boiled, drained, ½ cup... | 140 | 15 | .23 | .14 | 1.13 | n.a. | n.a. | 0 |
| **Soybean,** dried: | | | | | | | | |
| uncooked, 1 lb. ........ | 108 | 27 | 3.96 | 3.95 | 7.36 | 1.71 | 1701.5 | 0 |
| uncooked, ½ cup....... | 22 | 6 | .81 | .81 | 1.51 | .35 | 348.8 | 0 |
| boiled, ½ cup ......... | 8 | 6 | .13 | .25 | .34 | .20 | 46.2 | 0 |
| roasted, 1 lb........... | 907 | 10 | .95 | .66 | 6.40 | .94 | 957.1 | 0 |
| roasted, ½ cup ........ | 172 | 2 | .09 | .13 | 1.21 | .18 | 181.5 | 0 |
| dry-roasted, 1 lb........ | 105 | 21 | 1.94 | 3.43 | 4.79 | 1.02 | 927.9 | 0 |
| dry-roasted, ½ cup ..... | 20 | 4 | .37 | .65 | .91 | .19 | 175.9 | 0 |
| **Soybean, fermented,** see "Miso" and "Natto" | | | | | | | | |
| **Soybean, sprouted,** mature seeds: | | | | | | | | |
| raw, 1 lb.............. | 50 | 69 | 1.54 | .54 | 5.21 | .80 | 779.0 | 0 |
| raw, ½ cup ........... | 4 | 5 | .12 | .04 | .40 | .06 | 60.0 | 0 |
| steamed, ½ cup........ | 5 | 4 | .10 | .03 | .51 | n.a. | n.a. | 0 |
| **Soybean curd,** see "Tofu" | | | | | | | | |

| | Vitamin A | Vitamin C | Thiamin | Riboflavin | Niacin | B6 | Folacin | B12 |
|---|---|---|---|---|---|---|---|---|
| | (IU) | (Mg) | (Mg) | (Mg) | (Mg) | (Mg) | (Mcg) | (Mcg) |
| **Soybean kernels:** | | | | | | | | |
| roasted and toasted, 1 oz. | 57 | 1 | .03 | .04 | .50 | .09 | 64.0 | 0 |
| roasted and toasted, whole, 1 cup | 216 | 2.4 | .11 | .16 | 1.90 | .32 | 243.5 | 0 |
| **Spaghetti,** see "Pasta" | | | | | | | | |
| **Spaghetti sauce,** see "Tomato sauce" | | | | | | | | |
| **Spaghetti squash:** | | | | | | | | |
| raw, untrimmed, 1 lb. | 161 | 7 | .12 | .06 | 3.06 | .33 | 38.7 | 0 |
| raw, trimmed, cubed, ½ cup | 25 | 1 | .02 | .01 | .48 | .05 | 6.0 | 0 |
| baked or boiled, drained, ½ cup | 86 | 3 | .03 | .02 | .63 | .08 | 6.2 | 0 |
| **Spinach:** | | | | | | | | |
| fresh: | | | | | | | | |
| raw, untrimmed, 1 lb. | 21,932 | 92 | .26 | .62 | 2.37 | .64 | 634.8 | 0 |
| raw, 10-oz. pkg. | 13,699 | 57 | .16 | .39 | 1.48 | .40 | 396.5 | 0 |
| raw, trimmed, chopped, ½ cup | 1880 | 8 | .02 | .05 | .20 | .06 | 54.4 | 0 |
| boiled, drained, ½ cup | 7371 | 9 | .09 | .21 | .44 | .22 | 131.2 | 0 |
| canned, w/liquid, ½ cup | 7526 | 16 | .02 | .12 | .32 | .09 | 67.8 | 0 |
| canned, drained, ½ cup | 9390 | 15 | .02 | .15 | .42 | .11 | 104.6 | 0 |
| frozen, leaf, 10-oz. pkg. | 22,032 | 69 | .24 | .44 | 1.24 | .40 | 339.8 | 0 |
| frozen, boiled, drained, leaf, ½ cup | 7395 | 12 | .06 | .16 | .40 | .14 | 102.1 | 0 |
| **Spiny lobster,** mixed species, meat only: | | | | | | | | |
| raw, 1 lb. | n.a. | n.a. | .03 | .21 | 19.26 | n.a. | n.a. | n.a. |

---

[1] *Prepared without added ingredients.*

| | Vitamin A | Vitamin C | Thiamin | Riboflavin | Niacin | B6 | Folacin | B12 |
|---|---|---|---|---|---|---|---|---|
| | (IU) | (Mg) | (Mg) | (Mg) | (Mg) | (Mg) | (Mcg) | (Mcg) |
| boiled or steamed[1], 4 oz............. | n.a. | n.a. | .01 | .05 | 4.81 | n.a. | n.a. | n.a. |
| **Spleen,** braised[1]: | | | | | | | | |
| beef, 4 oz............ | 0 | 57 | .05 | .34 | 6.31 | .05 | n.a. | 5.69 |
| pork, 4 oz............ | 0 | 13 | .16 | .29 | 6.73 | .07 | n.a. | 3.13 |
| **Squash,** see specific listings | | | | | | | | |
| **Squash seeds,** see "Pumpkin seeds" | | | | | | | | |
| **Squid,** mixed species, meat only: | | | | | | | | |
| raw, 1 lb............. | n.a. | 21 | .09 | 1.87 | 9.87 | .25 | n.a. | 5.89 |
| dipped in flour, fried, 4 oz............... | n.a. | 5 | .06 | .52 | 2.95 | .07 | n.a. | 1.39 |
| **Star fruit,** see "Carambola" | | | | | | | | |
| **Steak,** see "Beef" and " 'Beef,' vegetarian" | | | | | | | | |
| **Stomach,** pork, raw, 1 oz............... | 0 | n.a. | .10 | .13 | 5.05 | .05 | n.a. | 1.12 |
| **Straightneck squash,** see "Crookneck squash" | | | | | | | | |
| **Strawberry:** | | | | | | | | |
| fresh: | | | | | | | | |
| untrimmed, 1 lb..... | 117 | 242 | .09 | .28 | .98 | .25 | 75.5 | 0 |
| untrimmed, 1 pint, approx. 12 oz..... | 87 | 182 | .06 | .21 | .74 | .19 | 56.6 | 0 |
| trimmed, ½ cup..... | 21 | 42 | .02 | .05 | .17 | .04 | 13.2 | 0 |
| canned, in heavy syrup, ½ cup............. | 33 | 40 | .03 | .04 | .07 | .06 | 35.6 | 0 |
| frozen: | | | | | | | | |
| unsweetened, ½ cup | 33 | 31 | .02 | .03 | .34 | .02 | 12.5 | 0 |
| sweetened, whole, 10-oz. pkg. ....... | 78 | 112 | .04 | .22 | .83 | .08 | 10.8 | 0 |
| sweetened, whole, ½ cup.......... | 35 | 50 | .02 | .10 | .37 | .04 | 4.9 | 0 |
| sweetened, sliced, 10-oz. pkg. ....... | 68 | 118 | .05 | .15 | 1.14 | .09 | 42.2 | 0 |
| sweetened, sliced, ½ cup.......... | 31 | 53 | .02 | .07 | .51 | .04 | 19.0 | 0 |

[1] *Prepared without added ingredients.*

| | Vitamin A | Vitamin C | Thiamin | Riboflavin | Niacin | B6 | Folacin | B12 |
|---|---|---|---|---|---|---|---|---|
| | (IU) | (Mg) | (Mg) | (Mg) | (Mg) | (Mg) | (Mcg) | (Mcg) |
| **Strawberry flavor drink mix:** | | | | | | | | |
| powder, 2–3 heaping tsp. | n.a. | <1 | <.01 | .02 | .02 | tr. | n.a. | 0 |
| (*Carnation* Instant Breakfast), 1 pkt. | 1750 | 27 | .30 | .17 | 5.00 | .40 | 100.0 | .60 |
| **Strawberry topping,** 2 tbsp. | 8 | 11 | tr. | .01 | .10 | 1 | 0 | 1 |
| **String beans,** see "Green beans" | | | | | | | | |
| **Stroganoff sauce mix,** vegetarian (*Natural Touch*), .8 oz. | 0 | 0 | .14 | .17 | .38 | .12 | n.a. | .54 |
| **Strudel, apple,** 2.5-oz. piece | 21 | 1 | .03 | .02 | n.a. | n.a. | n.a. | n.a. |
| **Stuffing mix, dry type:** | | | | | | | | |
| ½ cup prepared | n.a. | n.a. | .17 | .12 | 1.64 | .04 | 24.0 | .01 |
| corn bread, ½ cup prepared | 44 | 1.0 | .14 | .10 | 1.38 | .04 | 12.0 | 0 |
| **Succotash:** | | | | | | | | |
| canned: | | | | | | | | |
| w/liquid, 8 oz. | 332 | 10 | .07 | .13 | 1.45 | .11 | 71.9 | 0 |
| w/liquid, ½ cup | 187 | 6 | .04 | .07 | .82 | .06 | 40.5 | 0 |
| w/cream-style corn, 8 oz. | 319 | 14 | .06 | .15 | .38 | .29 | 100.4 | 0 |
| w/cream-style corn, ½ cup | 187 | 9 | .04 | .09 | .81 | .17 | 58.9 | 0 |
| frozen, 10-oz. pkg. | 729 | 24 | .25 | .20 | 3.91 | .28 | 118.0 | 0 |
| frozen, boiled, drained, ½ cup | 196 | 5 | .06 | .06 | 1.11 | .08 | 28.3 | 0 |
| **Sugar:** | | | | | | | | |
| brown, 1 cup packed | 0 | 0 | .02 | .07 | .20 | n.a. | n.a. | 0 |
| granulated or powdered, 1 tbsp. | 0 | 0 | 0 | 0 | 0 | 0 | 0 | 0 |
| **Sugar apple:** | | | | | | | | |
| untrimmed, 1 lb. | 15 | 91 | .27 | .28 | 2.20 | .50 | n.a. | 0 |
| 1 medium, 2⅞" × 3¼", 9.9 oz. | 9 | 56 | .17 | .18 | 1.37 | .31 | n.a. | 0 |

| | Vitamin A | Vitamin C | Thiamin | Riboflavin | Niacin | B6 | Folacin | B12 |
|---|---|---|---|---|---|---|---|---|
| | (IU) | (Mg) | (Mg) | (Mg) | (Mg) | (Mg) | (Mcg) | (Mcg) |
| pulp, ½ cup . . . . . . . . . . | 8 | 45 | .14 | .14 | 1.10 | .25 | n.a. | 0 |
| **Summer sausage,** see "Thuringer cervelat" | | | | | | | | |
| **Summer squash,** see specific listings | | | | | | | | |
| **Sunflower seed kernels:** | | | | | | | | |
| dried, 1 oz. . . . . . . . . . . | 14 | 0 | .65 | .07 | 1.28 | n.a. | n.a. | 0 |
| dried, 1 cup. . . . . . . . . . | 72 | 0 | 3.30 | .36 | 6.48 | n.a. | n.a. | 0 |
| dry-roasted, 1 oz. . . . . . . | n.a. | 0 | .03 | .07 | 2.00 | n.a. | n.a. | 0 |
| oil-roasted, 1 oz. . . . . . . . | n.a. | <1 | .09 | .08 | 1.17 | n.a. | n.a. | 0 |
| **Swamp cabbage:** | | | | | | | | |
| raw, untrimmed, 1 lb. . . . | 22,006 | 192 | .11 | .35 | 3.14 | n.a. | n.a. | 0 |
| raw, trimmed, chopped, | | | | | | | | |
|   1 cup . . . . . . . . . . . . . | 3528 | 31 | .02 | .06 | .50 | n.a. | n.a. | 0 |
| boiled, drained, chopped, | | | | | | | | |
|   1 cup . . . . . . . . . . . . . | 5096 | 16 | .02 | .08 | .49 | n.a. | n.a. | 0 |
| **Sweet potato** (see also "Yam"), fresh: | | | | | | | | |
| raw, untrimmed, 1 lb. . . . | 65,526 | 74 | .22 | .48 | 2.20 | .84 | 45.2 | 0 |
| raw, 1 medium, 5" long, | | | | | | | | |
|   6.3 oz. . . . . . . . . . . . . | 26,082 | 30 | .09 | .19 | .88 | .33 | 18.0 | 0 |
| baked in skin, peeled, | | | | | | | | |
|   1 medium, 5" long, | | | | | | | | |
|   4 oz. . . . . . . . . . . . . . . | 24,877 | 28 | .08 | .15 | .69 | .28 | 25.7 | 0 |
| baked in skin, peeled, | | | | | | | | |
|   mashed, ½ cup . . . . . | 21,822 | 25 | .07 | .13 | .60 | .24 | 22.6 | 0 |
| boiled w/out skin, | | | | | | | | |
|   mashed, ½ cup . . . . . | 27,968 | 28 | .09 | .23 | 1.05 | .40 | 18.2 | 0 |
| **Sweet potato, canned:** | | | | | | | | |
| mashed, ½ cup . . . . . . . | 19,268 | 7 | .03 | .12 | 1.22 | n.a. | n.a. | 0 |
| vacuum pack: | | | | | | | | |
|   pieces, 8 oz. . . . . . . . | 18,105 | 60 | .08 | .13 | 1.68 | .43 | 37.7 | 0 |
|   pieces, ½ cup . . . . . . | 7983 | 26 | .04 | .06 | .74 | .19 | 16.6 | 0 |
|   mashed, ½ cup . . . . . | 10,178 | 34 | .05 | .07 | .95 | .24 | 21.2 | 0 |
| syrup pack: | | | | | | | | |
|   w/liquid, 8 oz. . . . . . . | 12,971 | 24 | .05 | .10 | 1.03 | .12 | n.a. | 0 |
|   w/liquid, ½ cup . . . . . | 6520 | 12 | .03 | .05 | .52 | .58 | n.a. | 0 |
|   drained, ½ cup . . . . . | 7014 | 11 | .03 | .04 | .33 | .06 | n.a. | 0 |

| | Vitamin A | Vitamin C | Thiamin | Riboflavin | Niacin | B6 | Folacin | B12 |
|---|---|---|---|---|---|---|---|---|
| | (IU) | (Mg) | (Mg) | (Mg) | (Mg) | (Mg) | (Mcg) | (Mcg) |
| **Sweet potato, frozen,** | | | | | | | | |
| baked, cubes, ½ cup . . . | 14,441 | 8 | .06 | .05 | .49 | .16 | 19.6 | 0 |
| **Sweet potato leaves,** | | | | | | | | |
| trimmed, chopped, | | | | | | | | |
| 1 cup . . . . . . . . . . . . | 360 | 4 | .06 | .12 | .40 | n.a. | n.a. | 0 |
| **Swiss chard,** fresh: | | | | | | | | |
| raw, untrimmed, 1 lb. . . . | 13,771 | 125 | .17 | .38 | 1.67 | n.a. | n.a. | 0 |
| raw, trimmed, chopped, | | | | | | | | |
| ½ cup . . . . . . . . . . . | 594 | 5 | .01 | .02 | .07 | n.a. | n.a. | 0 |
| boiled, drained, ½ cup . . . | 2762 | 16 | .03 | .08 | .32 | n.a. | n.a. | 0 |
| **Swordfish,** meat only: | | | | | | | | |
| raw, 1 lb.. . . . . . . . . . . . | 540 | 5 | .17 | .43 | 43.91 | 1.87 | n.a. | 7.94 |
| baked, broiled, or | | | | | | | | |
| microwaved[1], 4 oz. . . . | 155 | 1 | .05 | .13 | 13.37 | .43 | n.a. | 2.29 |
| **Syrup,** see specific | | | | | | | | |
| listings | | | | | | | | |
| **Syrup, table blends:** | | | | | | | | |
| corn and maple, | | | | | | | | |
| 2 tbsp. . . . . . . . . . . . | 0 | 0 | 0 | 0 | 0 | 0 | 0 | 0 |
| cane and 15% maple, | | | | | | | | |
| 1 tbsp. . . . . . . . . . . . | 0 | 0 | tr. | tr. | tr. | .01 | 0 | 0 |
| corn refiners and sugar, | | | | | | | | |
| 1 tbsp. . . . . . . . . . . . | 0 | 0 | tr. | .01 | tr. | n.a. | 1.0 | 0 |
| pancake, 1 tbsp. . . . . . . | 0 | 0 | n.a. | n.a. | n.a. | 0 | 0 | 0 |
| pancake, w/butter, | | | | | | | | |
| 1 tbsp. . . . . . . . . . . . | 12 | 0 | n.a. | n.a. | n.a. | 0 | 0 | .03 |
| pancake, w/2% maple, | | | | | | | | |
| 1 tbsp. . . . . . . . . . . . | 0 | 0 | tr. | tr. | n.a. | 0 | 0 | 0 |
| pancake, light, 1 oz.. . . . . | 0 | 0 | n.a. | n.a. | n.a. | 0 | 0 | 0 |

---

[1] *Prepared without added ingredients.*

# T

| | Vitamin A | Vitamin C | Thiamin | Riboflavin | Niacin | B₆ | Folacin | B₁₂ |
|---|---|---|---|---|---|---|---|---|
| | (IU) | (Mg) | (Mg) | (Mg) | (Mg) | (Mg) | (Mcg) | (Mcg) |
| **Taco mix,** vegetarian (*Natural Touch*), 3 tbsp., .6 oz. | 122 | 0 | .06 | .03 | 0 | .06 | n.a. | .01 |
| **Tahini,** see "Sesame butter" | | | | | | | | |
| **Tamari sauce,** see "Soy sauce" | | | | | | | | |
| **Tamarind,** fresh: | | | | | | | | |
| untrimmed, 1 lb. | 46 | 5 | .66 | .23 | 2.99 | .10 | n.a. | 0 |
| pulp, ½ cup | 18 | 2 | .26 | .09 | 1.16 | .04 | n.a. | 0 |
| **Tangerine:** | | | | | | | | |
| fresh: | | | | | | | | |
| untrimmed, 1 lb. | 3005 | 101 | .34 | .07 | .52 | .22 | 66.5 | 0 |
| 1 medium, 2⅜" diam., approx. 4 oz. | 773 | 26 | .09 | .02 | .13 | .06 | 17.1 | 0 |
| sections w/out membrane, ½ cup | 897 | 30 | .10 | .02 | .16 | .07 | 19.9 | 0 |
| canned, in juice, ½ cup | 1056 | 43 | .10 | .04 | n.a. | n.a. | n.a. | 0 |
| canned, in light syrup, ½ cup | 1058 | 25 | .07 | .06 | .56 | n.a. | n.a. | 0 |
| **Tangerine juice:** | | | | | | | | |
| fresh, 6 fl. oz. | 780 | 58 | .11 | .04 | .19 | n.a. | n.a. | 0 |
| canned, sweetened, 6 fl. oz. | 786 | 41 | .11 | .04 | .19 | .06 | n.a. | 0 |
| frozen, sweetened, diluted, 6 fl. oz. | 1038 | 44 | .10 | .04 | .17 | .08 | 8.4 | 0 |
| **Tapioca,** pearl, dry, 1 oz. | n.a. | 0 | <.01 | 0 | 0 | <.01 | 1.1 | 0 |
| **Taro:** | | | | | | | | |
| raw, untrimmed, 1 lb. | 0 | 18 | .37 | .10 | 2.34 | n.a. | n.a. | 0 |
| raw, trimmed, sliced, ½ cup | 0 | 2 | .05 | .01 | .31 | n.a. | n.a. | 0 |
| cooked, sliced, ½ cup | 0 | 3 | .07 | .02 | .34 | n.a. | n.a. | 0 |
| **Taro, Tahitian:** | | | | | | | | |
| raw, trimmed, sliced, ½ cup | 1268 | 60 | .04 | .15 | .62 | n.a. | n.a. | 0 |

| | Vitamin A | Vitamin C | Thiamin | Riboflavin | Niacin | B6 | Folacin | B12 |
|---|---|---|---|---|---|---|---|---|
| | (IU) | (Mg) | (Mg) | (Mg) | (Mg) | (Mg) | (Mcg) | (Mcg) |
| **Taro, Tahitian,** *continued* | | | | | | | | |
| cooked, sliced, ½ cup . . . | 1200 | 26 | .03 | .14 | .33 | n.a. | n.a. | 0 |
| **Taro chips:** | | | | | | | | |
| 1 oz. . . . . . . . . . . . . . . . | 0 | 1 | .05 | .01 | .15 | n.a. | n.a. | 0 |
| 10 chips, .8 oz. . . . . . . . . | 0 | 1 | .04 | .01 | .12 | n.a. | n.a. | 0 |
| **Taro leaves:** | | | | | | | | |
| raw, untrimmed, 1 lb. . . . | 13,134 | 142 | .60 | 1.24 | 4.12 | n.a. | n.a. | 0 |
| raw, trimmed, 1 cup . . . . | 1351 | 15 | .06 | .13 | .42 | n.a. | n.a. | 0 |
| steamed, ½ cup. . . . . . . . | 3136 | 26 | .10 | .28 | .94 | n.a. | n.a. | 0 |
| **Taro shoots,** raw, sliced, | | | | | | | | |
| ½ cup. . . . . . . . . . . . . | 22 | 9 | .02 | .02 | .34 | n.a. | n.a. | n.a. |
| **Tarragon,** ground, 1 tsp. | 67 | n.a. | <.01 | .02 | .14 | n.a. | n.a. | 0 |
| **Tartar sauce,** 1 tbsp. . . . . | 30 | tr. | tr. | tr. | 0 | n.a. | n.a. | n.a. |
| **Tea:** | | | | | | | | |
| brewed, 6 fl. oz. . . . . . . . | 0 | 0 | 0 | .03 | 0 | 0 | 9.2 | 0 |
| instant, powder: | | | | | | | | |
| 1 tsp. . . . . . . . . . . . . | 0 | 0 | tr. | .01 | .09 | .01 | .7 | 0 |
| lemon flavor, | | | | | | | | |
| 1 rounded tsp. . . . . | 0 | 0 | 0 | .02 | .09 | n.a. | n.a. | 0 |
| lemon flavor, | | | | | | | | |
| saccharin | | | | | | | | |
| sweetened, 2 tsp. | 0 | 0 | 0 | .01 | .06 | n.a. | 4.6 | 0 |
| lemon flavor, sugar | | | | | | | | |
| sweetened, | | | | | | | | |
| 3 rounded tsp. . . . . | 0 | 0 | 0 | .05 | .09 | n.a. | 9.6 | 0 |
| **Tea, herbal,** brewed: | | | | | | | | |
| all flavors, except | | | | | | | | |
| chamomile, 6 fl. oz. . . . | 0 | 0 | .02 | .01 | 0 | 0 | 1.0 | 0 |
| chamomile, 6 fl. oz. . . . . . | 36 | 0 | .02 | .01 | 0 | 0 | 1.0 | 0 |
| **Tempeh:** | | | | | | | | |
| 1 lb. . . . . . . . . . . . . . . . | 3112 | 0 | .59 | .50 | 21.00 | 1.36 | 235.9 | 3.80 |
| ½ cup. . . . . . . . . . . . . . . | 569 | 0 | .11 | .09 | 3.84 | .25 | 43.2 | 0 |
| **Teriyaki sauce,** 1 tbsp. | 0 | 0 | .01 | .01 | .23 | .02 | 3.6 | 0 |
| **Thirst quencher drink,** | | | | | | | | |
| bottled, 8 fl. oz. . . . . . . | 0 | 0 | .01 | 0 | 0 | 0 | 0 | 0 |

| | Vitamin A | Vitamin C | Thiamin | Riboflavin | Niacin | B6 | Folacin | B12 |
|---|---|---|---|---|---|---|---|---|
| | (IU) | (Mg) | (Mg) | (Mg) | (Mg) | (Mg) | (Mcg) | (Mcg) |
| **Thuringer cervelat[1]**, beef and pork, 1 oz. . . . . . | 0 | 7 | .05 | .09 | 1.16 | .09 | n.a. | 1.31 |
| **Thyme:** | | | | | | | | |
| fresh chopped, 1 tsp. . . . . | 38 | 1 | 0 | tr. | .02 | tr. | 0 | 0 |
| dried, ground, 1 tsp. . . . . | 53 | n.a. | .01 | .01 | .07 | n.a. | n.a. | 0 |
| **Toaster pastry:** | | | | | | | | |
| all flavors (*Kellogg's Pop-Tarts*), 1 piece . . . . . . . | 500 | tr. | .15 | .17 | 2 | .20 | tr. | n.a. |
| brown sugar w/cinnamon, 1.8-oz. piece . . . . . . . . | 493 | n.a. | .19 | .29 | 2.29 | .21 | 40.0 | n.a. |
| fruit, 1.8-oz. piece . . . . . . | 502 | n.a. | .15 | .19 | 2.05 | .20 | 42.0 | n.a. |
| **Tofu,** raw: | | | | | | | | |
| firm: | | | | | | | | |
| 1 lb. . . . . . . . . . . . . . | 753 | 1 | .72 | .46 | 1.73 | .42 | 132.9 | 0 |
| ½ cup . . . . . . . . . . . | 209 | <1 | .20 | .13 | .48 | .12 | 36.9 | 0 |
| (*Azumaya*), 3.5 oz. . . . | n.a. | n.a. | .04 | .03 | .22 | n.a. | n.a. | n.a. |
| extra firm (*Azumaya*), 3.5 oz. . . . . . . . . . . . . | n.a. | <1 | .03 | .03 | .22 | n.a. | n.a. | n.a. |
| regular, 1 lb. . . . . . . . . . | 386 | 1 | .37 | .24 | .89 | .21 | 68.0 | 0 |
| regular, ½ cup. . . . . . . . | 105 | <1 | .10 | .06 | .24 | .06 | 18.6 | 0 |
| soft (*Azumaya*), 3.5 oz. . . . | n.a. | n.a. | .04 | .03 | .28 | n.a. | n.a. | n.a. |
| **Tofu, dried-frozen** (koyadofu), 1 lb. . . . . . | 2351 | 3 | 2.24 | 1.44 | 5.39 | 1.30 | 414.9 | 0 |
| **Tomatillo,** raw: | | | | | | | | |
| untrimmed, 1lb. . . . . . . . . | 515 | 53 | .20 | .16 | 8.39 | .25 | 31.0 | 0 |
| 1 medium, 1.2 oz. . . . . . . | 39 | 4 | .02 | .01 | .63 | .02 | 2.0 | 0 |
| chopped, ½ cup . . . . . . . | 75 | 8 | .03 | .02 | 1.22 | .04 | 4.0 | 0 |
| **Tomato, green:** | | | | | | | | |
| raw, untrimmed, 1 lb. . . . | 2649 | 97 | .25 | .17 | 2.06 | n.a. | n.a. | 0 |
| raw, 1 medium, 2⅗" diam., approx. 4.75 oz. . . . . . . . . . . . | 789 | 29 | .07 | .05 | .62 | n.a. | n.a. | 0 |

[1] With added sodium ascorbate; vitamin C value for product without additives would be negligible.

| | Vitamin A | Vitamin C | Thiamin | Riboflavin | Niacin | B6 | Folacin | B12 |
|---|---|---|---|---|---|---|---|---|
| | (IU) | (Mg) | (Mg) | (Mg) | (Mg) | (Mg) | (Mcg) | (Mcg) |

**Tomato, red**, ripe:
fresh:

| | | | | | | | | |
|---|---|---|---|---|---|---|---|---|
| raw, untrimmed, 1 lb. | 2571 | 79 | .24 | .20 | 2.54 | .33 | 61.0 | 0 |
| raw, 1 medium, 2⅗" diam., approx. 4.75 oz. | 766 | 24 | .07 | .06 | .77 | .10 | 18.0 | 0 |
| raw, chopped, ½ cup | 561 | 17 | .05 | .04 | .57 | .07 | 13.5 | 0 |
| boiled, ½ cup | 892 | 27 | .08 | .07 | .90 | .11 | 16.0 | 0 |

canned (see also "Tomato paste," and "Tomato puree"):

| | | | | | | | | |
|---|---|---|---|---|---|---|---|---|
| whole, 8 oz. | 1370 | 34 | .10 | .07 | 1.67 | .20 | n.a. | 0 |
| whole, ½ cup | 725 | 18 | .05 | .04 | .88 | .11 | n.a. | 0 |
| wedges, in tomato juice, 8 oz. | 1310 | 34 | .13 | .06 | 1.53 | n.a. | n.a. | 0 |
| wedges, in tomato juice, ½ cup | 757 | 19 | .07 | .04 | .88 | n.a. | n.a. | 0 |
| stewed, 8 oz. | 1259 | 30 | .10 | .08 | 1.67 | n.a. | n.a. | 0 |
| stewed, ½ cup | 710 | 17 | .06 | .05 | .91 | n.a. | n.a. | 0 |
| w/green chilies, 8 oz. | 885 | 14 | .07 | .04 | 1.45 | n.a. | n.a. | 0 |
| w/green chilies, ½ cup | 468 | 8 | .04 | .02 | .77 | n.a. | n.a. | 0 |

dried, see "Tomato, sun-dried"

**Tomato, sun-dried:**
plain:

| | | | | | | | | |
|---|---|---|---|---|---|---|---|---|
| 1 lb. | 3966 | 178 | 2.40 | 2.22 | 41.05 | 1.51 | 309.0 | 0 |
| 1 cup, approx. 32 pieces | 472 | 21 | .29 | .26 | 4.89 | .18 | 37.0 | 0 |
| 1 piece, .07 oz. | 17 | 1 | .01 | .01 | .18 | .01 | 1.0 | 0 |

oil-packed, drained:

| | | | | | | | | |
|---|---|---|---|---|---|---|---|---|
| 1 lb. | 5835 | 492 | .88 | 1.74 | 16.47 | 1.45 | 103.0 | 0 |
| 1 cup | 1415 | 112 | .21 | .42 | 4.00 | .35 | 25.0 | 0 |
| 1 piece, .1 oz. | 39 | 3 | .01 | .01 | .11 | .01 | 1.0 | 0 |

**Tomato juice**, canned,

| | | | | | | | | |
|---|---|---|---|---|---|---|---|---|
| 6 fl. oz. | 1012 | 33 | .09 | .06 | 1.23 | .20 | 36.1 | 0 |

**Tomato paste**, canned:

| | | | | | | | | |
|---|---|---|---|---|---|---|---|---|
| 6-oz. can. | 4196 | 72 | .26 | .32 | 5.48 | .64 | n.a. | 0 |
| ½ cup | 3234 | 55 | .20 | .25 | 4.22 | .50 | n.a. | 0 |

| | Vitamin A | Vitamin C | Thiamin | Riboflavin | Niacin | B6 | Folacin | B12 |
|---|---|---|---|---|---|---|---|---|
| | (IU) | (Mg) | (Mg) | (Mg) | (Mg) | (Mg) | (Mcg) | (Mcg) |
| **Tomato puree,** canned: | | | | | | | | |
| 8 oz. | 3087 | 80 | 16 | .12 | 3.89 | .34 | n.a. | 0 |
| ½ cup | 1701 | 44 | .09 | .07 | 2.14 | .19 | n.a. | 0 |
| **Tomato sauce,** canned: | | | | | | | | |
| plain, 8 oz. | 2221 | 30 | .15 | .13 | 2.61 | n.a | n.a. | 0 |
| plain, ½ cup | 1195 | 16 | .08 | .07 | 1.40 | n.a. | n.a. | 0 |
| w/herbs and cheese, 8 oz. | 2240 | 23 | .17 | .28 | 2.74 | n.a. | n.a. | n.a. |
| w/herbs and cheese, ½ cup | 1205 | 12 | .09 | .15 | 1.48 | n.a. | n.a. | n.a. |
| marinara sauce, 8 oz. | 2180 | 29 | .10 | .13 | 3.61 | n.a. | n.a. | 0 |
| marinara sauce, ½ cup | 1202 | 16 | .06 | .07 | 1.99 | n.a. | n.a. | 0 |
| w/mushrooms, 8 oz. | 2165 | 28 | .16 | .25 | 2.87 | n.a. | n.a. | 0 |
| w/mushrooms, ½ cup | 1165 | 15 | .09 | .13 | 1.54 | n.a. | n.a. | 0 |
| w/onions, 8 oz. | 1929 | 29 | .17 | .30 | 2.82 | n.a. | n.a. | 0 |
| w/onions, ½ cup | 1038 | 16 | .09 | .16 | 1.52 | n.a. | n.a. | 0 |
| w/onions, green peppers, and celery, 8 oz. | 1837 | 30 | .15 | .27 | 2.48 | n.a. | n.a. | 0 |
| w/onions, green peppers, and celery, ½ cup | 988 | 16 | .08 | .15 | 1.34 | n.a. | n.a. | 0 |
| spaghetti or pasta sauce: | | | | | | | | |
| 15.5-oz. jar | 5387 | 49 | .24 | .26 | 6.61 | n.a. | n.a. | 0 |
| 8 oz. | 2783 | 25 | .12 | .13 | 3.41 | n.a. | n.a. | 0 |
| ½ cup | 1528 | 14 | .07 | .07 | 1.87 | n.a. | n.a. | 0 |
| Spanish style, 8 oz. | 2234 | 20 | .17 | .14 | 2.93 | n.a. | n.a. | 0 |
| Spanish style, ½ cup | 1202 | 11 | .09 | .08 | 1.58 | n.a. | n.a. | 0 |
| w/tomato tidbits, 8 oz. | 1816 | 49 | .17 | .22 | 2.68 | n.a. | n.a. | 0 |
| w/tomato tidbits, ½ cup | 977 | 26 | .09 | .12 | 1.44 | n.a. | n.a. | 0 |
| **Tomato-beef cocktail,** canned, 6 fl. oz. | 234 | 2 | tr. | .05 | .30 | n.a. | n.a. | n.a. |
| **Tongue**[1]: | | | | | | | | |
| beef, simmered, 4 oz. | n.a. | 1 | .03 | .40 | 2.44 | .18 | 5.7 | 6.69 |

[1] *Prepared without added ingredients.*

| | Vitamin A | Vitamin C | Thiamin | Riboflavin | Niacin | B6 | Folacin | B12 |
|---|---|---|---|---|---|---|---|---|
| | (IU) | (Mg) | (Mg) | (Mg) | (Mg) | (Mg) | (Mcg) | (Mcg) |
| Tongue, *continued* | | | | | | | | |
| lamb, braised, 4 oz. . . . . . | 0 | 8 | .09 | .48 | 4.18 | .19 | 3.4 | 7.14 |
| pork, braised, 4 oz. . . . . . | 0 | 2 | .36 | .58 | 6.06 | .26 | n.a. | 2.71 |
| veal, braised, 4 oz. . . . . . . | 0 | 7 | .08 | .40 | 1.67 | .17 | 10.2 | 6.01 |
| **Toppings,** dessert, see specific listings | | | | | | | | |
| **Tortilla,** ready-to-bake or -fry: | | | | | | | | |
| corn, 7"-diam. piece, | | | | | | | | |
| .9 oz. . . . . . . . . . . . . | n.a. | 0 | .03 | .02 | .37 | .06 | 4.0 | 0 |
| flour, 8"-diam. piece, | | | | | | | | |
| 1.2 oz. . . . . . . . . . . . | 0 | 0 | .19 | .10 | 1.25 | .02 | 4.0 | 0 |
| **Tortilla chips:** | | | | | | | | |
| (*Buenitos* Regular/No Salt | | | | | | | | |
| Added), 1 oz. . . . . . . . | 109 | 2 | .08 | .02 | .42 | .05 | 5.2 | 0 |
| plain, 1 oz. . . . . . . . . . . | 56 | 0 | .02 | .05 | .36 | .08 | n.a. | 0 |
| nacho flavor, 1 oz. . . . . . . | 105 | 1 | .04 | .05 | .41 | .08 | 4.0 | n.a. |
| nacho flavor, light, | | | | | | | | |
| 1 oz. . . . . . . . . . . . . . | 108 | tr. | .06 | .08 | .12 | n.a. | n.a. | n.a. |
| ranch flavor, 1 oz. . . . . . . | 73 | tr. | .03 | .07 | .41 | n.a. | n.a. | 0 |
| taco flavor, 1 oz. . . . . . . . | 257 | n.a. | .07 | .06 | .57 | .08 | n.a. | 0 |
| **Tortilla flour mix,** see "Wheat flour" | | | | | | | | |
| **Trail mix,** regular, 1 oz. | 5 | tr. | .13 | .06 | 1.3 | .08 | 20.0 | 0 |
| **Tree fern,** cooked, | | | | | | | | |
| chopped, ½ cup . . . . . | 142 | 21 | 0 | .21 | 2.49 | n.a. | n.a | 0 |
| **Tripe,** beef, raw, 1 oz. . . . | 0 | 1 | <.01 | .05 | .02 | n.a. | .6 | .44 |
| **Triticale,** whole grain, | | | | | | | | |
| 1 cup . . . . . . . . . . . . | n.a. | 0 | .80 | .26 | 2.75 | .27 | 140.0 | 0 |
| **Triticale flour,** whole | | | | | | | | |
| grain, 1 cup. . . . . . . . | n.a. | 0 | .49 | .17 | 3.72 | .52 | 96.0 | 0 |
| **Trout,** meat only: | | | | | | | | |
| mixed species: | | | | | | | | |
| raw, 1 lb. . . . . . . . . | 263 | 2 | 1.59 | 1.50 | n.a. | n.a. | 60.0 | 35.34 |
| baked, broiled, or | | | | | | | | |
| microwaved[1], 4 oz. . . . | 71 | 1 | .48 | .48 | n.a. | n.a. | 17.0 | 8.49 |

---

[1] *Prepared without added ingredients.*

| | Vitamin A | Vitamin C | Thiamin | Riboflavin | Niacin | B6 | Folacin | B12 |
|---|---|---|---|---|---|---|---|---|
| | (IU) | (Mg) | (Mg) | (Mg) | (Mg) | (Mg) | (Mcg) | (Mcg) |
| rainbow: | | | | | | | | |
|   wild, raw, 1 lb. ..... | 282 | 11 | .56 | .48 | 24.42 | 1.84 | 53.0 | 20.20 |
|   wild, baked, broiled, or microwaved[1], 4 oz. .......... | 57 | 2 | .17 | .11 | 6.54 | .39 | 21.5 | 7.14 |
|   farmed, raw, 1 lb. .... | 1263 | 13 | .92 | .33 | 37.33 | 2.81 | 50.0 | 17.09 |
|   farmed, baked, broiled, or microwaved[1], 4 oz. | 325 | 4 | .27 | .91 | 9.97 | .45 | 27.2 | 5.64 |
| **Tuna,** meat only: | | | | | | | | |
| bluefin: | | | | | | | | |
|   raw, 1 lb.. ......... | 9905 | (0) | 1.09 | 1.34 | 39.26 | 2.06 | n.a. | 42.77 |
|   baked, broiled, or microwaved[1], 4 oz. | 2858 | (0) | .32 | .35 | 11.95 | .60 | n.a. | 12.34 |
| skipjack: | | | | | | | | |
|   raw, 1 lb.. ......... | 236 | (0) | .15 | n.a. | n.a. | 3.86 | n.a. | n.a. |
|   baked, broiled, or microwaved[1], 4 oz. | 68 | (0) | .04 | n.a. | n.a. | 1.11 | n.a. | n.a. |
| yellowfin: | | | | | | | | |
|   raw, 1 lb.. ......... | 268 | (0) | 1.97 | .21 | 44.43 | n.a. | n.a. | n.a. |
|   baked, broiled, or microwaved[1], 4 oz. | 77 | (0) | .57 | .06 | 13.54 | n.a. | n.a. | n.a. |
| **Tuna,** canned: | | | | | | | | |
| in soybean oil, drained: | | | | | | | | |
|   light, 4 oz.. ........ | 88 | (0) | .04 | n.a. | n.a. | .12 | 6.0 | n.a. |
|   light, yield from 6¼-oz. can ...... | 134 | (0) | .07 | n.a. | n.a. | .19 | 9.0 | n.a. |
|   white, 4 oz. ........ | n.a. | (0) | .02 | .09 | 13.27 | n.a. | 5.2 | n.a. |
| white, yield from 6¼-oz. can ............... | n.a. | (0) | .03 | .14 | 20.82 | n.a. | 8.1 | n.a. |
| in water, drained: | | | | | | | | |
|   light, 4 oz. ......... | 64 | 0 | .04 | .08 | 15.06 | .40 | 4.5 | 3.39 |
|   light, yield from 6¼ oz.-can ...... | 92 | 0 | .05 | .12 | 21.91 | .58 | 6.0 | 4.93 |

---

[1] *Prepared without added ingredients.*

|  | Vitamin A | Vitamin C | Thiamin | Riboflavin | Niacin | B6 | Folacin | B12 |
|---|---|---|---|---|---|---|---|---|
|  | (IU) | (Mg) | (Mg) | (Mg) | (Mg) | (Mg) | (Mcg) | (Mcg) |
| **Tuna**, canned, in water, drained, *continued* |  |  |  |  |  |  |  |  |
| white, 4 oz. . . . . . . . | 22 | 0 | .01 | .05 | 6.58 | .25 | 2.3 | 1.33 |
| white, yield from |  |  |  |  |  |  |  |  |
| 6¼-oz. can . . . . . . | 33 | 0 | .01 | .08 | 9.97 | .37 | 3.0 | 2.01 |
| **"Tuna," vegetarian,** |  |  |  |  |  |  |  |  |
| frozen, ½ cup drained |  |  |  |  |  |  |  |  |
| (*Worthington Tuno*), |  |  |  |  |  |  |  |  |
| 2 oz. . . . . . . . . . . . . | 0 | 0 | .14 | .04 | 1.23 | .32 | n.a. | 1.99 |
| **Turbot,** European, meat only: |  |  |  |  |  |  |  |  |
| raw, 1 lb. . . . . . . . . . . . | 159 | (0) | .30 | .36 | 9.98 | n.a. | n.a. | 9.98 |
| baked, broiled, or |  |  |  |  |  |  |  |  |
| microwaved[1], 4 oz. . . . | 45 | (0) | .09 | .11 | 3.04 | n.a. | n.a. | n.a. |
| **Turkey,** all classes, roasted[1], 4 oz., except as noted: |  |  |  |  |  |  |  |  |
| meat w/skin . . . . . . . . . . | 0 | 0 | .06 | .20 | 5.77 | .46 | 7.9 | .40 |
| meat only . . . . . . . . . . . | 0 | 0 | .07 | .21 | 6.17 | .52 | 7.9 | .42 |
| skin only, 1 oz. . . . . . . . | 0 | 0 | .01 | .04 | .75 | .02 | 1.1 | .07 |
| dark meat w/skin . . . . . . | 0 | 0 | .07 | .27 | 4.00 | .36 | 10.2 | .41 |
| light meat w/skin . . . . . . | 0 | 0 | .06 | .15 | 7.13 | .53 | 6.8 | .40 |
| back, meat w/skin . . . . . . | 0 | 0 | .06 | .25 | 3.91 | .34 | 9.1 | .39 |
| breast, meat w/skin . . . . . | 0 | 0 | .06 | .15 | 7.22 | .72 | 6.8 | .41 |
| leg, meat w/skin . . . . . . . | 0 | 0 | .07 | .27 | 4.04 | .37 | 10.2 | .41 |
| wing, meat w/skin . . . . . . | 0 | 0 | .06 | .15 | 6.50 | .48 | 6.8 | .39 |
| **Turkey, canned,** boned, |  |  |  |  |  |  |  |  |
| w/broth, 5-oz. can . . . . | 0 | 3 | .02 | .24 | 9.40 | n.a. | n.a. | n.a. |
| **Turkey, frozen or** |  |  |  |  |  |  |  |  |
| **refrigerated**, prebasted |  |  |  |  |  |  |  |  |
| w/broth, breast meat |  |  |  |  |  |  |  |  |
| w/skin, roasted, 4 oz. | 0 | 0 | .06 | .15 | 10.28 | .36 | n.a. | .36 |
| **Turkey, ground:** |  |  |  |  |  |  |  |  |
| raw, 4 oz. . . . . . . . . . | 6 | 0 | .06 | .15 | 3.98 | .40 | 8.0 | .39 |
| cooked, 4 oz. . . . . . . . . . | 0 | 0 | .04 | .14 | 3.95 | .32 | 5.0 | .27 |
| **"Turkey," vegetarian:** |  |  |  |  |  |  |  |  |
| canned (*Worthington* |  |  |  |  |  |  |  |  |
| *Turkee*), 3 slices, |  |  |  |  |  |  |  |  |
| 3.3 oz. . . . . . . . . . . . . | 0 | 0 | 3.21 | .14 | 1.10 | .24 | n.a. | 1.67 |

---

[1] *Prepared without added ingredients.*

| | Vitamin A | Vitamin C | Thiamin | Riboflavin | Niacin | B6 | Folacin | B12 |
|---|---|---|---|---|---|---|---|---|
| | (IU) | (Mg) | (Mg) | (Mg) | (Mg) | (Mg) | (Mcg) | (Mcg) |
| frozen, smoked (*Worthington*), 3 slices, 2 oz. . . . . . . . . . . . . . . | 0 | 0 | 10.18 | .16 | 2.00 | .29 | n.a. | 2.09 |
| **Turkey entree,** frozen, gravy and, 5-oz. pkg. | 59 | n.a. | .03 | .18 | 2.56 | .14 | n.a. | n.a. |
| **Turkey giblets,** simmered[1], 4 oz. . . . . . . | 6845 | 2 | .05 | 1.03 | 5.11 | .37 | 391.2 | 27.30 |
| **Turkey gizzard,** simmered[1], 4 oz. . . . . . | 210 | 2 | .04 | .37 | 3.48 | .14 | 59.0 | 2.20 |
| **Turkey heart,** see "Heart" | | | | | | | | |
| **Turkey liver,** see "Liver" | | | | | | | | |
| **Turkey luncheon meat,** breast, 1 oz. . . . . . . . . | 0 | 0 | .01 | .03 | 2.36 | .11 | n.a. | .57 |
| **Turmeric,** ground, 1 tsp. | n.a. | 1 | tr. | .01 | .11 | n.a. | n.a. | 0 |
| **Turnip,** fresh: | | | | | | | | |
| raw, untrimmed, 1 lb. . . . | 0 | 77 | .15 | .11 | 1.47 | .33 | 53.4 | 0 |
| raw, trimmed, cubed, ½ cup . . . . . . . . . . . . | 0 | 14 | .03 | .02 | .26 | .06 | 9.5 | 0 |
| boiled, drained, cubed, ½ cup . . . . . . . . . . . . | 0 | 9 | .02 | .02 | .23 | .05 | 7.1 | 0 |
| boiled, drained, mashed, ½ cup . . . . . . . . . . . . | 0 | 13 | .03 | .03 | .34 | .08 | 10.5 | 0 |
| frozen, mashed, 10-oz. pkg. . . . . . . . . | 74 | 13 | .09 | .06 | 1.14 | n.a. | n.a. | 0 |
| **Turnip greens:** | | | | | | | | |
| fresh: | | | | | | | | |
| raw, untrimmed, 1 lb. . . . . . . . . . . | 24,130 | 191 | .22 | .32 | 1.91 | .84 | 617.3 | 0 |
| raw, trimmed, chopped, ½ cup . . | 2128 | 17 | .02 | .03 | .17 | .07 | 54.4 | 0 |
| boiled, drained, chopped, ½ cup . . | 3959 | 20 | .03 | .05 | .30 | .30 | 85.3 | 0 |
| canned, w/liquid, ½ cup . . . . . . . . . . . . | 4196 | 18 | .01 | .07 | .42 | .42 | 48.2 | 0 |

---

[1] *Prepared without added ingredients.*

| | Vitamin A | Vitamin C | Thiamin | Riboflavin | Niacin | B6 | Folacin | B12 |
|---|---|---|---|---|---|---|---|---|
| | (IU) | (Mg) | (Mg) | (Mg) | (Mg) | (Mg) | (Mcg) | (Mcg) |

Turnip greens, *continued*
frozen, chopped:

| | | | | | | | | |
|---|---|---|---|---|---|---|---|---|
| 10-oz. pkg. . . . . . . . | 17,564 | 76 | .13 | 26 | 1.09 | .28 | 209.1 | 0 |
| boiled, drained, ⅓ of | | | | | | | | |
| 10-oz. pkg. . . . . . . | 5849 | 16 | .04 | .05 | .34 | .05 | 28.9 | 0 |
| boiled, drained, | | | | | | | | |
| ½ cup . . . . . . . . . | 6540 | 18 | .04 | .06 | .38 | .38 | 32.3 | 0 |
| frozen, w/turnips, | | | | | | | | |
| 10-oz. pkg. . . . . . . . | 17,345 | 73 | .13 | .25 | 1.10 | n.a. | n.a. | 0 |

# V

| | Vitamin A | Vitamin C | Thiamin | Riboflavin | Niacin | B6 | Folacin | B12 |
|---|---|---|---|---|---|---|---|---|
| | (IU) | (Mg) | (Mg) | (Mg) | (Mg) | (Mg) | (Mcg) | (Mcg) |
| **Vanilla extract:** | | | | | | | | |
| real, 1 tsp.............. | 0 | 0 | 0 | tr. | .02 | tr. | 0 | 0 |
| real (*Virginia Dare*), | | | | | | | | |
| 1 tsp. .............. | 0 | 0 | 0 | 0 | 0 | 0 | 0 | 0 |
| imitation, 1 tsp......... | 0 | 0 | 0 | tr. | .01 | tr. | 0 | 0 |
| **Vanilla flavor drink mix** | | | | | | | | |
| (*Carnation Instant* | | | | | | | | |
| *Breakfast*), 1 pkt...... | 1750 | 27 | .30 | .17 | 5.00 | .40 | 100.0 | .60 |
| **Veal**[1], meat only, 4 oz.: | | | | | | | | |
| cubed, for stew, leg and | | | | | | | | |
| shoulder, braised, lean | | | | | | | | |
| only. . . . . . . . . . . . . | 0 | 0 | .08 | .45 | 9.41 | .43 | 18.1 | 1.89 |
| ground, broiled . . . . . . . . | 0 | 0 | .08 | .31 | 9.11 | .44 | 12.5 | 1.44 |
| leg (top round): | | | | | | | | |
| braised, lean w/fat . . . | 0 | 0 | .07 | .40 | 11.98 | .41 | 20.4 | 1.33 |
| braised, lean only. . . . | 0 | 0 | .07 | .41 | 12.16 | .42 | 20.4 | 1.35 |
| pan-fried in vegetable | | | | | | | | |
| oil, lean w/fat. . . . . | 0 | 0 | .07 | .36 | 11.26 | .35 | 18.1 | 1.33 |
| pan-fried in vegetable | | | | | | | | |
| oil, lean only . . . . . | 0 | 0 | .07 | .37 | 11.43 | .35 | 18.1 | 1.34 |
| roasted, lean w/fat . . . | 0 | 0 | .08 | .40 | 13.66 | .56 | 17.0 | 1.64 |
| roasted, lean only . . . | 0 | 0 | .08 | .42 | 14.33 | .58 | 18.1 | 1.71 |
| loin: | | | | | | | | |
| braised, lean w/fat . . . | 0 | 0 | .05 | .34 | 10.24 | .29 | 15.9 | 1.37 |
| braised, lean only. . . . | 0 | 0 | .06 | .39 | 11.40 | .32 | 17.0 | 1.50 |
| roasted, lean w/fat . . . | 0 | 0 | .06 | .32 | 10.05 | .39 | 17.0 | 1.41 |
| roasted, lean only . . . | 0 | 0 | .07 | .34 | 10.73 | .42 | 18.1 | 1.49 |
| rib: | | | | | | | | |
| braised, lean w/fat . . . | 0 | 0 | .06 | .33 | 8.51 | .36 | 18.1 | 1.64 |
| braised, lean only. . . . | 0 | 0 | .07 | .35 | 8.97 | .39 | 18.1 | 1.74 |
| roasted, lean w/fat . . . | 0 | 0 | .06 | .31 | 7.92 | .28 | 14.7 | 1.66 |
| roasted, lean only . . . | 0 | 0 | .07 | .33 | 8.51 | .31 | 15.9 | 1.79 |

[1] *Prepared without added ingredients, except as noted.*

| | Vitamin A | Vitamin C | Thiamin | Riboflavin | Niacin | B6 | Folacin | B12 |
|---|---|---|---|---|---|---|---|---|
| | (IU) | (Mg) | (Mg) | (Mg) | (Mg) | (Mg) | (Mcg) | (Mcg) |
| **Veal,** _continued_ | | | | | | | | |
| shoulder, whole: | | | | | | | | |
| braised, lean w/fat ... | 0 | 0 | .07 | .39 | 7.28 | .28 | 17.0 | 2.09 |
| braised, lean only.... | 0 | 0 | .07 | .40 | 7.58 | .29 | 18.1 | 2.20 |
| roasted, lean w/fat ... | 0 | 0 | .08 | .39 | 7.18 | .29 | 13.6 | 2.06 |
| roasted, lean only ... | 0 | 0 | .08 | .39 | 7.30 | .29 | 14.7 | 2.11 |
| shoulder, arm: | | | | | | | | |
| braised, lean w/fat ... | 0 | 0 | .07 | .35 | 11.43 | .33 | 20.4 | 1.95 |
| braised, lean only.... | 0 | 0 | .07 | .37 | 12.15 | .34 | 21.5 | 2.06 |
| roasted, lean w/fat ... | 0 | 0 | .07 | .36 | 9.09 | .33 | 19.3 | 1.74 |
| roasted, lean only ... | 0 | 0 | .08 | .37 | 9.34 | .34 | 19.3 | 1.78 |
| shoulder, blade: | | | | | | | | |
| braised, lean w/fat ... | 0 | 0 | .07 | .40 | 6.24 | .27 | 17.0 | 2.19 |
| braised, lean only.... | 0 | 0 | .07 | .41 | 6.44 | .28 | 17.0 | 2.28 |
| roasted, lean w/fat ... | 0 | 0 | .08 | .40 | 6.50 | .27 | 12.5 | 2.28 |
| roasted, lean only ... | 0 | 0 | .08 | .41 | 6.60 | .27 | 12.5 | 2.34 |
| sirloin: | | | | | | | | |
| braised, lean w/fat ... | 0 | 0 | .06 | .40 | 7.46 | .40 | 17.0 | 1.68 |
| braised, lean only.... | 0 | 0 | .07 | .43 | 7.99 | .43 | 18.1 | 1.80 |
| roasted, lean w/fat ... | 0 | 0 | .07 | .40 | 10.06 | .36 | 17.0 | 1.61 |
| roasted, lean only ... | 0 | 0 | .07 | .42 | 10.58 | .39 | 18.1 | 1.69 |
| **"Veal," vegetarian,** frozen (_Worthington Veelets_), 2.5-oz. patty | 0 | 0 | 1.79 | .17 | 1.60 | .33 | n.a. | 2.98 |
| **Vegetable juice cocktail,** canned, 6 fl. oz........ | 2130 | 50 | .08 | .05 | 1.32 | .26 | n.a. | 0 |
| **Vegetables,** see specific listings | | | | | | | | |
| **Vegetables, mixed:** | | | | | | | | |
| canned, w/liquid, ½ cup............. | 6199 | 5 | .04 | .05 | .59 | .09 | 21.9 | 0 |
| canned, drained, ½ cup............. | 9551 | 4 | .04 | .04 | .47 | .07 | 19.4 | 0 |
| frozen[1]: 10-oz. pkg. .........14,421 | | 30 | .35 | .24 | 3.58 | .27 | 83.0 | 0 |

[1]Includes corn, lima beans, snap beans, green peas, and carrots.

| | Vitamin A | Vitamin C | Thiamin | Riboflavin | Niacin | B6 | Folacin | B12 |
|---|---|---|---|---|---|---|---|---|
| | (IU) | (Mg) | (Mg) | (Mg) | (Mg) | (Mg) | (Mcg) | (Mcg) |
| boiled, drained, ⅓ of 10-oz. pkg. . . . . . | 3920 | 3 | .07 | .11 | .78 | .07 | 17.4 | 0 |
| boiled, drained, ½ cup . . . . . . . . . | 3892 | 3 | .07 | .11 | .77 | .07 | 17.3 | 0 |
| **Vegetarian entree** (see also " 'Beef,' vegetarian" and other specific listings): | | | | | | | | |
| frozen: | | | | | | | | |
| (*Natural Touch* Dinner Entree), 3-oz. patty . . . . . . . | 0 | 0 | 0 | .19 | 0 | .01 | n.a. | 0 |
| lentil-rice loaf (*Natural Touch*), 3.2-oz. slice . . | 775 | 0 | .05 | .12 | 0 | .03 | n.a. | .07 |
| nine-bean loaf (*Natural Touch*), 1" slice, 3 oz. | 1509 | 1 | .06 | .11 | 0 | n.a. | n.a. | n.a. |
| mix, loaf (*Natural Touch*), 4 tbsp., 1.1 oz. . . . . . . | 0 | 0 | .10 | .15 | 0 | .01 | n.a. | .56 |
| mix, savory dinner loaf (*Loma Linda*), ⅓ cup, .9 oz.. . . . . . . . . . . . . | 0 | 0 | .45 | .05 | 2.30 | .39 | n.a. | 2.33 |
| **Vienna sausage,** canned, beef and pork, 1 oz.. . . | 0 | 0 | .02 | .03 | .46 | .03 | n.a. | .29 |
| **Vinegar,** cider, 1 tbsp.. . . | 0 | 0 | 0 | 0 | 0 | n.a. | n.a. | 0 |

# W

| | Vitamin A | Vitamin C | Thiamin | Riboflavin | Niacin | B6 | Folacin | B12 |
|---|---|---|---|---|---|---|---|---|
| | (IU) | (Mg) | (Mg) | (Mg) | (Mg) | (Mg) | (Mcg) | (Mcg) |
| **Waffle,** frozen: | | | | | | | | |
| plain, 1.2 oz.......... | 448 | 0 | .16 | .18 | 1.64 | .33 | 17.0 | .83 |
| plain, toasted, 1.2 oz..... | 400 | 0 | .13 | .16 | 1.46 | .30 | 12.0 | .83 |
| all flavors (*Eggo*), | | | | | | | | |
| 1 piece ............ | 500 | 0 | .15 | .17 | 2.0 | .20 | tr. | n.a. |
| **Wakame,** see "Seaweed" | | | | | | | | |
| **Walnut:** | | | | | | | | |
| black, dried: | | | | | | | | |
| in shell, 1 lb........ | 322 | n.a. | 2.36 | .12 | .75 | n.a. | n.a. | 0 |
| shelled, 1 oz........ | 1.03 | n.a. | .06 | .03 | 20 | n.a. | n.a. | 0 |
| shelled, chopped, | | | | | | | | |
| 1 cup ............ | 4.54 | n.a. | .27 | .14 | .86 | n.a. | n.a. | 0 |
| English or Persian, dried: | | | | | | | | |
| in shell, 1 lb........ | 252 | 7 | .78 | .31 | 2.13 | 1.29 | 134.7 | 0 |
| shelled, 1 oz........ | 35 | 1 | .11 | .04 | .30 | .18 | 18.7 | 0 |
| shelled, pieces or | | | | | | | | |
| chips, 1 cup ..... | 148 | 4 | .46 | .18 | 1.25 | .76 | 79.2 | 0 |
| **Water chestnuts,** | | | | | | | | |
| Chinese: | | | | | | | | |
| raw, sliced, ½ cup...... | 0 | 3 | .09 | .12 | .62 | n.a. | n.a. | 0 |
| canned, 4 medium, | | | | | | | | |
| 1 oz.............. | 0 | 1 | .05 | .07 | .36 | n.a. | n.a. | 0 |
| canned, w/liquid, sliced, | | | | | | | | |
| ½ cup............ | 3 | 1 | .01 | .02 | .25 | n.a. | n.a. | 0 |
| **Watercress,** raw: | | | | | | | | |
| untrimmed, 1 lb........ | 19,613 | 179 | .38 | .50 | .84 | .54 | n.a. | 0 |
| trimmed, chopped, | | | | | | | | |
| ½ cup............ | 799 | 7 | .02 | .02 | .03 | .02 | n.a. | 0 |
| **Watermelon:** | | | | | | | | |
| untrimmed, 1 lb........ | 862 | 23 | .19 | .05 | .47 | .34 | 5.1 | 0 |
| ¹⁄₁₆ of 10"-diam. melon, | | | | | | | | |
| 1"-thick slice, about | | | | | | | | |
| 2 lbs. w/rind ........ | 1762 | 47 | .39 | .10 | .96 | .69 | 10.4 | 0 |

| | Vitamin A | Vitamin C | Thiamin | Riboflavin | Niacin | B6 | Folacin | B12 |
|---|---|---|---|---|---|---|---|---|
| | (IU) | (Mg) | (Mg) | (Mg) | (Mg) | (Mg) | (Mcg) | (Mcg) |
| pulp, diced, ½ cup ..... | 293 | 8 | .06 | .02 | .16 | .12 | 1.7 | 0 |
| **Watermelon seed kernels:** | | | | | | | | |
| dried, 1 oz. ........... | 0 | 0 | .05 | .04 | 1.01 | n.a. | 16.4 | 0 |
| dried, 1 cup ........... | 0 | 0 | .21 | .16 | 3.83 | n.a. | 62.6 | 0 |
| **Waxgourd:** | | | | | | | | |
| raw, untrimmed, 1 lb. .... | 0 | 42 | .13 | .35 | 1.29 | n.a. | n.a. | 0 |
| raw, trimmed, cubed, | | | | | | | | |
| ½ cup ............. | 0 | 17 | .05 | .15 | .53 | n.a. | n.a. | 0 |
| boiled, drained, cubed, | | | | | | | | |
| ½ cup ............. | 0 | 18 | .06 | tr. | .67 | n.a. | n.a. | 0 |
| **Wheat, whole grain:** | | | | | | | | |
| durum, 1 cup ......... | (0) | 0 | .81 | .23 | 12.94 | .81 | n.a. | 0 |
| hard red spring, 1 cup ... | (0) | 0 | .97 | .21 | 10.96 | .64 | 83.0 | 0 |
| hard red winter, 1 cup ... | (0) | 0 | .74 | .22 | 10.49 | .58 | 72.0 | 0 |
| soft red winter, 1 cup ... | (0) | 0 | .66 | .16 | 8.06 | .46 | 68.0 | 0 |
| hard white, 1 cup ...... | (0) | 0 | .74 | .21 | 8.41 | .71 | n.a. | 0 |
| soft white, 1 cup ...... | (0) | 0 | .69 | .18 | 8.01 | .63 | n.a. | 0 |
| **Wheat, sprouted,** 1 cup | (0) | 3 | .24 | .17 | 3.33 | .29 | n.a. | 0 |
| **Wheat bran** (see also "Cereal, ready-to-eat"): | | | | | | | | |
| unprocessed, 2 tbsp..... | 0 | 0 | .04 | .03 | 1.54 | .04 | 9.0 | 0 |
| crude, 1 cup ......... | (0) | 0 | .31 | .35 | 8.15 | .78 | 48.0 | 0 |
| **Wheat flour:** | | | | | | | | |
| whole grain, 1 cup...... | (0) | 0 | .54 | .26 | 7.64 | .41 | 52.0 | 0 |
| white, enriched: | | | | | | | | |
| all-purpose, 1 cup ... | (0) | 0 | .98 | .62 | 7.38 | .06 | 33.0 | 0 |
| bread, 1 cup ....... | (0) | 0 | 1.11 | .70 | 10.35 | .05 | 40.0 | 0 |
| cake, 1 cup ........ | (0) | 0 | .97 | .47 | 7.40 | .04 | 21.0 | 0 |
| self-rising, 1 cup .... | (0) | 0 | .84 | .52 | 7.29 | .06 | 53.0 | 0 |
| tortilla mix, 1 cup ... | (0) | 0 | .82 | .55 | 6.46 | .04 | n.a. | 0 |
| **Wheat germ:** | | | | | | | | |
| (*Kretschmer*), 1 oz. or | | | | | | | | |
| ¼ cup ............. | 33 | 0 | .48 | .21 | 1.41 | .16 | 106.0 | .05 |
| crude, 1 oz. ........ | (0) | 0 | .53 | .14 | 1.93 | .37 | 79.7 | 0 |
| toasted, 1 oz., | | | | | | | | |
| approx. ¼ cup .... | (0) | 2 | .47 | .23 | 1.59 | .28 | 100.0 | 0 |

| | Vitamin A | Vitamin C | Thiamin | Riboflavin | Niacin | B6 | Folacin | B12 |
|---|---|---|---|---|---|---|---|---|
| | (IU) | (Mg) | (Mg) | (Mg) | (Mg) | (Mg) | (Mcg) | (Mcg) |
| **Wheat grass** (*Pines Instant Vegetable Nutrition*), 3 tsp. or 21 tablets .......... | 5005 | 32 | .03 | .20 | .75 | .13 | 109.0 | 3.00 |
| **Whelk,** unspecified, meat only: | | | | | | | | |
| raw, 1 lb.............. | 733 | (0) | .22 | .97 | 9.05 | 2.95 | 51.6 | 82.28 |
| boiled, poached, or steamed[1], 4 oz. ...... | 184 | (0) | .06 | .24 | 2.26 | .74 | 12.9 | 20.57 |
| **Whey:** | | | | | | | | |
| acid, fluid, 1 cup ....... | 17 | <1 | .10 | .34 | .19 | .10 | 5.0 | .44 |
| acid, dry, 1 oz. ......... | 16 | <1 | .18 | .58 | .32 | .18 | 9.4 | .71 |
| sweet, fluid, 1 cup ...... | 39 | <1 | .09 | .39 | .18 | .08 | 2.0 | .68 |
| sweet, dry, 1 oz. ........ | 12 | <1 | .15 | .63 | .36 | .17 | 3.4 | .67 |
| **Whiskey sour mix,** bottled, 1 fl. oz....... | 7 | 1 | <.01 | <.01 | 0 | 0 | 0 | 0 |
| **White beans,** dried: | | | | | | | | |
| regular: | | | | | | | | |
| uncooked, 1 lb. ........ | 0 | 0 | 1.98 | .66 | 2.17 | 1.44 | 1758.9 | 0 |
| uncooked, ½ cup.... | 0 | 0 | .44 | .15 | .48 | .32 | 391.6 | 0 |
| boiled, ½ cup ...... | 0 | 0 | .11 | .04 | .13 | .08 | 72.7 | 0 |
| canned, w/liquid, 8 oz............. | 0 | 0 | .22 | .08 | .26 | .17 | 148.3 | 0 |
| canned, w/liquid, ½ cup .......... | 0 | 0 | .13 | .05 | .15 | .10 | 85.6 | 0 |
| small: | | | | | | | | |
| uncooked, 1 lb. ...... | 0 | 0 | 3.37 | .94 | 6.09 | 1.99 | 1751.3 | 0 |
| uncooked, ½ cup.... | 0 | 0 | .80 | .22 | 1.45 | .47 | 417.0 | 0 |
| boiled, ½ cup ...... | 0 | 0 | .21 | .05 | .25 | .11 | 123.2 | 0 |
| **Whitefish,** mixed species, smoked, 4 oz. ........ | 215 | (0) | .04 | .11 | 2.72 | .44 | 8.3 | 3.70 |
| **Whiting,** mixed species, meat only: | | | | | | | | |
| raw, lb................ | 450 | (0) | .25 | .21 | 5.90 | .71 | 59.0 | 10.43 |

---

[1] *Prepared without added ingredients.*

| | Vitamin A | Vitamin C | Thiamin | Riboflavin | Niacin | B6 | Folacin | B12 |
|---|---|---|---|---|---|---|---|---|
| | (IU) | (Mg) | (Mg) | (Mg) | (Mg) | (Mg) | (Mcg) | (Mcg) |
| baked, broiled, or | | | | | | | | |
| microwaved[1], 4 oz. . . . | 129 | 0 | .08 | .07 | 1.89 | .20 | 17.0 | 2.95 |
| **Wild rice:** | | | | | | | | |
| uncooked, ½ cup. . . . . . . | 15 | 0 | .09 | .21 | 5.39 | .31 | 76.0 | 0 |
| cooked, ½ cup . . . . . . . . | 0 | 0 | .04 | .07 | 1.06 | .11 | 22.0 | 0 |
| **Wine:** | | | | | | | | |
| dessert, 18.8% alcohol, | | | | | | | | |
| 2 fl. oz.. . . . . . . . . . | 0 | 0 | <.01 | .01 | .02 | .01 | .6 | 0 |
| table, 11.5% alcohol: | | | | | | | | |
| red, 4 fl. oz. . . . . . . . | 0 | 0 | <.01 | .01 | .02 | .01 | .6 | 0 |
| rosé, 4 fl. oz.. . . . . . . | 0 | 0 | <.01 | .01 | .02 | .01 | .3 | 0 |
| white, 4 fl. oz. . . . . . . | 0 | 0 | <.01 | <.01 | .02 | <.01 | .1 | 0 |
| **Winged beans:** | | | | | | | | |
| raw, untrimmed, 1 lb. . . . | 569 | n.a. | .62 | .45 | 4.00 | .50 | n.a. | 0 |
| raw, trimmed, sliced, | | | | | | | | |
| ½ cup. . . . . . . . . . . . | 28 | n.a. | .03 | .02 | .20 | .03 | n.a. | 0 |
| boiled, drained, ½ cup. . . | 27 | 3 | .03 | 02 | .20 | .03 | n.a. | 0 |
| **Winged beans, dried:** | | | | | | | | |
| raw, 1 lb.. . . . . . . . . . . . | 0 | 0 | 4.67 | 2.04 | 14.02 | .79 | 202.1 | 0 |
| raw, ½ cup . . . . . . . . . . . | 0 | 0 | .94 | .41 | 2.81 | .16 | 40.5 | 0 |
| boiled, ½ cup . . . . . . . . . | 0 | 0 | .25 | .11 | .71 | .04 | 8.9 | 0 |
| **Winter squash,** see specific listings | | | | | | | | |
| **Wolffish,** Atlantic, meat only: | | | | | | | | |
| raw, 1 lb.. . . . . . . . . . . . | 1701 | (0) | .82 | .36 | 9.68 | n.a. | n.a. | 9.22 |
| baked, broiled, or | | | | | | | | |
| microwaved[1], 4 oz. . . . | 491 | (0) | .24 | .11 | 2.95 | n.a. | n.a. | 2.66 |
| **Wonton wrapper,** | | | | | | | | |
| .3-oz. piece . . . . . . . . . | 1 | 0 | .04 | .03 | .43 | tr. | 1.0 | 0 |

---

[1] *Prepared without added ingredients.*

# Y

| | Vitamin A | Vitamin C | Thiamin | Riboflavin | Niacin | B6 | Folacin | B12 |
|---|---|---|---|---|---|---|---|---|
| | (IU) | (Mg) | (Mg) | (Mg) | (Mg) | (Mg) | (Mcg) | (Mcg) |
| **Yam** (see also "Sweet potato"): | | | | | | | | |
| raw, untrimmed, 1 lb. ... | 0 | 67 | .44 | .13 | 2.96 | 1.14 | 89.7 | 0 |
| raw, trimmed, cubed, | | | | | | | | |
| ½ cup . . . . . . . . . . . . | 0 | 13 | .08 | .02 | .57 | .22 | 17.3 | 0 |
| boiled, drained, cubed, | | | | | | | | |
| ½ cup . . . . . . . . . . . . | 0 | 8 | .07 | .02 | .38 | .16 | 10.9 | 0 |
| **Yam, canned or frozen,** see "Sweet potato" | | | | | | | | |
| **Yam beans,** fresh: | | | | | | | | |
| raw, untrimmed, 1 lb. ... | 88 | 84 | .09 | .12 | .84 | .18 | 51.0 | 0 |
| raw, trimmed, sliced, | | | | | | | | |
| 1 cup . . . . . . . . . . . . | 25 | 24 | .03 | .04 | .24 | .05 | 15.0 | 0 |
| **Yard-long beans,** fresh: | | | | | | | | |
| raw, untrimmed, 1 lb. ... | 3725 | 81 | .46 | .47 | 1.77 | n.a. | n.a. | 0 |
| raw, trimmed, sliced, | | | | | | | | |
| ½ cup . . . . . . . . . . . . | 394 | 86 | .05 | .05 | .19 | n.a. | n.a. | 0 |
| boiled, drained, sliced, | | | | | | | | |
| ½ cup . . . . . . . . . . . . | 234 | 8 | .04 | .05 | .33 | n.a. | n.a. | 0 |
| **Yard-long beans,** dried: | | | | | | | | |
| uncooked, 1 lb. . . . . . . . . | 236 | 7 | 4.02 | 1.07 | 9.79 | 1.68 | 2984.2 | 0 |
| uncooked, ½ cup. . . . . . . | 44 | 1 | .75 | .20 | 1.81 | .31 | 552.6 | 0 |
| boiled, ½ cup . . . . . . . . . | 14 | <1 | .18 | .06 | .47 | .08 | 125.3 | 0 |
| **Yeast:** | | | | | | | | |
| baker's active, dry, | | | | | | | | |
| .2-oz. pkg. . . . . . . . . . . | n.a. | n.a. | n.a. | n.a. | 2.78 | n.a. | n.a. | n.a. |
| baker's, compressed, | | | | | | | | |
| .6-oz. cake. . . . . . . . . . | n.a. | n.a. | .32 | .19 | 2.09 | .07 | 133.0 | n.a. |
| brewer's, dry, 1 tbsp. | tr. | tr. | 1.25 | .34 | 3.00 | n.a. | n.a. | 0 |
| **Yellow beans,** dried: | | | | | | | | |
| uncooked, 1 lb. . . . . . . . . | 25 | 0 | 3.13 | 1.50 | 11.02 | 2.01 | 1763.3 | 0 |
| uncooked, ½ cup. . . . . . . | 5 | 0 | .68 | .32 | 2.38 | .43 | 381.0 | 0 |
| boiled, ½ cup . . . . . . . . . | 2 | 2 | .17 | .09 | .62 | .11 | 71.2 | 0 |
| **Yellowtail,** meat only: | | | | | | | | |
| raw, 1 lb.. . . . . . . . . . . . | 431 | 13 | .65 | .18 | 30.85 | .73 | 16.6 | 5.90 |

| | Vitamin A | Vitamin C | Thiamin | Riboflavin | Niacin | B6 | Folacin | B12 |
|---|---|---|---|---|---|---|---|---|
| | (IU) | (Mg) | (Mg) | (Mg) | (Mg) | (Mg) | (Mcg) | (Mcg) |
| baked, broiled, or microwaved[1], 4 oz. .... | 118 | 3 | .20 | .06 | 9.87 | .21 | 4.5 | 1.42 |
| **Yogurt:** | | | | | | | | |
| plain, 8 fl. oz.: | | | | | | | | |
| whole milk......... | 279 | 1 | .07 | .32 | .17 | .07 | 17.0 | .84 |
| low fat............ | 150 | 2 | .10 | .49 | .26 | .11 | 25.0 | 1.28 |
| skim ............. | 16 | 2 | .11 | .53 | .28 | .12 | 28.0 | 1.39 |
| coffee or vanilla, low fat, 8 fl. oz............. | 123 | 2 | .10 | .46 | .24 | .10 | 24.0 | 1.20 |
| **Yogurt, frozen,** soft serve: | | | | | | | | |
| chocolate, ½ cup....... | n.a. | tr. | .03 | .15 | .22 | .05 | 8.0 | .21 |
| vanilla, ½ cup ......... | 152 | 1 | .03 | .16 | .21 | .06 | 4.0 | .21 |

[1] *Prepared without added ingredients.*

# Z

| | Vitamin A | Vitamin C | Thiamin | Riboflavin | Niacin | B6 | Folacin | B12 |
|---|---|---|---|---|---|---|---|---|
| | (IU) | (Mg) | (Mg) | (Mg) | (Mg) | (Mg) | (Mcg) | (Mcg) |
| **Zucchini,** w/peel: | | | | | | | | |
| fresh: | | | | | | | | |
| raw, untrimmed, | | | | | | | | |
| 1 lb. . . . . . . . . . . | 1465 | 39 | .30 | .13 | 1.72 | .38 | 95.4 | 0 |
| raw, ends trimmed, | | | | | | | | |
| sliced, ½ cup . . . . . | 221 | 6 | .05 | .02 | .26 | .06 | 14.4 | 0 |
| boiled, drained, | | | | | | | | |
| sliced, ½ cup . . . . . | 216 | 4 | .04 | .04 | .39 | .07 | 15.1 | 0 |
| fresh, baby, raw: | | | | | | | | |
| untrimmed, 1 lb. . . . . | 1933 | 135 | .17 | .14 | 2.78 | .56 | 79.0 | 0 |
| 1 large, 2⅝" long, | | | | | | | | |
| .6 oz. . . . . . . . . . . | 78 | 6 | .01 | .01 | .11 | .02 | 3.0 | 0 |
| 1 medium, 3⅛" long, | | | | | | | | |
| .4 oz. . . . . . . . . . . | 54 | 4 | .01 | <.01 | .08 | .02 | 2.0 | 0 |
| canned, Italian style[1], | | | | | | | | |
| 8 oz. . . . . . . . . . . . | 1224 | 5 | .10 | .09 | 1.20 | n.a. | n.a. | 0 |
| canned, Italian style[1], | | | | | | | | |
| ½ cup . . . . . . . . . . . | 615 | 3 | .05 | .05 | .60 | n.a. | n.a. | 0 |
| frozen, 10-oz. pkg. . . . . . | 1373 | 15 | .14 | .12 | 1.23 | .14 | 28.0 | 0 |
| frozen, boiled, drained, | | | | | | | | |
| sliced, ½ cup . . . . . . . | 483 | 4 | .05 | .05 | .43 | .05 | 8.8 | 0 |

---

[1] Packed in tomato juice.

# Minerals

# Minerals

The importance of minerals in our diet has recently been receiving more attention. Fairly new and significant discoveries have resulted in further studies to ascertain the full impact these substances (at least the ones known at this time) have on our physical and mental well-being. What we do know for certain is that minerals work with vitamins and other nutrients—as well as with each other—to ensure the efficient performance of vital processes in our bodies. As with vitamins, a shortage of one essential mineral may disrupt the balance of others, and possibly render them ineffective altogether.

Minerals are inorganic substances which the human body cannot manufacture. However, with few exceptions (notably iron) and depending on specific dietary limitations or physical disorders, we can generally get all the minerals we need through the food we eat. Even under conditions of great physical and emotional stress, which sap the body of nutrients, supplementing the missing minerals can frequently make up the loss.

Minerals generally fall into one of two categories: *macrominerals* (which include calcium, phosphorus, potassium, magnesium, and sodium), and *trace minerals* (including iron, zinc, manganese, selenium, and copper). Macrominerals, so called because they are found in body tissue in relatively high amounts, are measured in milligrams. Trace minerals, measured in micrograms, are present in *very* minute quantities, but they are no less vital for healthy body functioning.

Listed below is an overview of the major nutritional minerals.

## Calcium

Though it is the most abundant mineral in the body, 99% of it is found in bones and teeth. The remaining 1%, which is scattered throughout the body, is essential for a wide variety of important functions. Calcium is one of the two minerals most deficient in the diets of women in America (iron is the other). It is not easily absorbed (vitamin D aids in its absorption), and consistent shortages of this important mineral can lead to osteoporosis (brittle bones) and a host of other bone-related problems in adults.

*Main Functions:* Works with phosphorus to build and strengthen bones and teeth; regulates heartbeat, alleviates insomnia (calcium is known to be a natural tranquilizer), and assists in blood clotting.

*Best Natural Sources:* Milk and milk products, cheese, sardines, soybeans, salmon, peanuts, sunflower seeds, dried beans, and green leafy vegetables.

*Recommended Daily Dosage:* 1000 milligrams for an average, healthy adult; more for pregnant and lactating women. Higher doses are also suggested for the elderly—it appears that the body absorbs calcium less efficiently as we age.

*Toxicity:* High daily doses can result in bone and tissue calcification throughout the body, can interfere with the function of the nervous and muscular systems, and may cause drowsiness.

## Copper

A trace mineral found in all body tissues, it is essential for the utilization of vitamin C.

*Main Function:* Important in formation of red blood cells; boosts energy levels by enhancing iron absorption; involved in protein metabolism and healing; promotes healthy functioning of the central nervous system.

*Best Natural Sources:* Dried beans and peas, whole wheat, prunes, calf and beef liver, shrimp and most seafood, green leafy vegetables, and almonds. Drinking tap water may be a good source if plumbing consists of copper piping.

*Recommended Daily Dosage:* 2 to 3 milligrams for adults.

*Toxicity:* Rare, but excess copper in the body may accumulate in the blood and deplete the supply of zinc in the brain. Symptoms of toxicity include insomnia, depression, vomiting, diarrhea, hair loss, and irregular menstruation.

## Iodine

This is a trace mineral, two thirds of which is found in the thyroid gland.

*Main Functions:* Promotes proper functioning of the thyroid gland, which in turn stimulates metabolism to assist in burning fat; enriches skin, hair, and nails.

*Best Natural Sources:* All seafood, seaweed, or kelp, sea salt, and iodized salt.

*Recommended Daily Dosage:* 150 micrograms for adults; 175 micrograms during pregnancy and 200 micrograms during lactation.

*Toxicity:* None known from natural food or water sources; however, an excess can cause iodine sensitivity or poisoning in certain individuals. When prepared as a drug, iodine levels should be carefully monitored; overdoses can be serious.

## Iron

Iron is a mineral concentrate in the blood that is present in all living cells. Along with calcium, iron is one of the minerals most often deficient in the diets of American women. Also, because less than 10% of our total iron intake is absorbed into the bloodstream, a condition called "iron-deficiency anemia" is one of our most common nutritional shortages.

*Main Functions:* Builds up blood quality by aiding in the production of hemoglobin, which transports oxygen through the bloodstream; promotes efficient muscle contraction; works with other nutrients to improve respiratory function; increases resistance to stress and disease.

*Best Natural Sources:* Liver and other organ meats, oysters, lean meat, green leafy vegetables, whole grains, dried fruits, molasses, egg yolks, oatmeal, and nuts. (*Note*: Iron from foods of animal origin is more easily absorbed than iron present in vegetable products.)

*Recommended Daily Dosage:* 10 milligrams for men and 15 for women, though more is suggested for pregnant women. The need for iron increases during periods of rapid growth, menstruation, surgery, and whenever there is a loss of blood.

*Toxicity:* Rare in normal, healthy people; however, an overabundance, sometimes found in elderly men, may result in damage to the heart, liver, and pancreas. Coffee and tea in large quantities can contribute to the inhibition of proper iron absorption.

### Magnesium

An essential mineral, 70% of magnesium is located in the bones and 30% in the soft body tissues and fluids. It is sometimes called the "antistress mineral" because of its beneficial effect on the nervous system. Deficiencies of magnesium are fairly common among alcoholics and in individuals with kidney disease, diabetes, and other physical disorders.

*Main Functions:* Works most efficiently with calcium; important for proper functioning of nerves and muscles; can promote a healthy heart; aids in lessening depression; helps prevent calcium deposits, kidney stones, and gallstones; assists in bone formation.

*Best Natural Sources:* Raw green leafy vegetables, almonds and cashews, soybeans, whole grains, figs, corn, and apples.

*Recommended Daily Dosage:* 280 to 350 milligrams, the higher dosage for men and pregnant and lactating women. Higher dosage recommended with use of alcohol and diuretics.

*Toxicity:* Rare, but it can occur when there is a decrease in normal urinary function or when there is a marked increase in the body's absorption of the mineral. May result in depression of the central nervous system.

## Manganese

This is a trace mineral that plays a vital part in activating numerous enzymes.

*Main Functions:* Assists in the digestion of food and the utilization of vitamins and other minerals; helps maintain healthy bone structure; valuable in production of sex hormones; provides "food" for the brain and central nervous system.

*Best Natural Sources:* Whole grains, nuts and seeds, egg yolks, green leafy vegetables, and fruits. A substantial portion of this mineral is generally lost in the processing of foods.

*Recommended Daily Dosage:* 2.5 to 5 milligrams are suggested for adults.

*Toxicity:* Very high doses can result in inefficient storage and utilization of iron, weakness and motor coordination difficulties, or irritability.

## Phosphorus

The second most abundant mineral in the body, phosphorus is found in every living cell.

*Main Functions:* Works efficiently with calcium; important in the proper utilization of carbohydrates by the body for growth, maintenance, and repair of cells and for the production of energy;

promotes regular heart function, bone growth, tooth development, and normal kidney function; important in the metabolism of many nutrients.

*Best Natural Sources:* High-protein foods, such as meat, fish, poultry, and eggs; whole grains, seeds and nuts.

*Recommended Daily Dosage:* 800 to 1200 milligrams for adults.

*Toxicity:* None known, but if phosphorus intake is high, calcium may have to be increased to ensure proper balance. (*Note*: Diets high in fat increase phosphorus absorption and lower calcium levels; adjustments must be made for proper balance.)

### Potassium

Found mainly in intracellular fluid, it is an essential mineral. Potassium works with sodium, so a proper balance of these two minerals is very important.

*Main Functions:* Helps regulate the body's water balance and heartbeat; important for normal growth; promotes healthy skin and proper kidney function to eliminate waste; sends oxygen to the brain (boosts clear thinking).

*Best Natural Sources:* Citrus fruits, especially oranges, bananas, potatoes, all green leafy vegetables, whole grains, and sunflower seeds.

*Recommended Daily Dosage:* No official RDA established, but approximate recommended dosage ranges from 1600 to 2000 milligrams for adults.

*Toxicity:* Excessive amounts in the blood may cause abnormal heartbeat. Certain medications, such as cortisone, deplete potassium supplies and can cause sodium retention; an adjustment may be necessary to maintain proper balance.

## Selenium

Discovered less than thirty years ago, this essential mineral acts as an antioxidant and works closely with vitamin E. Deficiencies are rare, but some early studies indicate that a lack of selenium might result in infertility and premature aging.

*Main Functions:* Helps to promote normal growth and fertility; functions as an antioxidant to prevent the breakdown of tissues, maintains elasticity, and delays aging.

*Best Natural Sources:* Brewer's yeast, organ meats, egg yolks, dairy products, fish and shellfish, whole grains, and onions. (*Note*: Selenium levels in food will vary depending on its presence in soil and in animal feed.)

*Recommended Daily Dosage:* 55 to 70 micrograms for adults; slightly higher amounts are recommended for lactating women.

*Toxicity:* Very high levels can be toxic (possible symptoms are hair, tooth, and nail loss or dermatitis). Since the role of selenium in nutrition has not yet been fully explored, only moderate supplements are advised.

## Zinc

This is an essential trace mineral. With the exception of iron, zinc is present in the body in larger amounts than any other trace mineral. It is a component of insulin and plays a major role in the efficiency of most bodily functions.

*Main Functions:* Promotes growth and mental alertness; helps wounds heal; aids in cell formation.

*Best Natural Sources:* Protein-rich foods, such as liver, meat, and eggs; natural unprocessed foods, such as whole grains, brewer's yeast, wheat bran, wheat germ, and raw seeds.

*Recommended Daily Dosage:* 12 to 15 milligrams for adults; slightly higher amounts for pregnant and lactating women.

*Toxicity:* Excessive amounts may result in iron and copper losses; may cause nausea, vomiting, or diarrhea. Increased amounts of zinc in the diet may require the addition of vitamin A for balance.

# A

| | Calcium (Mg) | Iron (Mg) | Magnesium (Mg) | Phosphorus (Mg) | Potassium (Mg) | Zinc (Mg) | Copper (Mg) | Manganese (Mg) |
|---|---|---|---|---|---|---|---|---|
| **Abalone,** mixed species, meat only: | | | | | | | | |
| raw, 1 lb. . . . . . . . . . . . | 142 | 14.47 | 219 | n.a. | n.a. | 3.70 | .89 | .18 |
| dipped in flour, fried, | | | | | | | | |
|   4 oz. . . . . . . . . . . . . . | 42 | 4.31 | 64 | n.a. | n.a. | 1.08 | .25 | n.a. |
| **Acerola,** fresh: | | | | | | | | |
| untrimmed, 1 lb. . . . . . . . | 44 | .73 | 66 | 40 | 530 | n.a. | n.a. | n.a. |
| trimmed, ½ cup. . . . . . . . | 6 | .10 | 9 | 6 | 72 | n.a. | n.a. | n.a. |
| **Acerola juice,** fresh, | | | | | | | | |
|   6 fl. oz. . . . . . . . . . . . | 18 | .90 | 24 | 18 | 174 | n.a. | n.a. | n.a. |
| **Acorn squash:** | | | | | | | | |
| raw, untrimmed, 1 lb. . . . | 114 | 2.41 | 110 | 124 | 1196 | .45 | .22 | n.a. |
| raw, trimmed, cubed, | | | | | | | | |
|   ½ cup. . . . . . . . . . . . | 23 | .49 | 23 | 25 | 243 | .09 | .05 | n.a. |
| baked or boiled, drained, | | | | | | | | |
|   cubed, ½ cup . . . . . . . | 45 | .95 | 43 | 46 | 446 | .18 | .09 | n.a. |
| boiled, drained, mashed, | | | | | | | | |
|   ½ cup . . . . . . . . . . . . | 32 | .68 | 31 | 33 | 321 | .13 | .06 | n.a. |
| **Adzuki beans,** dried: | | | | | | | | |
| uncooked, 1 lb. . . . . . . . . | 300 | 22.59 | 576 | 1726 | 5686 | 22.84 | 4.96 | 7.84 |
| uncooked, ½ cup. . . . . . . | 65 | 4.88 | 124 | 373 | 1229 | 4.93 | 1.07 | 1.70 |
| boiled, ½ cup . . . . . . . . . | 32 | 2.30 | 60 | 193 | 612 | 2.03 | .34 | .66 |
| canned, sweetened, | | | | | | | | |
|   ½ cup. . . . . . . . . . . . | 33 | 1.67 | 46 | 110 | 176 | n.a. | n.a. | n.a. |
| **Agar,** see "Seaweed" | | | | | | | | |
| **Alfalfa seeds,** sprouted, | | | | | | | | |
|   raw: | | | | | | | | |
| untrimmed, 1 lb. . . . . . . . | 144 | 4.35 | 120 | 317 | 357 | 4.19 | .71 | .85 |
| trimmed, 1 cup . . . . . . . . | 10 | .32 | 9 | 23 | 26 | .30 | .05 | .06 |
| **Allspice,** ground, | | | | | | | | |
|   1 tsp. . . . . . . . . . . . . | 13 | .13 | 3 | 2 | 20 | .02 | .01 | .06 |
| **Almond,** shelled, except as noted: | | | | | | | | |
| dried, unblanched: | | | | | | | | |
|   in shell, 1 lb. . . . . . . . | 482 | 6.63 | 538 | 943 | 1327 | 5.29 | 1.71 | 4.12 |

| | Calcium | Iron | Magnesium | Phosphorus | Potassium | Zinc | Copper | Manganese |
|---|---|---|---|---|---|---|---|---|
| | (Mg) | (Mg) | (Mg) | (Mg) | (Mg) | (Mg) | (Mg) | (Mg) |
| Almond, dried, unblanched, *continued* | | | | | | | | |
| 1 oz.............. | 75 | 1.04 | 84 | 148 | 208 | .83 | .27 | .65 |
| whole kernels, 1 cup | 377 | 5.19 | 421 | 738 | 1039 | 4.14 | 1.34 | 3.23 |
| dried, blanched, | | | | | | | | |
| 1 oz............... | 70 | 1.03 | 81 | 151 | 213 | .90 | .30 | .41 |
| dried, blanched, whole | | | | | | | | |
| kernels, 1 cup ....... | 358 | 5.26 | 415 | 771 | 1088 | 4.58 | 1.55 | 2.11 |
| dry-roasted, 1 oz. ...... | 80 | 1.08 | 86 | 156 | 219 | 1.39 | .35 | .56 |
| dry-roasted, whole | | | | | | | | |
| kernels, 1 cup ....... | 389 | 5.25 | 419 | 756 | 1063 | 6.76 | 1.69 | 2.73 |
| honey-roasted, 1 oz. .... | 75 | .80 | 68 | 113 | 159 | .74 | .35 | n.a. |
| honey-roasted, whole | | | | | | | | |
| kernels, 1 cup ....... | 379 | 4.08 | 346 | 576 | 806 | 3.74 | 1.40 | n.a. |
| oil-roasted: | | | | | | | | |
| unblanched, 1 oz. ... | 66 | 1.09 | 86 | 155 | 194 | 1.39 | .35 | .56 |
| unblanched, whole | | | | | | | | |
| kernels, 1 cup .... | 367 | 6.02 | 477 | 859 | 1073 | 7.69 | 1.92 | 3.10 |
| blanched, 1 oz. ...... | 55 | 1.51 | 82 | 164 | 197 | .40 | .26 | .42 |
| blanched, whole | | | | | | | | |
| kernels, 1 cup .... | 276 | 7.53 | 412 | 819 | 984 | 2.01 | 1.32 | 2.09 |
| toasted, 1 oz............ | 80 | 1.40 | 87 | 156 | 220 | 1.40 | .35 | .57 |
| **Almond butter:** | | | | | | | | |
| plain, 1 tbsp........... | 43 | .59 | 48 | 84 | 121 | .49 | .14 | .38 |
| honey and cinnamon, | | | | | | | | |
| 1 tbsp. ............. | 43 | .59 | 48 | 83 | 120 | .48 | .16 | .37 |
| **Almond extract** (*Virginia* | | | | | | | | |
| *Dare*), 1 tsp. ........ | tr. | tr. | tr. | 0 | 0 | tr. | tr. | n.a. |
| **Almond paste:** | | | | | | | | |
| 1 oz................. | 65 | .90 | 73 | 127 | 184 | .73 | .24 | .57 |
| ½ cup packed ......... | 262 | 3.58 | 294 | 507 | 734 | 2.93 | .95 | 2.28 |
| **Almond powder:** | | | | | | | | |
| full fat, 1 cup.......... | 142 | 1.82 | 200 | 395 | 461 | .14 | .45 | .92 |
| partially defatted, 1 cup .. | 154 | 2.26 | 178 | 331 | 467 | 1.97 | .67 | .90 |
| **Amaranth,** fresh: | | | | | | | | |
| raw, untrimmed, 1 lb. ... | 919 | 9.90 | 236 | 213 | 2604 | 3.82 | .69 | n.a. |

| | Calcium (Mg) | Iron (Mg) | Magnesium (Mg) | Phosphorus (Mg) | Potassium (Mg) | Zinc (Mg) | Copper (Mg) | Manganese (Mg) |
|---|---|---|---|---|---|---|---|---|
| raw, ½ cup .......... | 30 | .32 | 8 | 7 | 85 | .13 | .02 | n.a. |
| boiled, drained, ½ cup... | 138 | 1.49 | 36 | 47 | 423 | n.a. | n.a. | n.a. |
| **Amaranth,** whole grain, 1 cup ............. | 298 | 14.81 | 518 | 887 | 714 | 6.21 | 1.52 | 4.41 |
| **Anchovy,** European, fresh, meat only, raw, 1 lb. ............... | 668 | 14.73 | 185 | 788 | 1737 | 7.80 | .96 | n.a. |
| **Anchovy, canned,** in olive oil, drained: | | | | | | | | |
| yield from 2-oz. can..... | 104 | 2.08 | 31 | 113 | 245 | 1.10 | .15 | n.a. |
| 5 medium ............ | 46 | .93 | 14 | 50 | 109 | .49 | .07 | n.a. |
| **Anise extract** (*Virginia Dare*), 1 tsp. ........ | tr. | tr. | tr. | 0 | 0 | tr. | tr. | n.a. |
| **Anise seed,** 1 tsp....... | 14 | .78 | 6 | 7 | 48 | .08 | .02 | .04 |
| **Apple:** | | | | | | | | |
| fresh, cored, unpeeled: | | | | | | | | |
| raw, untrimmed, 1 lb. ............ | 30 | .74 | 19 | 30 | 480 | .15 | .17 | .19 |
| raw, 1 medium, 2¾" diam., approx. 3 per lb. ........ | 10 | .25 | 6 | 10 | 159 | .05 | .06 | .06 |
| raw, sliced, ½ cup... | 4 | .10 | 3 | 4 | 63 | .02 | .02 | .03 |
| fresh, cored, peeled: | | | | | | | | |
| raw, 1 medium, 2¾" diam., approx. 3 per lb. ........ | 5 | .09 | 4 | 9 | 144 | .05 | .04 | .03 |
| raw, sliced, ½ cup... | 2 | .04 | 2 | 4 | 62 | .02 | .02 | .01 |
| boiled, sliced, ½ cup | 4 | .16 | 3 | 7 | 76 | .04 | .03 | .10 |
| microwaved, sliced, ½ cup .......... | 4 | .14 | 3 | 7 | 79 | .03 | .04 | .12 |
| canned, sweetened, sliced: | | | | | | | | |
| unheated, ½ cup .... | 4 | .23 | 2 | 6 | 69 | .03 | .05 | .16 |
| heated, ½ cup ...... | 4 | .24 | 3 | 6 | 71 | .05 | .05 | .17 |
| dehydrated, sulfured: | | | | | | | | |
| uncooked, ½ cup.... | 6 | .60 | 7 | 16 | 192 | .09 | .08 | .04 |
| cooked, ½ cup ..... | 4 | .41 | 5 | 11 | 132 | .06 | .06 | .03 |

| | Calcium (Mg) | Iron (Mg) | Magnesium (Mg) | Phosphorus (Mg) | Potassium (Mg) | Zinc (Mg) | Copper (Mg) | Manganese (Mg) |
|---|---|---|---|---|---|---|---|---|
| **Apple,** *continued* | | | | | | | | |
| dried, sulfured: | | | | | | | | |
|   uncooked, 10 rings, | | | | | | | | |
|     2.3 oz.......... | 9 | .90 | 10 | 25 | 288 | .13 | .12 | .06 |
|   uncooked, ½ cup.... | 6 | .61 | 7 | 17 | 194 | .09 | .08 | .04 |
| frozen, unsweetened, sliced: | | | | | | | | |
|   unheated, ½ cup.... | 4 | .16 | 3 | 7 | 67 | .04 | .05 | .15 |
|   heated, ½ cup...... | 5 | .19 | 3 | 8 | 78 | .05 | .07 | .15 |
| **Apple butter,** 1 tbsp..... | 1 | .02 | 0 | 1 | 16 | .01 | .01 | n.a. |
| **Apple juice:** | | | | | | | | |
| canned or bottled, | | | | | | | | |
|   6 fl. oz............. | 12 | .66 | 6 | 12 | 222 | .06 | .04 | .21 |
| frozen, undiluted, 6-fl.-oz. | | | | | | | | |
|   container.......... | 43 | 1.92 | 37 | 52 | 945 | .27 | .11 | .48 |
| frozen, diluted, 8 fl. oz. ... | 14 | .61 | 12 | 16 | 301 | .09 | .03 | .15 |
| **Applesauce,** canned: | | | | | | | | |
| unsweetened, ½ cup .... | 4 | .15 | 4 | 9 | 91 | .03 | .03 | .09 |
| sweetened, ½ cup ...... | 5 | .45 | 4 | 9 | 78 | .05 | .06 | .10 |
| **Apricot:** | | | | | | | | |
| fresh: | | | | | | | | |
|   untrimmed, 1 lb. .... | 61 | 2.29 | 32 | 82 | 1246 | 1.11 | .38 | .33 |
|   3 medium, approx. | | | | | | | | |
|     4 oz............ | 15 | .58 | 8 | 21 | 313 | .28 | .09 | .08 |
|   pitted, halves, ½ cup | 11 | .84 | 12 | 30 | 458 | .41 | .14 | .12 |
| canned, unpeeled, halves: | | | | | | | | |
|   in water, ½ cup..... | 10 | .39 | 9 | 16 | 233 | .14 | .10 | .06 |
|   in juice, ½ cup ..... | 15 | .37 | 12 | 25 | 205 | .14 | .07 | .06 |
|   in light syrup, ½ cup | 14 | .50 | 11 | 17 | 175 | .14 | .10 | .07 |
|   in heavy syrup, | | | | | | | | |
|     ½ cup.......... | 11 | .39 | 9 | 16 | 181 | .14 | .10 | .07 |
| canned, peeled, whole: | | | | | | | | |
|   in water, ½ cup..... | 10 | .62 | 11 | 19 | 175 | .13 | .08 | .06 |
|   in heavy syrup, | | | | | | | | |
|     ½ cup.......... | 11 | .55 | 10 | 17 | 173 | .14 | .08 | .07 |
|   in extra heavy syrup, | | | | | | | | |
|     ½ cup.......... | 10 | .77 | 10 | 18 | 155 | .13 | .08 | .06 |

|  | Calcium | Iron | Magnesium | Phosphorus | Potassium | Zinc | Copper | Manganese |
|---|---|---|---|---|---|---|---|---|
|  | (Mg) | (Mg) | (Mg) | (Mg) | (Mg) | (Mg) | (Mg) | (Mg) |
| dehydrated, sulfured: |  |  |  |  |  |  |  |  |
| uncooked, ½ cup.... | 37 | 3.79 | 38 | 94 | 1110 | .60 | .35 | .22 |
| cooked, ½ cup ..... | 30 | 3.08 | 31 | 77 | 902 | .49 | .28 | .18 |
| dried, sulfured, halves: |  |  |  |  |  |  |  |  |
| uncooked, 10 halves, |  |  |  |  |  |  |  |  |
| 1.2 oz........... | 16 | 1.65 | 16 | 41 | 482 | .26 | .15 | .10 |
| uncooked, ½ cup.... | 30 | 3.10 | 31 | 76 | 896 | .49 | .28 | .18 |
| cooked, unsweetened, |  |  |  |  |  |  |  |  |
| ½ cup.......... | 20 | 2.08 | 21 | 52 | 611 | .33 | .19 | .12 |
| cooked, sweetened, |  |  |  |  |  |  |  |  |
| ½ cup.......... | 20 | 2.05 | 20 | 51 | 598 | .32 | .19 | .12 |
| frozen, sweetened, |  |  |  |  |  |  |  |  |
| ½ cup............ | 12 | 1.09 | 11 | 23 | 277 | .12 | .08 | .06 |
| **Apricot nectar,** canned, |  |  |  |  |  |  |  |  |
| 8 fl. oz............. | 17 | .96 | 13 | 23 | 286 | .23 | .18 | n.a. |
| **Arrowroot flour,** 1 cup... | 51 | .42 | 4 | 7 | 14 | .09 | .05 | .60 |
| **Artichoke,** globe: |  |  |  |  |  |  |  |  |
| fresh: |  |  |  |  |  |  |  |  |
| raw, untrimmed, 1 lb. | 80 | 2.32 | 108 | 163 | 671 | .88 | .42 | .46 |
| boiled, drained, |  |  |  |  |  |  |  |  |
| 1 medium, |  |  |  |  |  |  |  |  |
| 10.6 oz.......... | 54 | 1.55 | 72 | 103 | 425 | .59 | .28 | .31 |
| hearts, boiled, |  |  |  |  |  |  |  |  |
| drained, ½ cup ... | 38 | 1.09 | 51 | 72 | 297 | .41 | .20 | .22 |
| frozen, hearts: |  |  |  |  |  |  |  |  |
| 9-oz. pkg. ........ | 48 | 1.27 | 70 | 147 | 632 | .82 | .14 | .62 |
| boiled, drained, ⅓ of |  |  |  |  |  |  |  |  |
| 9-oz. pkg. ....... | 17 | .45 | 25 | 49 | 211 | .29 | .05 | .22 |
| **Arugula,** raw: |  |  |  |  |  |  |  |  |
| untrimmed, 1 lb. ...... | 436 | n.a. | 129 | 140 | 1003 | 1.27 | .21 | .87 |
| trimmed, ½ cup........ | 3 | n.a. | 1 | 1 | 7 | .01 | tr. | .01 |
| **Asparagus:** |  |  |  |  |  |  |  |  |
| fresh: |  |  |  |  |  |  |  |  |
| raw, untrimmed, |  |  |  |  |  |  |  |  |
| 1 lb. ........... | 50 | 2.10 | 44 | 135 | 657 | 1.10 | .42 | .63 |

| | Calcium | Iron | Magnesium | Phosphorus | Potassium | Zinc | Copper | Manganese |
|---|---|---|---|---|---|---|---|---|
| | (Mg) | (Mg) | (Mg) | (Mg) | (Mg) | (Mg) | (Mg) | (Mg) |
| Asparagus, fresh, *continued* | | | | | | | | |
| raw, trimmed, 4 spears, ½"-diam. base | 12 | .51 | 11 | 33 | 158 | .27 | .10 | .15 |
| raw, trimmed, cuts and spears, ½ cup | 14 | .58 | 12 | 38 | 183 | .31 | .12 | .18 |
| boiled, drained, 4 spears | 12 | .44 | 6 | 32 | 96 | .25 | .07 | .09 |
| boiled, drained, ½ cup | 18 | .66 | 9 | 48 | 144 | .38 | .10 | .14 |
| canned w/liquid, ½ cup | 17 | .71 | 11 | 46 | 186 | .57 | .13 | .19 |
| frozen: | | | | | | | | |
| 10-oz. pkg. | 72 | 2.07 | 41 | 181 | 718 | 1.69 | .39 | .58 |
| boiled, drained, ⅓ of 10-oz. pkg. | 23 | .62 | 13 | 54 | 213 | .54 | .17 | .18 |
| boiled, drained, 4 spears | 14 | .38 | 8 | 33 | 131 | .33 | .10 | .11 |
| **Avocado:** | | | | | | | | |
| California: | | | | | | | | |
| untrimmed, 1 lb. | 37 | 4.06 | 140 | 145 | 2185 | 1.45 | .91 | .84 |
| 1 medium, approx. 8 oz. | 19 | 2.04 | 70 | 73 | 1097 | .73 | .46 | .42 |
| pureed, ½ cup | 13 | 1.36 | 47 | 49 | 729 | .49 | .31 | .28 |
| Florida, 1 medium, approx. 1 lb. untrimmed | 33 | 1.60 | 104 | 119 | 1484 | 1.28 | .76 | .52 |
| Florida, pureed, ½ cup | 13 | .61 | 39 | 45 | 561 | .49 | .29 | .20 |

# B

| | Calcium | Iron | Magnesium | Phosphorus | Potassium | Zinc | Copper | Manganese |
|---|---|---|---|---|---|---|---|---|
| | (Mg) | (Mg) | (Mg) | (Mg) | (Mg) | (Mg) | (Mg) | (Mg) |
| **Bacon,** cooked, 3 medium slices, 20 per lb. . . . . . . . . . | 2 | .31 | 5 | 64 | 92 | .62 | .03 | .01 |
| **Bacon, substitute:** | | | | | | | | |
| beef, heated, 3 strips, 1.2 oz. . . . . . . . . . . . . | n.a. | 1.07 | 9 | 80 | 140 | 2.17 | n.a. | n.a. |
| pork, cured, heated, 3 strips, 15 per 20-oz. pkg. . . . . . . . . . | 5 | .67 | 9 | 90 | 158 | 1.25 | .05 | .02 |
| turkey (*Louis Rich*), 1 heated slice . . . . . . . | 1 | .19 | 3 | 41 | 36 | .27 | n.a. | n.a. |
| **"Bacon," vegetarian,** frozen: | | | | | | | | |
| .3-oz. strip. . . . . . . . . . . | 2 | .19 | 2 | 6 | 14 | .03 | .01 | .02 |
| (*Morningstar Farms* Breakfast Strips), .6-oz. strip. . . . . . . . . | 7 | .27 | n.a. | 42 | 15 | .05 | n.a. | n.a. |
| (*Worthington Stripples*), .6-oz. strip. . . . . . . . . | 7 | .27 | n.a. | 42 | 15 | .05 | n.a. | n.a. |
| **Bacon bits** (*Oscar Mayer*), ¼ oz. . . . . . . . | 1 | .14 | 2 | 41 | 38 | .33 | n.a. | n.a. |
| **Bagel,** 3½"-diam. piece: | | | | | | | | |
| plain or water . . . . . . . . . | 53 | 2.53 | 21 | 68 | 72 | .62 | .12 | .38 |
| plain or water, toasted . . . . . . . . . . . | 53 | 2.52 | 21 | 68 | 72 | .62 | .12 | .38 |
| cinnamon-raisin . . . . . . . . | 13 | 2.7 | n.a. | n.a. | n.a. | n.a. | n.a. | n.a. |
| cinnamon-raisin, toasted . . . . . . . . . . . . | 13 | 2.7 | n.a. | n.a. | n.a. | n.a. | n.a. | n.a. |
| egg . . . . . . . . . . . . . . . . | 9 | 2.8 | 18 | 59 | 48 | .55 | .06 | .29 |
| egg, toasted. . . . . . . . . . | 9 | 2.8 | 18 | 59 | 48 | .55 | .06 | .29 |
| oat bran . . . . . . . . . . . . | 9 | 2.2 | n.a. | n.a. | n.a. | n.a. | n.a. | n.a. |
| oat bran, toasted . . . . . . . | 9 | 2.2. | n.a. | n.a. | n.a. | n.a. | n.a. | n.a. |

| | Calcium | Iron | Magnesium | Phosphorus | Potassium | Zinc | Copper | Manganese |
|---|---|---|---|---|---|---|---|---|
| | (Mg) | (Mg) | (Mg) | (Mg) | (Mg) | (Mg) | (Mg) | (Mg) |
| **Baked beans,** canned: | | | | | | | | |
| (*Grandma Brown's*), | | | | | | | | |
| ½ cup............. | 74 | 2.04 | 58 | 149 | 371 | .90 | .30 | .60 |
| (*Grandma Brown's* | | | | | | | | |
| Saucepan), ½ cup .... | 70 | 1.95 | 46 | 135 | 298 | .84 | .24 | .55 |
| plain or vegetarian, | | | | | | | | |
| 8 oz.............. | 114 | .66 | 73 | 236 | 671 | 3.17 | .47 | .78 |
| plain or vegetarian, | | | | | | | | |
| ½ cup............. | 64 | .37 | 41 | 132 | 376 | 1.78 | .26 | .44 |
| w/beef, 8 oz.......... | 102 | 3.63 | 57 | 164 | 726 | 2.72 | .68 | 1.36 |
| w/beef, ½ cup........ | 60 | 2.13 | 33 | 108 | 426 | 1.60 | .40 | .80 |
| w/franks, 8 oz........ | 109 | 3.93 | 63 | 236 | 533 | 4.23 | .48 | .95 |
| w/franks, ½ cup ...... | 61 | 2.22 | 35 | 133 | 301 | 2.39 | .27 | .54 |
| w/pork: | | | | | | | | |
| 8 oz.............. | 119 | 3.67 | 77 | 246 | 700 | 3.31 | .49 | .82 |
| ½ cup............ | 66 | 2.15 | 42 | 137 | 389 | 1.84 | .27 | .46 |
| and sweet sauce, | | | | | | | | |
| 8 oz............ | 139 | 3.77 | 78 | 239 | 603 | 3.40 | .23 | .84 |
| and sweet sauce, | | | | | | | | |
| ½ cup.......... | 77 | 2.01 | 43 | 132 | 335 | 1.89 | .13 | .47 |
| and tomato sauce, | | | | | | | | |
| 8 oz............ | 127 | 7.44 | 79 | 267 | 681 | 13.30 | .58 | 1.11 |
| and tomato sauce, | | | | | | | | |
| ½ cup.......... | 70 | 4.13 | 44 | 148 | 378 | 7.38 | .32 | .62 |
| **Baking powder,** all types, | | | | | | | | |
| 1 tsp. ............. | 270 | .51 | 1 | 101 | 1 | n.a. | n.a. | n.a |
| **Baking soda,** 1 tsp...... | 0 | 0 | 0 | 0 | 0 | 0 | 0 | 0 |
| **Balsam pear,** fresh: | | | | | | | | |
| leafy tips: | | | | | | | | |
| raw, untrimmed, | | | | | | | | |
| 1 lb. ........... | 145 | 3.52 | 146 | 171 | 1047 | n.a. | n.a. | n.a. |
| raw, trimmed, | | | | | | | | |
| ½ cup.......... | 20 | .49 | 20 | 24 | 146 | n.a. | n.a. | n.a. |
| boiled, drained, | | | | | | | | |
| ½ cup.......... | 12 | .30 | 27 | 22 | 174 | n.a. | n.a. | n.a. |

| | Calcium | Iron | Magnesium | Phosphorus | Potassium | Zinc | Copper | Manganese |
|---|---|---|---|---|---|---|---|---|
| | (Mg) | (Mg) | (Mg) | (Mg) | (Mg) | (Mg) | (Mg) | (Mg) |
| pods: | | | | | | | | |
| raw, untrimmed, | | | | | | | | |
| 1 lb. . . . . . . . . . . | 72 | 1.60 | 64 | 118 | 1114 | 3.01 | n.a. | n.a. |
| raw, trimmed, | | | | | | | | |
| ½" pieces, ½ cup | 18 | .40 | 16 | 29 | 275 | .74 | n.a. | n.a. |
| boiled, drained, | | | | | | | | |
| ½" pieces, ½ cup | 6 | .24 | 10 | 22 | 198 | n.a. | n.a. | n.a. |
| **Bamboo shoots:** | | | | | | | | |
| fresh: | | | | | | | | |
| raw, untrimmed, | | | | | | | | |
| 1 lb. . . . . . . . . . . | 17 | .66 | 4 | 78 | 701 | n.a. | n.a. | n.a. |
| raw, trimmed, | | | | | | | | |
| ½" slices, ½ cup | 10 | .38 | 2 | 45 | 405 | n.a. | n.a. | n.a. |
| boiled, drained, | | | | | | | | |
| ½" slices, ½ cup | 7 | .15 | 2 | 12 | 320 | n.a. | n.a. | n.a. |
| canned, drained, | | | | | | | | |
| ⅛" slices, ½ cup . . . . . | 5 | .21 | 3 | 17 | 52 | n.a. | n.a. | n.a. |
| **Banana:** | | | | | | | | |
| fresh: | | | | | | | | |
| untrimmed, 1 lb. . . . . | 17 | .90 | 84 | 58 | 1166 | .48 | .31 | .45 |
| 1 medium; 8¾" long, | | | | | | | | |
| 6.2 oz. untrimmed | 7 | .35 | 33 | 22 | 451 | .19 | .12 | .17 |
| peeled, mashed, | | | | | | | | |
| ½ cup . . . . . . . . . | 7 | .35 | 32 | 22 | 445 | .19 | .12 | .17 |
| dehydrated or powdered, | | | | | | | | |
| 1 oz. . . . . . . . . . . . . . | 6 | .33 | 31 | 21 | 423 | .17 | .11 | .16 |
| dehydrated or powdered, | | | | | | | | |
| 1 tbsp. . . . . . . . . . . | 1 | .07 | 7 | 5 | 92 | .04 | .02 | .04 |
| **Banana, baking,** see "Plantain" | | | | | | | | |
| **Banana chips,** 1 oz. . . . . | 5 | .35 | 22 | 16 | 152 | .21 | .06 | .44 |
| **Barbecue loaf,** pork and | | | | | | | | |
| beef, 1 oz. . . . . . . . . . . | 15 | .33 | 5 | 38 | 93 | .70 | .02 | .01 |
| **Barbecue sauce:** | | | | | | | | |
| 1 tbsp. . . . . . . . . . . . . . | 3 | .14 | n.a. | 3 | 28 | n.a. | n.a. | n.a. |
| 1 cup . . . . . . . . . . . . . . | 48 | 2.25 | n.a. | 50 | 435 | n.a. | n.a. | n.a. |

| | Calcium | Iron | Magnesium | Phosphorus | Potassium | Zinc | Copper | Manganese |
|---|---|---|---|---|---|---|---|---|
| | (Mg) | (Mg) | (Mg) | (Mg) | (Mg) | (Mg) | (Mg) | (Mg) |
| **Barbecue seasoning** | | | | | | | | |
| (*Tone's Perc*), ¼ tsp. | 3 | .16 | 2 | 3 | 13 | .03 | tr. | .02 |
| **Barley,** 1 cup: | | | | | | | | |
| uncooked............ | 61 | 6.63 | 244 | 485 | 831 | 5.10 | .92 | 3.58 |
| pearled, uncooked ...... | 57 | 5.00 | 158 | 442 | 560 | 4.25 | .84 | 2.64 |
| pearled, cooked ........ | 17 | 2.09 | 35 | 85 | 145 | 1.29 | .17 | .41 |
| **Basil,** ground, 1 tsp..... | 30 | .59 | 6 | 7 | 48 | .08 | .02 | .04 |
| **Bass,** meat only: | | | | | | | | |
| freshwater, mixed species: | | | | | | | | |
| raw, 1 lb........... | 363 | 6.77 | 136 | 906 | 1615 | 2.97 | .42 | 4.03 |
| baked, broiled, or | | | | | | | | |
| microwaved[1], | | | | | | | | |
| 4 oz............ | 116 | 2.17 | 43 | 290 | 517 | .94 | .13 | 1.29 |
| striped: | | | | | | | | |
| raw, 1 lb........... | n.a. | 3.79 | n.a. | n.a. | n.a. | 1.83 | .14 | .07 |
| baked, broiled, or | | | | | | | | |
| microwaved[1], | | | | | | | | |
| 4 oz............ | n.a. | 1.22 | n.a. | n.a. | n.a. | .58 | .05 | .02 |
| **Bass, sea,** see "Sea bass" | | | | | | | | |
| **Bay leaf,** crumbled, | | | | | | | | |
| 1 tsp. ............. | 5 | .26 | 1 | 1 | 3 | .02 | tr. | .05 |
| **Bean sprouts,** see specific listings | | | | | | | | |
| **Beans,** see specific listings | | | | | | | | |
| **Beef,** retail trim[2], meat only[3], 4 oz.: | | | | | | | | |
| brisket, whole, all grades, braised: | | | | | | | | |
| lean and fat (trimmed | | | | | | | | |
| to ¼") .......... | 9 | 2.54 | 20 | 212 | 262 | 5.78 | .11 | .02 |

---

[1] *Prepared without added ingredients.*
[2] *Meat trimmed to 0" or ¼" fat refers to the amount of fat present during cooking. For "lean only" listings, all visible fat is trimmed after cooking. (Bear in mind that a small amount of fat is always present, even in meat trimmed to 0" fat before cooking.)*
[3] *Prepared without added ingredients, except as noted.*

| | Calcium (Mg) | Iron (Mg) | Magnesium (Mg) | Phosphorus (Mg) | Potassium (Mg) | Zinc (Mg) | Copper (Mg) | Manganese (Mg) |
|---|---|---|---|---|---|---|---|---|
| lean and fat (trimmed to 0").......... | 8 | 2.87 | 24 | 245 | 294 | 6.76 | .12 | .02 |
| lean only......... | 7 | 3.19 | 26 | 273 | 323 | 7.81 | .13 | .02 |
| brisket, flat half, all grades, braised: | | | | | | | | |
| lean and fat (trimmed to ¼")......... | 9 | 2.60 | 22 | 228 | 276 | 5.47 | .11 | .02 |
| lean and fat (trimmed to 0").......... | 6 | 3.12 | 27 | 281 | 328 | 6.93 | .14 | .02 |
| lean only......... | 6 | 3.22 | 28 | 291 | 338 | 7.21 | .14 | .02 |
| brisket, point half, all grades, braised: | | | | | | | | |
| lean and fat (trimmed to ¼")......... | 10 | 2.49 | 19 | 198 | 251 | 6.07 | .10 | .02 |
| lean and fat (trimmed to 0").......... | 9 | 2.65 | 20 | 212 | 264 | 6.61 | .11 | .02 |
| lean only......... | 7 | 3.16 | 25 | 256 | 310 | 8.38 | .13 | .02 |
| chuck, arm pot roast, choice grade, braised: | | | | | | | | |
| lean and fat (trimmed to ¼")......... | 11 | 3.46 | 22 | 245 | 276 | 7.60 | .15 | .02 |
| lean and fat (trimmed to 0").......... | 11 | 3.80 | 24 | 269 | 297 | 8.51 | .16 | .02 |
| lean only......... | 10 | 4.30 | 27 | 304 | 328 | 9.82 | .19 | .02 |
| chuck, arm pot roast, select grade, braised: | | | | | | | | |
| lean and fat (trimmed to ¼")......... | 11 | 3.58 | 23 | 254 | 284 | 7.93 | .16 | .02 |
| lean and fat (trimmed to 0").......... | 11 | 3.90 | 25 | 276 | 303 | 8.75 | .17 | .02 |
| lean only......... | 10 | 4.30 | 27 | 304 | 328 | 9.82 | .19 | .02 |
| chuck, blade roast, choice grade, braised: | | | | | | | | |
| lean and fat (trimmed to ¼")......... | 15 | 3.46 | 22 | 223 | 259 | 9.23 | .14 | .02 |
| lean and fat (trimmed to 0").......... | 15 | 3.58 | 23 | 230 | 265 | 9.64 | .14 | .02 |
| lean only......... | 15 | 4.17 | 26 | 266 | 298 | 11.65 | .17 | .02 |

| | Calcium | Iron | Magnesium | Phosphorus | Potassium | Zinc | Copper | Manganese |
|---|---|---|---|---|---|---|---|---|
| | (Mg) | (Mg) | (Mg) | (Mg) | (Mg) | (Mg) | (Mg) | (Mg) |

Beef, *continued*

chuck, blade roast, select grade, braised:

| | | | | | | | | |
|---|---|---|---|---|---|---|---|---|
| lean and fat (trimmed to ¼") .......... | 15 | 3.58 | 23 | 230 | 265 | 9.64 | .14 | .02 |
| lean and fat (trimmed to 0") .......... | 15 | 3.66 | 23 | 236 | 271 | 9.93 | .15 | .02 |
| lean only .......... | 15 | 4.17 | 26 | 266 | 298 | 11.65 | .17 | .02 |

flank, choice grade:

| | | | | | | | | |
|---|---|---|---|---|---|---|---|---|
| braised, lean and fat (trimmed to 0") ... | 7 | 3.78 | 26 | 290 | 382 | 6.54 | .13 | .02 |
| braised, lean only.... | 7 | 3.93 | 27 | 303 | 398 | 6.86 | .14 | .02 |
| broiled, lean and fat (trimmed to 0") ... | 8 | 2.85 | 26 | 261 | 456 | 5.28 | .11 | .02 |
| broiled, lean only.... | 8 | 2.91 | 27 | 268 | 469 | 5.44 | .11 | .02 |

ground, extra lean:

| | | | | | | | | |
|---|---|---|---|---|---|---|---|---|
| baked, medium ..... | 8 | 2.59 | 19 | 141 | 254 | 6.06 | .09 | .02 |
| baked, well-done .... | 10 | 3.36 | 25 | 184 | 330 | 7.87 | .11 | .02 |
| broiled, medium..... | 8 | 2.66 | 24 | 183 | 355 | 6.18 | .08 | .02 |
| broiled, well-done ... | 10 | 3.14 | 28 | 215 | 418 | 7.29 | .09 | .02 |
| pan-fried, medium ... | 8 | 2.68 | 24 | 181 | 354 | 6.15 | .10 | .02 |
| pan-fried, well-done | 9 | 3.10 | 27 | 210 | 408 | 7.11 | .11 | .02 |

ground, lean:

| | | | | | | | | |
|---|---|---|---|---|---|---|---|---|
| baked, medium ..... | 10 | 2.37 | 19 | 145 | 254 | 5.78 | .08 | .02 |
| baked, well-done .... | 14 | 3.02 | 24 | 186 | 324 | 7.38 | .10 | .02 |
| broiled, medium..... | 12 | 2.39 | 24 | 179 | 341 | 6.08 | .07 | .02 |
| broiled, well-done ... | 14 | 2.78 | 27 | 206 | 396 | 7.03 | .09 | .02 |
| pan-fried, medium ... | 11 | 2.47 | 23 | 180 | 339 | 5.90 | .09 | .02 |
| pan-fried, well-done | 12 | 2.81 | 26 | 205 | 386 | 6.70 | .10 | .02 |

ground, regular:

| | | | | | | | | |
|---|---|---|---|---|---|---|---|---|
| baked, medium ..... | 11 | 2.73 | 17 | 155 | 251 | 5.55 | .08 | .02 |
| baked, well-done .... | 14 | 3.39 | 22 | 193 | 311 | 6.88 | .10 | .02 |
| broiled, medium..... | 12 | 2.77 | 23 | 193 | 331 | 5.87 | .09 | .02 |
| broiled, well-done ... | 14 | 3.11 | 25 | 217 | 371 | 6.59 | .10 | .02 |
| pan-fried, medium ... | 12 | 2.78 | 23 | 194 | 340 | 5.75 | .09 | .02 |

| | Calcium | Iron | Magnesium | Phosphorus | Potassium | Zinc | Copper | Manganese |
|---|---|---|---|---|---|---|---|---|
| | (Mg) | (Mg) | (Mg) | (Mg) | (Mg) | (Mg) | (Mg) | (Mg) |
| pan-fried, well-done | 15 | 3.07 | 25 | 214 | 376 | 6.37 | .10 | .02 |
| ground, frozen patties, | | | | | | | | |
| broiled, medium...... | 12 | 2.38 | 23 | 179 | 333 | 6.12 | .07 | .02 |
| porterhouse steak (short loin), choice grade, broiled: | | | | | | | | |
| lean and fat (trimmed | | | | | | | | |
| to ¼")........... | 9 | 2.98 | 28 | 212 | 399 | 5.26 | .14 | .01 |
| lean only.......... | 8 | 3.40 | 33 | 242 | 462 | 6.12 | .16 | .02 |
| rib, whole (ribs 6–12), choice grade: | | | | | | | | |
| broiled, lean and fat | | | | | | | | |
| (trimmed to ¼")... | 14 | 2.44 | 22 | 198 | 349 | 5.82 | .09 | .01 |
| broiled, lean only.... | 12 | 2.91 | 28 | 242 | 432 | 7.45 | .11 | .02 |
| roasted, lean and fat | | | | | | | | |
| (trimmed to ¼")... | 12 | 2.62 | 22 | 195 | 336 | 5.94 | .09 | .01 |
| roasted, lean only ... | 11 | 3.24 | 28 | 243 | 424 | 7.88 | .11 | .02 |
| rib, whole (ribs 6–12), prime grade: | | | | | | | | |
| broiled, lean and fat | | | | | | | | |
| (trimmed to ¼")... | 12 | 2.39 | 23 | 189 | 347 | 5.79 | .09 | .01 |
| broiled, lean only.... | 11 | 2.86 | 28 | 230 | 430 | 7.43 | .11 | .02 |
| roasted, lean and fat | | | | | | | | |
| (trimmed to ¼")... | 12 | 2.43 | 22 | 195 | 339 | 5.98 | .09 | .01 |
| roasted, lean only ... | 11 | 2.96 | 28 | 242 | 426 | 7.87 | .11 | .02 |
| rib, whole (ribs 6–12), select grade: | | | | | | | | |
| broiled, lean and fat | | | | | | | | |
| (trimmed to ¼")... | 12 | 2.49 | 23 | 203 | 358 | 6.01 | .09 | .01 |
| broiled, lean only.... | 12 | 2.91 | 28 | 242 | 432 | 7.45 | .11 | .02 |
| roasted, lean and fat | | | | | | | | |
| (trimmed to ¼")... | 12 | 2.70 | 23 | 202 | 347 | 6.21 | .10 | .02 |
| roasted, lean only ... | 11 | 3.24 | 28 | 243 | 424 | 7.88 | .11 | .02 |
| rib, large end (ribs 6–9), choice grade: | | | | | | | | |
| broiled, lean and fat | | | | | | | | |
| (trimmed to ¼")... | 11 | 2.42 | 20 | 200 | 338 | 5.52 | .09 | .01 |
| broiled, lean only.... | 10 | 2.91 | 26 | 246 | 422 | 7.12 | .10 | .02 |
| roasted, lean and fat | | | | | | | | |
| (trimmed to ¼")... | 11 | 2.57 | 22 | 191 | 321 | 6.33 | .10 | .01 |

| | Calcium | Iron | Magnesium | Phosphorus | Potassium | Zinc | Copper | Manganese |
|---|---|---|---|---|---|---|---|---|
| | (Mg) | (Mg) | (Mg) | (Mg) | (Mg) | (Mg) | (Mg) | (Mg) |
| Beef, rib, large end, choice grade, *continued* | | | | | | | | |
| roasted, lean and fat | | | | | | | | |
| (trimmed to 0") . . . | 11 | 2.64 | 23 | 195 | 329 | 6.52 | .10 | .01 |
| roasted, lean only . . . | 9 | 3.20 | 28 | 237 | 405 | 8.46 | .12 | .02 |
| rib, large end (ribs 6–9), prime grade: | | | | | | | | |
| broiled, lean and fat | | | | | | | | |
| (trimmed to ¼") . . . | 11 | 2.31 | 20 | 183 | 330 | 5.39 | .09 | .01 |
| broiled, lean only . . . . | 9 | 2.81 | 27 | 226 | 418 | 7.09 | .10 | .02 |
| roasted, lean and fat | | | | | | | | |
| (trimmed to ¼") . . . | 11 | 2.60 | 22 | 192 | 324 | 6.40 | .10 | .01 |
| roasted, lean only . . . | 9 | 3.20 | 28 | 237 | 405 | 8.46 | .12 | .02 |
| rib, large end (ribs 6–9), select grade: | | | | | | | | |
| broiled, lean and fat | | | | | | | | |
| (trimmed to ¼") . . . | 11 | 2.48 | 22 | 206 | 349 | 5.74 | .09 | .01 |
| broiled, lean only . . . . | 10 | 2.91 | 26 | 246 | 422 | 7.12 | .10 | .02 |
| roasted, lean and fat | | | | | | | | |
| (trimmed to ¼") . . . | 11 | 2.68 | 23 | 197 | 335 | 6.67 | .10 | .02 |
| roasted, lean and fat | | | | | | | | |
| (trimmed to 0") . . . | 10 | 2.72 | 23 | 201 | 340 | 6.82 | .10 | .02 |
| roasted, lean only . . . | 9 | 3.20 | 28 | 237 | 405 | 8.46 | .12 | .02 |
| rib, shortrib, choice grade: | | | | | | | | |
| braised, lean and fat | 14 | 2.62 | 17 | 184 | 254 | 5.53 | .11 | .01 |
| braised, lean only . . . . | 12 | 3.81 | 25 | 266 | 355 | 8.85 | .12 | .02 |
| rib, small end (ribs 10–12), choice grade: | | | | | | | | |
| broiled, lean and fat | | | | | | | | |
| (trimmed to ¼") . . . | 15 | 2.47 | 25 | 197 | 365 | 6.28 | .10 | .02 |
| broiled, lean and fat | | | | | | | | |
| (trimmed to 0") . . . | 15 | 2.59 | 26 | 208 | 388 | 6.72 | .10 | .02 |
| broiled, lean only . . . . | 15 | 2.91 | 31 | 236 | 447 | 7.93 | .11 | .02 |
| roasted, lean and fat | | | | | | | | |
| (trimmed to ¼") . . . | 15 | 2.66 | 22 | 202 | 356 | 5.41 | .09 | .01 |
| roasted, lean only . . . | 14 | 3.30 | 28 | 252 | 451 | 7.04 | .10 | .02 |
| rib, small end (ribs 10–12), prime grade: | | | | | | | | |
| broiled, lean and fat | | | | | | | | |
| (trimmed to ¼") . . . | 15 | 2.51 | 25 | 200 | 372 | 6.41 | .10 | .02 |

| | Calcium | Iron | Magnesium | Phosphorus | Potassium | Zinc | Copper | Manganese |
|---|---|---|---|---|---|---|---|---|
| | (Mg) | (Mg) | (Mg) | (Mg) | (Mg) | (Mg) | (Mg) | (Mg) |
| broiled, lean only.... | 15 | 2.91 | 31 | 236 | 447 | 7.93 | .11 | .02 |
| roasted, lean and fat (trimmed to ¼")... | 15 | 2.19 | 22 | 200 | 361 | 5.39 | .09 | .01 |
| roasted, lean only ... | 15 | 2.61 | 28 | 248 | 458 | 7.02 | .10 | .02 |
| **rib, small end (ribs 10–12), select grade:** | | | | | | | | |
| broiled, lean and fat (trimmed to ¼")... | 15 | 2.51 | 25 | 200 | 372 | 6.41 | .10 | .02 |
| broiled, lean and fat (trimmed to 0") ... | 15 | 2.61 | 26 | 209 | 390 | 6.78 | .10 | .02 |
| broiled, lean only.... | 15 | 2.91 | 31 | 236 | 447 | 7.93 | .11 | .02 |
| roasted, lean and fat (trimmed to ¼")... | 15 | 2.73 | 23 | 208 | 366 | 5.57 | .09 | .01 |
| roasted, lean only ... | 14 | 3.30 | 28 | 252 | 451 | 7.04 | .10 | .02 |
| **rib eye, small end (ribs 10–12), choice grade:** | | | | | | | | |
| broiled, lean and fat (trimmed to 0") ... | 15 | 2.61 | 26 | 209 | 390 | 6.78 | .10 | .02 |
| broiled, lean only.... | 15 | 2.91 | 31 | 236 | 447 | 7.93 | .11 | .02 |
| **round, full cut, choice grade:** | | | | | | | | |
| broiled, lean and fat (trimmed to ¼")... | 7 | 2.87 | 28 | 270 | 445 | 4.90 | .11 | .02 |
| broiled, lean only.... | 6 | 3.06 | 32 | 290 | 479 | 5.26 | .12 | .02 |
| **round, full cut, select grade:** | | | | | | | | |
| broiled, lean and fat (trimmed to ¼")... | 7 | 2.88 | 29 | 270 | 445 | 4.91 | .11 | .02 |
| broiled, lean only.... | 6 | 3.07 | 32 | 290 | 480 | 5.28 | .12 | .02 |
| **round, bottom, choice grade:** | | | | | | | | |
| braised, lean and fat (trimmed to ¼")... | 7 | 3.54 | 25 | 278 | 320 | 5.57 | .14 | .02 |
| braised, lean and fat (trimmed to 0") ... | 6 | 3.84 | 27 | 302 | 342 | 6.08 | .15 | .02 |
| braised, lean only.... | 6 | 3.92 | 28 | 308 | 349 | 6.21 | .15 | .02 |
| roasted, lean and fat (trimmed to ¼")... | 7 | 3.24 | 28 | 247 | 403 | 4.76 | .11 | .02 |
| roasted, lean and fat (trimmed to 0") ... | 6 | 3.50 | 32 | 268 | 437 | 5.16 | .12 | .02 |

| | Calcium | Iron | Magnesium | Phosphorus | Potassium | Zinc | Copper | Manganese |
|---|---|---|---|---|---|---|---|---|
| | (Mg) | (Mg) | (Mg) | (Mg) | (Mg) | (Mg) | (Mg) | (Mg) |
| **Beef, round, bottom, choice grade, *continued*** | | | | | | | | |
| roasted, lean only ... | 6 | 3.55 | 32 | 271 | 443 | 5.24 | .12 | .02 |
| **round, bottom, select grade:** | | | | | | | | |
| braised, lean and fat | | | | | | | | |
| (trimmed to ¼")... | 7 | 3.57 | 26 | 280 | 321 | 5.61 | .14 | .02 |
| braised, lean and fat | | | | | | | | |
| (trimmed to 0") ... | 6 | 3.87 | 28 | 304 | 345 | 6.12 | .15 | .02 |
| braised, lean only.... | 6 | 3.92 | 28 | 308 | 350 | 6.21 | .15 | .02 |
| roasted, lean and fat | | | | | | | | |
| (trimmed to ¼")... | 7 | 3.29 | 29 | 251 | 409 | 4.83 | .12 | .02 |
| roasted, lean and fat | | | | | | | | |
| (trimmed to 0") ... | 6 | 3.53 | 32 | 270 | 440 | 5.21 | .12 | .02 |
| roasted, lean only ...... | 6 | 3.55 | 32 | 271 | 443 | 5.24 | .12 | .02 |
| **round, eye of, choice grade, roasted:** | | | | | | | | |
| lean and fat (trimmed | | | | | | | | |
| to ¼") .......... | 7 | 2.08 | 27 | 234 | 407 | 4.89 | .11 | .02 |
| lean and fat (trimmed | | | | | | | | |
| to 0")........... | 6 | 2.20 | 31 | 254 | 445 | 5.34 | .11 | .02 |
| lean only .......... | 6 | 2.21 | 31 | 256 | 448 | 5.38 | .11 | .02 |
| **round, eye of, select grade, roasted:** | | | | | | | | |
| lean and fat (trimmed | | | | | | | | |
| to ¼") .......... | 7 | 2.10 | 28 | 237 | 414 | 4.96 | .11 | .02 |
| lean and fat (trimmed | | | | | | | | |
| to 0")........... | 6 | 2.20 | 31 | 254 | 445 | 5.34 | .11 | .02 |
| lean only .......... | 6 | 2.21 | 31 | 256 | 448 | 5.38 | .11 | .02 |
| **round, tip, choice grade, roasted:** | | | | | | | | |
| lean and fat (trimmed | | | | | | | | |
| to ¼") .......... | 7 | 3.07 | 27 | 252 | 401 | 7.25 | .13 | .02 |
| lean and fat (trimmed | | | | | | | | |
| to 0")........... | 6 | 3.24 | 29 | 267 | 425 | 7.76 | .14 | .02 |
| lean only .......... | 6 | 3.33 | 31 | 274 | 438 | 8.02 | .14 | .02 |
| **round, tip, prime grade, roasted:** | | | | | | | | |
| lean and fat (trimmed | | | | | | | | |
| to ¼") .......... | 7 | 3.06 | 27 | 249 | 398 | 7.18 | .13 | .02 |
| lean only .......... | 6 | 3.33 | 31 | 274 | 438 | 8.02 | .14 | .02 |

| | Calcium | Iron | Magnesium | Phosphorus | Potassium | Zinc | Copper | Manganese |
|---|---|---|---|---|---|---|---|---|
| | (Mg) | (Mg) | (Mg) | (Mg) | (Mg) | (Mg) | (Mg) | (Mg) |
| round, tip, select grade, roasted: | | | | | | | | |
| lean and fat (trimmed to ¼") . . . . . . . . . . | 7 | 3.14 | 28 | 257 | 411 | 7.44 | .13 | .02 |
| lean and fat (trimmed to 0") . . . . . . . . . . | 6 | 3.27 | 29 | 269 | 429 | 7.82 | .14 | .02 |
| lean only . . . . . . . . . . | 6 | 3.33 | 31 | 274 | 438 | 8.02 | .14 | .02 |
| round, top, choice grade: | | | | | | | | |
| braised, lean and fat (trimmed to ¼") . . . | 6 | 3.50 | 27 | 239 | 354 | 4.81 | .13 | .05 |
| braised, lean and fat (trimmed to 0") . . . | 5 | 3.71 | 28 | 253 | 374 | 5.10 | .14 | .06 |
| braised, lean only . . . . | 5 | 3.76 | 29 | 256 | 379 | 5.17 | .14 | .06 |
| broiled, lean and fat (trimmed to ¼") . . . | 8 | 3.12 | 33 | 265 | 475 | 5.98 | .13 | .02 |
| broiled, lean only . . . . | 7 | 3.27 | 35 | 279 | 501 | 6.32 | .14 | .02 |
| pan-fried in vegetable oil, lean and fat (trimmed to ¼") . . . | 7 | 3.31 | 36 | 304 | 533 | 4.84 | .14 | .02 |
| pan-fried in vegetable oil, lean only . . . . . | 6 | 3.57 | 40 | 331 | 582 | 5.24 | .15 | .02 |
| round, top, prime grade: | | | | | | | | |
| broiled, lean and fat (trimmed to ¼") . . . | 7 | 3.21 | 34 | 273 | 490 | 6.17 | .14 | .02 |
| broiled, lean only . . . . | 7 | 3.27 | 35 | 279 | 501 | 6.32 | .14 | .02 |
| round, top, select grade: | | | | | | | | |
| braised, lean and fat (trimmed to ¼") . . . | 6 | 3.56 | 27 | 243 | 359 | 4.89 | .13 | .05 |
| braised, lean and fat (trimmed to 0") . . . | 5 | 3.71 | 28 | 253 | 374 | 4.50 | .14 | .06 |
| braised, lean only . . . . | 5 | 3.76 | 29 | 256 | 379 | 5.17 | .14 | .06 |
| broiled, lean and fat (trimmed to ¼") . . . | 8 | 3.12 | 33 | 265 | 475 | 5.98 | .13 | .02 |
| broiled, lean only . . . . | 7 | 3.27 | 35 | 279 | 501 | 6.32 | .14 | .02 |
| shank, crosscuts, choice grade: | | | | | | | | |
| simmered, lean and fat (trimmed to ¼") | 34 | 3.97 | 31 | 271 | 458 | 10.56 | .18 | .02 |

| | Calcium | Iron | Magnesium | Phosphorus | Potassium | Zinc | Copper | Manganese |
|---|---|---|---|---|---|---|---|---|
| | (Mg) | (Mg) | (Mg) | (Mg) | (Mg) | (Mg) | (Mg) | (Mg) |
| Beef, shank, crosscuts, choice grade, *continued* | | | | | | | | |
| simmered, lean only | 36 | 4.38 | 34 | 298 | 507 | 11.90 | .20 | .02 |
| short loin, see "porterhouse steak," above, and "T-bone steak" and "top loin," below | | | | | | | | |
| sirloin, top, choice grade: | | | | | | | | |
| broiled, lean and fat | | | | | | | | |
| (trimmed to ¼")... | 12 | 3.45 | 32 | 249 | 412 | 6.58 | .15 | .02 |
| broiled, lean and fat | | | | | | | | |
| (trimmed to 0") ... | 12 | 3.65 | 34 | 265 | 438 | 7.04 | .16 | .02 |
| broiled, lean only .... | 12 | 3.81 | 36 | 277 | 457 | 7.39 | .17 | .02 |
| pan-fried in vegetable oil, lean and fat | | | | | | | | |
| (trimmed to ¼")... | 14 | 3.78 | 32 | 260 | 449 | 6.12 | .15 | .02 |
| pan-fried in vegetable oil, lean only ..... | 12 | 4.42 | 37 | 303 | 527 | 7.26 | .17 | .02 |
| sirloin, top, select grade: | | | | | | | | |
| broiled, lean and fat | | | | | | | | |
| (trimmed to ¼")... | 12 | 3.49 | 33 | 254 | 418 | 6.70 | .15 | .02 |
| broiled, lean and fat | | | | | | | | |
| (trimmed to 0") ... | 12 | 3.72 | 35 | 271 | 446 | 7.20 | .16 | .02 |
| broiled, lean only.... | 12 | 3.81 | 36 | 277 | 457 | 7.39 | .17 | .02 |
| T-bone steak (short loin), choice grade: | | | | | | | | |
| broiled, lean and fat | | | | | | | | |
| (trimmed to ¼")... | 9 | 3.01 | 28 | 209 | 403 | 5.31 | .14 | .01 |
| broiled, lean only.... | 8 | 3.40 | 33 | 236 | 462 | 6.12 | .16 | .02 |
| tenderloin, choice grade: | | | | | | | | |
| broiled, lean and fat | | | | | | | | |
| (trimmed to ¼")... | 9 | 3.55 | 29 | 237 | 414 | 5.49 | .18 | .02 |
| broiled, lean and fat | | | | | | | | |
| (trimmed to 0") ... | 8 | 3.86 | 32 | 257 | 451 | 6.01 | .19 | .02 |
| broiled, lean only.... | 8 | 4.06 | 34 | 270 | 475 | 6.34 | .20 | .02 |
| roasted, lean and fat | | | | | | | | |
| (trimmed to ¼")... | 10 | 3.47 | 29 | 263 | 454 | 4.50 | .14 | .02 |
| roasted, lean only ... | 9 | 4.18 | 36 | 3.19 | 555 | 5.43 | .16 | .02 |

| | Calcium | Iron | Magnesium | Phosphorus | Potassium | Zinc | Copper | Manganese |
|---|---|---|---|---|---|---|---|---|
| | (Mg) | (Mg) | (Mg) | (Mg) | (Mg) | (Mg) | (Mg) | (Mg) |
| tenderloin, prime grade: | | | | | | | | |
| broiled, lean and fat | | | | | | | | |
| (trimmed to ¼")... | 9 | 3.52 | 28 | 235 | 411 | 5.43 | .17 | .02 |
| broiled, lean only.... | 8 | 4.06 | 34 | 270 | 475 | 6.34 | .20 | .02 |
| roasted, lean and fat | | | | | | | | |
| (trimmed to ¼")... | 10 | 3.47 | 25 | 226 | 374 | 4.89 | .16 | .02 |
| roasted, lean only ... | 8 | 4.15 | 31 | 268 | 446 | 5.86 | .19 | .02 |
| tenderloin, select grade: | | | | | | | | |
| broiled, lean and fat | | | | | | | | |
| (trimmed to ¼")... | 9 | 3.63 | 29 | 243 | 424 | 5.62 | .18 | .02 |
| broiled, lean and fat | | | | | | | | |
| (trimmed to 0") ... | 8 | 3.89 | 33 | 259 | 455 | 6.06 | .19 | .02 |
| broiled, lean only.... | 8 | 4.06 | 34 | 270 | 475 | 6.34 | .20 | .02 |
| roasted, lean and fat | | | | | | | | |
| (trimmed to ¼")... | 10 | 3.47 | 25 | 227 | 370 | 4.50 | .14 | .02 |
| roasted, lean only ... | 8 | 4.18 | 31 | 271 | 443 | 5.43 | .16 | .02 |
| top loin (short loin), choice grade: | | | | | | | | |
| broiled, lean and fat | | | | | | | | |
| (trimmed to ¼")... | 10 | 2.52 | 26 | 218 | 392 | 5.14 | .11 | .02 |
| broiled, lean and fat | | | | | | | | |
| (trimmed to 0") ... | 9 | 2.73 | 29 | 240 | 437 | 5.75 | .12 | .02 |
| broiled, lean only.... | 9 | 2.80 | 31 | 247 | 449 | 5.92 | .12 | .02 |
| top loin (short loin), prime grade: | | | | | | | | |
| broiled, lean and fat | | | | | | | | |
| (trimmed to ¼")... | 10 | 2.52 | 26 | 218 | 392 | 5.14 | .11 | .02 |
| broiled, lean only.... | 9 | 2.80 | 31 | 247 | 449 | 5.92 | .12 | .02 |
| top loin (short loin), select grade: | | | | | | | | |
| broiled, lean and fat | | | | | | | | |
| (trimmed to ¼")... | 10 | 2.56 | 27 | 223 | 401 | 5.27 | .11 | .02 |
| broiled, lean and fat | | | | | | | | |
| (trimmed to 0") ... | 9 | 2.76 | 29 | 243 | 440 | 5.79 | .12 | .02 |
| broiled, lean only.... | 9 | 2.80 | 31 | 247 | 449 | 5.92 | .12 | .02 |
| **Beef, corned:** | | | | | | | | |
| brisket, cured, cooked, | | | | | | | | |
| 4 oz.............. | 9 | 2.11 | 14 | 142 | 164 | 5.19 | .17 | .02 |

| | Calcium (Mg) | Iron (Mg) | Magnesium (Mg) | Phosphorus (Mg) | Potassium (Mg) | Zinc (Mg) | Copper (Mg) | Manganese (Mg) |
|---|---|---|---|---|---|---|---|---|
| Beef, corned, *continued* | | | | | | | | |
| loaf, jellied, 1-oz. slice | 3 | .58 | 3 | 21 | 29 | 1.16 | .02 | .01 |
| **"Beef," vegetarian** (see also "Hamburger, vegetarian"): | | | | | | | | |
| canned: | | | | | | | | |
| (*Worthington* Savory Slices), 3 slices, 3 oz. . . . . . . . . . | 1 | 1.40 | n.a. | 88 | 41 | .25 | n.a. | n.a. |
| steak (*Worthington Prime Stakes*), 3.25-oz. piece . . . . | 12 | .38 | n.a. | 86 | 82 | .38 | n.a. | n.a. |
| steak (*Worthington Vegetable Steaks*), 2.5 oz. . . . . . . . . . | 5 | 3.20 | n.a. | n.a. | 18 | .65 | n.a. | n.a. |
| stew (*Worthington* Country Stew), 1 cup, 8.5 oz. . . . . | 51 | 5.09 | n.a. | 188 | 270 | 1.03 | n.a. | n.a. |
| Swiss steak, w/gravy (*Loma Linda Swiss Stake*), 3.2-oz. piece . . . . . | 24 | .31 | n.a. | 122 | 226 | .41 | n.a. | n.a. |
| frozen: | | | | | | | | |
| (*Worthington* Beef Style Meatless), ⅜" slice, 1.9 oz. . . . | 4 | 2.63 | n.a. | n.a. | 44 | .22 | n.a. | n.a. |
| (*Worthington Stakelets*), 2.5-oz. piece . . . . . | 49 | .99 | n.a. | n.a. | 95 | .50 | n.a. | n.a. |
| corned (*Worthington*), 4 slices, 2 oz. . . . . | 6 | 1.17 | n.a. | 91 | 58 | .26 | n.a. | n.a. |
| pie (*Worthington*), 8-oz. pie . . . . . . . . | 19 | 1.31 | n.a. | n.a. | 107 | .52 | n.a. | n.a. |
| smoked (*Worthington*), 6 slices, 2 oz. . . . . | 5 | 1.25 | n.a. | n.a. | 153 | .14 | n.a. | n.a. |

| | Calcium | Iron | Magnesium | Phosphorus | Potassium | Zinc | Copper | Manganese |
|---|---|---|---|---|---|---|---|---|
| | (Mg) | (Mg) | (Mg) | (Mg) | (Mg) | (Mg) | (Mg) | (Mg) |
| steak (*Loma Linda* Griddle Steaks), 1.9-oz. piece . . . . . | 15 | 1.75 | n.a. | 172 | 319 | .37 | n.a. | n.a. |
| **Beef gravy,** canned, ¼ cup. . . . . . . . . . . . | 4 | .41 | n.a. | 18 | 47 | .58 | .06 | .12 |
| **Beef jerky,** chopped, formed, 1 oz. . . . . . . . | n.a. | 1.56 | 14 | 108 | n.a. | 2.30 | .06 | .03 |
| **Beef luncheon meat:** | | | | | | | | |
| loaf, 1-oz. slice . . . . . . . | 3 | .66 | 4 | 34 | 59 | .72 | .03 | .01 |
| thin-sliced, 5 slices, approx. ¾ oz. . . . . . . . | n.a. | .45 | 4 | 35 | 86 | .84 | .02 | .01 |
| **Beef seasoning** (*Tone's Perc*), ¼ tsp. . . . . . . . . | 4 | .09 | 1 | 3 | 10 | .02 | tr. | .01 |
| **Beer,** alcoholic: | | | | | | | | |
| regular, 12 fl. oz. . . . . . . | 18 | .18 | 23 | 44 | 89 | .06 | .03 | .04 |
| light, 12 fl. oz. . . . . . . . . | 18 | .12 | 17 | 43 | 64 | .11 | .09 | .06 |
| **Beet,** root: | | | | | | | | |
| fresh: | | | | | | | | |
| raw, untrimmed, 1 lb. . . . . . . . . . . | 50 | 2.44 | 71 | 123 | 988 | 1.07 | .23 | 1.00 |
| raw, 2 beets, 2" diam., approx. 8.5 oz. . . . . . . . . . | 27 | 1.31 | 38 | 66 | 530 | .57 | .12 | .54 |
| raw, sliced, ½ cup . . . | 11 | .55 | 16 | 27 | 221 | .24 | .05 | .22 |
| boiled, drained, 2 beets, 2" diam. | 16 | .79 | 23 | 38 | 305 | .35 | .07 | .33 |
| boiled, drained, sliced, ½ cup. . . . . | 14 | .67 | 20 | 32 | 259 | .29 | .06 | .28 |
| canned, w/liquid, ½ cup: | | | | | | | | |
| sliced . . . . . . . . . . . . | 17 | .82 | 20 | 20 | 175 | .28 | .12 | .30 |
| Harvard, sliced. . . . . . | 13 | .44 | 24 | 21 | 201 | n.a. | n.a. | n.a. |
| pickled, sliced . . . . . . | 13 | .47 | 18 | 20 | 169 | .30 | .13 | n.a. |

| | Calcium | Iron | Magnesium | Phosphorus | Potassium | Zinc | Copper | Manganese |
|---|---|---|---|---|---|---|---|---|
| | (Mg) | (Mg) | (Mg) | (Mg) | (Mg) | (Mg) | (Mg) | (Mg) |
| **Beet greens:** | | | | | | | | |
| raw, untrimmed, 1 lb. . . . | 303 | 8.38 | 183 | 102 | 1390 | .97 | .49 | n.a. |
| raw, trimmed, 1" pieces, | | | | | | | | |
| ½ cup . . . . . . . . . . . . . | 23 | .63 | 14 | 8 | 104 | .07 | .04 | n.a. |
| boiled, drained, 1" pieces, | | | | | | | | |
| ½ cup . . . . . . . . . . . . . | 82 | 1.37 | 49 | 29 | 654 | .36 | .18 | n.a. |
| **Berliner,** pork and beef, | | | | | | | | |
| 1 oz. . . . . . . . . . . . . . . | 3 | .33 | 4 | 37 | 80 | .70 | .02 | .01 |
| **Biscuit, ready-to-eat,** | | | | | | | | |
| plain or buttermilk, | | | | | | | | |
| 1 piece . . . . . . . . . . . | 17 | 1.2 | 6 | 151 | 78 | .17 | .03 | .14 |
| **Biscuit, refrigerated dough:** | | | | | | | | |
| plain or buttermilk, baked, | | | | | | | | |
| 1 piece . . . . . . . . . . . | 5 | .7 | 4 | 104 | 42 | .10 | .02 | .07 |
| mixed grain, 1 piece . . . . | 8 | 1.2 | n.a. | n.a. | 201 | n.a. | n.a. | n.a. |
| **Black beans,** dried: | | | | | | | | |
| uncooked, 1 lb. . . . . . . . | 560 | 22.75 | 777 | 1596 | 6726 | 16.55 | 3.82 | 4.81 |
| uncooked, ½ cup. . . . . . . | 120 | 4.87 | 166 | 341 | 1438 | 3.54 | .84 | 1.03 |
| boiled, ½ cup . . . . . . . . . | 24 | 1.80 | 60 | 120 | 306 | .96 | .18 | .38 |
| **Black turtle soup beans,** dried: | | | | | | | | |
| uncooked, 1 lb. . . . . . . . | 726 | 39.46 | 726 | 1996 | 6804 | 9.98 | 4.54 | 4.54 |
| uncooked, ½ cup. . . . . . . | 147 | 8.00 | 147 | 405 | 1380 | 2.02 | .92 | .92 |
| boiled, ½ cup . . . . . . . . . | 51 | 2.62 | 45 | 140 | 398 | .70 | .25 | .30 |
| canned, w/liquid, | | | | | | | | |
| ½ cup . . . . . . . . . . . . . | 42 | 2.28 | 42 | 130 | 370 | .65 | .23 | .28 |
| **Blackberry:** | | | | | | | | |
| fresh, untrimmed, 1 lb. . . . | 139 | 2.50 | 86 | 89 | 853 | 1.19 | .61 | 5.62 |
| fresh, trimmed, ½ cup . . . | 23 | .41 | 14 | 15 | 141 | .20 | .10 | .93 |
| canned, in heavy syrup, | | | | | | | | |
| ½ cup . . . . . . . . . . . . . | 27 | .83 | 22 | 18 | 127 | .23 | .17 | .89 |
| frozen, unsweetened, | | | | | | | | |
| ½ cup . . . . . . . . . . . . . | 22 | .61 | 17 | 23 | 106 | .19 | .09 | .92 |
| **Black-eyed peas,** see "Cowpeas" | | | | | | | | |
| **Blueberry:** | | | | | | | | |
| fresh, untrimmed, 1 lb. . . . | 28 | .73 | 22 | 46 | 394 | .48 | .27 | 1.25 |

| | Calcium | Iron | Magnesium | Phosphorus | Potassium | Zinc | Copper | Manganese |
|---|---|---|---|---|---|---|---|---|
| | (Mg) | (Mg) | (Mg) | (Mg) | (Mg) | (Mg) | (Mg) | (Mg) |
| fresh, trimmed, ½ cup | 5 | .12 | 4 | 8 | 65 | .08 | .04 | .20 |
| canned, in heavy syrup, | | | | | | | | |
| ½ cup............. | 7 | .42 | 4 | 13 | 51 | .09 | .07 | .26 |
| frozen: | | | | | | | | |
| unsweetened, ½ cup | 6 | .14 | 4 | 9 | 42 | .06 | .03 | .11 |
| sweetened, ⅓ of | | | | | | | | |
| 10-oz. pkg. ...... | 5 | .37 | 2 | 7 | 56 | .06 | .04 | .25 |
| sweetened, ½ cup ... | 7 | .45 | 3 | 8 | 69 | .07 | .05 | .30 |
| **Bluefish,** meat only: | | | | | | | | |
| raw, 1 lb.............. | 31 | 2.16 | 151 | 1031 | 1688 | 3.66 | .24 | .10 |
| baked, broiled, or | | | | | | | | |
| microwaved[1], 4 oz. .... | 10 | .70 | 48 | 330 | 541 | 1.18 | .08 | .03 |
| **Bologna:** | | | | | | | | |
| beef, 1-oz. slice ........ | 3 | .47 | 3 | 25 | 44 | .61 | .01 | .01 |
| beef and pork, | | | | | | | | |
| 1-oz. slice .......... | 3 | .43 | 3 | 26 | 51 | .55 | .02 | .01 |
| Lebanon, beef, 1 oz. .... | 4 | .70 | 5 | 43 | 85 | 1.13 | .03 | .02 |
| pork, 1-oz. slice........ | 3 | .22 | 4 | 39 | 80 | .57 | .02 | .01 |
| **"Bologna," vegetarian,** | | | | | | | | |
| frozen (*Worthington* | | | | | | | | |
| *Bolono*), 2 oz. ........ | 40 | 2.08 | n.a. | n.a. | 125 | .39 | n.a. | n.a. |
| **Borage,** raw, untrimmed, | | | | | | | | |
| 1 lb. .............. | 465 | 16.50 | 260 | 251 | 2226 | n.a. | n.a. | n.a. |
| **Bouillon,** dehydrated: | | | | | | | | |
| beef, 1 cube .......... | n.a. | .08 | 2 | 8 | 15 | .01 | n.a. | .01 |
| chicken, 1 cube ........ | n.a. | .09 | 3 | 9 | 18 | .01 | n.a. | .02 |
| **Boysenberry:** | | | | | | | | |
| fresh, see "Blackberry" | | | | | | | | |
| canned, in heavy | | | | | | | | |
| syrup, ½ cup........ | 23 | .55 | 14 | 13 | 115 | .24 | .09 | .32 |
| frozen, unsweetened, | | | | | | | | |
| ½ cup............. | 18 | .56 | 11 | 18 | 92 | .15 | .05 | .36 |

---

[1] *Prepared without added ingredients.*

| | Calcium | Iron | Magnesium | Phosphorus | Potassium | Zinc | Copper | Manganese |
|---|---|---|---|---|---|---|---|---|
| | (Mg) | (Mg) | (Mg) | (Mg) | (Mg) | (Mg) | (Mg) | (Mg) |

**Brain[1]:**

beef, pan-fried in

  vegetable oil, 4 oz..... | 10 | 2.52 | 17 | 438 | 401 | 1.53 | .25 | .04

beef, simmered, 4 oz. | 10 | 2.51 | 16 | 399 | 272 | 1.42 | .27 | .04

lamb, braised, 4 oz...... | 14 | 1.91 | 16 | 382 | 232 | 1.54 | .24 | .07

lamb, pan-fried in

  vegetable oil, 4 oz..... | 24 | 2.31 | 25 | 561 | 406 | 2.27 | .54 | .08

pork, braised, 4 oz. ..... | 10 | 2.06 | .14 | 249 | 221 | 1.68 | .30 | .10

veal, braised, 4 oz....... | 18 | 1.89 | 18 | 437 | 243 | 1.83 | .29 | .04

veal, pan-fried in

  vegetable oil, 4 oz..... | 11 | 1.21 | 20 | 492 | 535 | 2.06 | .34 | .05

**Bran,** see "Cereal" and specific bran listings

**Bratwurst,** 1 oz.:

pork, cooked ......... | 13 | .36 | 4 | 42 | 60 | .65 | .03 | .01

pork and beef[2]......... | 14 | .29 | 4 | 38 | 80 | .60 | .02 | .01

**Braunschweiger[2]** (see

  also "Liverwurst"),

  pork, 1 oz.......... | 2 | 2.65 | 3 | 48 | 57 | .80 | .07 | .04

**Brazil nut,** dried, unblanched:

in shell, 1 lb........... | 383 | 7.40 | 490 | 1306 | 1306 | 9.98 | 3.85 | 1.69

shelled, 1 oz., 8 medium

  or 6 large .......... | 50 | .97 | 64 | 170 | 170 | 1.30 | .50 | .22

shelled, 1 cup, approx.

  32 large............ | 246 | 4.76 | 315 | 840 | 840 | 6.42 | 2.48 | 1.08

**Bread,** 1 slice or piece, except as noted:

Boston brown[3], canned,

  1 oz............... | 20 | .6 | 18 | 32 | 90 | .14 | .02 | .29

egg................. | 37 | 1.21 | 7 | 42 | 46 | .31 | .07 | .2

egg, toasted.......... | 38 | 1.23 | 8 | 43 | 47 | .32 | .07 | .2

French.............. | 19 | .63 | 7 | 26 | 28 | .22 | .05 | .13

French, toasted ........ | 19 | .63 | 7 | 26 | 28 | .22 | .05 | .13

---

[1] *Prepared without added ingredients, except as noted.*

[2] *Nonfat dry milk added.*

[3] *Made with white cornmeal.*

| | Calcium (Mg) | Iron (Mg) | Magnesium (Mg) | Phosphorus (Mg) | Potassium (Mg) | Zinc (Mg) | Copper (Mg) | Manganese (Mg) |
|---|---|---|---|---|---|---|---|---|
| high calcium: | | | | | | | | |
| dark | 139 | .63 | n.a. | n.a. | 36 | n.a. | n.a. | n.a. |
| dark, toasted | 137 | .62 | n.a. | n.a. | 36 | n.a. | n.a. | n.a. |
| light | 130 | .64 | 7 | 15 | 34 | .19 | .02 | .08 |
| light, toasted | 128 | .63 | 7 | 14 | 34 | .19 | .02 | .08 |
| Indian (Navajo) fry, 5"-diam. piece | 210 | 3.24 | 15 | 141 | 67 | .45 | .09 | .42 |
| Italian | 23 | .88 | 8 | 31 | 33 | .26 | .06 | .14 |
| Italian, toasted | 23 | .87 | 8 | 31 | 33 | .26 | .06 | .14 |
| mixed grain | 24 | .90 | 14 | 46 | 53 | .33 | .07 | .39 |
| mixed grain, toasted | 24 | .90 | 14 | 46 | 53 | .33 | .07 | .39 |
| oat bran: | | | | | | | | |
| regular | 19 | .94 | n.a. | n.a. | n.a. | n.a. | n.a. | n.a. |
| regular, toasted | 19 | .93 | n.a. | n.a. | n.a. | n.a. | n.a. | n.a. |
| light | 13 | .72 | n.a. | n.a. | 24 | n.a. | n.a. | n.a. |
| light, toasted | 13 | .71 | n.a. | n.a. | 23 | n.a. | n.a. | n.a. |
| oatmeal: | | | | | | | | |
| regular | 18 | .73 | 10 | 34 | 38 | .28 | .06 | .25 |
| regular, toasted | 18 | .73 | 10 | 34 | 39 | .28 | .06 | .26 |
| light | 26 | .53 | n.a. | n.a. | n.a. | n.a. | n.a. | n.a. |
| light, toasted | 26 | .52 | n.a. | n.a. | n.a. | n.a. | n.a. | n.a. |
| pita, enriched, 6½"- diam. piece | 52 | 1.57 | 16 | 58 | 72 | .51 | .10 | .29 |
| pita, whole wheat, 6½"-diam. piece | 10 | n.a. | 44 | 115 | 108 | .97 | n.a. | 1.11 |
| protein | 24 | .79 | n.a. | n.a. | n.a. | n.a. | n.a. | n.a. |
| protein, toasted | 23 | .78 | n.a. | n.a. | n.a. | n.a. | n.a. | n.a. |
| pumpernickel, 1.1 oz. | 22 | .92 | 17 | 57 | 66 | .47 | .09 | .42 |
| pumpernickel, 1.1 oz., toasted | 22 | .91 | 17 | 57 | 66 | .47 | .09 | .42 |
| raisin, enriched | 17 | .75 | 7 | 28 | 59 | .19 | .05 | .13 |
| raisin, enriched, toasted | 17 | .76 | 7 | 28 | 59 | .19 | .05 | .13 |

|  | Calcium | Iron | Magnesium | Phosphorus | Potassium | Zinc | Copper | Manganese |
|---|---|---|---|---|---|---|---|---|
|  | (Mg) | (Mg) | (Mg) | (Mg) | (Mg) | (Mg) | (Mg) | (Mg) |
| Bread, *continued* | | | | | | | | |
| rice bran . . . . . . . . . . . . | 19 | .97 | n.a. | n.a. | n.a. | n.a. | n.a. | n.a. |
| rice bran, toasted. . . . . . | 19 | .98 | n.a. | n.a. | n.a. | n.a. | n.a. | n.a. |
| rye: | | | | | | | | |
| seeded or | | | | | | | | |
| unseeded. . . . . . . . | 23 | .90 | 13 | 40 | 53 | .36 | .06 | .26 |
| seeded or unseeded, | | | | | | | | |
| toasted . . . . . . . . | 23 | .90 | 13 | 40 | 53 | .36 | .06 | .26 |
| light, .9 oz. . . . . . . . . | 18 | .71 | n.a. | n.a. | 23 | n.a. | n.a. | n.a. |
| light, .9 oz., | | | | | | | | |
| toasted . . . . . . . . . | 17 | .70 | n.a. | n.a. | 22 | n.a. | n.a. | n.a. |
| Vienna, enriched, .9 oz. | 28 | .80 | n.a. | 21 | 23 | n.a. | n.a. | n.a. |
| wheat: | | | | | | | | |
| plain, .9 oz. . . . . . . . . | 26 | .83 | 12 | 38 | 50 | .26 | .05 | .27 |
| plain, .9 oz., | | | | | | | | |
| toasted . . . . . . . . . | 26 | .83 | 12 | 38 | 50 | .26 | .05 | .26 |
| bran, 1.3 oz. . . . . . . . | 27 | 1.10 | 29 | 67 | 82 | .49 | .08 | .6 |
| bran, 1.3 oz., | | | | | | | | |
| toasted . . . . . . . . . | 27 | 1.11 | 30 | 67 | 82 | .49 | .08 | .61 |
| cracked (18 slices | | | | | | | | |
| per lb.) . . . . . . . . . | 11 | .7 | 13 | 38 | 44 | .31 | .06 | .34 |
| cracked, toasted. . . . . | 11 | .7 | 13 | 38 | 44 | .31 | .06 | .34 |
| light, .8 oz. . . . . . . . . | 18 | .68 | n.a. | n.a. | n.a. | n.a. | n.a. | n.a. |
| light, .8 oz., | | | | | | | | |
| toasted . . . . . . . . . | 18 | .67 | n.a. | n.a. | n.a. | n.a. | n.a. | n.a. |
| whole . . . . . . . . . . . | 20 | .94 | 24 | 65 | 71 | .6 | .08 | .66 |
| whole, toasted . . . . . . | 20 | .93 | 24 | 64 | 71 | .54 | .08 | .65 |
| wheat germ . . . . . . . . . . | 25 | .98 | n.a. | n.a. | 72 | n.a. | n.a. | n.a. |
| wheat germ, toasted . . . . | 25 | .97 | n.a. | n.a. | 71 | n.a. | n.a. | n.a. |
| white, enriched: | | | | | | | | |
| regular, .9 oz. . . . . . . | 27 | .76 | 6 | 23 | 30 | .15 | .03 | .10 |
| regular, .9 oz., | | | | | | | | |
| toasted . . . . . . . . . | 27 | .77 | 6 | 24 | 30 | .16 | .03 | .10 |
| light, .8 oz. . . . . . . . . | 22 | .73 | n.a. | n.a. | 18 | .31 | .08 | n.a. |
| light, .8 oz., | | | | | | | | |
| toasted . . . . . . . . . | 21 | .72 | n.a. | n.a. | 17 | .30 | .08 | n.a. |

| | Calcium | Iron | Magnesium | Phosphorus | Potassium | Zinc | Copper | Manganese |
|---|---|---|---|---|---|---|---|---|
| | (Mg) | (Mg) | (Mg) | (Mg) | (Mg) | (Mg) | (Mg) | (Mg) |
| **Bread, sweet, mix**[1]**, corn bread,** 2½" x 2½" square piece ........ | 133 | .80 | n.a. | 209 | 61 | n.a. | n.a. | n.a. |
| **Bread crumbs,** enriched: | | | | | | | | |
| dry, grated, plain, 1 cup ............. | 64 | 1.74 | 13 | 42 | 63 | .35 | .05 | .23 |
| dry, grated, seasoned, 1 cup ............. | 119 | 3.82 | 45 | 160 | 324 | 1.09 | n.a. | n.a. |
| soft, 1 cup............ | 57 | 1.30 | n.a. | 49 | 50 | n.a. | n.a. | n.a. |
| **Bread cubes,** white, 1 cup ............. | 38 | .90 | n.a. | 32 | 34 | n.a. | n.a. | n.a. |
| **Bread stick,** plain, 1 stick, 9¼" x ⅜"..... | 1 | .26 | 2 | 7 | 7 | .05 | .01 | .03 |
| **Breadfruit:** | | | | | | | | |
| untrimmed, 1 lb........ | 61 | 1.92 | 89 | 106 | 1732 | .41 | .30 | .21 |
| trimmed, ½ cup........ | 19 | .60 | 28 | 33 | 539 | .13 | .09 | .07 |
| **Breakfast bar,** 1 bar: | | | | | | | | |
| chocolate chip (*Carnation*) | 20 | 4.50 | 60 | 60 | 110 | 3.00 | .50 | .05 |
| chocolate crunch (*Carnation*) ......... | 20 | 4.50 | 60 | 60 | 130 | 3.00 | .50 | .18 |
| peanut butter, w/ chocolate chips (*Carnation*) ......... | 20 | 4.50 | 60 | 60 | 110 | 3.00 | .50 | .18 |
| peanut butter crunch (*Carnation*) ......... | 20 | 4.50 | 60 | 60 | 110 | 3.00 | .50 | .21 |
| **Broad beans,** fresh, raw: | | | | | | | | |
| untrimmed, 1 lb........ | 97 | 8.36 | 167 | 418 | 1100 | n.a. | n.a. | n.a. |
| trimmed, ½ cup........ | 12 | 1.04 | 21 | 52 | 137 | n.a. | n.a. | n.a. |
| **Broad beans,** dried: | | | | | | | | |
| uncooked, 1 lb........ | 467 | 30.37 | 872 | 1908 | 4817 | 14.23 | 3.74 | 7.38 |
| uncooked, ½ cup....... | 77 | 5.02 | 144 | 315 | 796 | 2.35 | .62 | 1.22 |

[1] *Prepared according to package directions, with eggs and milk.*

| | Calcium | Iron | Magnesium | Phosphorus | Potassium | Zinc | Copper | Manganese |
|---|---|---|---|---|---|---|---|---|
| | (Mg) | (Mg) | (Mg) | (Mg) | (Mg) | (Mg) | (Mg) | (Mg) |
| **Broad beans,** *continued* | | | | | | | | |
| boiled, ½ cup . . . . . . . . | 31 | 1.27 | 36 | 106 | 228 | .86 | .22 | .36 |
| canned, w/liquid, 8 oz. . . . | 60 | 2.27 | 73 | 179 | 550 | 1.42 | .25 | .65 |
| canned, w/liquid, | | | | | | | | |
| ½ cup . . . . . . . . . . . . | 34 | 1.28 | 41 | 101 | 310 | .80 | .14 | .37 |
| **Broccoli:** | | | | | | | | |
| fresh: | | | | | | | | |
| raw, untrimmed, | | | | | | | | |
| 1 lb. . . . . . . . . . . | 134 | 2.44 | 70 | 182 | 898 | 1.10 | .13 | .63 |
| raw, trimmed, | | | | | | | | |
| 1 spear, 5.3 oz. . . . | 73 | 1.33 | 38 | 99 | 490 | .60 | .07 | .35 |
| raw, trimmed, | | | | | | | | |
| chopped, ½ cup . . | 21 | .39 | 11 | 29 | 143 | .18 | .02 | .10 |
| boiled, drained, | | | | | | | | |
| 1 spear, 6.3 oz. . . . | 82 | 1.50 | 43 | 107 | 526 | .68 | .08 | .39 |
| boiled, drained, | | | | | | | | |
| chopped, ½ cup . . | 36 | .65 | 19 | 46 | 228 | .30 | .03 | .17 |
| frozen: | | | | | | | | |
| chopped, 10-oz. pkg. | 159 | 2.30 | 50 | 142 | 602 | 1.37 | .11 | .84 |
| chopped or spears, | | | | | | | | |
| boiled, drained, | | | | | | | | |
| ½ cup . . . . . . . . . | 47 | .56 | 19 | 51 | 166 | .28 | .04 | .30 |
| spears, 10-oz. pkg. . . | 115 | 2.03 | 45 | 167 | 710 | .96 | .10 | .73 |
| spears, boiled, | | | | | | | | |
| drained, ⅓ of | | | | | | | | |
| 10-oz. pkg. . . . . . . | 42 | .51 | 17 | 46 | 150 | .25 | .04 | .27 |
| **Brown gravy mix[1]:** | | | | | | | | |
| ¼ cup . . . . . . . . . . . . . . | 17 | .06 | n.a. | 26 | 50 | n.a. | n.a. | n.a. |
| vegetarian (*Loma Linda* | | | | | | | | |
| *Gravy Quik*), .2 oz. . . . . | 4 | .07 | n.a. | n.a. | 7 | .02 | n.a. | n.a. |
| **Brownie,** 1 piece: | | | | | | | | |
| 1¾" × ¾", 1 oz. . . . . . . . | 8 | .64 | 9 | 29 | 42 | .2 | .06 | n.a. |

[1] *Prepared according to package directions, with water.*

| | Calcium | Iron | Magnesium | Phosphorus | Potassium | Zinc | Copper | Manganese |
|---|---|---|---|---|---|---|---|---|
| | (Mg) | (Mg) | (Mg) | (Mg) | (Mg) | (Mg) | (Mg) | (Mg) |
| w/nuts, .9 oz. . . . . . . . . | 13 | .60 | n.a. | 26 | 50 | n.a. | n.a. | n.a. |
| frozen, w/chocolate icing, | | | | | | | | |
| .9 oz. . . . . . . . . . . . . | 10 | .40 | n.a. | 31 | 44 | n.a. | n.a. | n.a. |
| **Brussels sprouts:** | | | | | | | | |
| fresh: | | | | | | | | |
| raw, untrimmed, | | | | | | | | |
| 1 lb. . . . . . . . . . . | 169 | 5.71 | 94 | 282 | 1589 | 1.71 | .29 | 1.38 |
| raw, 1 sprout, | | | | | | | | |
| .75 oz. . . . . . . . . . | 8 | .27 | 4 | 13 | 74 | .08 | .01 | .06 |
| raw, trimmed, ½ cup | 18 | .62 | 10 | 30 | 171 | .18 | .03 | .15 |
| boiled, drained, | | | | | | | | |
| 1 sprout, .75 oz. . . . | 7 | .25 | 4 | 12 | 67 | .07 | .02 | .05 |
| boiled, drained, | | | | | | | | |
| ½ cup . . . . . . . . . . | 28 | .94 | 16 | 44 | 247 | .25 | .07 | .18 |
| frozen, 10-oz. pkg. . . . . . | 75 | 2.65 | 57 | 176 | 1052 | .87 | .09 | .88 |
| frozen, boiled, drained, | | | | | | | | |
| ½ cup . . . . . . . . . . . . | 19 | .58 | .19 | 42 | 254 | .28 | .06 | .25 |
| **Buckwheat,** whole grain, | | | | | | | | |
| 1 cup . . . . . . . . . . . . | 31 | 3.74 | 392 | 590 | 782 | 4.08 | 1.87 | 2.21 |
| **Buckwheat flour,** | | | | | | | | |
| 1 cup . . . . . . . . . . . . | 49 | 4.88 | 301 | 404 | 692 | 3.75 | .62 | 2.44 |
| **Buckwheat groats,** | | | | | | | | |
| roasted: | | | | | | | | |
| uncooked, 1 oz. . . . . . . . | 5 | .70 | 63 | 90 | 91 | .69 | .18 | .46 |
| uncooked, ½ cup. . . . . . . | 14 | 2.02 | 181 | 261 | 263 | 1.98 | .51 | 1.33 |
| cooked, 1 cup . . . . . . . . | 14 | 1.58 | 101 | 139 | 175 | 1.21 | .29 | .80 |
| **Bulgar:** | | | | | | | | |
| uncooked, 1 oz. . . . . . . . | 10 | .70 | 46 | 85 | 116 | .55 | .09 | .86 |
| uncooked, ½ cup. . . . . . . | 25 | 1.72 | 115 | 210 | 287 | 1.35 | .24 | 2.13 |
| cooked, 1 cup . . . . . . . . | 18 | 1.75 | 58 | 73 | 124 | 1.04 | .14 | 1.11 |
| **Burbot,** meat only: | | | | | | | | |
| raw, 1 lb. . . . . . . . . . . | 227 | 4.08 | 143 | 907 | 1833 | 3.42 | .91 | 3.18 |
| baked, broiled, or | | | | | | | | |
| microwaved[1], 4 oz. . . . | 73 | 1.30 | 46 | 290 | 587 | 1.10 | .29 | 1.02 |

[1] *Prepared without added ingredients.*

| | Calcium | Iron | Magnesium | Phosphorus | Potassium | Zinc | Copper | Manganese |
|---|---|---|---|---|---|---|---|---|
| | (Mg) | (Mg) | (Mg) | (Mg) | (Mg) | (Mg) | (Mg) | (Mg) |
| **Burdock root:** | | | | | | | | |
| raw, untrimmed, 1 lb. | 139 | 2.72 | 130 | 174 | 1048 | n.a. | n.a. | n.a. |
| raw, trimmed, 1 root, 5.5 oz. | 64 | 1.25 | 59 | 80 | 480 | n.a. | n.a. | n.a. |
| boiled, drained, 1" pieces, 1 cup | 62 | .96 | 49 | 116 | 450 | n.a. | n.a. | n.a. |
| **Butter:** | | | | | | | | |
| regular, 1 stick | 27 | .18 | 2 | 26 | 29 | .06 | .02 | tr. |
| regular, 1 tbsp. | 3 | .02 | <1 | 3 | 4 | .01 | tr. | tr. |
| whipped, 1 stick | 18 | .12 | 2 | 17 | 20 | .40 | .01 | tr. |
| whipped, 1 tbsp. | 2 | .02 | <1 | 2 | 2 | tr. | tr. | tr. |
| **Butter beans** (*Van Camp's*), 1 cup | 0 | 0 | .09 | .08 | .53 | n.a. | n.a. | n.a. |
| **Butterbur:** | | | | | | | | |
| raw, untrimmed, 1 lb. | 411 | .40 | 57 | 48 | 2614 | n.a. | n.a. | n.a. |
| raw, trimmed, 1 cup | 97 | .09 | 13 | 11 | 616 | n.a. | n.a. | n.a. |
| canned, chopped, 1 cup | 42 | .78 | 3 | 5 | 15 | n.a. | n.a. | n.a. |
| **Butterfish,** meat only: | | | | | | | | |
| raw, 1 lb. | n.a. | 2.27 | n.a. | n.a. | 1699 | 3.47 | .25 | .07 |
| baked, broiled, or microwaved[1], 4 oz. | n.a. | .73 | n.a. | n.a. | 445 | 1.12 | .08 | .02 |
| **Butternut squash:** | | | | | | | | |
| fresh: | | | | | | | | |
| raw, untrimmed, 1 lb. | 183 | 2.67 | 130 | 126 | 1341 | .55 | .27 | n.a. |
| raw, trimmed, cubed, ½ cup | 34 | .49 | .24 | 23 | 246 | .10 | .05 | n.a. |
| boiled, drained, cubed, ½ cup | 42 | .61 | 30 | 27 | 290 | .13 | .07 | n.a. |
| frozen, 12-oz. pkg. | 97 | 2.99 | 46 | 75 | 722 | .58 | .17 | n.a. |
| frozen, boiled, mashed, ½ cup | 23 | .70 | 11 | 17 | 160 | .14 | .04 | n.a. |

---

[1] *Prepared without added ingredients.*

| | Calcium | Iron | Magnesium | Phosphorus | Potassium | Zinc | Copper | Manganese |
|---|---|---|---|---|---|---|---|---|
| | (Mg) | (Mg) | (Mg) | (Mg) | (Mg) | (Mg) | (Mg) | (Mg) |
| **Butternuts,** dried: | | | | | | | | |
| in shell, 1 lb........... | 65 | 4.92 | 290 | 546 | 515 | 3.83 | .55 | 8.01 |
| shelled, 1 oz........... | 15 | 1.14 | 67 | 127 | 119 | .89 | .13 | 1.86 |
| **Butterscotch topping,** | | | | | | | | |
| 2 tbsp. ............ | 22 | .08 | 3 | n.a. | n.a. | n.a. | n.a. | n.a. |

# C

| | Calcium | Iron | Magnesium | Phosphorus | Potassium | Zinc | Copper | Manganese |
|---|---|---|---|---|---|---|---|---|
| | (Mg) | (Mg) | (Mg) | (Mg) | (Mg) | (Mg) | (Mg) | (Mg) |
| **Cabbage:** | | | | | | | | |
| raw: | | | | | | | | |
| untrimmed, 1 lb. .... | 172 | 2.13 | 53 | 85 | 892 | .67 | .09 | .58 |
| trimmed, 1 head, | | | | | | | | |
| 5⅜"-diam. ....... | 424 | 5.09 | 134 | 211 | 2231 | 1.66 | .21 | 1.44 |
| trimmed, shredded, | | | | | | | | |
| ½ cup .......... | 17 | .21 | 5 | 8 | 86 | .06 | .01 | .06 |
| boiled, drained, shredded, | | | | | | | | |
| ½ cup ............ | 23 | .13 | 6 | 12 | 73 | .07 | .01 | .09 |
| **Cabbage, Chinese:** | | | | | | | | |
| bok-choy: | | | | | | | | |
| raw, untrimmed, | | | | | | | | |
| 1 lb. ........... | 419 | 3.19 | 74 | 148 | 1004 | n.a. | n.a. | n.a. |
| raw, trimmed, | | | | | | | | |
| shredded, ½ cup | 37 | .28 | 7 | 13 | 88 | n.a. | n.a. | n.a. |
| boiled, drained, | | | | | | | | |
| shredded, ½ cup | 79 | .88 | 9 | 25 | 315 | n.a. | n.a. | n.a. |
| pe-tsai: | | | | | | | | |
| raw, untrimmed, | | | | | | | | |
| 1 lb. ........... | 323 | 1.29 | 56 | 122 | 1004 | .96 | .15 | .80 |
| raw, trimmed, | | | | | | | | |
| shredded, ½ cup | 29 | .12 | 5 | 11 | 90 | .09 | .01 | .07 |
| boiled, drained, | | | | | | | | |
| .5-oz. leaf ....... | 4 | .04 | 1 | 5 | 31 | .03 | <.01 | .02 |
| boiled, drained, | | | | | | | | |
| shredded, ½ cup | 19 | .18 | 6 | 23 | 134 | .11 | .02 | .09 |
| **Cabbage, red:** | | | | | | | | |
| raw, untrimmed, 1 lb. | 185 | 1.79 | 56 | 152 | 746 | .77 | .35 | .65 |
| raw, trimmed, shredded, | | | | | | | | |
| ½ cup ............ | 18 | .17 | 5 | 15 | 72 | .07 | .03 | .06 |
| boiled, drained, .75-oz. | | | | | | | | |
| leaf .............. | 8 | .08 | 2 | 6 | 31 | .03 | .02 | .03 |

| | Calcium | Iron | Magnesium | Phosphorus | Potassium | Zinc | Copper | Manganese |
|---|---|---|---|---|---|---|---|---|
| | (Mg) | (Mg) | (Mg) | (Mg) | (Mg) | (Mg) | (Mg) | (Mg) |
| boiled, drained, shredded, ½ cup . . . . . . . . . . . . . | 28 | .27 | 8 | 21 | 105 | .11 | .05 | .10 |
| **Cabbage, savoy:** | | | | | | | | |
| raw, untrimmed, 1 lb. . . . | 127 | 1.45 | 102 | 152 | 835 | n.a. | n.a. | n.a. |
| raw, trimmed, shredded, ½ cup . . . . . . . . . . . . . | 12 | .14 | 10 | 15 | 81 | n.a. | n.a. | n.a. |
| boiled, drained, shredded, ½ cup . . . . . . . . . . . . . | 22 | .28 | 17 | 24 | 134 | n.a. | n.a. | n.a. |
| **Cake:** | | | | | | | | |
| angelfood, ¹⁄₁₂ of 9"-diam. cake . . . . . . . . . . . . . | 40 | .15 | 3 | n.a. | 26 | .02 | .02 | .02 |
| Boston creme pie, ⅙ of 19.5-oz. cake. . . . . . . . | 21 | .35 | 6 | 46 | 36 | .15 | n.a. | .05 |
| cheesecake, 1 oz.. . . . . . . | 14 | .18 | 3 | 26 | 25 | .14 | .01 | .04 |
| chocolate w/chocolate frosting, ⅛ of 18-oz. cake . . . . . . . . . . . . . | 28 | 1.41 | 22 | 78 | 128 | .44 | .16 | .21 |
| coffee cake: | | | | | | | | |
| cheese, 1 oz.. . . . . . . | 17 | .18 | 4 | 28 | n.a. | .17 | .02 | .05 |
| cinnamon w/crumb topping, 1 oz. . . . . | 15 | .54 | 6 | 31 | 35 | .23 | .04 | .13 |
| creme-filled w/chocolate frosting, 1 oz. . . . . . . . | 11 | .15 | 4 | 21 | n.a. | .12 | .02 | .05 |
| fruit, 1 oz.. . . . . . . . . . . . | 13 | .69 | 5 | 33 | 26 | .18 | .01 | .07 |
| fruitcake, 1.5-oz. piece . . . . . . . . . . . . . | 14 | .89 | 7 | 22 | 66 | .12 | .02 | .10 |
| pound, 1-oz. slice . . . . . . | 10 | .39 | 3 | 39 | 34 | .13 | .01 | .03 |
| pound, fat-free, 1-oz. slice . . . . . . . . . . . . . | 12 | .58 | 3 | 41 | 31 | .09 | .02 | .04 |
| sponge, ¹⁄₁₂ of 16-oz. cake . . . . . . . . . . . . . | 26 | 1.03 | 4 | 52 | 38 | .19 | .02 | .08 |
| yellow, w/chocolate frosting, 2.3-oz. slice. . . . . . . . | 24 | 1.33 | 19 | 103 | 114 | .4 | .12 | .17 |

| | Calcium | Iron | Magnesium | Phosphorus | Potassium | Zinc | Copper | Manganese |
|---|---|---|---|---|---|---|---|---|
| | (Mg) | (Mg) | (Mg) | (Mg) | (Mg) | (Mg) | (Mg) | (Mg) |

**Cake,** *continued*
yellow, w/vanilla frosting,

| | Calcium | Iron | Magnesium | Phosphorus | Potassium | Zinc | Copper | Manganese |
|---|---|---|---|---|---|---|---|---|
| 2.3-oz. slice . . . . . . . . | 39 | .68 | 4 | 92 | 34 | .16 | .02 | .06 |

**Cake, frozen,** devil's food:
w/chocolate frosting, ⅙ of 7½"-diam. cake . . . . . .

| | Calcium | Iron | Magnesium | Phosphorus | Potassium | Zinc | Copper | Manganese |
|---|---|---|---|---|---|---|---|---|
| | 46 | .70 | n.a. | 78 | 101 | n.a. | n.a. | n.a. |

w/whipped cream filling and chocolate frosting, 2 layer, ⅙ of 7¼"-diam. cake . . . . . .

| | Calcium | Iron | Magnesium | Phosphorus | Potassium | Zinc | Copper | Manganese |
|---|---|---|---|---|---|---|---|---|
| | 68 | .50 | n.a. | 104 | 96 | n.a. | n.a. | n.a. |

**Cake, snack:**
chocolate, cupcake, w/ frosting, lowfat, 1.5-oz. piece . . . . . . . .

| | Calcium | Iron | Magnesium | Phosphorus | Potassium | Zinc | Copper | Manganese |
|---|---|---|---|---|---|---|---|---|
| | 15 | .66 | 11 | 79 | 96 | .24 | .08 | .10 |

devil's food, w/creme filling, 1.8-oz. piece . . .

| | Calcium | Iron | Magnesium | Phosphorus | Potassium | Zinc | Copper | Manganese |
|---|---|---|---|---|---|---|---|---|
| | 37 | 1.68 | 20 | 47 | 61 | n.a. | n.a. | n.a. |

sponge, w/creme filling, 1.5-oz. piece . . . . . . . .

| | Calcium | Iron | Magnesium | Phosphorus | Potassium | Zinc | Copper | Manganese |
|---|---|---|---|---|---|---|---|---|
| | 19 | .55 | 3 | n.a. | n.a. | n.a. | n.a. | n.a. |

**Cake mix**[1]**:**
angel food, 1/12 of 9" cake . . . . . . . . . . . .

| | Calcium | Iron | Magnesium | Phosphorus | Potassium | Zinc | Copper | Manganese |
|---|---|---|---|---|---|---|---|---|
| | 44 | .20 | n.a. | 91 | 71 | n.a. | n.a. | n.a. |

brownie, see "Brownie"
coffee cake, crumb, 2.5-oz. piece . . . . . . . .

| | Calcium | Iron | Magnesium | Phosphorus | Potassium | Zinc | Copper | Manganese |
|---|---|---|---|---|---|---|---|---|
| | 44 | 1.20 | n.a. | 125 | 78 | n.a. | n.a. | n.a. |

devil's food, w/chocolate frosting, 2 layer, 2.4-oz. piece . . . . . . . .

| | Calcium | Iron | Magnesium | Phosphorus | Potassium | Zinc | Copper | Manganese |
|---|---|---|---|---|---|---|---|---|
| | 41 | 1.40 | n.a. | 72 | 90 | n.a. | n.a. | n.a. |

gingerbread, ⅑ of 8" square . . . . . . . . . . .

| | Calcium | Iron | Magnesium | Phosphorus | Potassium | Zinc | Copper | Manganese |
|---|---|---|---|---|---|---|---|---|
| | 57 | 1.20 | n.a. | 63 | 173 | n.a. | n.a. | n.a. |

[1] *Prepared according to package directions.*

| | Calcium | Iron | Magnesium | Phosphorus | Potassium | Zinc | Copper | Manganese |
|---|---|---|---|---|---|---|---|---|
| | (Mg) | (Mg) | (Mg) | (Mg) | (Mg) | (Mg) | (Mg) | (Mg) |
| yellow, w/chocolate frosting, 2 layer, 2.4-oz. piece . . . . . . . . | 63 | 1.00 | n.a. | 126 | 75 | n.a. | n.a. | n.a. |
| **Candy:** | | | | | | | | |
| almond, chocolate coated, 1 oz. . . . . . . . . . . . . . . | 58 | .80 | n.a. | 97 | 155 | n.a. | n.a. | n.a. |
| almond, sugar coated, 1 oz. . . . . . . . . . . . . . . | 28 | .50 | n.a. | 47 | 72 | n.a. | n.a. | n.a. |
| (*Baby Ruth*), 2.1-oz. bar | 24 | .49 | 43 | n.a. | 129 | .41 | n.a. | n.a. |
| (*Bar None*), 1.5-oz. bar | 62 | .52 | 31 | 86 | 168 | .53 | .11 | .22 |
| (*Butterfinger*), 2.16-oz. bar . . . . . . . . | 15 | .64 | 28 | 58 | 130 | .44 | .12 | .24 |
| butterscotch, 1 oz. . . . . . . | 1 | .02 | 0 | 1 | 1 | tr. | .01 | .01 |
| candy corn, 1 oz. . . . . . . . | 2 | .10 | n.a. | tr. | 1 | n.a. | n.a. | n.a. |
| caramel: | | | | | | | | |
| plain, .3-oz. piece. . . . | 11 | .01 | 1 | 9 | 17 | .04 | tr. | tr. |
| chocolate coated, w/cookie (*Twix*), 2-oz. pkg. . . . . . . . | 68 | .38 | 17 | n.a. | 118 | .39 | .07 | n.a. |
| milk chocolate coated (*Rolo*), 1.93-oz. pkg. . . . . | 74 | .27 | 16 | 88 | 143 | .38 | .06 | .11 |
| w/peanut, chocolate coated (*Oh! Henry*), 2-oz. bar . . . . . . . . | 62 | .32 | n.a. | n.a. | 185 | n.a. | n.a. | n.a. |
| carob, 1 oz. . . . . . . . . . . . | 130 | n.a. | 13 | n.a. | 255 | .40 | n.a. | .04 |
| chocolate, w/almonds: | | | | | | | | |
| (*Hershey's* Golden Almond), 3-oz. bar | 279 | 1.27 | 94 | 229 | 400 | 1.44 | .33 | .71 |
| (*Hershey's Solitaires*), 3-oz. pkg. . . . . . . . | 305 | 1.19 | 100 | 255 | 428 | 1.56 | .32 | .71 |
| candy coated (*M&M's*), 1.69-oz. pkg. . . . . . | 81 | .73 | 32 | 94 | 187 | .61 | .17 | .20 |

| | Calcium | Iron | Magnesium | Phosphorus | Potassium | Zinc | Copper | Manganese |
|---|---|---|---|---|---|---|---|---|
| | (Mg) | (Mg) | (Mg) | (Mg) | (Mg) | (Mg) | (Mg) | (Mg) |
| Candy, chocolate, w/almonds, *continued* | | | | | | | | |
| w/caramel (*Cara-mello*), 1.6-oz. bar | 89 | .49 | 19 | 72 | n.a. | .43 | .08 | .07 |
| chocolate, dark, sweet (*Hershey's Special Dark*), 1.45 oz....... | 8 | .86 | 47 | 66 | 139 | .61 | .33 | .33 |
| chocolate, milk: | | | | | | | | |
| 1 oz.............. | 50 | .40 | 16 | 61 | 96 | n.a. | n.a. | n.a. |
| 1.55-oz. bar........ | 84 | .61 | 27 | 95 | 169 | .61 | .17 | .13 |
| w/almonds, 1.55 oz. bar...... | 99 | .72 | 40 | 116 | 195 | .59 | .19 | .28 |
| creamy (*Hershey's Symphony*), 1.4-oz. bar....... | 94 | .40 | 22 | 100 | 154 | .45 | .12 | .07 |
| w/crisps (*Krackel*), 1.6-oz. bar....... | 84 | .38 | 26 | 104 | 161 | .57 | .18 | .15 |
| w/crisps (*Nestlé Crunch*), 1.4-oz. bar....... | 68 | .26 | 18 | 71 | 138 | .44 | .10 | .13 |
| w/crisps and peanuts (*Nestlé 100 Grand*), 1.5-oz. bar....... | 50 | .29 | 14 | 59 | 107 | .26 | .06 | .08 |
| w/fruit and nuts (*Chunky*), 1.4-oz. bar....... | 57 | .50 | 29 | 83 | 213 | n.a. | n.a. | n.a. |
| w/peanuts (*Mr. Goodbar*), 1.75-oz. bar...... | 56 | .60 | 48 | 140 | 225 | .90 | .25 | .40 |
| w/pecan and caramel (*Demet's Turtles*), .6-oz. piece ...... | 27 | .23 | n.a. | n.a. | 52 | n.a. | n.a. | n.a. |
| w/peanuts, candy coated (*M&M's*), 1.74-oz. pkg...... | 65 | .73 | 40 | 134 | 191 | .74 | .20 | .33 |

| | Calcium (Mg) | Iron (Mg) | Magnesium (Mg) | Phosphorus (Mg) | Potassium (Mg) | Zinc (Mg) | Copper (Mg) | Manganese (Mg) |
|---|---|---|---|---|---|---|---|---|
| chocolate, semisweet, 1 oz.... | 9 | .89 | 32 | 37 | 104 | .46 | .20 | .23 |
| chocolate, white, w/ almonds (*Nestlé Alpine*), 1.25-oz. bar .. | 81 | .2 | n.a. | n.a. | 146 | n.a. | n.a. | n.a. |
| chocolate chips, see "Chocolate, baking" | | | | | | | | |
| coconut, chocolate coated: | | | | | | | | |
| (*Mound's*), 1.9-oz. bar...... | 12 | 2.03 | 37 | 65 | n.a. | .56 | .30 | .41 |
| w/almonds (*Almond Joy*), 1.76-oz. bar | 40 | .6 | 33 | 70 | n.a. | .40 | .14 | .29 |
| (*5th Avenue*), 2.6-oz. bar......... | 42 | .60 | 38 | 90 | 197 | .65 | .13 | .22 |
| fondant, mint, 1 oz..... | 2 | .10 | n.a. | tr. | 1 | n.a. | n.a. | n.a. |
| fruit flavored: | | | | | | | | |
| (*Skittles*), 2.3-oz. pkg. | 2 | .06 | 1 | n.a. | 15 | .01 | .02 | n.a. |
| chews (*Starburst*), 2.07-oz. pkg...... | 2 | .08 | 1 | 4 | 1 | 0 | .01 | .01 |
| fudge: | | | | | | | | |
| chocolate, 1 oz...... | 22 | .30 | n.a. | 24 | 42 | n.a. | n.a. | n.a. |
| chocolate, w/nuts, 1 oz............ | 22 | .30 | n.a. | 32 | 50 | n.a. | n.a. | n.a. |
| vanilla, 1 oz. ....... | 32 | .10 | n.a. | 24 | 36 | n.a. | n.a. | n.a. |
| vanilla, w/nuts, 1 oz. | 31 | .20 | n.a. | 32 | 32 | n.a. | n.a. | n.a. |
| fudge, chocolate coated: | | | | | | | | |
| chocolate, 1 oz...... | 29 | .40 | n.a. | 31 | 55 | n.a. | n.a. | n.a. |
| chocolate w/nuts, 1 oz. | 29 | .40 | n.a. | 39 | 62 | n.a. | n.a. | n.a. |
| w/caramel and peanuts, 1 oz. ..... | 51 | .40 | n.a. | 53 | 85 | n.a. | n.a. | n.a. |
| w/peanuts and caramel, 1 oz. ..... | 36 | .30 | n.a. | 54 | 63 | n.a. | n.a. | n.a. |
| gum, chewing, 1 stick ... | n.a. | n.a. | n.a. | n.a. | 0 | n.a. | n.a. | n.a. |
| gumdrops, 10 small, 1.2 oz.............. | 1 | .14 | 0 | 0 | 2 | 0 | tr. | tr. |

| | Calcium | Iron | Magnesium | Phosphorus | Potassium | Zinc | Copper | Manganese |
|---|---|---|---|---|---|---|---|---|
| | (Mg) | (Mg) | (Mg) | (Mg) | (Mg) | (Mg) | (Mg) | (Mg) |
| Candy, *continued* | | | | | | | | |
| hard, 1 oz............. | 1 | .09 | 1 | 1 | 1 | 0 | .01 | tr. |
| honey (*Bit-O-Honey*), 1.7-oz. bar.......... | 27 | .14 | n.a. | n.a. | 60 | n.a. | n.a. | n.a. |
| honeycomb, w/peanut butter, chocolate coated, 1 oz......... | 23 | .50 | n.a. | 38 | 64 | n.a. | n.a. | n.a. |
| jelly beans, 10 large..... | 1 | .31 | 0 | 1 | 11 | .02 | .01 | .01 |
| licorice: | | | | | | | | |
| cherry (*Y&S Nibs*), 1 oz............. | 18 | .17 | 2 | 88 | 18 | .05 | .26 | .04 |
| strawberry (*Y&S Twizzlers*) 2.5-oz. pkg....... | 25 | .35 | n.a. | n.a. | n.a. | n.a. | n.a. | n.a. |
| (*Mars*), 1.76-oz. bar..... | 84 | .55 | 36 | n.a. | 162 | .55 | .13 | n.a.. |
| marshmallow, .25-oz. piece ........ | 0 | .02 | 0 | 1 | 0 | 0 | .01 | tr. |
| (*Milky Way*), 2.15-oz. bar......... | 79 | .46 | 21 | 98 | 147 | .43 | .09 | .12 |
| mint, chocolate coated: (*York* Peppermint Pattie), 1.5-oz. piece ..... | 7 | .64 | 27 | 41 | n.a. | .33 | .19 | .17 |
| dark (*After Eight*), 2 pieces, .3 oz. ... | 2 | .12 | n.a. | n.a. | 13 | n.a. | n.a. | n.a. |
| nougat and caramel, chocolate coated, 1 oz............... | 36 | .50 | n.a. | 35 | 60 | n.a. | n.a. | n.a. |
| peanut, chocolate coated: 1 oz............... | 33 | .40 | n.a. | 84 | 143 | n.a. | n.a. | n.a. |
| (*Goobers*), 1.38 oz. pkg...... | 49 | .52 | n.a. | n.a. | 196 | n.a. | n.a. | .32 |
| peanut bar, 1 oz........ | 12 | .50 | n.a. | 77 | 127 | n.a. | n.a. | n.a. |
| peanut brittle, 1 oz...... | 10 | .70 | n.a. | 27 | 43 | n.a. | n.a. | n.a. |

| | Calcium | Iron | Magnesium | Phosphorus | Potassium | Zinc | Copper | Manganese |
|---|---|---|---|---|---|---|---|---|
| | (Mg) | (Mg) | (Mg) | (Mg) | (Mg) | (Mg) | (Mg) | (Mg) |
| peanut butter: | | | | | | | | |
| candy coated (*Reese's Pieces*), 1.95-oz. pkg...... | 73 | .82 | 44 | 126 | 242 | .61 | .07 | .24 |
| chocolate coated, w/ cookies (*Twix*), 2-oz. pkg. ....... | 68 | .38 | 17 | 77 | 118 | .39 | .07 | .07 |
| peanut butter cup, chocolate coated (*Reese's*), 1.6 oz. pkg. | 35 | .49 | 38 | 108 | 180 | .63 | .18 | .36 |
| raisins, chocolate coated (*Raisinets*), 1.56 oz.... | 48 | .54 | 20 | 65 | 231 | n.a. | n.a. | n.a. |
| raisins, milk chocolate coated, 10 pieces, .35 oz............. | 9 | .17 | 5 | 14 | 51 | n.a. | n.a. | n.a. |
| sesame crunch, 1 oz............... | n.a. | 1.21 | 71 | n.a. | n.a. | 1.07 | .27 | n.a. |
| (*Snicker's*), 2.16-oz. bar......... | 70 | .48 | 36 | 129 | 199 | .70 | .15 | .30 |
| (*3 Musketeers*), 2.13-oz. bar......... | 50 | .44 | 17 | 55 | 80 | .33 | .09 | .10 |
| toffee (*Skor*), 1.4-oz. bar.......... | 45 | .16 | 14 | 60 | 95 | .30 | .05 | .06 |
| wafer, bar, chocolate coated (*Kit Kat*), 2.8-oz. pkg.......... | 142 | .67 | 34 | 137 | 243 | .79 | .19 | .24 |
| (*Whatchamacallit*), 1.8-oz. bar.......... | 62 | .46 | 29 | 102 | 177 | .57 | .07 | .22 |
| **Cantaloupe:** | | | | | | | | |
| untrimmed, 1 lb........ | 24 | .49 | 25 | 39 | 714 | .36 | .10 | .11 |
| ½ of 5"-diam. melon .... | 28 | .57 | 28 | 45 | 825 | .41 | .11 | .13 |
| pulp, cubed, ½ cup ..... | 9 | .17 | 9 | 14 | 247 | .13 | .03 | .04 |
| **Carambola,** trimmed, cubed, ½ cup ....... | 3 | .18 | 7 | 11 | 112 | .08 | .08 | .06 |

|  | Calcium (Mg) | Iron (Mg) | Magnesium (Mg) | Phosphorus (Mg) | Potassium (Mg) | Zinc (Mg) | Copper (Mg) | Manganese (Mg) |
|---|---|---|---|---|---|---|---|---|
| **Caramel**, see "Candy" | | | | | | | | |
| **Caramel topping,** | | | | | | | | |
| 2 tbsp. . . . . . . . . . . . | 22 | .08 | 3 | n.a. | n.a. | n.a. | n.a. | n.a. |
| **Caraway seed,** 1 tsp. . . . | 14 | .34 | 5 | 12 | 28 | .12 | .02 | .03 |
| **Cardamom,** ground, | | | | | | | | |
| 1 tsp. . . . . . . . . . . . | 8 | .28 | 5 | 4 | 22 | .15 | .01 | .56 |
| **Cardoon,** raw: | | | | | | | | |
| untrimmed, 1 lb. . . . . . . | 156 | 1.56 | 93 | 51 | 889 | n.a. | n.a. | n.a. |
| trimmed, shredded, | | | | | | | | |
| ½ cup . . . . . . . . . . . . | 62 | .62 | 37 | 20 | 356 | n.a. | n.a. | n.a. |
| **Carissa:** | | | | | | | | |
| untrimmed, 1 lb. . . . . . . | 44 | 5.11 | 62 | 27 | 1015 | n.a. | .82 | n.a. |
| trimmed, sliced, | | | | | | | | |
| ½ cup . . . . . . . . . . . . | 9 | .99 | 12 | 6 | 195 | n.a. | .16 | n.a. |
| **Carob flour,** 1 cup . . . . . . | 359 | 3.03 | 56 | 81 | 852 | .94 | .59 | .52 |
| **Carp,** meat only: | | | | | | | | |
| raw, 1 lb. . . . . . . . . . . . | 184 | 5.61 | 133 | 1880 | 1511 | 6.72 | .26 | n.a. |
| baked, broiled, or | | | | | | | | |
| microwaved[1], 4 oz. . . . | 59 | 1.80 | 43 | 602 | 484 | 2.15 | .08 | n.a. |
| **Carrot,** fresh, w/out greens: | | | | | | | | |
| fresh: | | | | | | | | |
| raw, untrimmed, | | | | | | | | |
| 1 lb. . . . . . . . . . . | 107 | 2.00 | 61 | 179 | 1305 | .80 | .19 | .57 |
| raw, 7½"-long carrot, | | | | | | | | |
| 2.8 oz. . . . . . . . . . | 19 | .36 | 11 | 32 | 233 | .14 | .03 | .10 |
| raw, shredded, ½ cup | 15 | .27 | 8 | 24 | 178 | .11 | .03 | .03 |
| boiled, drained, | | | | | | | | |
| sliced, ½ cup. . . . . | 24 | .48 | 10 | 24 | 177 | .23 | .11 | .59 |
| fresh, baby, raw: | | | | | | | | |
| trimmed, 1 lb. . . . . . . | 104 | n.a. | 53 | 170 | 1263 | .67 | .22 | .36 |
| 1 large, 3¼" long, | | | | | | | | |
| .5 oz. . . . . . . . . . . | 3 | n.a. | 2 | 6 | 42 | .02 | .01 | .01 |

[1] *Prepared without added ingredients.*

| | Calcium | Iron | Magnesium | Phosphorus | Potassium | Zinc | Copper | Manganese |
|---|---|---|---|---|---|---|---|---|
| | (Mg) | (Mg) | (Mg) | (Mg) | (Mg) | (Mg) | (Mg) | (Mg) |
| 1 medium, 2¾" long, .4 oz. | 2 | n.a. | 1 | 4 | 28 | .01 | .01 | .01 |
| canned, w/liquid, sliced, ½ cup | 31 | .75 | 11 | 25 | 213 | .35 | .13 | .55 |
| canned, drained, sliced, ½ cup | 19 | .47 | 6 | 17 | 131 | .19 | .08 | .33 |
| frozen, sliced, 10-oz. pkg. | 92 | 1.72 | 30 | 64 | 515 | .72 | .21 | 1.11 |
| frozen, boiled, drained, sliced, ½ cup | 21 | .35 | 7 | 19 | 115 | .18 | .05 | .30 |
| **Carrot juice**, canned, 6 fl. oz. | 44 | .85 | 26 | 77 | 538 | .33 | .09 | .24 |
| **Casaba melon:** | | | | | | | | |
| untrimmed, 1 lb. | 14 | 1.09 | 22 | 19 | 572 | n.a. | n.a. | n.a. |
| pulp, cubed, ½ cup | 5 | .34 | 7 | 6 | 179 | n.a. | n.a. | n.a. |
| **Cashew:** | | | | | | | | |
| dry-roasted, 1 oz. | 13 | 1.70 | 74 | 139 | 160 | 1.59 | .63 | n.a. |
| dry-roasted, wholes and halves, 1 cup | 62 | 8.22 | 356 | 671 | 774 | 7.67 | 3.04 | n.a. |
| oil-roasted, 1 oz. | 12 | 1.16 | 72 | 121 | 151 | 1.35 | .62 | .23 |
| oil-roasted, wholes and halves, 1 cup | 53 | 5.33 | 332 | 554 | 689 | 6.18 | 2.81 | 1.05 |
| **Cashew butter:** | | | | | | | | |
| 1 oz. | 12 | 1.43 | 73 | 130 | 155 | 1.47 | .62 | n.a. |
| 1 tbsp. | 7 | .80 | 41 | 73 | 87 | .83 | .35 | n.a. |
| **Catfish**, channel, meat only: | | | | | | | | |
| wild: | | | | | | | | |
| raw, 1 lb. | 65 | 1.35 | 105 | 947 | 1624 | 2.30 | .15 | .11 |
| baked, broiled, or microwaved[1], 4 oz. | 12 | .40 | 32 | 345 | 475 | .69 | .04 | .03 |
| farmed: | | | | | | | | |
| raw, 1 lb. | 41 | 2.25 | 103 | 915 | 1358 | 3.35 | .46 | .08 |

[1] *Prepared without added ingredients.*

| | Calcium | Iron | Magnesium | Phosphorus | Potassium | Zinc | Copper | Manganese |
|---|---|---|---|---|---|---|---|---|
| | (Mg) | (Mg) | (Mg) | (Mg) | (Mg) | (Mg) | (Mg) | (Mg) |
| Catfish, farmed, *continued* | | | | | | | | |
| baked, broiled, or | | | | | | | | |
| microwaved[1], 4 oz. | 10 | .93 | 29 | 278 | 364 | 1.19 | .14 | .02 |
| **Catfish, ocean,** see "Wolffish" | | | | | | | | |
| **Catsup,** 1 tbsp. . . . . . . . . | 3 | .10 | 3 | 6 | 72 | .03 | .03 | .02 |
| **Cauliflower:** | | | | | | | | |
| fresh: | | | | | | | | |
| raw, untrimmed, 1 lb. | 39 | .77 | 27 | 78 | 536 | .50 | .08 | .28 |
| raw, trimmed, | | | | | | | | |
| 3 florets, 2 oz. . . . . | 12 | .24 | 9 | 25 | 170 | .16 | .02 | .09 |
| raw, trimmed, | | | | | | | | |
| 1" pieces, ½ cup . . | 11 | .22 | 8 | 22 | 151 | .14 | .02 | .08 |
| boiled, drained, | | | | | | | | |
| 3 florets . . . . . . . . | 9 | .18 | 5 | 17 | 76 | .10 | .01 | .07 |
| boiled, drained, | | | | | | | | |
| 1" pieces, ½ cup | 10 | .20 | 6 | 20 | 88 | .11 | .02 | .09 |
| frozen, 10-oz. pkg. . . . . . . | 63 | 1.54 | 34 | 100 | 548 | .49 | .09 | .56 |
| frozen, boiled, drained, | | | | | | | | |
| 1" pieces, ½ cup . . . . . | 15 | .37 | 8 | 22 | 125 | .12 | .02 | .14 |
| **Cauliflower, green:** | | | | | | | | |
| raw: | | | | | | | | |
| untrimmed, 1 lb. . . . . | 90 | 2.02 | 54 | 171 | 830 | 1.77 | .11 | .68 |
| trimmed, ⅕ head, | | | | | | | | |
| 3.3 oz. . . . . . . . . . . | 30 | .68 | 18 | 57 | 279 | .60 | .04 | .23 |
| trimmed, 1" pieces, | | | | | | | | |
| ½ cup . . . . . . . . . . | 16 | .37 | 10 | 31 | 150 | .32 | .02 | .12 |
| boiled, drained, ⅕ head | 29 | .64 | 17 | 51 | 251 | .56 | .04 | .22 |
| boiled, drained, 1" pieces, | | | | | | | | |
| ½ cup . . . . . . . . . . . . . | 20 | .44 | 12 | 35 | 173 | .39 | .03 | .15 |
| **Celeriac,** raw: | | | | | | | | |
| untrimmed, 1 lb. . . . . . . . | 168 | 2.73 | 78 | 449 | 1170 | n.a. | n.a. | n.a. |
| trimmed, ½ cup. . . . . . . . | 34 | .55 | 16 | 90 | 234 | n.a. | n.a. | n.a. |

---

[1] *Prepared without added ingredients.*

| | Calcium | Iron | Magnesium | Phosphorus | Potassium | Zinc | Copper | Manganese |
|---|---|---|---|---|---|---|---|---|
| | (Mg) | (Mg) | (Mg) | (Mg) | (Mg) | (Mg) | (Mg) | (Mg) |

**Celery:**

raw:

| untrimmed, 1 lb. . . . . | 163 | 1.61 | 45 | 103 | 1160 | .53 | .14 | .41 |

trimmed, 7½"-long

| stalk, 1.6 oz. . . . . . | 16 | .16 | 4 | 10 | 115 | .05 | .01 | .04 |

trimmed, diced,

| ½ cup. . . . . . . . . . | 24 | .24 | 7 | 15 | 172 | .08 | .02 | .06 |

boiled, drained, diced,

| ½ cup. . . . . . . . . . . . | 32 | .31 | 9 | 19 | 213 | .10 | .03 | .08 |

| **Celery seed,** 1 tsp. . . . . . | 35 | .90 | 9 | 11 | 28 | .14 | .03 | .15 |

**Celtuce,** raw:

| untrimmed, 1 lb. . . . . . . . | 131 | 1.87 | 94 | 131 | 1123 | n.a. | n.a. | n.a. |
| trimmed, .3-oz. leaf . . . . . | 3 | .04 | 2 | 3 | 26 | n.a. | n.a. | n.a. |

**Cereal, ready-to-eat:**

bran (see also "oat bran," and "wheat bran" below, and "rice bran"):

| (*All Bran*), ½ cup. . . . | 100 | 4.50 | 120 | 294 | n.a. | 3.75 | .36 | n.a. |

(*All Bran* Extra Fiber),

| ½ cup. . . . . . . . . | 100 | 4.50 | 120 | 287 | n.a. | 3.75 | .30 | n.a. |

| (*Bran Buds*), ⅓ cup | 20 | 4.50 | 80 | 166 | n.a. | 3.75 | .21 | n.a. |

(*Frosted Bran*),

| ¾ cup. . . . . . . . . | 0 | 4.50 | 40 | 100 | n.a. | 3.75 | .08 | n.a. |

(*Fruitful Bran*),

| 1¼ cup. . . . . . . . . | 20 | 4.50 | 60 | 161 | n.a. | 1.20 | .16 | n.a. |

(*Kellogg's* Raisin

| Bran), 1 cup . . . . . | 40 | 4.50 | 80 | 191 | n.a. | 3.75 | .28 | n.a. |

corn:

(*Corn Pops*),

| 1 cup . . . . . . . . . | 0 | 1.80 | 0 | 0 | n.a. | 1.50 | .03 | n.a. |

(*Kellogg's Corn

Flakes*), 1 cup . . . . | 0 | 8.40 | 0 | 0 | n.a. | 0 | .02 | n.a. |

(*Kellogg's Frosted

Flakes*), ¾ cup. . . . | 0 | 4.50 | 0 | 0 | n.a. | 0 | .01 | n.a. |

(*Nut & Honey Crunch*),

| 1¼ cup. . . . . . . . . | 0 | 4.50 | 0 | 40 | n.a. | .30 | .04 | n.a. |

| | Calcium | Iron | Magnesium | Phosphorus | Potassium | Zinc | Copper | Manganese |
|---|---|---|---|---|---|---|---|---|
| | (Mg) | (Mg) | (Mg) | (Mg) | (Mg) | (Mg) | (Mg) | (Mg) |

Cereal, ready-to-eat, corn, *continued*

| | | | | | | | | |
|---|---|---|---|---|---|---|---|---|
| (*Nut & Honey Crunch O's*), ¾ cup . . . . . . | 0 | 1.80 | 24 | 86 | n.a. | 1.50 | .04 | n.a. |
| (*Nutri-Grain Corn*), 1 oz. . . . . . . . . . . | 1 | .60 | 26 | 67 | 80 | 3.75 | .08 | n.a. |
| granola, see "mixed grain" below | | | | | | | | |
| mixed grain: | | | | | | | | |
| (*Apple Jacks*), 1 cup . . . . | 0 | 4.50 | 8 | 24 | n.a. | 3.75 | .08 | n.a. |
| (*Cap'n Crunch*), 1 oz. | 6 | 4.81 | 10 | 30 | 36 | 2.37 | .04 | .19 |
| (*Cap'n Crunch Crunchberries*), 1 oz. . . . . | 7 | 4.74 | 11 | 33 | 43 | 2.83 | .01 | .19 |
| (*Cap'n Crunch Peanut Butter Crunch*), 1 oz. . . . . . . . . . . | 5 | 5.00 | 14 | 38 | 52 | 2.56 | .05 | .18 |
| (*Cinnamon Mini Buns*), ¾ cup . . . . | 0 | 4.50 | 8 | 24 | n.a. | 3.75 | .02 | n.a. |
| (*Crispix*), 1 cup . . . . . | 0 | 1.80 | 0 | 22 | n.a. | 1.50 | .04 | n.a. |
| (*Doouble Dip Crunch*), ¾ cup . . . | 0 | 1.80 | 0 | 0 | n.a. | 1.50 | .01 | n.a. |
| (*Froot Loops*), 1 cup | 0 | 4.50 | 8 | 21 | n.a. | 3.75 | .02 | n.a. |
| (*Healthy Choice Flakes*), 1 cup . . . . | 0 | 6.30 | 32 | 86 | n.a. | 1.50 | .08 | n.a. |
| (*Healthy Choice Squares*), 1¼ cup | 0 | 6.30 | 60 | 194 | n.a. | 1.50 | .13 | n.a. |
| (*Kellogg's* Low Fat Granola), ½ cup . . | 20 | 1.80 | 40 | 135 | n.a. | 3.75 | .08 | n.a. |
| (*Kellogg's Mueslix* Crispy Blend), ⅔ cup . . . . . . . . . | 20 | 4.50 | 40 | 108 | n.a. | 3.75 | .12 | n.a. |
| (*Kellogg's Mueslix* Golden Crunch), ¾ cup . . . . . . . . . | 40 | 4.50 | 60 | 149 | n.a. | 3.00 | .16 | n.a. |
| (*King Vitamin*), 1 oz. | 6 | 8.10 | 14 | 40 | 50 | .30 | .04 | .22 |
| (*Pop-Tarts Crunch*), ¾ cup . . . . . . . . . | 0 | 4.50 | 8 | n.a. | n.a. | 3.75 | n.a. | n.a. |

| | Calcium | Iron | Magnesium | Phosphorus | Potassium | Zinc | Copper | Manganese |
|---|---|---|---|---|---|---|---|---|
| | (Mg) | (Mg) | (Mg) | (Mg) | (Mg) | (Mg) | (Mg) | (Mg) |
| (*Product 19*), 1 cup . . . . . . . . . | 0 | 18.00 | 16 | 43 | n.a. | 15.00 | .04 | n.a. |
| (*Special K*), 1 cup . . . | 0 | 8.40 | 16 | 61 | n.a. | 3.75 | .13 | n.a. |
| w/almonds (*Kellogg's Temptations*), 1 cup . . . . . . . . . | 0 | 4.50 | n.a. | 8 | n.a. | n.a. | n.a. | n.a. |
| almond raisin (*Nutri-Grain*), 1¼ cup . . . | 20 | 1.10 | 16 | 102 | n.a. | 3.75 | .08 | n.a. |
| w/fiber nuggets or fruit and nuts (*Just Right*), 1 cup . . . . . | 0 | 16.20 | 32 | 108 | n.a. | .90 | .08 | n.a. |
| w/pecans (*Kellogg's Temptations*), 1 cup . . . . . . . . . | 0 | 4.50 | n.a. | n.a. | n.a. | n.a. | n.a. | n.a. |
| w/raisins (*Kellogg's Low Fat Granola*), ⅔ cup . . . . . . . . | 20 | 1.80 | 40 | 127 | n.a. | 3.75 | .12 | n.a. |
| w/raisins, oat clusters, and almonds (*Healthy Choice*), 1 cup . . . . . . . | 20 | 6.30 | 40 | 138 | n.a. | 1.50 | .12 | n.a. |
| oat: (*Life*), 1 oz. . . . . . . . . | 93 | 8.10 | 46 | 162 | 171 | .84 | .17 | 1.03 |
| cinnamon (*Life*), 1 oz. . . . . . . . . . . . | 89 | 8.10 | 47 | 159 | 167 | 1.07 | .16 | 1.30 |
| oat bran: (*Common Sense*), ¾ cup . . . . . . . . . | 0 | 8.40 | 40 | 153 | n.a. | 3.75 | .08 | n.a. |
| (*Cracklin' Oat Bran*), ¾ cup . . . . . . . . . | 20 | 1.80 | 80 | 187 | n.a. | 1.50 | .15 | n.a. |
| rice: (*Apple Raisin Crisp*), 1 cup . . . . . . . . . | 0 | 1.80 | 8 | 86 | n.a. | 1.50 | .04 | n.a. |
| (*Cocoa Krispies*), ¾ cup . . . . . . . . . | 0 | 1.80 | 8 | 24 | n.a. | 1.50 | .05 | n.a. |
| (*Frosted Krispies*), ¾ cup . . . . . . . . . | 0 | 1.80 | 0 | 24 | n.a. | .30 | 0 | n.a. |

| | Calcium | Iron | Magnesium | Phosphorus | Potassium | Zinc | Copper | Manganese |
|---|---|---|---|---|---|---|---|---|
| | (Mg) | (Mg) | (Mg) | (Mg) | (Mg) | (Mg) | (Mg) | (Mg) |
| Cereal, ready-to-eat, *continued* | | | | | | | | |
| (*Fruity Marshmallow* | | | | | | | | |
| *Krispies*), ¾ cup . . | 0 | 1.80 | 0 | 0 | n.a. | .30 | .04 | n.a. |
| (*Rice Krispies*), | | | | | | | | |
| 1¼ cup . . . . . . . . | 0 | 1.80 | 8 | 36 | n.a. | .60 | .05 | n.a. |
| (*Rice Krispie Treats*), | | | | | | | | |
| ¾ cup . . . . . . . . . | 0 | 1.80 | 0 | 20 | n.a. | 0 | 0 | n.a. |
| w/apple cinnamon | | | | | | | | |
| (*Rice Krispies*), | | | | | | | | |
| ¾ cup . . . . . . . . . | 0 | 1.80 | 0 | 25 | n.a. | .30 | .02 | n.a. |
| wheat: | | | | | | | | |
| (*Apple Cinnamon* | | | | | | | | |
| *Squares*), ¾ cup . . | 20 | 16.20 | 40 | 154 | n.a. | 1.50 | .12 | n.a. |
| (*Blueberry Squares*), | | | | | | | | |
| ¾ cup . . . . . . . . . | 0 | 16.20 | 60 | 162 | n.a. | 1.50 | .12 | n.a. |
| (*Frosted Mini-* | | | | | | | | |
| *Wheats*), 1 cup . . . | 0 | 16.20 | 60 | 160 | n.a. | 1.50 | .20 | n.a. |
| (*Frosted Mini-Wheats* | | | | | | | | |
| Bite-Size), 1 cup . . | 0 | 16.20 | 60 | 160 | n.a. | 1.50 | .20 | n.a. |
| (*Kellogg's Smacks*), | | | | | | | | |
| ¾ cup . . . . . . . . . | 0 | 1.80 | 16 | 37 | n.a. | .30 | .04 | n.a. |
| (*Nutri-Grain* Wheat), | | | | | | | | |
| ¾ cup . . . . . . . . . | 0 | 1.10 | 40 | 117 | n.a. | 3.75 | .09 | n.a. |
| (*Nutri-Grain* Wheat & | | | | | | | | |
| Raisins), 1¼ cup . . | 20 | 2.70 | 60 | 157 | n.a. | 3.75 | .16 | n.a. |
| (*Raisin Squares*), | | | | | | | | |
| ¾ cup . . . . . . . . . | 0 | 16.20 | 40 | 160 | n.a. | 1.50 | .12 | n.a. |
| (*Strawberry Squares*), | | | | | | | | |
| ¾ cup . . . . . . . . . | 20 | 16.20 | 60 | 144 | n.a. | 1.50 | .16 | n.a. |
| w/wheat bran | | | | | | | | |
| (*Kellogg's Complete*), | | | | | | | | |
| ¾ cup . . . . . . . . . | 0 | 8.40 | 60 | 144 | n.a. | 3.75 | .13 | n.a. |
| **Cereal, cooking,** uncooked, except as noted: | | | | | | | | |
| corn grits, yellow, | | | | | | | | |
| enriched, regular or | | | | | | | | |
| quick, 1 pkt. . . . . . . . | 1 | 1.11 | 8 | 21 | 39 | .12 | .02 | .03 |

| | Calcium | Iron | Magnesium | Phosphorus | Potassium | Zinc | Copper | Manganese |
|---|---|---|---|---|---|---|---|---|
| | (Mg) | (Mg) | (Mg) | (Mg) | (Mg) | (Mg) | (Mg) | (Mg) |
| oat and oatmeal: | | | | | | | | |
| (*Instant Quaker*), | | | | | | | | |
| 1 pkt. . . . . . . . . . | 170 | 8.35 | 39 | 140 | 103 | .88 | .14 | 1.20 |
| (*Quaker* Quick/Old | | | | | | | | |
| Fashioned), ⅓ cup | | | | | | | | |
| or ⅔ cup cooked | 15 | 1.08 | 38 | 130 | 109 | .87 | .09 | 1.22 |
| apple and cinnamon | | | | | | | | |
| (*Instant Quaker*), | | | | | | | | |
| 1 pkt. . . . . . . . . . | 168 | 5.89 | 39 | 102 | 108 | .66 | .13 | .01 |
| cinnamon and spice | | | | | | | | |
| (*Instant Quaker*), | | | | | | | | |
| 1 pkt. . . . . . . . . . | 178 | 8.08 | 40 | 143 | 117 | .84 | .13 | 1.10 |
| maple and brown | | | | | | | | |
| sugar (*Instant* | | | | | | | | |
| *Quaker*), 1 pkt.. . . . . | 170 | 8.35 | 42 | 149 | 116 | .85 | .14 | 1.15 |
| raisins and spice | | | | | | | | |
| (*Instant Quaker*), | | | | | | | | |
| 1 pkt. . . . . . . . . . | 165 | 6.23 | 39 | 135 | 152 | .91 | .15 | 1.20 |
| wheat, farina, | | | | | | | | |
| enriched, 1 pkt. . . . | 4 | 1.05 | 4 | 25 | 26 | .15 | .02 | n.a. |
| **Cervelat,** see "Thuringer cervelat" | | | | | | | | |
| **Chard,** see "Swiss chard" | | | | | | | | |
| **Chayote:** | | | | | | | | |
| raw, untrimmed, 1 lb. . . . | 85 | 1.80 | 63 | 117 | 674 | n.a. | n.a. | n.a. |
| raw, trimmed, 1 medium, | | | | | | | | |
| 7.2 oz.. . . . . . . . . . . . . | 39 | .81 | 28 | 53 | 305 | n.a. | n.a. | n.a. |
| boiled, drained, 1" pieces, | | | | | | | | |
| ½ cup . . . . . . . . . . . . . | 10 | .18 | 9 | 23 | 138 | n.a. | n.a. | n.a. |
| **Cheese:** | | | | | | | | |
| American, pasteurized | | | | | | | | |
| processed, 1 oz. . . . . . | 174 | .11 | 6 | 211 | 46 | .85 | .01 | tr. |
| blue, 1 oz.. . . . . . . . . . . . | 150 | .09 | 7 | 110 | 73 | .75 | .01 | tr. |
| brick, 1 oz. . . . . . . . . . . | 191 | .12 | 7 | 128 | 38 | .74 | .01 | tr. |
| Brie, 1 oz.. . . . . . . . . . . . | 52 | .14 | n.a. | 53 | 43 | n.a. | .01 | .01 |
| Camembert, 1 oz. . . . . . . | 110 | .09 | 6 | 98 | 53 | .68 | .01 | .01 |
| cheddar, 1 oz.. . . . . . . . . | 204 | .19 | 8 | 145 | 28 | .88 | .01 | tr. |

| | Calcium | Iron | Magnesium | Phosphorus | Potassium | Zinc | Copper | Manganese |
|---|---|---|---|---|---|---|---|---|
| | (Mg) | (Mg) | (Mg) | (Mg) | (Mg) | (Mg) | (Mg) | (Mg) |

Cheese, *continued*

cheddar, low fat,

| | | | | | | | | |
|---|---|---|---|---|---|---|---|---|
| 1 oz. . . . . . . . . . . . . . | 118 | .12 | 5 | 137 | 19 | .52 | .01 | tr. |
| cheddar, low sodium, | | | | | | | | |
| 1 oz. . . . . . . . . . . . . . | 200 | .20 | 8 | 137 | 32 | .88 | .01 | tr. |
| Colby, 1 oz. . . . . . . . . . | 194 | .22 | 7 | 129 | 36 | .87 | .01 | tr. |
| cottage, ½ cup not packed: | | | | | | | | |
| creamed, large curd | 68 | .16 | 6 | 149 | 95 | .42 | .03 | tr. |
| creamed, small curd | 63 | .15 | 5 | 139 | 88 | .39 | .03 | tr. |
| creamed, w/fruit. . . . . | 54 | .12 | 5 | 118 | 76 | .33 | .03 | tr. |
| dry curd . . . . . . . . . | 23 | .17 | 3 | 75 | 23 | .34 | .02 | tr. |
| low fat 2% . . . . . . . . | 77 | .18 | 7 | 170 | 109 | .48 | .03 | tr. |
| low fat 1% . . . . . . . . | 69 | .16 | 6 | 151 | 97 | .43 | .03 | tr. |
| cream, 1 oz. . . . . . . . . . | 23 | .34 | 2 | 30 | 34 | .15 | .01 | tr. |
| Edam, 1 oz. . . . . . . . . . . | 207 | .12 | 8 | 152 | 53 | 1.06 | .01 | tr. |
| feta, 1 oz. . . . . . . . . . . . | 140 | .18 | 5 | 96 | 18 | .82 | .01 | .01 |
| fontina, 1 oz. . . . . . . . . . | 156 | .06 | 4 | n.a. | n.a. | .99 | .01 | tr. |
| goat, hard, 1 oz. . . . . . . . | 254 | .53 | 15 | 207 | 14 | .45 | .18 | .07 |
| goat, semisoft, 1 oz. . . . . | 84 | .46 | 8 | 106 | 45 | .19 | .16 | .03 |
| goat, soft, 1 oz. . . . . . . . . | 40 | .54 | 4 | 73 | 7 | .26 | .21 | .03 |
| Gouda, 1 oz. . . . . . . . . . | 198 | .07 | 8 | 155 | 34 | 1.11 | .01 | tr. |
| Gruyère, 1 oz. . . . . . . . . | 287 | n.a. | n.a. | 172 | 23 | n.a. | .01 | .01 |
| Limburger, 1 oz. . . . . . . . | 141 | .04 | 6 | 111 | 36 | .60 | .01 | .01 |
| Mexican, queso anejo, | | | | | | | | |
| 1 oz. . . . . . . . . . . . . . | 193 | .13 | 8 | 126 | 25 | .84 | tr. | .01 |
| Mexican, queso asadero, | | | | | | | | |
| 1 oz. . . . . . . . . . . . . . | 188 | .15 | 7 | 126 | 25 | .86 | .01 | .01 |
| Mexican, queso | | | | | | | | |
| chihuahua, 1 oz. . . . . . | 185 | .13 | 6 | 125 | 15 | .99 | .01 | .02 |
| mozzarella: | | | | | | | | |
| whole milk, 1 oz. . . . . | 147 | .05 | 5 | 105 | 19 | .63 | .01 | tr. |
| whole milk, low | | | | | | | | |
| moisture, 1 oz. . . . | 163 | .06 | 6 | 117 | 21 | .70 | .01 | tr. |
| part skim, 1 oz. . . . . . | 183 | .06 | 7 | 131 | 24 | .78 | .01 | tr. |
| part skim, low | | | | | | | | |
| moisture, 1 oz. . . . | 207 | .07 | 7 | 149 | 27 | .89 | .01 | tr. |

| | Calcium | Iron | Magnesium | Phosphorus | Potassium | Zinc | Copper | Manganese |
|---|---|---|---|---|---|---|---|---|
| | (Mg) | (Mg) | (Mg) | (Mg) | (Mg) | (Mg) | (Mg) | (Mg) |
| Muenster, 1 oz......... | 203 | .12 | 8 | 133 | 38 | .80 | .01 | tr. |
| Neufchâtel, 1 oz....... | 21 | .08 | 2 | 39 | 32 | .15 | tr. | tr. |
| Parmesan: | | | | | | | | |
|    grated, 1 oz........ | 390 | .27 | 14 | 229 | 30 | .90 | .01 | .01 |
|    grated, 1 tbsp....... | 69 | .05 | 3 | 40 | 5 | .16 | tr. | tr. |
|    hard, 1 oz.......... | 336 | .23 | 12 | 197 | 26 | .78 | .01 | .01 |
| pimiento, pasteurized | | | | | | | | |
|    processed, 1 oz. ..... | 174 | .12 | 6 | 211 | 46 | .84 | .01 | tr. |
| provolone, 1 oz......... | 214 | .15 | 8 | 141 | 39 | .92 | .01 | tr. |
| ricotta: | | | | | | | | |
|    whole milk, ½ cup... | 257 | .47 | 14 | 196 | 130 | 1.40 | .03 | .01 |
|    part skim, ½ cup.... | 337 | .55 | 18 | 226 | 155 | 1.70 | .04 | .01 |
| Roquefort, 1 oz........ | 188 | .16 | 8 | 111 | 26 | .59 | .01 | .01 |
| Swiss, 1 oz............ | 272 | .05 | 10 | 171 | 31 | 1.11 | .01 | tr. |
| Swiss, pasteurized | | | | | | | | |
|    processed, 1 oz. ..... | 219 | .17 | 8 | 216 | 61 | 1.02 | .01 | tr. |
| Tilsit, 1 oz. ........... | 198 | .06 | 4 | 142 | 18 | .99 | .01 | tr. |
| **Cheese food:** | | | | | | | | |
| American, cold pack, | | | | | | | | |
|    1 oz.............. | 141 | .24 | 8 | 113 | 103 | .85 | .01 | tr. |
| American, pasteurized | | | | | | | | |
|    processed, 1 oz. ..... | 163 | .24 | 9 | 130 | 79 | .85 | .01 | tr. |
| Swiss, pasteurized | | | | | | | | |
|    processed, 1 oz. ..... | 205 | .17 | 8 | 149 | 81 | 1.01 | .01 | tr. |
| **Cheese sauce mix,** | | | | | | | | |
|    ½ cup[1] ............ | 285 | .14 | 24 | 219 | 277 | .49 | n.a. | n.a. |
| **Cheese spread,** American | | | | | | | | |
|    pasteurized processed, | | | | | | | | |
|    1 oz.............. | 159 | .09 | 8 | 202 | 69 | .73 | .01 | .01 |
| **Cheese stick or straw,** 5" | | | | | | | | |
|    long, 10 pieces, 2.1 oz. | 155 | .40 | n.a. | 124 | 38 | n.a. | n.a. | n.a. |

[1] *Prepared according to package directions, with whole milk.*

| | Calcium | Iron | Magnesium | Phosphorus | Potassium | Zinc | Copper | Manganese |
|---|---|---|---|---|---|---|---|---|
| | (Mg) | (Mg) | (Mg) | (Mg) | (Mg) | (Mg) | (Mg) | (Mg) |
| **Cheese substitute,** | | | | | | | | |
| mozzarella, 1 oz. . . . . . | 173 | n.a. | 12 | 165 | 129 | .55 | .03 | .01 |
| **Cherry:** | | | | | | | | |
| fresh, sour red: | | | | | | | | |
| untrimmed, 1 lb. . . . . | 63 | 1.32 | 36 | 61 | 705 | .41 | .43 | .46 |
| pitted, ½ cup. . . . . . . | 12 | .25 | 7 | 12 | 134 | .08 | .08 | .09 |
| w/pits, ½ cup . . . . . . | 8 | .17 | 5 | 8 | 89 | .05 | .05 | .06 |
| fresh, sweet: | | | | | | | | |
| untrimmed, 1 lb. . . . . | 60 | 1.58 | 46 | 78 | 914 | .24 | .39 | .38 |
| w/pits, ½ cup . . . . . . | 11 | .28 | 8 | 14 | 163 | .05 | .07 | .07 |
| 10 medium, approx. 2.6 oz. . . . . . . . . . | 10 | .26 | 8 | 13 | 152 | .04 | .07 | .06 |
| canned, sour, red: | | | | | | | | |
| in water, ½ cup. . . . . | 13 | 1.67 | 7 | 12 | 120 | .08 | .09 | .09 |
| in light syrup, ½ cup. . . . . . . . . . . . | 13 | 1.66 | 7 | 12 | 119 | .08 | .09 | .09 |
| in heavy syrup, ½ cup . . . . . . . . . | 13 | 1.66 | 7 | 12 | 119 | .08 | .08 | .09 |
| canned, sweet: | | | | | | | | |
| in water, ½ cup. . . . . | 13 | .45 | 11 | 19 | 162 | .09 | .09 | .08 |
| in juice, ½ cup . . . . . | 17 | .73 | 16 | 27 | 163 | .12 | .09 | .08 |
| in light syrup, ½ cup . . . . . . . . . | 12 | .45 | 11 | 23 | 186 | .13 | .18 | .08 |
| in heavy syrup, ½ cup . . . . . . . . . | 12 | .46 | 11 | 23 | 187 | .13 | .18 | .08 |
| frozen: | | | | | | | | |
| sour, red, unsweetened, ½ cup . . . . . . . . . | 10 | .41 | 7 | 13 | 96 | .08 | .07 | .04 |
| sweet, sweetened, 10-oz. pkg. . . . . . | 34 | .99 | 28 | 45 | 564 | .11 | .07 | .31 |
| sweet, sweetened, ½ cup . . . . . . . . . | 16 | .45 | 13 | 21 | 257 | .05 | .03 | .14 |
| **Chestnut, Chinese,** shelled, except as noted: | | | | | | | | |
| raw, in shell, 1 lb. . . . . . . | 68 | 5.37 | 321 | 364 | 1703 | 3.31 | 1.38 | 6.10 |

| | Calcium | Iron | Magnesium | Phosphorus | Potassium | Zinc | Copper | Manganese |
|---|---|---|---|---|---|---|---|---|
| | (Mg) | (Mg) | (Mg) | (Mg) | (Mg) | (Mg) | (Mg) | (Mg) |
| raw, 1 oz. . . . . . . . . . . . | 5 | .40 | 24 | 27 | 127 | .25 | .10 | .46 |
| boiled or steamed, 1 oz. | 3 | .27 | 16 | 19 | 87 | .17 | .07 | .31 |
| dried, 1 oz. . . . . . . . . . . | 8 | .65 | 39 | 44 | 206 | .40 | .17 | .74 |
| roasted, in shell, 1 lb. . . . | 65 | 5.12 | 306 | 347 | 1622 | 3.15 | 1.32 | n.a. |
| roasted, 1 oz. . . . . . . . . . | 5 | .43 | 26 | 29 | 135 | .26 | .11 | n.a. |
| **Chestnut, European,** shelled, except as noted: | | | | | | | | |
| raw: | | | | | | | | |
| in shell, 1 lb. . . . . . . . | 91 | 3.38 | 108 | 312 | 1738 | 1.76 | 1.50 | 3.20 |
| unpeeled, 1 oz. . . . . . | 8 | .29 | 9 | 26 | 147 | .15 | .13 | .27 |
| unpeeled, 1 cup, | | | | | | | | |
| approx. 13 kernels | 40 | 1.46 | 47 | 135 | 751 | .76 | .65 | 1.38 |
| peeled, 1 oz. . . . . . . . | 5 | .27 | 9 | 11 | 137 | .14 | .12 | .10 |
| boiled or steamed, 1 oz. | 13 | .49 | 15 | 28 | 203 | .07 | .13 | .24 |
| dried, unpeeled, | | | | | | | | |
| 1 oz. . . . . . . . . . . . . . . | 19 | .68 | 21 | 50 | 280 | .10 | .19 | .37 |
| dried, peeled, 1 oz. . . . . . | 18 | .68 | 21 | 39 | 281 | .10 | .19 | .34 |
| roasted: | | | | | | | | |
| in shell, 1 lb. . . . . . . . | 84 | 2.59 | 94 | 305 | 1690 | 1.62 | .45 | 3.37 |
| peeled, 1 oz. . . . . . . . | 8 | .26 | 9 | 30 | 168 | .16 | .14 | .34 |
| peeled, 1 cup, | | | | | | | | |
| approx. 17 kernels | 42 | 1.30 | 47 | 153 | 846 | .81 | .73 | 1.69 |
| **Chestnut, Japanese,** shelled, except as noted: | | | | | | | | |
| raw, in shell, 1 lb. . . . . . . | 92 | 4.34 | 148 | 217 | 986 | 3.30 | 1.68 | 4.76 |
| raw, 1 oz. . . . . . . . . . . . | 9 | .41 | 14 | 21 | 94 | .31 | .16 | .45 |
| boiled or steamed, | | | | | | | | |
| 1 oz. . . . . . . . . . . . . . . | 3 | .15 | 5 | 7 | 34 | .11 | .06 | .16 |
| dried, in shell, 1 lb. . . . . . | 215 | 10.12 | 344 | 506 | 2300 | 7.69 | 3.93 | 11.11 |
| dried, 1 oz. . . . . . . . . . . | 20 | .96 | 33 | 48 | 218 | .73 | .37 | 1.05 |
| roasted, 1 oz. . . . . . . . . . | 10 | .60 | 18 | 26 | n.a. | .41 | .21 | .59 |
| **Chia seeds,** dried, 1 oz. | 150 | 2.84 | n.a. | 174 | n.a. | 1.51 | .47 | n.a. |
| **Chicken**[1], fresh, 4 oz., except as noted: | | | | | | | | |
| broiler-fryer, flour-coated, fried: | | | | | | | | |
| meat w/skin . . . . . . . . | 19 | 1.56 | 28 | 217 | 265 | 2.31 | .09 | .04 |

[1] *Prepared without added ingredients.*

| | Calcium | Iron | Magnesium | Phosphorus | Potassium | Zinc | Copper | Manganese |
|---|---|---|---|---|---|---|---|---|
| | (Mg) | (Mg) | (Mg) | (Mg) | (Mg) | (Mg) | (Mg) | (Mg) |
| **Chicken, broiler-fryer, fried,** *continued* | | | | | | | | |
| dark meat w/skin . . . . | 19 | 1.70 | 27 | 200 | 261 | 2.95 | .10 | .04 |
| light meat w/skin . . . . | 18 | 1.37 | 31 | 242 | 271 | 1.43 | .07 | .03 |
| back meat w/skin . . . . | 27 | 1.84 | 26 | 188 | 256 | 2.80 | .10 | .06 |
| breast meat w/skin . . . | 18 | 1.35 | 34 | 264 | 294 | 1.25 | .06 | .03 |
| drumstick, meat w/skin, 1.7 oz. (2.6 oz. raw w/bone) . . . . . | 6 | .66 | 11 | 86 | 112 | 1.42 | .04 | .01 |
| leg, meat w/skin, 4 oz. (5.5 oz. raw w/bone) . . . . . . . . | 15 | 1.60 | 27 | 204 | 261 | 3.00 | .10 | .04 |
| thigh, meat w/skin, 2.2 oz. (2.9 oz. raw w/bone) . . . . . | 8 | .93 | 5 | 116 | 147 | 1.56 | .06 | .02 |
| wing, meat w/skin, 1.1 oz. (2.2 oz. raw w/bone) . . . . . | 5 | .40 | 6 | 48 | 57 | .56 | .02 | .01 |
| **broiler-fryer, roasted:** | | | | | | | | |
| meat w/skin . . . . . . . . | 17 | 1.43 | 26 | 206 | 253 | 2.20 | .07 | .02 |
| meat only . . . . . . . . . | 17 | 1.37 | 28 | 221 | 276 | 2.38 | .08 | .02 |
| skin only, 1 oz. . . . . . | 4 | .43 | 4 | 35 | 39 | .35 | .02 | .01 |
| dark meat w/skin . . . . | 17 | 1.54 | 25 | 191 | 249 | 2.82 | .09 | .02 |
| dark meat only . . . . . . | 17 | 1.51 | 26 | 203 | 272 | 3.18 | .09 | .02 |
| light meat w/skin . . . . | 17 | 1.29 | 28 | 227 | 257 | 1.39 | .06 | .02 |
| light meat only . . . . . . | 17 | 1.20 | 31 | 245 | 280 | 1.39 | .06 | .02 |
| **roaster, roasted:** | | | | | | | | |
| meat w/skin . . . . . . . . | 14 | 1.43 | 23 | 203 | 239 | 1.64 | .07 | .02 |
| meat only . . . . . . . . . | 14 | 1.37 | 24 | 218 | 260 | 1.72 | .06 | .02 |
| dark meat only . . . . . . | 12 | 1.51 | 23 | 194 | 254 | 2.42 | .08 | .02 |
| light meat only . . . . . . | 15 | 1.22 | 26 | 246 | 268 | .88 | .05 | .02 |
| **stewing, stewed:** | | | | | | | | |
| meat w/skin . . . . . . . . | 15 | 1.55 | 23 | 204 | 206 | 2.01 | .11 | .02 |
| meat only . . . . . . . . . | 15 | 1.62 | 25 | 231 | 229 | 2.34 | .13 | .02 |
| dark meat only . . . . . . | 14 | 1.86 | 25 | 212 | 231 | 3.54 | .16 | .03 |
| light meat only . . . . . . | 16 | 1.35 | 26 | 255 | 226 | .94 | .10 | .02 |

| | Calcium | Iron | Magnesium | Phosphorus | Potassium | Zinc | Copper | Manganese |
|---|---|---|---|---|---|---|---|---|
| | (Mg) | (Mg) | (Mg) | (Mg) | (Mg) | (Mg) | (Mg) | (Mg) |
| capon, roasted, meat w/ skin. . . . . . . . . . . . . . | 16 | 1.69 | 27 | 279 | 289 | 1.97 | .08 | .02 |
| Cornish hen, see "Cornish game hen" | | | | | | | | |
| **Chicken giblets,** simmered[1], 4 oz. . . . . . | 14 | 7.30 | 23 | 260 | 179 | 5.18 | .29 | .19 |
| **Chicken gizzard,** simmered[1], 4 oz. . . . . . | 11 | 4.71 | 23 | 176 | 203 | 4.97 | .12 | .07 |
| **"Chicken," vegetarian:** | | | | | | | | |
| canned: | | | | | | | | |
| (*Worthington Fri-Chik*), 2 pieces, 3.2 oz. . . . . . . . . . | 15 | .96 | n.a. | 83 | 146 | .38 | n.a. | n.a. |
| diced (*Worthington*), ¼ cup, 1.9 oz. . . . . | 8 | .67 | n.a. | 51 | 102 | .24 | n.a. | n.a. |
| fried, w/gravy (*Loma Linda*), 2 pieces, 5.2 oz. . . . . . . . . . | 15 | .89 | n.a. | n.a. | 62 | .62 | n.a. | n.a. |
| sliced (*Worthington*), 3 slices, 3.2 oz. . . . | 13 | 1.09 | n.a. | 112 | 167 | .40 | n.a. | n.a. |
| frozen: | | | | | | | | |
| (*Worthington Chicketts*), 2 slices, 1.9 oz. . . . . . . . . . | 16 | 1.74 | n.a. | n.a. | 31 | .54 | n.a. | n.a. |
| (*Worthington Chik-Stiks*), 1.7-oz. piece . . . . . | 10 | .84 | n.a. | n.a. | 59 | .31 | n.a. | n.a. |
| diced (*Worthington Meatless*), ¼ cup, 2 oz. . . . . . . . . . . | 8 | .67 | n.a. | 51 | 102 | .24 | n.a. | n.a. |
| fried (*Loma Linda Chik'n*), 2-oz. piece | 2 | .63 | n.a. | n.a. | 76 | .20 | n.a. | n.a. |
| nuggets (*Loma Linda*), 5 pieces, 3 oz. . . . . . . . . . | 41 | 1.39 | n.a. | n.a. | 153 | .43 | n.a. | n.a. |

[1] *Prepared without added ingredients.*

|  | Calcium (Mg) | Iron (Mg) | Magnesium (Mg) | Phosphorus (Mg) | Potassium (Mg) | Zinc (Mg) | Copper (Mg) | Manganese (Mg) |
|---|---|---|---|---|---|---|---|---|
| **"Chicken," vegetarian, frozen,** *continued* | | | | | | | | |
| patty (*Morningstar* | | | | | | | | |
| *Farms*), 2.5-oz. patty | 11 | 1.02 | n.a. | 121 | 163 | .31 | n.a. | n.a. |
| patty (*Worthington* | | | | | | | | |
| *Crispy Chik*), | | | | | | | | |
| 2.5-oz. patty ..... | 10 | 1.26 | n.a. | n.a. | 201 | .33 | n.a. | n.a. |
| pie (*Worthington*), | | | | | | | | |
| 8-oz. pie ........ | 17 | 1.41 | n.a. | n.a. | 114 | .59 | n.a. | n.a. |
| sliced (*Worthington*), | | | | | | | | |
| 2 slices, 2 oz. .... | 12 | 2.08 | n.a. | 111 | 276 | .26 | n.a. | n.a. |
| mix, supreme (*Loma* | | | | | | | | |
| *Linda*), ⅓ cup, .9 oz. | 29 | 1.42 | n.a. | n.a. | 448 | .48 | n.a. | n.a. |
| **Chicken gravy,** canned, | | | | | | | | |
| ¼ cup ......... | 12 | .28 | n.a. | 17 | 65 | .48 | .06 | .12 |
| **"Chicken" gravy mix,** | | | | | | | | |
| vegetarian, (*Loma* | | | | | | | | |
| *Linda Gravy Quik*), | | | | | | | | |
| .2 oz.............. | 4 | .18 | n.a. | 24 | 31 | .06 | n.a. | n.a. |
| **Chicken heart,** see "Heart" | | | | | | | | |
| **Chicken liver,** see "Liver" | | | | | | | | |
| **Chicken seasoning** | | | | | | | | |
| (*Tone's Perc*), ¼ tsp. | 5 | .13 | 1 | 3 | 9 | .03 | tr. | .02 |
| **Chickpeas:** | | | | | | | | |
| uncooked, 1 lb........ | 478 | 28.31 | 523 | 1661 | 3969 | 15.54 | 3.84 | 10.0 |
| uncooked, ½ cup....... | 105 | 6.24 | 115 | 366 | 875 | 3.43 | .85 | 2.20 |
| boiled, ½ cup ......... | 40 | 2.37 | 39 | 137 | 239 | 1.25 | .29 | .85 |
| canned, w/liquid, 8 oz.... | 74 | 3.06 | 66 | 204 | 390 | 2.40 | .39 | 1.37 |
| canned, w/liquid, | | | | | | | | |
| ½ cup............. | 39 | 1.62 | 35 | 108 | 206 | 1.27 | .21 | .73 |
| **Chicory, witloof,** raw: | | | | | | | | |
| untrimmed, 1 lb........ | 77 | .97 | 40 | 105 | 850 | .66 | .21 | .41 |
| 1 head, 5" to 7", approx. | | | | | | | | |
| 2 oz............... | 10 | .13 | 5 | 14 | 112 | .09 | .03 | .05 |
| chopped, ½ cup ....... | 9 | .11 | 4 | 12 | 95 | .07 | .02 | .05 |
| **Chicory greens,** fresh, | | | | | | | | |
| raw: | | | | | | | | |
| untrimmed, 1 lb........ | 372 | 3.35 | 112 | 175 | 1562 | n.a. | n.a. | n.a. |

| | Calcium | Iron | Magnesium | Phosphorus | Potassium | Zinc | Copper | Manganese |
|---|---|---|---|---|---|---|---|---|
| | (Mg) | (Mg) | (Mg) | (Mg) | (Mg) | (Mg) | (Mg) | (Mg) |
| trimmed, chopped, ½ cup............. | 90 | .81 | 27 | 42 | 378 | n.a. | n.a. | n.a. |
| **Chicory root,** raw: | | | | | | | | |
| untrimmed, 1 lb. ....... | 153 | 2.98 | 82 | 227 | 1079 | n.a. | n.a. | n.a. |
| trimmed, 1 root, 2.2 oz.............. | 25 | .48 | 13 | 37 | 174 | n.a. | n.a. | n.a. |
| trimmed, 1" pieces, ½ cup............. | 18 | .36 | 10 | 27 | 131 | n.a. | n.a. | n.a. |
| **Chili,** canned: | | | | | | | | |
| w/beans, 8 oz.......... | 106 | 7.78 | 102 | 350 | 829 | 4.53 | n.a. | n.a. |
| w/beans, ½ cup........ | 60 | 4.39 | 58 | 197 | 468 | 2.56 | n.a. | n.a. |
| vegetarian (*Worthington*), 8.1 oz.............. | 43 | 3.24 | n.a. | n.a. | 424 | 1.24 | n.a. | n.a. |
| vegetarian (*Natural Touch*), 8.1 oz. ...... | 37 | 2.46 | n.a. | n.a. | 487 | 1.36 | n.a. | n.a. |
| **Chili powder,** 1 tsp. .... | 7 | .37 | 4 | 8 | 50 | .07 | .01 | .06 |
| **Chitterlings,** pork, simmered[1], 4 oz. ..... | 31 | 4.20 | 11 | 53 | 9 | 5.74 | .26 | n.a. |
| **Chives:** | | | | | | | | |
| fresh, 1 lb. ........... | 415 | 7.26 | 190 | 263 | 1341 | 2.52 | .71 | 1.69 |
| fresh, chopped, 1 tbsp. ... | 3 | .05 | 1 | 2 | 9 | .02 | .01 | .01 |
| freeze-dried, 1 tbsp...... | 2 | .04 | n.a. | 1 | 6 | n.a. | n.a. | n.a. |
| **Chocolate,** see "Candy" | | | | | | | | |
| **Chocolate,** baking: | | | | | | | | |
| chips, semisweet, ¼ cup............. | 13 | 1.45 | n.a. | 45 | 148 | n.a. | n.a. | n.a. |
| unsweetened, 1 oz. square ........ | 21 | 1.79 | 88 | 118 | 236 | 1.14 | .62 | .54 |
| **Chocolate flavor drink mix,** powder: | | | | | | | | |
| 2–3 heaping tsp. or ¾ cup.............. | 8 | .68 | 21 | 28 | 128 | .33 | .15 | .15 |
| (*Carnation* Instant Breakfast), 1 pkt...... | 150 | 4.50 | 80 | 150 | 410 | 3.00 | .50 | n.a. |

[1] *Prepared without added ingredients.*

| | Calcium | Iron | Magnesium | Phosphorus | Potassium | Zinc | Copper | Manganese |
|---|---|---|---|---|---|---|---|---|
| | (Mg) | (Mg) | (Mg) | (Mg) | (Mg) | (Mg) | (Mg) | (Mg) |
| **Chocolate flavor drink mix,** *continued* | | | | | | | | |
| malt (*Carnation* Instant | | | | | | | | |
| Breakfast), 1 pkt...... | 80 | 4.50 | 80 | 100 | 260 | 3.00 | .50 | n.a. |
| **Chocolate milk:** | | | | | | | | |
| whole, 1 cup......... | 280 | .60 | 33 | 251 | 417 | 1.02 | .16 | .19 |
| low fat 2%, 1 cup...... | 284 | .60 | 33 | 254 | 422 | 1.02 | .16 | .19 |
| low fat 1%, 1 cup...... | 287 | .60 | 33 | 256 | 426 | 1.02 | .16 | .19 |
| **Chocolate syrup:** | | | | | | | | |
| thin type, w/out added | | | | | | | | |
| nutrients, 2 tbsp. or | | | | | | | | |
| 1 fl. oz............. | 5 | .79 | 24 | 48 | 84 | .27 | .19 | .14 |
| thin type, w/added | | | | | | | | |
| nutrients, 1 tbsp...... | n.a. | 2.55 | n.a. | n.a. | 90 | n.a. | n.a. | n.a. |
| **Chocolate topping,** fudge | | | | | | | | |
| type, 1 tbsp......... | 21 | .25 | 10 | 36 | 45 | .17 | .06 | .06 |
| **Chrysanthemum garland:** | | | | | | | | |
| raw: | | | | | | | | |
| untrimmed, 1 lb..... | 242 | 13.64 | 76 | 139 | 2488 | n.a. | n.a. | n.a. |
| trimmed, .5-oz. stem | 8 | .44 | 2 | 4 | 80 | n.a. | n.a. | n.a. |
| trimmed, 1" pieces, | | | | | | | | |
| 1 cup | 14 | .78 | 4 | 8 | 143 | n.a. | n.a. | n.a. |
| boiled, drained, 1" pieces, | | | | | | | | |
| ½ cup............. | 34 | 1.87 | 9 | 22 | 284 | n.a. | n.a. | n.a. |
| **Cilantro,** see "Coriander" | | | | | | | | |
| **Cinnamon,** ground, 1 tsp. | 28 | .88 | 1 | 1 | 11 | .05 | .01 | .38 |
| **Cisco,** smoked, 4 oz. ... | 2 | .05 | 2 | 14 | 27 | .03 | .02 | tr. |
| **Citrus fruit juice drink,** | | | | | | | | |
| frozen, diluted, 6 fl. oz. | 17 | 2.08 | 11 | 19 | 208 | .09 | .06 | .14 |
| **Clam,** mixed species, meat only: | | | | | | | | |
| raw, 1 lb............. | 209 | 63.41 | 42 | 766 | 1425 | 6.19 | 1.56 | 2.27 |
| raw, 9 large or 20 small, | | | | | | | | |
| 6.3 oz.............. | 83 | 25.16 | 17 | 304 | 565 | 2.46 | .62 | .90 |
| boiled, poached, or | | | | | | | | |
| steamed[1], 4 oz....... | 104 | 31.71 | 20 | 383 | 712 | 3.10 | .78 | n.a. |

---

[1] *Prepared without added ingredients.*

| | Calcium | Iron | Magnesium | Phosphorus | Potassium | Zinc | Copper | Manganese |
|---|---|---|---|---|---|---|---|---|
| | (Mg) | (Mg) | (Mg) | (Mg) | (Mg) | (Mg) | (Mg) | (Mg) |
| boiled, poached, or | | | | | | | | |
| steamed[1], 20 small ... | 83 | 25.16 | 17 | 304 | 565 | 2.46 | .62 | n.a. |
| breaded, fried, 20 small | 119 | 26.16 | 27 | 353 | 612 | 2.74 | .67 | n.a. |
| **Clam, canned,** mixed species: | | | | | | | | |
| drained, 4 oz. ......... | 104 | 31.71 | 20 | 383 | 712 | 3.10 | .78 | n.a. |
| drained, 1 cup......... | 148 | 44.47 | 30 | 540 | 1005 | 4.37 | 1.01 | n.a. |
| **Clam juice,** canned, ½ cup | 15 | n.a. | 13 | n.a. | n.a. | .12 | .47 | .09 |
| **Clove,** ground, 1 tsp..... | 14 | .18 | 6 | 2 | 23 | .02 | .01 | .63 |
| **Cocoa mix, powder:** | | | | | | | | |
| unsweetened, 1 tbsp..... | 6 | .69 | 25 | 37 | 76 | .34 | .19 | .19 |
| (*Carnation* 70 Calorie), | | | | | | | | |
| 1 pkt. ............. | 97 | .43 | 20 | 82 | 220 | .30 | .01 | n.a. |
| (*Hershey's* European | | | | | | | | |
| Style), 1 tbsp. ....... | 7 | 1.73 | 27 | 42 | 256 | .36 | .20 | .29 |
| w/out added nutrients, | | | | | | | | |
| 1-oz. pkt. or 3–4 | | | | | | | | |
| heaping tsp.......... | 93 | .34 | 24 | 89 | 202 | .41 | .08 | .08 |
| w/added nutrients, | | | | | | | | |
| 1.1-oz. pkt. ......... | 100 | 1.80 | 22 | 111 | 404 | .22 | .10 | .09 |
| chocolate: | | | | | | | | |
| fudge (*Carnation*), | | | | | | | | |
| 1 pkt. .......... | 44 | .63 | 20 | 66 | 260 | .27 | .24 | n.a. |
| milk (*Carnation*), | | | | | | | | |
| 1 pkt. .......... | 76 | .43 | 20 | 90 | 260 | .36 | .15 | n.a. |
| rich (*Carnation*), 1 pkt. | 60 | .45 | 20 | 84 | 260 | .30 | .15 | tr. |
| w/marshmallows | | | | | | | | |
| (*Carnation*), 1 pkt. | | | | | | | | |
| or 4 heaping tsp. | 57 | .45 | 19 | 80 | 240 | .28 | .15 | tr. |
| **Coconut,** shelled, except as noted: | | | | | | | | |
| raw: | | | | | | | | |
| in shell, 1 lb........ | 34 | 5.72 | 76 | 266 | 840 | 2.59 | 1.03 | 3.54 |
| 1 piece, 2" × 2" × | | | | | | | | |
| ½", 1.6 oz........ | 6 | 1.09 | 14 | 51 | 160 | .57 | .23 | .78 |

[1] *Prepared without added ingredients.*

| | Calcium | Iron | Magnesium | Phosphorus | Potassium | Zinc | Copper | Manganese |
|---|---|---|---|---|---|---|---|---|
| | (Mg) | (Mg) | (Mg) | (Mg) | (Mg) | (Mg) | (Mg) | (Mg) |
| **Coconut, raw,** *continued* | | | | | | | | |
| shredded or grated, | | | | | | | | |
| 1 cup . . . . . . . . . | 12 | 1.94 | 26 | 90 | 285 | .88 | .35 | 1.20 |
| dried, shredded: | | | | | | | | |
| unsweetened, 1 oz. . . | 7 | .94 | 26 | 59 | 154 | .52 | .09 | .13 |
| sweetened 1 oz. . . . . . | 4 | .54 | 14 | 30 | 96 | .68 | .43 | .57 |
| sweetened 1 cup . . . . | 14 | 1.78 | 47 | 99 | 313 | 1.69 | .29 | 2.30 |
| dried, creamed, 1 oz. . . . . | 7 | .95 | 26 | 59 | 156 | .58 | .23 | .79 |
| dried, toasted, 1 oz. . . . . | 8 | .96 | 26 | 60 | 157 | .58 | .23 | .80 |
| **Coconut cream,** canned: | | | | | | | | |
| ½ cup. . . . . . . . . . . . . . | 2 | .75 | n.a. | 33 | 150 | .89 | .35 | 1.21 |
| 1 tbsp. . . . . . . . . . . . . . | 0 | .10 | n.a. | 4 | 19 | .11 | .05 | .16 |
| **Coconut milk**[1], 1 cup . . . . | 39 | 3.94 | 89 | 240 | 630 | 1.61 | .64 | 2.20 |
| **Coconut water**[2], 1 cup . . . | 58 | .69 | 60 | 49 | 600 | .25 | .10 | n.a. |
| **Cod,** meat only: | | | | | | | | |
| Atlantic: | | | | | | | | |
| raw, 1 lb. . . . . . . . . . | 72 | 1.72 | 144 | 922 | 1873 | 2.04 | .13 | .07 |
| baked, broiled, or | | | | | | | | |
| microwaved[3], 4 oz. | 16 | .56 | 48 | 156 | 277 | .66 | .04 | n.a. |
| dried, salted, 1 oz. . . . | 45 | .70 | 37 | 266 | 408 | .44 | .05 | n.a. |
| Pacific: | | | | | | | | |
| raw, 1 lb. . . . . . . . . . | 33 | 1.19 | 110 | 789 | 1827 | 1.81 | .12 | .05 |
| baked, broiled, or | | | | | | | | |
| microwaved[3], 4 oz. | 10 | .37 | 35 | 253 | 586 | .58 | .04 | .02 |
| **Cod, canned,** Atlantic: | | | | | | | | |
| w/liquid, 11-oz. can . . . . . | 66 | 1.52 | 128 | 811 | 1647 | 1.79 | .01 | n.a. |
| w/liquid, 4 oz. . . . . . . . . | 24 | .56 | 46 | 295 | 599 | .66 | .04 | n.a. |
| **Coffee,** brewed, 6 fl. oz. | 3 | .08 | 10 | 2 | 96 | .03 | .01 | .05 |
| **Coffee, flavored,** instant, prepared: | | | | | | | | |
| cappuccino flavor, | | | | | | | | |
| 6 fl. oz. . . . . . . . . . . . | 7 | .15 | 9 | 26 | 119 | .08 | .03 | .03 |

---

[1] *Liquid expressed from mixture of grated coconut and water.*

[2] *Liquid from coconuts.*

[3] *Prepared without added ingredients.*

| | Calcium | Iron | Magnesium | Phosphorus | Potassium | Zinc | Copper | Manganese |
|---|---|---|---|---|---|---|---|---|
| | (Mg) | (Mg) | (Mg) | (Mg) | (Mg) | (Mg) | (Mg) | (Mg) |
| mocha flavor[1], 6 fl. oz.... | 7 | .24 | 9 | 29 | 119 | .15 | .06 | .05 |
| **Coffee flavor drink mix** (*Carnation* Instant Breakfast), 1 pkt...... | 150 | 4.50 | 80 | 150 | 340 | 3.00 | .50 | n.a. |
| **Coffee substitute**, cereal grain, (*Kaffree Roma*), 1 tsp.............. | 1 | .08 | n.a. | n.a. | 20 | .01 | n.a. | n.a. |
| **Coffee liqueur,** 1 fl. oz............. | tr. | .02 | 1 | 2 | 10 | .01 | .01 | n.a. |
| **Coffee w/cream liqueur,** 1 fl. oz.............. | 5 | .04 | 1 | 15 | 10 | .05 | .01 | n.a. |
| **Collards:** | | | | | | | | |
| fresh: | | | | | | | | |
| raw, untrimmed, 1 lb. | 74 | .50 | 24 | 27 | 437 | .35 | .10 | .71 |
| raw, trimmed, chopped, ½ cup .. | 5 | .03 | 2 | 2 | 30 | .02 | .01 | .05 |
| boiled, drained, chopped, ½ cup .. | 15 | .10 | 5 | 5 | 84 | .07 | .02 | .15 |
| frozen, chopped, 10-oz. pkg. ......... | 570 | 3.03 | 82 | 77 | 719 | .73 | .15 | 1.80 |
| frozen, boiled, drained, chopped, ½ cup ..... | 179 | .95 | 26 | 23 | 214 | .23 | .05 | .56 |
| **Cookie:** | | | | | | | | |
| animal crackers, 1 oz., about 11 pieces...... | 12 | .78 | 5 | 32 | 28 | .18 | .05 | .12 |
| butter, 2" diam., 1 piece | 1 | .11 | 1 | 5 | 6 | .02 | .01 | .01 |
| chocolate chip, 2¼" diam., .4-oz. piece .... | 2 | .28 | 3 | 11 | 14 | .06 | .02 | .05 |
| chocolate chip, soft type, .5-oz. piece ......... | 2 | .36 | 5 | 8 | 14 | .07 | .02 | .06 |
| coconut bar, 10 pieces, 3.2 oz................ | 65 | 1.30 | n.a. | 108 | 205 | n.a. | n.a. | n.a. |

---

[1]*With added calcium.*

| | Calcium | Iron | Magnesium | Phosphorus | Potassium | Zinc | Copper | Manganese |
|---|---|---|---|---|---|---|---|---|
| | (Mg) | (Mg) | (Mg) | (Mg) | (Mg) | (Mg) | (Mg) | (Mg) |
| Cookie, *continued* | | | | | | | | |
| fig bar, square, | | | | | | | | |
| .6-oz. piece . . . . . . . . | 10 | .46 | 4 | 10 | 33 | .06 | .02 | .06 |
| fortune, .3-oz. piece . . . . . | 1 | .12 | 1 | 3 | 3 | .01 | .01 | .02 |
| fudge, cake-type, | | | | | | | | |
| .7-oz. piece . . . . . . . . | 7 | .52 | 7 | 17 | 29 | .12 | .06 | .07 |
| gingersnap, .2-oz. piece | 5 | .45 | 3 | 6 | 24 | .04 | .02 | .11 |
| graham cracker: | | | | | | | | |
| plain or honey, | | | | | | | | |
| 2½"-square piece | 2 | .26 | 2 | 7 | 9 | .06 | .01 | .06 |
| chocolate coated, | | | | | | | | |
| 2½"-square | | | | | | | | |
| piece . . . . . . . . . . | 8 | .5 | 8 | 19 | 29 | .14 | .06 | .10 |
| sugar honey, | | | | | | | | |
| 2 square pieces . . . | 12 | .20 | n.a. | 47 | 38 | n.a. | n.a. | n.a. |
| ladyfinger, .4-oz. piece . . . | 5 | .39 | 1 | 19 | 12 | .13 | .01 | .03 |
| macaroon, 2 pieces, | | | | | | | | |
| 1.3 oz. . . . . . . . . . . . . | 10 | .30 | n.a. | 32 | 176 | n.a. | n.a. | n.a. |
| marshmallow, chocolate | | | | | | | | |
| coated, .5-oz. piece . . . | 6 | .33 | 5 | 13 | 24 | .08 | .03 | .04 |
| molasses, .5-oz. piece . . . | 11 | .96 | 8 | 14 | 52 | .07 | .06 | .19 |
| oatmeal raisin, | | | | | | | | |
| .6-oz. piece . . . . . . . . | 7 | .46 | 6 | 25 | 26 | .14 | .02 | .15 |
| oatmeal raisin, light, | | | | | | | | |
| 2 pieces, 1 oz. . . . . . . . | 11 | .62 | 10 | 30 | 60 | .18 | .06 | .23 |
| oatmeal raisin, soft-type, | | | | | | | | |
| .5-oz. piece . . . . . . . . | 13 | .42 | 4 | 31 | 20 | .07 | .08 | .06 |
| peanut butter, regular, | | | | | | | | |
| .5-oz. piece . . . . . . . . | 5 | .38 | 7 | 13 | 25 | .08 | .03 | .04 |
| peanut butter, soft-type, | | | | | | | | |
| .5-oz. piece . . . . . . . . | 2 | .13 | 5 | 13 | 16 | .08 | .01 | .06 |
| peanut butter sandwich, | | | | | | | | |
| .5-oz. piece . . . . . . . . | 7 | .36 | 7 | 26 | 27 | .15 | .03 | .13 |
| raisin, soft-type, | | | | | | | | |
| .5-oz. piece . . . . . . . . | 7 | .34 | 3 | 12 | 21 | .05 | .06 | n.a. |

| | Calcium | Iron | Magnesium | Phosphorus | Potassium | Zinc | Copper | Manganese |
|---|---|---|---|---|---|---|---|---|
| | (Mg) | (Mg) | (Mg) | (Mg) | (Mg) | (Mg) | (Mg) | (Mg) |
| sandwich, chocolate: | | | | | | | | |
|    regular, .4-oz. piece | 3 | .39 | 4 | 10 | 18 | .08 | .04 | .05 |
|    chocolate coated, | | | | | | | | |
|      .6-oz. piece ...... | 6 | .53 | 7 | 15 | 41 | .10 | .05 | .06 |
|    w/extra creme, | | | | | | | | |
|      .5-oz. piece ...... | 3 | .37 | 4 | 12 | 16 | .08 | .05 | .05 |
| sandwich, vanilla, | | | | | | | | |
|    .4-oz. piece ......... | 3 | .22 | 1 | 8 | 9 | .04 | .01 | .03 |
| shortbread: | | | | | | | | |
|    plain, .3-oz. piece.... | 3 | .22 | 1 | 9 | 8 | .04 | .01 | .03 |
|    w/pecans, .5-oz. piece | 4 | .34 | 3 | 12 | 10 | .08 | .02 | .09 |
| sugar, .5-oz. piece ...... | 3 | .32 | 2 | 12 | 9 | .07 | n.a. | n.a. |
| sugar wafer, creme-filled, | | | | | | | | |
|    .1-oz. piece ......... | 1 | .07 | 0 | 2 | 2 | .01 | tr. | .01 |
| tofu (*The Great Tofu* | | | | | | | | |
|    *Cookie*), 2 pieces..... | 9 | 1.80 | 3 | 18 | 24 | .02 | n.a. | n.a. |
| wafer: | | | | | | | | |
|    chocolate, | | | | | | | | |
|      .2-oz. piece ...... | 2 | .24 | 3 | 8 | 13 | .07 | .03 | .04 |
|    vanilla, regular, | | | | | | | | |
|      .2-oz. piece ...... | 2 | .13 | 1 | 4 | 6 | .02 | .01 | .02 |
|    vanilla, light, | | | | | | | | |
|      1-oz. piece....... | 2 | .10 | 1 | 4 | 4 | .01 | tr. | .01 |
|    vanilla, brown-edge, | | | | | | | | |
|      10 pieces, 2 oz.... | 24 | .20 | n.a. | 37 | 42 | n.a. | n.a. | n.a.. |
| wheat free (*The Great* | | | | | | | | |
|    *Wheat Free Cookie*), | | | | | | | | |
|    4 pieces ............ | 36 | 3.50 | 4 | 21 | 35 | .03 | n.a. | n.a. |
| **Cookie, refrigerated dough:** | | | | | | | | |
| chocolate chip, 1 oz. ..... | 7 | .64 | 7 | 19 | 51 | .14 | .05 | n.a. |
| oatmeal, 1 oz.......... | 5 | .34 | 5 | 17 | 24 | .10 | .02 | n.a. |
| peanut butter, 1 oz...... | 16 | .27 | 6 | 38 | 49 | .11 | .02 | n.a. |
| sugar, 1 oz............. | 13 | .26 | 1 | 27 | 23 | .04 | .01 | n.a. |
| **Coriander:** | | | | | | | | |
| fresh, raw: | | | | | | | | |
|    untrimmed, 1 lb..... | 378 | 7.52 | 101 | 140 | 2090 | n.a. | n.a. | n.a. |

| | Calcium | Iron | Magnesium | Phosphorus | Potassium | Zinc | Copper | Manganese |
|---|---|---|---|---|---|---|---|---|
| | (Mg) | (Mg) | (Mg) | (Mg) | (Mg) | (Mg) | (Mg) | (Mg) |
| Coriander, *continued* | | | | | | | | |
| trimmed, 9 plants, | | | | | | | | |
| .8 oz.. . . . . . . . . . . | 20 | .39 | 5 | 7 | 108 | n.a. | n.a. | n.a. |
| trimmed, ¼ cup. . . . . | 4 | .08 | 1 | 1 | 22 | n.a. | n.a. | n.a. |
| dried, leaf, 1 tsp.. . . . . . . . | 7 | .25 | 4 | 3 | 27 | n.a. | .01 | .04 |
| **Coriander seeds,** 1 tsp. | 13 | .29 | 6 | 7 | 23 | .08 | .02 | .03 |
| **Corn,** yellow or white: | | | | | | | | |
| fresh: | | | | | | | | |
| raw, untrimmed (in | | | | | | | | |
| husk), 1 lb. . . . . . . | 3 | .84 | 61 | 146 | 441 | .74 | .09 | .26 |
| raw, trimmed, 1 ear, | | | | | | | | |
| 3.2 oz. . . . . . . . . . | 2 | .46 | 34 | 80 | 243 | .41 | .05 | .15 |
| raw, kernels, ½ cup | 2 | .40 | 29 | 69 | 208 | .35 | .04 | .12 |
| boiled, drained, 1 ear | 2 | .47 | 24 | 79 | 192 | .37 | .04 | .15 |
| boiled, drained, | | | | | | | | |
| kernels, ½ cup. . . . | 2 | .50 | 26 | 84 | 204 | .39 | .04 | .16 |
| canned, kernels: | | | | | | | | |
| w/liquid, ½ cup . . . . . | 5 | .44 | 20 | 65 | 196 | .46 | .07 | .04 |
| cream style, ½ cup | 4 | .49 | 22 | 65 | 172 | .68 | .07 | .05 |
| vacuum pack, ½ cup | 5 | .44 | 24 | 67 | 195 | .48 | .05 | .07 |
| w/red and green | | | | | | | | |
| peppers, ½ cup . . . | 5 | .90 | 29 | 71 | 174 | .42 | .07 | n.a. |
| frozen, kernels, except as noted: | | | | | | | | |
| 10-oz. pkg. . . . . . . . . | 12 | 1.20 | 51 | 197 | 596 | 1.04 | .10 | .36 |
| ½ cup. . . . . . . . . . . . | 4 | .35 | 15 | 57 | 172 | .30 | .03 | .10 |
| on cob, boiled, | | | | | | | | |
| 4-oz. ear . . . . . . . . | 2 | .39 | 18 | 47 | 158 | .40 | .03 | .09 |
| boiled, drained, ⅓ of | | | | | | | | |
| 10-oz. pkg. . . . . . . | 4 | .33 | 18 | 54 | 139 | .38 | .04 | .12 |
| boiled, drained, | | | | | | | | |
| ½ cup. . . . . . . . . . | 3 | .29 | 16 | 47 | 121 | .33 | .03 | .11 |
| **Corn, whole grain,** 1 cup | 12 | 4.50 | 211 | 349 | 476 | 3.66 | .52 | .81 |
| **Corn bran,** crude, 1 cup | 32 | 2.12 | 48 | 55 | 33 | 1.18 | .19 | .11 |
| **Corn bread,** see "Bread, sweet, mix" | | | | | | | | |
| **Corn chips and similar snacks:** | | | | | | | | |
| plain, 1 oz. . . . . . . . . . . . | 36 | .37 | 21 | 52 | 40 | .36 | .05 | .11 |

| | Calcium | Iron | Magnesium | Phosphorus | Potassium | Zinc | Copper | Manganese |
|---|---|---|---|---|---|---|---|---|
| | (Mg) | (Mg) | (Mg) | (Mg) | (Mg) | (Mg) | (Mg) | (Mg) |
| barbecue, 1 oz. . . . . . . . . | 37 | .44 | 22 | 59 | 67 | .30 | .05 | .22 |
| onion flavor, 1 oz. . . . . . . | 8 | 1.06 | 8 | 20 | 40 | .09 | .03 | .06 |
| puffs/twists, cheese, | | | | | | | | |
|   1 oz. . . . . . . . . . . . . . | 16 | .67 | 5 | 31 | 47 | .11 | .02 | .02 |
| tortilla, see "Tortilla chips" | | | | | | | | |
| **Corn flour:** | | | | | | | | |
| whole grain, 1 cup. . . . . . | 8 | 2.78 | 109 | 318 | 369 | 2.02 | .27 | .54 |
| masa, enriched, 1 cup | 161 | 8.22 | 125 | 255 | 340 | 2.03 | .19 | .55 |
| **Corn grits, enriched:** | | | | | | | | |
| uncooked, 1 cup . . . . . . . | 3 | 6.10 | 42 | 114 | 213 | .64 | .12 | .17 |
| cooked, 1 cup . . . . . . . . . | 1 | 1.55 | 11 | 29 | 54 | .17 | .03 | .04 |
| **Corn syrup:** | | | | | | | | |
| dark, 1 tbsp. . . . . . . . . . | 4 | .07 | 2 | 2 | 9 | .01 | .01 | .02 |
| high fructose, 1 tbsp. . . . . | 0 | .01 | 0 | n.a. | 0 | 0 | 0 | .01 |
| light, 1 tbsp. . . . . . . . . . . | 1 | .01 | 0 | 0 | 1 | 0 | tr. | .02 |
| malt, 1 tbsp. . . . . . . . . . . | 15 | .23 | 17 | 57 | 77 | .03 | .05 | .02 |
| blended, see "Syrup, table blends" | | | | | | | | |
| **Cornish game hen:** | | | | | | | | |
| raw, meat w/skin, 1 bird, | | | | | | | | |
|   11.8 oz. . . . . . . . . . . . | 37 | 2.60 | 60 | 470 | 792 | 3.84 | .17 | .05 |
| raw, meat only, 1 bird, | | | | | | | | |
|   8.4 oz. . . . . . . . . . . . . . | 29 | 1.77 | 51 | 382 | 643 | 3.14 | .13 | .04 |
| roasted[1], meat w/skin, | | | | | | | | |
|   1 bird, 8.1 oz. . . . . . . . . | 31 | 2.08 | 40 | 334 | 562 | 3.41 | .14 | .04 |
| roasted[1], meat only, | | | | | | | | |
|   1 bird, 3.8 oz. . . . . . . . . | 14 | .83 | 20 | 159 | 268 | 1.63 | .06 | .02 |
| **Cornmeal,** dry: | | | | | | | | |
| whole grain, 1 cup. . . . . . | 7 | 4.21 | 155 | 294 | 350 | 2.21 | .24 | .61 |
| degermed, enriched, | | | | | | | | |
|   1 cup . . . . . . . . . . . . . | 7 | 5.70 | 56 | 116 | 224 | .99 | .11 | .14 |
| self-rising, enriched[2]: | | | | | | | | |
|   bolted, 1 cup. . . . . . . | 440 | 7.03 | 105 | 981 | 331 | 2.44 | .18 | n.a. |

---

[1] *Prepared without added ingredients.*

[2] *With added nutrients.*

| | Calcium | Iron | Magnesium | Phosphorus | Potassium | Zinc | Copper | Manganese |
|---|---|---|---|---|---|---|---|---|
| | (Mg) | (Mg) | (Mg) | (Mg) | (Mg) | (Mg) | (Mg) | (Mg) |
| Cornmeal, self-rising, *continued* | | | | | | | | |
| bolted, w/wheat flour, | | | | | | | | |
| 1 cup . . . . . . . . . | 508 | 8.41 | 91 | 1106 | 352 | 2.36 | .24 | n.a. |
| degermed, 1 cup . . . . | 482 | 6.53 | 68 | 859 | 235 | 1.38 | .18 | n.a. |
| **Cornstarch,** 1 cup . . . . . . | 2 | .61 | 3 | 16 | 4 | .08 | .06 | .07 |
| **Cottonseed flour:** | | | | | | | | |
| partially defatted, 1 cup | 449 | 11.90 | 677 | 1501 | 1666 | 10.98 | 1.11 | n.a. |
| low fat, 1 oz. . . . . . . . . . | 135 | 3.57 | 203 | 451 | 500 | 3.30 | .33 | n.a. |
| **Cottonseed kernels,** roasted: | | | | | | | | |
| 1 cup . . . . . . . . . . . . . . | 149 | 8.05 | 656 | 1192 | 2012 | 8.94 | 1.79 | n.a. |
| 1 tbsp. . . . . . . . . . . . . | 10 | .54 | 44 | 80 | 135 | .60 | .12 | n.a. |
| **Cottonseed meal,** | | | | | | | | |
| partially defatted, 1 oz. | 143 | 3.79 | 216 | 478 | 531 | 3.50 | .35 | n.a. |
| **Country gravy mix,** | | | | | | | | |
| vegetarian (*Loma Linda* | | | | | | | | |
| *Gravy Quik*), 1 tbsp., | | | | | | | | |
| .2 oz. . . . . . . . . . . . . . | 1 | .03 | n.a. | n.a. | 7 | .02 | n.a. | n.a. |
| **Couscous:** | | | | | | | | |
| uncooked: | | | | | | | | |
| 1 cup . . . . . . . . . . . | 44 | 1.99 | 81 | 313 | 305 | 1.52 | .45 | 1.44 |
| (*Casbah*), 3.5 oz. . . . . | 42 | 3.40 | n.a. | 370 | 370 | n.a. | n.a. | n.a. |
| whole wheat | | | | | | | | |
| (*Casbah*), 3.5 oz. | 37 | 4.30 | n.a. | 386 | 435 | n.a. | n.a. | n.a. |
| cooked, 1 cup . . . . . . . . | 15 | .69 | 15 | 39 | 104 | .46 | .07 | .15 |
| **Cowpeas:** | | | | | | | | |
| fresh: | | | | | | | | |
| raw, untrimmed (in | | | | | | | | |
| pods), 1 lb. . . . . . . | 290 | 2.54 | 117 | 123 | 998 | 2.34 | .3.0 | 1.30 |
| raw, trimmed, | | | | | | | | |
| ½ cup . . . . . . . . . . | 90 | .79 | 37 | 38 | 311 | .73 | .09 | .40 |
| boiled, drained, | | | | | | | | |
| ½ cup . . . . . . . . . . | 105 | .92 | 42 | 42 | 342 | .85 | .11 | .47 |
| fresh, leafy tips: | | | | | | | | |
| raw, untrimmed, | | | | | | | | |
| 1 lb. . . . . . . . . . . | 147 | 4.53 | 102 | 21 | 1074 | n.a. | n.a. | n.a. |

| | Calcium | Iron | Magnesium | Phosphorus | Potassium | Zinc | Copper | Manganese |
|---|---|---|---|---|---|---|---|---|
| | (Mg) | (Mg) | (Mg) | (Mg) | (Mg) | (Mg) | (Mg) | (Mg) |
| raw, trimmed, chopped, 1 cup . . . | 23 | .69 | 16 | 3 | 164 | n.a. | n.a. | n.a. |
| boiled, drained, choppd, ½ cup . . . | 18 | .28 | 16 | 11 | 91 | n.a. | n.a. | n.a. |
| fresh, young pods, w/seeds: | | | | | | | | |
| raw, untrimmed, 1 lb. . . . . . . . . . . | 268 | 4.13 | n.a. | 268 | 888 | n.a. | n.a. | n.a. |
| raw, trimmed, ½ cup | 31 | .47 | n.a. | 31 | 101 | n.a. | n.a. | n.a. |
| boiled, drained, ½ cup . . . . . . . . . | 26 | .33 | m.a. | 23 | 92 | n.a. | n.a. | n.a. |
| frozen, 10-oz. pkg. . . . . . . | 73 | 6.69 | 158 | 348 | 1252 | 4.50 | .58 | 2.50 |
| frozen, boiled, drained, ½ cup . . . . . . . . . . . . | 20 | 1.80 | 42 | 104 | 319 | 1.21 | .16 | .67 |
| **Cowpeas, dried:** | | | | | | | | |
| uncooked, 1 lb. . . . . . . . . | 497 | 37.53 | 834 | 1925 | 5046 | 15.28 | 3.83 | 6.93 |
| uncooked, ½ cup. . . . . . . | 92 | 6.95 | 154 | 357 | 934 | 2.83 | .71 | 1.28 |
| boiled, ½ cup . . . . . . . . . | 21 | 2.16 | 46 | 134 | 239 | 1.11 | .23 | .41 |
| canned: | | | | | | | | |
| plain, w/liquid, 8 oz. | 45 | 2.21 | 63 | 158 | 390 | 1.59 | .27 | .64 |
| plain, w/liquid, ½ cup | 24 | 1.17 | 33 | 83 | 206 | .84 | .14 | .34 |
| w/pork, 8 oz. . . . . . . . | 39 | 3.23 | 98 | 219 | 404 | 2.35 | .39 | .89 |
| w/pork, ½ cup. . . . . . | 21 | 1.71 | 52 | 116 | 213 | 1.24 | .20 | .47 |
| **Cowpeas, Catjang,** dried: | | | | | | | | |
| uncooked, 1 lb. . . . . . . . | 384 | 45.14 | 1512 | 1986 | 6235 | 27.69 | 4.80 | 7.00 |
| uncooked, ½ cup. . . . . . | 71 | 8.36 | 280 | 368 | 1155 | 5.13 | .89 | 1.30 |
| cooked, boiled, ½ cup . . . | 22 | 2.62 | 83 | 122 | 322 | 1.61 | .23 | .41 |
| **Crab, Alaska king,** meat only: | | | | | | | | |
| raw, 1 lb.. . . . . . . . . . . . . | 210 | 2.68 | n.a. | 992 | 925 | 26.97 | 4.18 | .16 |
| raw, 6 oz., yield from 1-lb. whole leg. . . . . . . | 80 | 1.01 | n.a. | 376 | 351 | 10.23 | 1.57 | .06 |
| boiled or steamed[1], 4 oz. . . . . . . . . . . . . . | 67 | .86 | n.a. | 318 | 297 | 8.64 | 1.34 | n.a. |
| boiled or steamed[1], 4.7 oz. (1-lb. raw leg) . . . . | 80 | 1.01 | n.a. | 376 | 350 | 10.21 | 1.58 | n.a. |

---

[1] *Prepared without added ingredients.*

| | Calcium (Mg) | Iron (Mg) | Magnesium (Mg) | Phosphorus (Mg) | Potassium (Mg) | Zinc (Mg) | Copper (Mg) | Manganese (Mg) |
|---|---|---|---|---|---|---|---|---|
| **Crab, blue,** meat only: | | | | | | | | |
| raw, 1 lb.. . . . . . . . . . . . | 404 | 3.34 | 154 | 1039 | 1494 | 16.03 | 3.04 | .68 |
| raw, .75 oz., yield from | | | | | | | | |
| ⅓ lb. whole crab . . . . . | 19 | .15 | 7 | 48 | 69 | .74 | .14 | .03 |
| canned, drained, 4 oz. . . . | 115 | .95 | 44 | 295 | 424 | 4.56 | .86 | n.a. |
| canned, drained, 1 cup . . | 137 | 1.13 | 52 | 351 | 505 | 5.42 | 1.03 | n.a. |
| **Crab, Dungeness,** meat only: | | | | | | | | |
| raw, 1 lb.. . . . . . . . . . . . | 210 | 1.66 | 206 | 824 | 1605 | 19.35 | 3.06 | .36 |
| raw, 5.7 oz., yield from | | | | | | | | |
| 1.5-lb. whole crab . . . . | 75 | .59 | 74 | 296 | 577 | 6.95 | 1.10 | .13 |
| boiled or steamed[1], | | | | | | | | |
| 4 oz.. . . . . . . . . . . . . | 67 | .48 | 66 | 198 | 463 | 6.20 | .83 | .11 |
| boiled or steamed[1], 4.5 oz. | | | | | | | | |
| (1.5-lb. crab, raw) . . . . | 75 | .54 | 73 | 222 | 519 | 6.95 | .93 | .12 |
| **Crab, queen,** meat only: | | | | | | | | |
| raw, 1 lb.. . . . . . . . . . . . | 118 | n.a. | n.a. | 603 | 785 | n.a. | n.a. | n.a. |
| boiled or steamed[1], | | | | | | | | |
| 4 oz.. . . . . . . . . . . . . . | 37 | n.a. | n.a. | 145 | 227 | n.a. | n.a. | n.a. |
| **Crabapple:** | | | | | | | | |
| untrimmed, 1 lb. . . . . . . . | 76 | 1.49 | 28 | 63 | 810 | n.a. | .28 | .48 |
| w/skin, sliced, ½ cup . . . . | 10 | .20 | 4 | 9 | 107 | n.a. | .04 | .06 |
| **Cracker:** | | | | | | | | |
| butter, 10 round or | | | | | | | | |
| 1.2 oz.. . . . . . . . . . . . | 49 | .20 | n.a. | 86 | 37 | n.a. | n.a. | n.a. |
| cheese, plain, 1"-square | | | | | | | | |
| piece . . . . . . . . . . . . | 2 | .05 | 0 | 2 | 1 | .01 | tr. | .01 |
| cheese–peanut butter | | | | | | | | |
| sandwich, .3-oz. piece | 6 | .20 | 4 | 23 | 17 | .08 | .02 | .05 |
| crispbread, rye, | | | | | | | | |
| .4-oz. piece . . . . . . . . . | 3 | .24 | 8 | 27 | 32 | .24 | .03 | .25 |
| graham, see "Cookie" | | | | | | | | |
| matzo: | | | | | | | | |
| plain, 1-oz. piece . . . . | 4 | .9 | 7 | 25 | 32 | .19 | .02 | .18 |
| egg, 1-oz. piece . . . . . | 11 | .77 | n.a. | n.a. | 43 | .21 | n.a. | .17 |

---

[1] *Prepared without added ingredients.*

| | Calcium (Mg) | Iron (Mg) | Magnesium (Mg) | Phosphorus (Mg) | Potassium (Mg) | Zinc (Mg) | Copper (Mg) | Manganese (Mg) |
|---|---|---|---|---|---|---|---|---|
| egg and onion, 1-oz. piece . . . . . . | 10 | 1.24 | 8 | 25 | 24 | .21 | .02 | .23 |
| whole wheat, 1-oz. piece . . . . . . | 7 | 1.32 | 38 | 86 | 89 | .74 | .10 | .99 |
| melba toast: | | | | | | | | |
| plain, .2-oz. piece . . . . | 5 | .19 | 3 | 10 | 10 | .10 | .01 | .06 |
| rye, .2-oz. piece . . . . . | 4 | .18 | 2 | 9 | 10 | .07 | .02 | .04 |
| wheat, .2-oz. piece . . . | 2 | .22 | 3 | 8 | 7 | .07 | .01 | .05 |
| milk, .4-oz. piece . . . . . . . | 21 | .43 | 3 | 36 | 14 | .08 | .93 | .07 |
| rusk toast, .4-oz. piece . . . | 3 | .27 | 4 | 15 | 25 | .11 | .02 | .04 |
| rye: | | | | | | | | |
| plain, 1 triple cracker, .9 oz. . . . . . . . . . . . | 10 | 1.48 | 30 | 84 | 124 | .70 | .12 | n.a. |
| sandwich type, w/ cheese filling, .3-oz. piece . . . . . . | 16 | .17 | 3 | 24 | 24 | .05 | .01 | .04 |
| seasoned, 1 triple cracker, .8 oz. . . . . | 10 | .67 | 23 | 68 | 100 | .56 | .11 | n.a. |
| saltine, .1-oz. piece . . . . . | 4 | .16 | 1 | 3 | 4 | .02 | .01 | .02 |
| saltine, no fat/low sodium, 3 pieces, .5 oz. . . . . . . . . . . . . . | 3 | 1.16 | 4 | 17 | 17 | .14 | .02 | .10 |
| snack type: | | | | | | | | |
| 1 round .1-oz. piece | 4 | .11 | 1 | 7 | 4 | .02 | .01 | .02 |
| sandwich, w/cheese filling, .3-oz. piece . . . . . . . | 18 | .17 | 2 | 28 | 30 | .04 | .01 | .02 |
| sandwich, w/peanut butter filling, .3-oz. piece . . . . . . | 7 | .21 | 4 | 17 | 16 | .07 | .02 | .05 |
| soda biscuit, 10 pieces, 1.8 oz. . . . . . . . . . . . . | 11 | .80 | n.a. | 45 | 60 | n.a. | n.a. | n.a. |
| soup or oyster, 10 pieces. . . . . . . . . . | 2 | .10 | n.a. | 7 | 9 | n.a. | n.a. | n.a. |
| wheat: | | | | | | | | |
| plain, .1-oz. piece . . . . . | 1 | .09 | 1 | 4 | 4 | .03 | .01 | .04 |

|  | Calcium | Iron | Magnesium | Phosphorus | Potassium | Zinc | Copper | Manganese |
|---|---|---|---|---|---|---|---|---|
|  | (Mg) | (Mg) | (Mg) | (Mg) | (Mg) | (Mg) | (Mg) | (Mg) |
| **Cracker, wheat,** *continued* | | | | | | | | |
| sandwich, w/cheese filling, | | | | | | | | |
| .3-oz. piece . . . . . . | 14 | .18 | 4 | 27 | 21 | .06 | .01 | n.a. |
| sandwich, w/peanut butter filling, | | | | | | | | |
| .3-oz. piece . . . . . . | 12 | .19 | 3 | 24 | 21 | .06 | tr. | .05 |
| whole, .1-oz. piece. . . | 2 | .12 | 4 | 12 | 12 | .09 | .02 | .09 |
| **Cracker meal,** 1 cup . . . . | 27 | 5.33 | 28 | 120 | 132 | .79 | .26 | 1.09 |
| **Cranberry,** fresh: | | | | | | | | |
| untrimmed, 1 lb. . . . . . . . | 32 | .85 | 22 | 37 | 305 | .56 | .25 | .68 |
| whole, ½ cup . . . . . . . . . | 4 | .10 | 3 | 4 | 34 | .06 | .03 | .07 |
| chopped, ½ cup . . . . . . . | 4 | .11 | 3 | 5 | 39 | .07 | .03 | .09 |
| **Cranberry beans,** dried: | | | | | | | | |
| uncooked, 1 lb. . . . . . . . . | 576 | 22.69 | 706 | 1689 | 6041 | 16.48 | 3.60 | 4.17 |
| uncooked, ½ cup. . . . . . . | 124 | 4.90 | 152 | 365 | 1305 | 3.56 | .78 | .90 |
| boiled, ½ cup . . . . . . . . . | 44 | 1.84 | 44 | 119 | 340 | 1.00 | .20 | .33 |
| canned, w/liquid, 8 oz. | 76 | 3.51 | 73 | 195 | 589 | 1.90 | .32 | .45 |
| canned, w/liquid, ½ cup. . . . . . . . . . . . . | 44 | 2.01 | 41 | 112 | 337 | 1.09 | .19 | .26 |
| **Cranberry juice cocktail:** | | | | | | | | |
| bottled, 6 fl. oz. . . . . . . . . | 7 | .28 | 4 | 4 | 34 | .14 | .03 | .37 |
| frozen, diluted, 6 fl. oz. | 9 | .17 | 4 | 3 | 27 | .07 | .02 | .08 |
| **Cranberry sauce,** canned, sweetened, ½ cup . . . . | 5 | .30 | 4 | 8 | 35 | .07 | .03 | .08 |
| **Cranberry-apple juice drink,** bottled, 6 fl. oz. | 13 | .11 | 3 | 5 | 50 | .08 | .01 | n.a. |
| **Cranberry-apricot juice drink,** bottled, 6 fl. oz. | 17 | .28 | 6 | 10 | 113 | .07 | .03 | n.a. |
| **Cranberry-grape juice drink,** bottled, 6 fl. oz. | 15 | .02 | 6 | 7 | 44 | .07 | .01 | n.a. |
| **Cranberry-orange relish,** canned, ½ cup . . . . . | 15 | .28 | 6 | 11 | 53 | n.a. | .06 | n.a. |
| **Crayfish,** mixed species, meat only: | | | | | | | | |
| wild: | | | | | | | | |
| raw, 1 lb. . . . . . . . . . . | 120 | 3.81 | 122 | 1160 | 1371 | 5.91 | 1.90 | 1.02 |

| | Calcium | Iron | Magnesium | Phosphorus | Potassium | Zinc | Copper | Manganese |
|---|---|---|---|---|---|---|---|---|
| | (Mg) | (Mg) | (Mg) | (Mg) | (Mg) | (Mg) | (Mg) | (Mg) |
| raw, 8 crayfish, approx. 1 oz...... | 7 | .23 | 7 | 69 | 82 | .35 | .11 | .06 |
| boiled or steamed[1], 4 oz............ | 68 | .94 | 37 | 306 | 336 | 2.00 | .78 | .59 |
| **farmed:** | | | | | | | | |
| raw, 1 lb............ | 114 | 2.48 | 137 | 987 | 1186 | 4.58 | 1.08 | .66 |
| raw, 8 crayfish, approx. 1 oz...... | 7 | .15 | 8 | 59 | 71 | .27 | .06 | .04 |
| boiled or steamed[1], 4 oz............ | 58 | 1.26 | 37 | 273 | 270 | 1.68 | .66 | .25 |
| **Cream:** | | | | | | | | |
| half and half, 1 cup..... | 254 | .17 | 25 | 230 | 314 | 1.23 | .02 | tr. |
| half and half, 1 tbsp..... | 16 | .01 | 2 | 14 | 19 | .08 | tr. | tr. |
| light, coffee or table, 1 cup ............. | 231 | .10 | 21 | 192 | 292 | .65 | .02 | tr. |
| light, coffee or table, 1 tbsp. ............ | 14 | .01 | 1 | 12 | 18 | .04 | tr. | tr. |
| medium (25% fat), 1 cup ............. | 216 | .10 | 20 | 169 | 274 | .62 | .02 | tr. |
| medium (25% fat), 1 tbsp. ............ | 14 | .01 | 1 | 11 | 17 | .04 | tr. | tr. |
| **whipping:** | | | | | | | | |
| light, 1 cup, approx. 2 cups whipped... | 166 | .07 | 17 | 146 | 231 | .60 | .02 | tr. |
| light, 1 tbsp........ | 10 | tr. | 1 | 9 | 15 | .04 | tr. | tr. |
| heavy, 1 cup, approx. 2 cups whipped... | 154 | .07 | 17 | 149 | 179 | .55 | .01 | tr. |
| heavy, 1 tbsp....... | 10 | tr. | 1 | 9 | 11 | .03 | tr. | tr. |
| whipped topping, pressurized, 1 cup .... | 61 | .03 | 6 | 54 | 88 | .22 | .06 | tr. |
| whipped topping, pressurized, 1 tbsp.... | 3 | tr. | tr. | 3 | 4 | .01 | tr. | tr. |

---

[1] *Prepared without added ingredients.*

| | Calcium | Iron | Magnesium | Phosphorus | Potassium | Zinc | Copper | Manganese |
|---|---|---|---|---|---|---|---|---|
| | (Mg) | (Mg) | (Mg) | (Mg) | (Mg) | (Mg) | (Mg) | (Mg) |
| **Cream, sour, cultured:** | | | | | | | | |
| 1 cup .............. | 268 | .14 | 26 | 195 | 331 | .62 | .04 | .01 |
| 1 tbsp. ............. | 14 | .01 | 1 | 10 | 17 | .03 | tr. | tr. |
| half and half, 1 tbsp. .... | 16 | .01 | 2 | 14 | 19 | .08 | tr. | tr. |
| **Cream, sour, nondairy,** | | | | | | | | |
| 1 oz.............. | 1 | n.a. | n.a. | 13 | 46 | n.a. | .02 | .03 |
| **Cream of tartar,** | | | | | | | | |
| 1 tsp. ............. | 0 | .11 | 0 | 0 | 2 | .01 | .01 | .01 |
| **Cream topping, nondairy:** | | | | | | | | |
| frozen: | | | | | | | | |
| semisolid, 1 tbsp. ... | tr. | tr. | tr. | tr. | 1 | tr. | tr. | tr. |
| (*Rich's*), 3.5 oz...... | 3 | .06 | 2 | 1 | 3 | 0 | 0 | n.a. |
| powdered, 1.5 oz. ...... | 458 | 0 | 0 | 0 | 0 | 0 | 0 | 0 |
| powdered, prepared w/ | | | | | | | | |
| whole milk, 1 tbsp. ... | 4 | tr. | tr. | 3 | 6 | .01 | tr. | tr. |
| pressurized, 1 tbsp...... | tr. | tr. | tr. | 1 | 1 | tr. | tr. | tr. |
| **Creamer, nondairy:** | | | | | | | | |
| liquid: | | | | | | | | |
| (*Coffee-mate*), | | | | | | | | |
| .5 fl. oz.......... | <1 | .01 | tr. | 7 | 20 | .01 | 0 | n.a. |
| (*Rich's Coffee Rich* | | | | | | | | |
| Light), 3.5 oz. .... | 4 | .03 | 2 | 45 | 100 | 0 | 0 | n.a. |
| (*Rich's Farm Rich*), | | | | | | | | |
| 3.5 oz. ........ | 4 | .03 | 2 | 59 | 135 | 0 | 0 | n.a. |
| (*Rich's Farm Rich Fat* | | | | | | | | |
| Free), 3.5 oz...... | 4 | .02 | 2 | 58 | 137 | 0 | 0 | n.a. |
| (*Rich's Farm Rich* | | | | | | | | |
| Light), 3.5 oz. .... | 4 | .01 | 2 | 59 | 135 | 0 | 0 | n.a. |
| **Creme de menthe,** | | | | | | | | |
| 1 fl. oz............. | 0 | .02 | 0 | 0 | 0 | n.a. | .03 | .01 |
| **Cress, garden:** | | | | | | | | |
| raw, untrimmed, 1 lb. ... | 261 | 4.19 | n.a. | 245 | 1952 | n.a. | n.a. | n.a. |
| raw, trimmed, ½ cup.... | 20 | .33 | n.a. | 19 | 152 | n.a. | n.a. | n.a. |
| boiled, drained, ½ cup... | 41 | .54 | n.a. | 33 | 240 | n.a. | n.a. | n.a. |

| | Calcium | Iron | Magnesium | Phosphorus | Potassium | Zinc | Copper | Manganese |
|---|---|---|---|---|---|---|---|---|
| | (Mg) | (Mg) | (Mg) | (Mg) | (Mg) | (Mg) | (Mg) | (Mg) |
| **Croaker,** Atlantic, meat | | | | | | | | |
| only, raw, 1 lb. . . . . . . | 68 | 1.68 | 181 | 951 | 1565 | 1.88 | .19 | .11 |
| **Croissant,** 2-oz. piece: | | | | | | | | |
| plain . . . . . . . . . . . . . . . | 21 | 1.16 | 9 | 60 | 67 | .43 | .05 | .19 |
| apple filled. . . . . . . . . . | 17 | .63 | 7 | 33 | 51 | .6 | .02 | .12 |
| cheese filled . . . . . . . . . | 30 | 1.23 | 14 | 74 | 76 | .54 | .06 | .19 |
| **Crookneck squash:** | | | | | | | | |
| fresh: | | | | | | | | |
| raw, untrimmed, | | | | | | | | |
| 1 lb. . . . . . . . . . . | 95 | 2.14 | 94 | 146 | 952 | 1.32 | .46 | .71 |
| raw, trimmed, sliced, | | | | | | | | |
| ½ cup . . . . . . . . . | 14 | .31 | 14 | 21 | 138 | .19 | .07 | .10 |
| boiled, drained, | | | | | | | | |
| sliced, ½ cup. . . . . | 24 | .32 | .22 | 35 | 173 | .35 | .09 | .19 |
| canned, drained, sliced, | | | | | | | | |
| ½ cup . . . . . . . . . . . . | 13 | .7 | 14 | 22 | 104 | .32 | .09 | .11 |
| frozen, boiled, drained, | | | | | | | | |
| sliced, ½ cup. . . . . . . | 19 | .49 | 26 | 40 | 243 | .32 | .07 | .25 |
| **Croutons:** | | | | | | | | |
| plain, 1 cup. . . . . . . . . . | 23 | 1.22 | 9 | 35 | 37 | .27 | .05 | .15 |
| seasoned, 1 cup . . . . . . | 38 | 1.13 | 17 | 56 | 72 | .38 | .07 | .21 |
| (*Kellogg's Croutettes*), | | | | | | | | |
| 1 cup . . . . . . . . . . . . | 30 | 1.50 | 9 | 37 | 40 | .30 | .06 | n.a. |
| **Cucumber,** w/peel: | | | | | | | | |
| untrimmed, 1 lb. . . . . . . | 63 | 1.15 | 48 | 88 | 634 | .90 | .15 | .33 |
| 1 medium, 8¼" long, | | | | | | | | |
| 10.6 oz. . . . . . . . . . . | 43 | .78 | 33 | 60 | 434 | .61 | .10 | .23 |
| sliced, ½ cup . . . . . . . . | 7 | .14 | 6 | 10 | 75 | .11 | .02 | .04 |
| **Cumin seed,** 1 tsp. . . . . . | 20 | 1.39 | 8 | 10 | 38 | .10 | .02 | .07 |
| **Currant:** | | | | | | | | |
| fresh: | | | | | | | | |
| black, untrimmed, | | | | | | | | |
| 1 lb. . . . . . . . . . . | 244 | 6.82 | 108 | 261 | 1432 | 1.19 | .38 | 1.14 |
| black, trimmed, | | | | | | | | |
| ½ cup. . . . . . . . . | 31 | .86 | 14 | 33 | 180 | .15 | .05 | .14 |

|  | Calcium (Mg) | Iron (Mg) | Magnesium (Mg) | Phosphorus (Mg) | Potassium (Mg) | Zinc (Mg) | Copper (Mg) | Manganese (Mg) |
|---|---|---|---|---|---|---|---|---|
| Currant, fresh, *continued* | | | | | | | | |
| red or white, untrimmed, 1 lb... | 146 | 4.42 | 57 | 194 | 1221 | 1.02 | .48 | .83 |
| red or white, trimmed, ½ cup... | 18 | .56 | 7 | 24 | 154 | .13 | .06 | .10 |
| dried, Zante, ½ cup..... | 62 | 2.34 | 30 | 90 | 642 | .47 | .34 | .34 |
| **Curry powder,** 1 tsp..... | 10 | .59 | 5 | 7 | 31 | .08 | .02 | .09 |
| **Cusk,** meat only: | | | | | | | | |
| raw, 1 lb............. | 46 | 3.76 | 142 | 924 | 1779 | 1.73 | .08 | .07 |
| baked, broiled, or microwaved[1], 4 oz. ... | 15 | 1.20 | 45 | 297 | 570 | .56 | .03 | .02 |
| **Custard mix,** dry: | | | | | | | | |
| egg, 3-oz. pkg. ........ | 193 | 1.64 | 37 | 239 | 395 | .90 | .06 | n.a. |
| flan/caramel, 3-oz. pkg. | 20 | .07 | 0 | 1 | 130 | .04 | .01 | n.a. |
| **Custard apple:** | | | | | | | | |
| untrimmed, 1 lb........ | 80 | 1.85 | 47 | 56 | 1004 | n.a. | n.a. | n.a. |
| trimmed, 1 oz......... | 9 | .20 | 5 | 6 | 108 | n.a. | n.a. | n.a. |
| **Cuttlefish,** mixed species, meat only: | | | | | | | | |
| raw, 1 lb............. | 410 | 27.29 | n.a. | 1755 | 1607 | 7.84 | 2.66 | n.a. |
| boiled or steamed[1], 4 oz............... | 204 | 12.29 | n.a. | 658 | 722 | 3.92 | 1.13 | n.a. |

---

[1] *Prepared without added ingredients.*

# D

| | Calcium | Iron | Magnesium | Phosphorus | Potassium | Zinc | Copper | Manganese |
|---|---|---|---|---|---|---|---|---|
| | (Mg) | (Mg) | (Mg) | (Mg) | (Mg) | (Mg) | (Mg) | (Mg) |
| **Daikon,** see "Radish, Oriental" | | | | | | | | |
| **Dandelion greens:** | | | | | | | | |
| raw, untrimmed, 1 lb. . . . | 848 | 14.06 | 163 | 299 | 1801 | n.a. | n.a. | n.a. |
| raw, chopped, ½ cup. . . . | 52 | .87 | 10 | 18 | 111 | n.a. | n.a. | n.a. |
| boiled, drained, chopped, | | | | | | | | |
| ½ cup. . . . . . . . . . . . | 73 | .94 | n.a. | 22 | 121 | n.a. | n.a. | n.a. |
| **Danish pastry:** | | | | | | | | |
| plain, round, | | | | | | | | |
| 2-oz. piece. . . . . . . . . | 60 | 1.10 | n.a. | 58 | 53 | n.a. | n.a. | n.a. |
| cheese, 2.5-oz. piece . . . . | 25 | 1.14 | 11 | 77 | 70 | n.a. | n.a. | n.a. |
| cinnamon, | | | | | | | | |
| 2.3-oz. piece . . . . . . . . | 46 | 1.27 | 12 | 70 | 81 | .47 | .07 | .24 |
| w/fruit, 2.5-oz. piece . . . . | 33 | 1.26 | 11 | 63 | 59 | .38 | .05 | .18 |
| w/nuts, 2.3-oz. piece . . . . | 61 | 1.17 | 21 | 71 | 62 | .57 | .13 | .55 |
| **Date,** domestic, natural, dry: | | | | | | | | |
| w/pits, 1 lb.. . . . . . . . . . | 133 | 4.70 | 145 | 161 | 2662 | 1.19 | 1.18 | 1.22 |
| 10 dates, 2.9 oz. . . . . . . . | 27 | .96 | 29 | 33 | 541 | .24 | .24 | .25 |
| pitted, chopped, ½ cup . . | 29 | 1.03 | 32 | 35 | 581 | .26 | .26 | .27 |
| **Dill,** dried: | | | | | | | | |
| seeds, 1 tsp. . . . . . . . . . | 32 | .34 | 5 | 6 | 25 | .11 | .02 | .04 |
| weed, 1 cup sprigs . . . . . | 18 | n.a. | 5 | 6 | 66 | .08 | .01 | 11 |
| **Dock,** raw: | | | | | | | | |
| untrimmed, 1 lb. . . . . . . . | 140 | 7.62 | 327 | 200 | 1238 | n.a. | n.a. | n.a. |
| trimmed, chopped, | | | | | | | | |
| ½ cup. . . . . . . . . . . . | 29 | 1.61 | 69 | 42 | 261 | n.a. | n.a. | n.a. |
| **Dolphinfish,** meat only: | | | | | | | | |
| raw, 1 lb.. . . . . . . . . . . . | n.a. | 5.13 | n.a. | n.a. | 1887 | 2.07 | .19 | .07 |
| baked, broiled, or | | | | | | | | |
| microwaved[1], 4 oz. . . . | n.a. | 1.64 | n.a. | n.a. | 604 | .67 | .06 | .02 |
| **Donut:** | | | | | | | | |
| cake type: | | | | | | | | |
| plain, 1.7-oz. piece. . . | 21 | .92 | 9 | 127 | 60 | .26 | .05 | .16 |

[1] *Prepared without added ingredients.*

| | Calcium | Iron | Magnesium | Phosphorus | Potassium | Zinc | Copper | Manganese |
|---|---|---|---|---|---|---|---|---|
| | (Mg) | (Mg) | (Mg) | (Mg) | (Mg) | (Mg) | (Mg) | (Mg) |
| **Donut, cake type,** *continued* | | | | | | | | |
| plain, chocolate coated, 1.5-oz. piece | 15 | 1.06 | 17 | 87 | n.a. | .26 | .09 | .17 |
| plain, sugared or glazed, 1.6-oz. piece | 27 | .48 | 8 | 53 | 46 | .20 | .05 | .15 |
| chocolate, sugared or glazed, 1.5-oz. piece | 89 | .95 | 14 | 68 | n.a. | .24 | .08 | .16 |
| wheat, sugared or glazed, 1.6-oz. piece | 22 | .50 | 10 | 47 | 66 | .31 | .05 | n.a. |
| French cruller, glazed, 1.4-oz. piece | 11 | n.a. | 5 | 50 | 32 | .11 | .03 | n.a. |
| yeast type: | | | | | | | | |
| glazed, 2.1-oz. piece | 26 | 1.22 | 13 | 56 | 65 | .46 | .10 | .16 |
| creme filled, 3-oz. piece | 22 | 1.56 | 17 | 65 | 68 | .68 | .10 | n.a. |
| jelly filled, 3-oz. piece | 21 | 1.50 | 17 | 72 | 67 | .64 | .12 | n.a. |
| **Drum,** freshwater, meat only: | | | | | | | | |
| raw, 1 lb.. | 272 | 4.08 | 136 | 816 | 1247 | 2.97 | 1.05 | 3.18 |
| baked, broiled, or microwaved[1], 4 oz. | 87 | 1.30 | 43 | 262 | 400 | .96 | .34 | 1.02 |
| **Duck,** domesticated: | | | | | | | | |
| roasted[1], meat w/skin, 4 oz. | 12 | 3.06 | 18 | 177 | 231 | 2.11 | .26 | n.a. |
| roasted[1], meat only, 4 oz. | 14 | 3.06 | 23 | 230 | 286 | 2.95 | .26 | n.a. |
| **Duck, wild,** raw, meat w/ skin, 1 oz. | 1 | 1.18 | 6 | 48 | 71 | .22 | .09 | n.a. |
| **Dutch brand loaf,** pork and beef, 1-oz. slice. | 24 | .35 | 6 | 46 | 107 | .49 | .02 | .01 |

[1] *Prepared without added ingredients.*

# E

| | Calcium | Iron | Magnesium | Phosphorus | Potassium | Zinc | Copper | Manganese |
|---|---|---|---|---|---|---|---|---|
| | (Mg) | (Mg) | (Mg) | (Mg) | (Mg) | (Mg) | (Mg) | (Mg) |
| **Eclair,** chocolate, frozen | | | | | | | | |
| (*Rich's*), 3.5 oz...... | 12 | .83 | 5 | 42 | 56 | .27 | .02 | n.a. |
| **Eel,** mixed species, meat only: | | | | | | | | |
| raw, 1 lb.............. | 91 | 2.27 | n.a. | 979 | 1236 | 7.34 | .10 | .16 |
| baked, broiled, or | | | | | | | | |
| microwaved[1], 4 oz. ... | 29 | .73 | n.a. | 314 | 396 | 2.36 | .03 | (0) |
| **Egg,** chicken: | | | | | | | | |
| raw: | | | | | | | | |
| whole, fresh or | | | | | | | | |
| frozen, 1 large, | | | | | | | | |
| approx. 1.75 oz.... | 25 | .72 | 5 | 89 | 60 | .55 | .01 | .01 |
| white, fresh or frozen, | | | | | | | | |
| from 1 large egg ..... | 2 | .01 | 4 | 4 | 48 | 0 | tr. | tr. |
| yolk, fresh, from 1 large | | | | | | | | |
| egg ............... | 23 | .59 | 1 | 81 | 16 | .52 | tr. | .01 |
| cooked, 1 large egg: | | | | | | | | |
| fried[2]............. | 25 | .72 | 5 | 89 | 61 | .55 | .01 | .01 |
| hard boiled ........ | 25 | .60 | 5 | 86 | 63 | .52 | .01 | .01 |
| omelet[3] ........... | 26 | .73 | 5 | 90 | 62 | .56 | .01 | .01 |
| poached .......... | 25 | .72 | 5 | 89 | 60 | .55 | .01 | .01 |
| scrambled[4] ........ | 44 | .73 | 7 | 104 | 84 | .61 | .01 | .01 |
| yolk, frozen[5], 1 oz....... | 33 | .86 | 3 | 118 | 28 | .75 | .01 | .02 |
| yolk, frozen, sugared, | | | | | | | | |
| 1 oz............... | 30 | .78 | 2 | 106 | 26 | .68 | .01 | .02 |
| dried, whole, 1 oz....... | 60 | 2.23 | 13 | 192 | 139 | 1.53 | .08 | .04 |
| dried, stabilized[6]: | | | | | | | | |
| whole, 1 oz......... | 63 | 2.35 | 14 | 203 | 146 | 1.62 | .08 | .04 |

[1] *Without added ingredients.*
[2] *Recipe: 95% egg, 5% margarine, and salt.*
[3] *Recipe: 74% egg, 22% water, 4% margarine, and salt.*
[4] *Recipe: 74% egg, 22% whole milk, 4% margarine, and salt.*
[5] *Includes approximately 17% white.*
[6] *Glucose reduced.*

| | Calcium | Iron | Magnesium | Phosphorus | Potassium | Zinc | Copper | Manganese |
|---|---|---|---|---|---|---|---|---|
| | (Mg) | (Mg) | (Mg) | (Mg) | (Mg) | (Mg) | (Mg) | (Mg) |
| Egg, chicken, dried, stabilized, *continued* | | | | | | | | |
| white, flakes, 1 oz.... | 24 | .07 | 19 | 24 | 295 | .04 | .07 | .02 |
| white, powder, 1 oz. | 25 | .07 | 20 | 25 | 316 | .05 | .05 | .01 |
| dried, yolk, 1 oz. ...... | 80 | 2.94 | 8 | 268 | 48 | 1.74 | .08 | .03 |
| **Egg, chicken,** substitute or imitation: | | | | | | | | |
| frozen, 1 oz. .......... | 21 | .56 | n.a. | 20 | 60 | .28 | .01 | tr. |
| frozen (*Morningstar Farms Better'n Eggs*), ¼ cup, 2 oz......... | 7 | .63 | n.a. | 29 | 68 | .51 | n.a. | n.a. |
| liquid, 1 oz............. | 15 | .60 | n.a. | 34 | 94 | .37 | .01 | tr. |
| powder, 1 oz. ......... | 92 | .90 | n.a. | 136 | 211 | n.a. | .06 | .02 |
| **Egg, duck,** fresh, whole, raw, 1 egg, approx. 2.5 oz............. | 45 | 2.70 | 12 | 154 | 156 | .99 | .04 | .03 |
| **Egg, quail,** fresh, whole, raw, 1 egg, approx. .3 oz.............. | 27 | 0 | .01 | .07 | .01 | .01 | n.a. | n.a. |
| **"Egg," breakfast, vegetarian,** frozen, (*Morningstar Farms Scramblers*), ¼ cup, 2 oz............... | 31 | 1.07 | n.a. | 50 | 50 | .80 | n.a. | n.a. |
| **Egg roll,** frozen, vegetarian (*Worthington*), 3-oz. roll ........... | 15 | .57 | n.a. | 70 | 96 | .31 | n.a. | n.a. |
| **Eggnog,** dairy, nonalcoholic, 1 cup ... | 330 | .51 | 47 | 278 | 420 | 1.17 | n.a. | n.a. |
| **Eggnog flavor mix,** 2 heaping tsp. prepared w/1 cup whole milk ... | 291 | .38 | 33 | 228 | 369 | .92 | .02 | .01 |
| **Eggplant:** | | | | | | | | |
| raw: | | | | | | | | |
| untrimmed, 1 lb. ..... | 27 | 1.01 | 51 | 81 | 796 | .52 | .20 | .48 |

| | Calcium | Iron | Magnesium | Phosphorus | Potassium | Zinc | Copper | Manganese |
|---|---|---|---|---|---|---|---|---|
| | (Mg) | (Mg) | (Mg) | (Mg) | (Mg) | (Mg) | (Mg) | (Mg) |
| trimmed, peeled, 1 eggplant, 1.9 lbs. untrimmed | 34 | 1.26 | 64 | 102 | 992 | .65 | .25 | .59 |
| trimmed, peeled, 1" pieces, ½ cup | 3 | .11 | 6 | 9 | 89 | .06 | .02 | .05 |
| boiled, drained, 1" cubes, ½ cup | 3 | .17 | 6 | 11 | 119 | .07 | .05 | .07 |
| **Elderberry,** 1 cup | 55 | 2.32 | n.a. | 57 | 406 | n.a. | n.a. | n.a. |
| **Endive:** | | | | | | | | |
| untrimmed, 1 lb. | 203 | 3.22 | 57 | 111 | 1225 | 3.08 | .39 | 1.64 |
| trimmed, 1 head, 1.3 lbs. | 267 | 4.23 | 74 | 145 | 1611 | 4.05 | .51 | 2.16 |
| trimmed, chopped, ½ cup | 13 | .21 | 4 | 7 | 79 | .20 | .03 | .11 |
| **Endive, Belgian,** see "Chicory, witloof" | | | | | | | | |
| **Eppaw,** raw, ½ cup | 55 | .58 | 16 | 83 | 170 | n.a. | n.a. | n.a. |

# F

| | Calcium | Iron | Magnesium | Phosphorus | Potassium | Zinc | Copper | Manganese |
|---|---|---|---|---|---|---|---|---|
| | (Mg) | (Mg) | (Mg) | (Mg) | (Mg) | (Mg) | (Mg) | (Mg) |
| **Falafel**[1]: | | | | | | | | |
| 1 lb. . . . . . . . . . . . . . . | 243 | 15.49 | 373 | 870 | 2654 | 6.80 | 1.17 | 3.13 |
| 1 patty, 2¼" diam., | | | | | | | | |
| .6 oz. . . . . . . . . . . . . | 9 | .58 | 14 | 33 | 99 | .26 | .04 | .12 |
| **Farina**, whole grain, enriched: | | | | | | | | |
| dry, 1 cup . . . . . . . . . . | 25 | 6.54 | 23 | 154 | 165 | .94 | .14 | n.a. |
| cooked, 1 cup . . . . . . . . | 4 | 1.16 | 4 | 28 | 30 | .16 | .03 | n.a. |
| **Fast foods** (unspecified), 1 serving: | | | | | | | | |
| breakfast: | | | | | | | | |
| biscuit, plain, 2.6 oz. | 90 | 1.63 | 9 | 260 | 86 | .29 | .04 | .30 |
| biscuit, w/egg: | | | | | | | | |
| 4.8 oz. . . . . . . . . . . | 154 | 3.13 | 20 | 184 | 160 | 1.10 | .08 | .30 |
| and bacon, 5.3 oz. | 189 | 3.73 | 23 | 238 | 250 | 1.64 | .11 | .28 |
| and ham, 6.8 oz. . . . | 221 | 4.55 | 30 | 317 | 319 | 2.23 | .14 | .30 |
| and sausage, | | | | | | | | |
| 6.3 oz. . . . . . . . . | 155 | 3.96 | 25 | 490 | 319 | 2.16 | .10 | .32 |
| and steak, 5.2 oz. . . | 138 | 5.30 | 24 | 225 | 306 | 2.80 | .11 | .25 |
| cheese and bacon, | | | | | | | | |
| 5.1 oz. . . . . . . . . | 164 | 2.55 | 20 | 459 | 230 | 1.54 | .08 | .26 |
| biscuit, w/ham, 4 oz. | 161 | 2.73 | 22 | 554 | 197 | 1.65 | .04 | .36 |
| biscuit, w/sausage, | | | | | | | | |
| 4.4 oz. . . . . . . . . . . | 128 | 2.59 | 20 | 446 | 198 | 1.56 | .05 | .36 |
| biscuit, w/steak, | | | | | | | | |
| 5 oz. . . . . . . . . . . | 115 | 4.31 | 27 | 205 | 233 | 2.66 | .12 | .42 |
| croissant, w/egg and cheese: | | | | | | | | |
| 4.5 oz. . . . . . . . . . . | 244 | 2.20 | 22 | 349 | 174 | 1.76 | .09 | .23 |
| and bacon, 4.6 oz. | 151 | 2.19 | 23 | 276 | 201 | 1.90 | .10 | .22 |
| and ham, 5.4 oz. . . . | 144 | 2.13 | 26 | 336 | 272 | 2.17 | .13 | .22 |
| and sausage, | | | | | | | | |
| 5.6 oz. . . . . . . . . | 144 | 3.04 | 25 | 290 | 283 | 2.15 | .11 | .25 |

[1] *Recipe: water, broad beans, soybean oil, onions, flour, salt, garlic, coriander, and cumin.*

| | Calcium | Iron | Magnesium | Phosphorus | Potassium | Zinc | Copper | Manganese |
|---|---|---|---|---|---|---|---|---|
| | (Mg) | (Mg) | (Mg) | (Mg) | (Mg) | (Mg) | (Mg) | (Mg) |
| danish pastry: | | | | | | | | |
| cheese, 3.2 oz. . . . . | 70 | 1.85 | 16 | 80 | 116 | .63 | .09 | .35 |
| cinnamon, 3.1 oz. | 37 | 1.80 | 14 | 74 | 96 | .49 | .08 | .37 |
| fruit, 3.3 oz. . . . . . . . | 22 | 1.40 | 14 | 69 | 110 | .48 | .06 | .19 |
| eggs, scrambled, | | | | | | | | |
| 2 eggs. . . . . . . . . | 54 | 2.43 | 13 | 228 | 138 | 1.56 | .06 | .04 |
| English muffin: | | | | | | | | |
| w/butter, 2.2 oz. . . . | 103 | 1.59 | 13 | 85 | 69 | .42 | .06 | .21 |
| w/cheese and | | | | | | | | |
| sausage, 4.1 oz. | 168 | 2.25 | 24 | 186 | 215 | 1.68 | .08 | .22 |
| w/egg, cheese, and | | | | | | | | |
| Canadian bacon, | | | | | | | | |
| 5.1 oz. . . . . . . . . | 207 | 3.28 | 33 | 319 | 213 | 1.80 | .13 | .26 |
| w/egg, cheese, and | | | | | | | | |
| sausage, 5.8 oz. | 196 | 3.46 | 30 | 288 | 294 | 2.36 | .12 | .30 |
| French toast, w/ | | | | | | | | |
| butter, 2 slices, | | | | | | | | |
| 4.8 oz. . . . . . . . . | 73 | 1.89 | 16 | 146 | 177 | .60 | .07 | .21 |
| French toast sticks, | | | | | | | | |
| 5 sticks, 5 oz. . . . . | 78 | 2.96 | 26 | 123 | 126 | .93 | .27 | .22 |
| pancakes, w/butter | | | | | | | | |
| and syrup, 3 | | | | | | | | |
| cakes, 8.2 oz. . . . . | 128 | 2.61 | 48 | 476 | 250 | 1.03 | .15 | .32 |
| potatoes, hashed | | | | | | | | |
| brown, ½ cup . . . . | 7 | .48 | 16 | 69 | 267 | .22 | .07 | .11 |
| sausage, 1-oz. patty | 9 | .34 | 5 | 50 | 97 | .68 | .04 | .02 |
| sausage, .5-oz. link . . | 4 | .16 | 2 | 24 | 47 | .33 | .02 | .01 |
| entrees: | | | | | | | | |
| chicken, breaded, fried: | | | | | | | | |
| dark meat, 1 thigh | | | | | | | | |
| and 1 drumstick, | | | | | | | | |
| 5.2 oz. . . . . . . . . | 36 | 1.60 | 37 | 240 | 446 | 3.24 | .12 | .13 |
| light meat, 2 pieces, | | | | | | | | |
| 5.7 oz. . . . . . . . . | 60 | 1.49 | 38 | 307 | 566 | 1.55 | .10 | .16 |
| chicken nuggets, breaded, fried, 6 pieces: | | | | | | | | |
| plain, 3.6 oz. . . . . . . | 16 | 1.27 | 20 | 204 | 251 | 1.06 | .17 | .13 |

| | Calcium | Iron | Magnesium | Phosphorus | Potassium | Zinc | Copper | Manganese |
|---|---|---|---|---|---|---|---|---|
| | (Mg) | (Mg) | (Mg) | (Mg) | (Mg) | (Mg) | (Mg) | (Mg) |

Fast foods, chicken nuggets, *continued*

| | Calcium | Iron | Magnesium | Phosphorus | Potassium | Zinc | Copper | Manganese |
|---|---|---|---|---|---|---|---|---|
| w/barbecue sauce, 4.6 oz. | 21 | 1.46 | 25 | 214 | 319 | 1.11 | .17 | .16 |
| w/honey, 4.1 oz. | 17 | 1.32 | 20 | 203 | 255 | 1.09 | .17 | .14 |
| w/mustard sauce, 4.6 oz. | 25 | 1.48 | 25 | 219 | 280 | 1.14 | .17 | .17 |
| w/sweet and sour sauce, 4.6 oz. | 20 | 1.48 | 23 | 211 | 277 | 1.10 | .17 | .15 |
| chili con carne, 1 cup | 67 | 5.19 | 45 | 198 | 691 | 3.56 | .60 | .40 |
| clams, breaded, fried, ¾ cup | 21 | 3.04 | 31 | 239 | 265 | 1.63 | .10 | .31 |
| crab, baked, 3.8 oz. | 415 | 1.38 | 82 | 336 | 598 | 7.02 | 1.08 | .79 |
| crab, soft shell, breaded, fried, 4.4 oz. crab | 55 | 1.81 | 25 | 132 | 163 | 1.06 | .19 | .31 |
| crab cake, 2.1-oz. cake | 202 | 1.12 | .25 | 227 | 162 | 2.12 | .37 | .28 |
| fish, battered or breaded, fried, 3.2-oz. fillet | 17 | 1.92 | 22 | 156 | 292 | .40 | .04 | .17 |
| oysters, battered or breaded, fried, 6 pieces, 4.9 oz. | 27 | 4.46 | 24 | 195 | 182 | 15.64 | .80 | .42 |
| scallops, breaded, fried, 6 pieces, 5.1 oz. | 18 | 2.04 | 32 | 292 | 294 | 1.08 | .22 | .30 |
| shrimp, breaded, fried, 6–8 pieces, 5.8 oz. | 84 | 2.94 | 39 | 345 | 184 | 1.21 | .14 | .33 |
| Mexican foods: | | | | | | | | |
| burrito, w/beans, 2 pieces: | | | | | | | | |
| 7.7 oz. | 113 | 4.52 | 86 | 97 | 653 | 1.53 | .38 | .87 |
| and cheese, 6.6 oz. | 214 | 2.27 | 80 | 180 | 496 | 1.64 | .35 | .43 |
| and chilies, 7.2 oz. | 100 | 4.54 | 72 | 114 | 580 | 3.40 | .33 | .78 |
| and meat, 8.1 oz. | 105 | 4.89 | 83 | 142 | 656 | 3.84 | .38 | .83 |

| | Calcium (Mg) | Iron (Mg) | Magnesium (Mg) | Phosphorus (Mg) | Potassium (Mg) | Zinc (Mg) | Copper (Mg) | Manganese (Mg) |
|---|---|---|---|---|---|---|---|---|
| cheese and beef, | | | | | | | | |
| 7.2 oz.......... | 131 | 3.73 | 50 | 140 | 410 | 2.35 | .33 | .40 |
| cheese and chilies, | | | | | | | | |
| 11.9 oz......... | 288 | 7.68 | 99 | 286 | 810 | 6.07 | .59 | .81 |
| burrito, w/beef, 2 pieces: | | | | | | | | |
| 7.8 oz............ | 84 | 6.09 | 81 | 175 | 739 | 4.73 | .41 | .79 |
| and chilies, 7.1 oz. | 87 | 4.43 | 60 | 141 | 499 | 4.32 | .32 | .75 |
| cheese and chilies, | | | | | | | | |
| 10.7 oz......... | 223 | 7.81 | 69 | 316 | 667 | 7.91 | .36 | .61 |
| chimichanga, w/beef, 1 piece: | | | | | | | | |
| 6.1 oz............ | 63 | 4.55 | 62 | 123 | 587 | 4.95 | .42 | .56 |
| and cheese, 6.5 oz. | 238 | 3.84 | 60 | 187 | 203 | 3.37 | .35 | .49 |
| and red chilies, | | | | | | | | |
| 6.7 oz.......... | 71 | 4.18 | 65 | 113 | 613 | 3.03 | .28 | .62 |
| cheese and red | | | | | | | | |
| chilies, 6.3 oz.... | 218 | 3.14 | 41 | 146 | 330 | 4.63 | .56 | .39 |
| enchilada, w/cheese, 1 piece: | | | | | | | | |
| 5.7 oz............ | 324 | 1.31 | 50 | 133 | 240 | 2.51 | .26 | .24 |
| and beef, 6.8 oz. | 228 | 3.08 | 82 | 168 | 574 | 2.69 | .52 | .58 |
| enchirito, w/cheese, | | | | | | | | |
| beef and beans, | | | | | | | | |
| 6.8-oz. piece ..... | 217 | 2.39 | 71 | 224 | 560 | 2.75 | .27 | .38 |
| frijoles, w/cheese, | | | | | | | | |
| 1 cup .......... | 188 | 2.24 | 85 | 175 | 605 | 1.73 | .34 | .50 |
| nachos, w/cheese, 6–8 pieces: | | | | | | | | |
| 4 oz............. | 272 | 1.27 | 55 | 276 | 172 | 1.78 | .14 | .22 |
| and jalapeños, | | | | | | | | |
| 7.2 oz.......... | 620 | 2.45 | 109 | 394 | 293 | 2.90 | .17 | .44 |
| and beans, ground | | | | | | | | |
| beef, and | | | | | | | | |
| peppers, 9 oz.... | 384 | 2.78 | 97 | 389 | 451 | 3.65 | .75 | .42 |
| taco, small, 6 oz..... | 221 | 2.42 | 71 | 203 | 473 | 3.93 | .21 | .44 |
| taco, large, 9.3 oz. | 339 | 3.72 | 109 | 313 | 728 | 6.05 | .32 | .68 |
| taco salad[1], 1½ cups | 192 | 2.28 | 52 | 143 | 416 | 2.68 | .22 | .33 |

[2] Recipe: chili con carne, lettuce, tomato, cheese, and taco shell.

| | Calcium | Iron | Magnesium | Phosphorus | Potassium | Zinc | Copper | Manganese |
|---|---|---|---|---|---|---|---|---|
| | (Mg) | (Mg) | (Mg) | (Mg) | (Mg) | (Mg) | (Mg) | (Mg) |
| Fast foods, Mexican foods, *continued* | | | | | | | | |
| taco salad, w/chili[1], | | | | | | | | |
| 1½ cups . . . . . . . . | 246 | 2.67 | 52 | 154 | 393 | 3.29 | .30 | .34 |
| tostado, 1 piece: | | | | | | | | |
| w/beans and cheese, | | | | | | | | |
| 5.1 oz. . . . . . . . . . | 211 | 1.88 | 59 | 116 | 403 | 1.90 | .21 | .37 |
| w/beans, beef, and | | | | | | | | |
| cheese, 7.9 oz. . . | 190 | 2.45 | 68 | 173 | 490 | 3.18 | .32 | .36 |
| w/beef and cheese, | | | | | | | | |
| 5.7 oz. . . . . . . . . . | 217 | 2.86 | 64 | 180 | 572 | 3.68 | .26 | .50 |
| w/guacamole, | | | | | | | | |
| 2.3 oz. . . . . . . . . . | 212 | .82 | 37 | 117 | 325 | 2.03 | .13 | .18 |
| pizza, ⅛ of 12" pie: | | | | | | | | |
| w/cheese . . . . . . . . . . | 116 | .58 | 16 | 113 | 110 | .82 | .08 | .23 |
| w/cheese, meat, | | | | | | | | |
| vegetables . . . . . . . | 101 | 1.53 | 18 | 131 | 178 | 1.12 | .12 | .12 |
| w/pepperoni. . . . . . . . | 65 | .94 | 8 | 75 | 153 | .52 | .06 | .10 |
| sandwiches, 1 piece: | | | | | | | | |
| cheeseburger, single meat patty: | | | | | | | | |
| plain, 3.6 oz. . . . . . . | 140 | 2.44 | 21 | 196 | 165 | 2.37 | .09 | .23 |
| w/condiments[2], | | | | | | | | |
| 4 oz. . . . . . . . . . . . | 111 | 2.43 | 21 | 177 | 223 | 2.09 | .10 | .18 |
| w/condiments and | | | | | | | | |
| vegetables[3], | | | | | | | | |
| 5.4 oz. . . . . . . . . . | 182 | 2.65 | 26 | 216 | 229 | 2.62 | .12 | .29 |
| cheeseburger, double meat patty: | | | | | | | | |
| plain, 5.5. oz. . . . . . . | 232 | 3.41 | 33 | 374 | 308 | 4.96 | .13 | .23 |
| w/condiments and | | | | | | | | |
| vegetables[3], | | | | | | | | |
| 5.9 oz. . . . . . . . . . | 171 | 3.42 | 31 | 242 | 335 | 3.49 | .15 | .30 |

---

[1] *Recipe: chili con carne, lettuce, tomato, cheese, and taco shell.*
[2] *Condiments include catsup, mustard, pickles, and onions.*
[3] *Condiments and vegetables include catsup, mustard, mayonnaise-style dressing, pickles, onions, lettuce, and tomatoes.*

| | Calcium | Iron | Magnesium | Phosphorus | Potassium | Zinc | Copper | Manganese |
|---|---|---|---|---|---|---|---|---|
| | (Mg) | (Mg) | (Mg) | (Mg) | (Mg) | (Mg) | (Mg) | (Mg) |
| double-decker bun, plain, 5.6 oz. . . . . | 224 | 3.70 | 33 | 338 | 285 | 4.35 | .14 | .30 |
| double-decker bun, w/ condiments and vegetables[1], 8 oz. . . . . . . . . . | 169 | 4.71 | 36 | 350 | 389 | 4.13 | .16 | .27 |
| cheeseburger, large, single meat patty: | | | | | | | | |
| plain, 6.5 oz. . . . . . . | 91 | 5.47 | 38 | 423 | 644 | 5.54 | .16 | .31 |
| w/bacon and condiments[2], 6.9 oz. . . . . . . . . | 162 | 4.73 | 44 | 399 | 331 | 6.82 | .16 | .33 |
| w/condiments and vegetables[1], 7.7 oz. . . . . . . . . | 205 | 4.66 | 43 | 312 | 445 | 4.60 | .19 | .31 |
| w/ham, condiments and vegetables[1], 9 oz. . . . . . . . . . | 301 | 5.04 | 51 | 530 | 539 | 6.63 | .25 | .37 |
| cheeseburger, large, double meat patty, w/condiments and vegetables[1], 9.1 oz. . . . . . . . . . | 240 | 5.91 | 52 | 396 | 596 | 6.68 | .21 | .32 |
| chicken fillet sandwich: | | | | | | | | |
| plain, 6.4 oz. . . . . . . | 60 | 4.68 | 35 | 233 | 353 | 1.87 | .23 | .47 |
| w/cheese, 8 oz. . . . . | 258 | 3.63 | 43 | 407 | 334 | 2.90 | .17 | .38 |
| fish sandwich, w/tartar sauce: | | | | | | | | |
| 5.6 oz. . . . . . . . . . . | 84 | 2.60 | 33 | 212 | 339 | .99 | .19 | .37 |
| and cheese, 6.5 oz. . . | 185 | 3.50 | 37 | 312 | 353 | 1.17 | .12 | .36 |
| hamburger, single meat patty: | | | | | | | | |
| plain, 3.2 oz. . . . . . . | 63 | 2.41 | 19 | 102 | 145 | 2.00 | .09 | .21 |

[1] Condiments and vegetables include catsup, mustard, mayonnaise-style dressing, pickles, onions, lettuce, and tomatoes.
[2] Condiments include catsup, mustard, pickles, and onions.

| | Calcium | Iron | Magnesium | Phosphorus | Potassium | Zinc | Copper | Manganese |
|---|---|---|---|---|---|---|---|---|
| | (Mg) | (Mg) | (Mg) | (Mg) | (Mg) | (Mg) | (Mg) | (Mg) |

Fast foods, sandwiches, hamburger, single meat patty, *continued*

| | Calcium | Iron | Magnesium | Phosphorus | Potassium | Zinc | Copper | Manganese |
|---|---|---|---|---|---|---|---|---|
| w/condiments[1], | | | | | | | | |
| 3.8 oz......... | 52 | 2.46 | 23 | 110 | 215 | 2.05 | .12 | .21 |
| w/condiments and vegetables[1], | | | | | | | | |
| 3.9 oz......... | 63 | 2.62 | 22 | 125 | 227 | 2.06 | .10 | .25 |
| hamburger, double meat patty: | | | | | | | | |
| plain, 6.2 oz...... | 87 | 4.55 | 36 | 234 | 363 | 5.71 | .17 | .28 |
| w/condiments[2], | | | | | | | | |
| 7.6 oz......... | 92 | 5.55 | 44 | 284 | 527 | 5.80 | .19 | .33 |
| hamburger, large, single meat patty: | | | | | | | | |
| plain, 4.8 oz...... | 74 | 3.57 | 28 | 176 | 268 | 4.11 | .13 | .24 |
| w/condiments and vegetables[2], | | | | | | | | |
| 7.7 oz......... | 96 | 4.92 | 43 | 233 | 479 | 4.98 | .20 | .35 |
| hamburger, large, double meat patty, w/condiments and vegetables[2], | | | | | | | | |
| 8 oz............ | 102 | 5.85 | 49 | 314 | 569 | 5.68 | .22 | .25 |
| ham and cheese, | | | | | | | | |
| 5.1 oz.......... | 130 | 3.25 | 16 | 152 | 290 | 1.38 | .18 | .14 |
| ham, egg, and cheese, 5 oz...... | 212 | 3.11 | 26 | 346 | 209 | 1.99 | .12 | .24 |
| hot dog: | | | | | | | | |
| plain, 3.5 oz...... | 24 | 2.31 | 13 | 97 | 143 | 1.98 | .08 | .09 |
| w/chili, 4 oz...... | 19 | 3.29 | 10 | 192 | 166 | .78 | .10 | .11 |
| coated (corn dog), 6.2 oz......... | 101 | 6.18 | 17 | 166 | 262 | 1.31 | .25 | .19 |
| roast beef, plain, 4.9 oz.......... | 54 | 4.23 | 31 | 239 | 316 | 3.39 | .10 | .13 |
| roast beef, w/cheese, 6.2 oz............. | 183 | 5.05 | 40 | 401 | 345 | 5.37 | .20 | .31 |

[1] *Condiments include catsup, mustard, pickles, and onions.*

[2] *Condiments and vegetables include catsup, mustard, mayonnaise-style dressing, pickles, onions, lettuce, and tomatoes.*

| | Calcium | Iron | Magnesium | Phosphorus | Potassium | Zinc | Copper | Manganese |
|---|---|---|---|---|---|---|---|---|
| | (Mg) | (Mg) | (Mg) | (Mg) | (Mg) | (Mg) | (Mg) | (Mg) |
| steak, chopped, w/ lettuce, tomato, and mayonnaise, 7.2 oz.......... | 91 | 5.17 | 49 | 297 | 525 | 4.54 | .22 | .37 |
| submarine: w/cold cuts[1], 8 oz........... | 189 | 2.51 | 68 | 287 | 394 | 2.58 | .30 | .53 |
| w/roast beef[2], 7.6 oz.......... | 41 | 2.81 | 67 | 193 | 330 | 4.39 | .36 | .43 |
| w/tuna salad[3], 9 oz........... | 74 | 2.65 | 79 | 219 | 335 | 1.88 | .43 | .51 |
| salad, w/out dressing, 1½ cups: plain[4]............ | 26 | 1.30 | 22 | 80 | 356 | .43 | .10 | .31 |
| w/added cheese and eggs[5]........... | 100 | .68 | 24 | 132 | 371 | .99 | .09 | .27 |
| w/added chicken[6].... | 37 | 1.09 | 33 | 169 | 447 | .90 | .09 | .25 |
| w/added pasta and seafood[7] ........ | 73 | 3.16 | 50 | 204 | 600 | 1.68 | .36 | .67 |
| w/added shrimp[8] .... | 60 | .91 | 38 | 159 | 404 | 1.27 | .16 | .14 |
| chef, w/added turkey, ham and cheese[9]...... | 235 | 1.96 | 48 | 401 | 402 | 3.15 | .17 | .36 |
| side dishes: coleslaw, ¾ cup .... | 34 | .73 | 9 | 36 | 177 | .19 | .04 | .12 |

[1] Recipe: bread, lettuce, cheese, salami, ham, tomato, onion, and oil.

[2] Recipe: bread, beef, tomato, lettuce, and mayonnaise.

[3] Recipe: tuna salad, bread, lettuce, oil.

[4] Recipe: lettuce, cabbage, cucumber, green pepper, tomato, radish, and carrot.

[5] Recipe: lettuce, tomato, egg, cheese, celery, cucumber, and radish.

[6] Recipe: lettuce, chicken, celery, tomato, green pepper, and carrot.

[7] Recipe: lettuce, macaroni, salad dressing, pollock, sweet pepper, carrot, celery, crab, turbot, olives, and onion.

[8] Recipe: lettuce, shrimp, celery, tomato, green pepper, and carrot.

[9] Recipe: lettuce, tomato, turkey, ham, cheese, egg, celery, cucumber, radish, and carrot.

| | Calcium | Iron | Magnesium | Phosphorus | Potassium | Zinc | Copper | Manganese |
|---|---|---|---|---|---|---|---|---|
| | (Mg) | (Mg) | (Mg) | (Mg) | (Mg) | (Mg) | (Mg) | (Mg) |

Fast foods, side dishes, *continued*

corn on the cob,

| | | | | | | | | |
|---|---|---|---|---|---|---|---|---|
| w/butter, 1 ear.... | 5 | .88 | 42 | 108 | 360 | .90 | .07 | .20 |
| hush puppies, | | | | | | | | |
| 5 pieces, 2.8 oz. .. | 69 | 1.43 | 16 | 190 | 188 | .43 | .21 | .27 |
| onion rings, | | | | | | | | |
| 8–9 rings, 2.9 oz. | 73 | .85 | 15 | 86 | 129 | .35 | .07 | .30 |
| potato, baked, w/cheese sauce: | | | | | | | | |
| 10.4 oz.......... | 310 | 3.02 | 66 | 320 | 1167 | 1.88 | .63 | .52 |
| and bacon, | | | | | | | | |
| 10.5 oz......... | 309 | 3.15 | 68 | 347 | 1179 | 2.16 | .65 | .51 |
| and broccoli, | | | | | | | | |
| 12 oz.......... | 334 | 3.33 | 77 | 347 | 1440 | 2.03 | .65 | .51 |
| and chili, 13.9 oz. .. | 409 | 6.13 | 111 | 498 | 1570 | 3.78 | .83 | .68 |
| potato, baked, w/sour cream and | | | | | | | | |
| chives, 10.1 oz. ... | 105 | 3.13 | 70 | 185 | 1383 | .90 | .69 | .58 |
| potato, french fried: | | | | | | | | |
| regular, 2.7 oz. .... | 12 | 1.02 | 25 | 101 | 541 | .39 | .10 | .19 |
| large, 4.1 oz....... | 18 | 1.55 | 38 | 153 | 819 | .60 | .16 | .29 |
| potato, mashed, w/milk and mar- | | | | | | | | |
| garine, ⅓ cup .... | 17 | .37 | 15 | 44 | 236 | .25 | .08 | .09 |
| potato chips, 1 oz.... | 7 | .46 | 19 | 47 | 361 | .31 | .09 | .13 |
| potato salad, ⅓ cup | 13 | .69 | 7 | 53 | 256 | .19 | .08 | .07 |

desserts:

| | | | | | | | | |
|---|---|---|---|---|---|---|---|---|
| animal crackers, | | | | | | | | |
| 2.4-oz. box ...... | 11 | 1.47 | 11 | 64 | 57 | .30 | .05 | .33 |
| brownie, 2-oz. piece | 16 | 1.26 | 17 | 57 | 84 | .40 | .13 | n.a. |
| chocolate chip cookies, 1.9-oz. box | 20 | 1.47 | 17 | 52 | 82 | .33 | .18 | .24 |
| fruit pie[1], fried, 3-oz. pie............ | 12 | .89 | 8 | 38 | 51 | .17 | .04 | .17 |

[1] *Apple, cherry, or lemon.*

| | Calcium | Iron | Magnesium | Phosphorus | Potassium | Zinc | Copper | Manganese |
|---|---|---|---|---|---|---|---|---|
| | (Mg) | (Mg) | (Mg) | (Mg) | (Mg) | (Mg) | (Mg) | (Mg) |
| ice milk cone, vanilla, soft-serve, 3.6 oz. | 153 | .15 | 16 | 139 | 169 | .57 | .02 | .02 |
| sundae: | | | | | | | | |
|   caramel, 5.5 oz. | 189 | .22 | 28 | 217 | 318 | .82 | .08 | .09 |
|   hot fudge, 5.6 oz. | 207 | .58 | 34 | 228 | 395 | .95 | .13 | .13 |
|   strawberry, 5.4 oz. | 161 | .32 | 25 | 154 | 270 | .66 | .08 | .17 |
| beverages: | | | | | | | | |
| beer, regular, 12 fl. oz. | 1 | .01 | 2 | 4 | 7 | 0 | tr. | tr. |
| beer, light, 12 fl. oz. | 1 | .01 | 1 | 4 | 5 | .01 | .01 | .01 |
| coffee, brewed, 6 fl. oz. | 1 | .01 | 2 | 0 | 16 | 0 | tr. | 0 |
| coffee, instant, decaffeinated, 6 fl. oz. | 6 | .08 | 7 | 5 | 63 | .05 | .01 | .02 |
| hot chocolate, 6 fl. oz. | 96 | .35 | 25 | 89 | 203 | .46 | .09 | .08 |
| juice, 6 fl. oz.: | | | | | | | | |
|   grapefruit | 15 | .25 | 20 | 26 | 252 | .09 | .06 | .04 |
|   orange | 17 | .19 | 19 | 30 | 355 | .09 | .08 | .03 |
|   tomato | 16 | 1.06 | 20 | 34 | 400 | .26 | .18 | .14 |
| lemonade, 8 fl. oz. | 8 | .41 | 5 | 5 | 38 | .09 | .05 | .01 |
| orange drink, 6 fl. oz. | 12 | .53 | 3 | 3 | 33 | .16 | .01 | .03 |
| shake, 10 fl. oz.: | | | | | | | | |
|   chocolate | 319 | .88 | 47 | 288 | 567 | 1.15 | .18 | .11 |
|   strawberry | 320 | .30 | 36 | 283 | 516 | 1.00 | .06 | .04 |
|   vanilla | 344 | .26 | 35 | 289 | 492 | 1.01 | .14 | .04 |
| soda, 12-fl. oz. can: | | | | | | | | |
|   cola | 9 | .13 | 3 | 46 | 4 | .05 | .04 | .13 |
|   ginger ale | 12 | .66 | 3 | 1 | 5 | .18 | .07 | n.a. |
|   lemon-lime | 9 | .25 | 2 | 1 | 4 | .18 | .04 | .05 |
|   orange | 19 | .23 | 4 | 4 | 9 | .38 | .06 | n.a. |
|   pepper type | 12 | .14 | 1 | 41 | 2 | .15 | .02 | n.a. |
|   root beer | 19 | .18 | 4 | 2 | 3 | .26 | .03 | n.a. |

| | Calcium | Iron | Magnesium | Phosphorus | Potassium | Zinc | Copper | Manganese |
|---|---|---|---|---|---|---|---|---|
| | (Mg) | (Mg) | (Mg) | (Mg) | (Mg) | (Mg) | (Mg) | (Mg) |
| **Fast foods, beverages,** *continued* | | | | | | | | |
| tea, brewed, 6 fl. oz. | 0 | .04 | 5 | 1 | 66 | .04 | .02 | n.a. |
| tea, iced, instant, sugar-sweetened, lemon flavor, 12 fl. oz ....... | 8 | .08 | 8 | 4 | 74 | .12 | .03 | 1.01 |
| **Fat,** see specific listings | | | | | | | | |
| **Fava beans,** see "Broad beans" | | | | | | | | |
| **Feijoa:** | | | | | | | | |
| untrimmed, 1 lb. ....... | 57 | .27 | 32 | 67 | 529 | .15 | .19 | .29 |
| 1 fruit, approx. 1.8 oz.... | 8 | .04 | 5 | 10 | 78 | .02 | .03 | .04 |
| pureed, ½ cup......... | 20 | .10 | 12 | 24 | 189 | .06 | .07 | .10 |
| **Fennel,** fresh, raw: | | | | | | | | |
| untrimmed, 1 lb........ | 162 | n.a. | 57 | 162 | 1352 | .66 | .22 | .63 |
| trimmed, 1 medium, 2¼" x 2½", 8.3 oz..... | 116 | n.a. | 40 | 116 | 969 | .47 | .16 | .45 |
| trimmed, sliced, 1 cup... | 43 | n.a. | 15 | 43 | 360 | .18 | .06 | .17 |
| **Fennel seeds,** 1 tsp..... | 24 | .37 | 8 | 10 | 34 | .07 | .02 | .13 |
| **Fenugreek seeds,** 1 tsp. | 6 | 1.24 | 7 | 11 | 28 | .09 | .04 | .05 |
| **Fig:** | | | | | | | | |
| fresh: | | | | | | | | |
| untrimmed, 1 lb. ..... | 157 | 1.64 | 75 | 62 | 1042 | .66 | .31 | .58 |
| 1 medium, 1.8 oz.... | 18 | .18 | 8 | 7 | 116 | .07 | .04 | .06 |
| 1 large, 2.3 oz. ...... | 22 | .23 | 11 | 9 | 148 | .09 | .05 | .08 |
| canned: | | | | | | | | |
| in water or heavy syrup, ½ cup..... | 35 | .37 | 13 | 13 | 128 | .15 | .14 | .11 |
| in light or extra heavy syrup, ½ cup..... | 35 | .37 | 13 | 13 | 128 | .14 | .14 | .11 |
| dried: | | | | | | | | |
| uncooked, 1 lb...... | 646 | 10.03 | 266 | 307 | 3199 | 2.27 | 1.41 | 1.74 |
| uncooked, 10 figs, approx. 6.6 oz. ... | 269 | 4.18 | 111 | 128 | 1332 | .94 | .59 | .73 |
| uncooked, ½ cup.... | 143 | 2.23 | 59 | 68 | 709 | .50 | .31 | .39 |

| | Calcium (Mg) | Iron (Mg) | Magnesium (Mg) | Phosphorus (Mg) | Potassium (Mg) | Zinc (Mg) | Copper (Mg) | Manganese (Mg) |
|---|---|---|---|---|---|---|---|---|
| cooked, ½ cup . . . . . | 79 | 1.23 | 33 | 38 | 391 | .28 | .17 | .21 |
| **Filbert,** dried, shelled, except as noted: | | | | | | | | |
| unblanched: | | | | | | | | |
| in shell, 1 lb. . . . . . . . | 391 | 6.82 | 595 | 650 | 929 | 5.01 | 3.15 | 4.21 |
| 1 oz. . . . . . . . . . . . . | 53 | .93 | 81 | 89 | 126 | .68 | .43 | .57 |
| chopped, 1 cup . . . . . | 216 | 3.76 | 328 | 359 | 512 | 2.76 | 1.74 | 2.32 |
| blanched, 1 oz. . . . . . . . | 55 | .96 | 84 | 92 | 131 | .71 | .44 | .59 |
| dry-roasted, 1 oz. . . . . . | 55 | .96 | 84 | 92 | 131 | .71 | .44 | .59 |
| oil-roasted, 1 oz. . . . . . . | 56 | .97 | 85 | 92 | 132 | .71 | .45 | .60 |
| **Fish,** see specific listings | | | | | | | | |
| **"Fish,"** vegetarian: | | | | | | | | |
| frozen (*Worthington* Fillets), 2 pieces, 3 oz. | 15 | 2.11 | n.a. | n.a. | 133 | .92 | n.a. | n.a. |
| mix (*Loma Linda* Ocean Platter), ⅓ cup, .9 oz. . . | 4 | 1.33 | n.a. | n.a. | 448 | .47 | n.a. | n.a. |
| **Fish fillet or portion,** breaded, fried, frozen, 2-oz. piece, 4" x 2" x ½" . . . . . . . . | 11 | .42 | 14 | 103 | 149 | .38 | .06 | .14 |
| **Fish stick,** breaded, fried, frozen, 1-oz. stick, 4" x 1" x ½" . . . . . . . . | 6 | .21 | 7 | 51 | 73 | .19 | .03 | .07 |
| **Flatfish,** meat only: | | | | | | | | |
| raw, 1 lb. . . . . . . . . . . . . | 80 | 1.62 | 142 | 834 | 1637 | 2.05 | .15 | .08 |
| baked, broiled, or microwaved[1], 4 oz. . . . | 20 | .39 | 66 | 328 | 390 | .71 | .03 | (0) |
| **Flounder,** see "Flatfish" | | | | | | | | |
| **Flour,** see "Wheat flour" and specific listings | | | | | | | | |
| **Frankfurter:** | | | | | | | | |
| beef, 1 link, 5" long x ⅞", approx. 2 oz. . . . . . . . . | 11 | .81 | 2 | 50 | 95 | 1.24 | .03 | .02 |

---

[1] *Prepared without added ingredients.*

|  | Calcium | Iron | Magnesium | Phosphorus | Potassium | Zinc | Copper | Manganese |
|---|---|---|---|---|---|---|---|---|
|  | (Mg) | (Mg) | (Mg) | (Mg) | (Mg) | (Mg) | (Mg) | (Mg) |
| Frankfurter, *continued* |  |  |  |  |  |  |  |  |
| beef and pork, 1 link, |  |  |  |  |  |  |  |  |
| 5" long x ⅞", approx. |  |  |  |  |  |  |  |  |
| 2 oz. . . . . . . . . . . . . | 6 | .66 | 6 | 49 | 95 | 1.05 | .05 | .02 |
| cheese (cheesefurter or |  |  |  |  |  |  |  |  |
| cheese smokie), 1 oz. | 16 | .30 | 4 | 50 | 58 | .64 | .02 | .01 |
| **"Frankfurter," vegetarian:** |  |  |  |  |  |  |  |  |
| canned: |  |  |  |  |  |  |  |  |
| (*Loma Linda* Big Franks), |  |  |  |  |  |  |  |  |
| 1.8-oz. link . . . . . . | 8 | .77 | n.a. | n.a. | 51 | .89 | n.a. | n.a. |
| (*Loma Linda* |  |  |  |  |  |  |  |  |
| *Linketts*), |  |  |  |  |  |  |  |  |
| 1.2-oz. link . . . . . . | 4 | .39 | n.a. | 41 | 29 | .46 | n.a. | n.a. |
| (*Worthington Super* |  |  |  |  |  |  |  |  |
| *Links*), 1.7-oz. link | 9 | .14 | n.a. | n.a. | 29 | .20 | n.a. | n.a. |
| (*Worthington Veja-* |  |  |  |  |  |  |  |  |
| *Links*), 1.1-oz. link | 4 | .73 | n.a. | n.a. | 18 | .10 | n.a. | n.a. |
| frozen: |  |  |  |  |  |  |  |  |
| (*Morningstar Farms* |  |  |  |  |  |  |  |  |
| Deli Franks), |  |  |  |  |  |  |  |  |
| 1.6-oz. link . . . . . . | 16 | .26 | n.a. | 36 | 50 | .38 | n.a. | n.a. |
| (*Worthington* |  |  |  |  |  |  |  |  |
| *Leanies*), |  |  |  |  |  |  |  |  |
| 1.4-oz. link . . . . . . | 25 | .90 | n.a. | n.a. | 43 | .23 | n.a. | n.a. |
| corn battered (*Loma* |  |  |  |  |  |  |  |  |
| *Linda* Corn Dogs), |  |  |  |  |  |  |  |  |
| 2.5-oz. piece . . . . . | 13 | .85 | n.a. | n.a. | 39 | .43 | n.a. | n.a. |
| **French beans,** dried: |  |  |  |  |  |  |  |  |
| uncooked, 1 lb. . . . . . . . . | 844 | 1542 | 851 | 1377 | 5969 | 8.62 | 2.00 | 5.44 |
| uncooked, ½ cup. . . . . . . | 171 | 3.13 | 173 | 279 | 1211 | 1.75 | .41 | 1.10 |
| boiled, drained, ½ cup | 54 | .93 | 48 | 88 | 318 | .55 | .10 | .33 |
| **French-cut beans,** see "Green beans" |  |  |  |  |  |  |  |  |
| **French toast, frozen,** |  |  |  |  |  |  |  |  |
| 2.1-oz. piece . . . . . . . . | 63 | 1.31 | 10 | 82 | 79 | .46 | .05 | .15 |
| **Frosting mix,** dry, ¹⁄₁₂ package: |  |  |  |  |  |  |  |  |
| chocolate, creamy . . . . . . | n.a. | .38 | n.a. | n.a. | 58 | n.a. | n.a. | n.a. |

| | Calcium | Iron | Magnesium | Phosphorus | Potassium | Zinc | Copper | Manganese |
|---|---|---|---|---|---|---|---|---|
| | (Mg) | (Mg) | (Mg) | (Mg) | (Mg) | (Mg) | (Mg) | (Mg) |
| vanilla, creamy......... | 1 | 0 | 1 | 1 | 2 | n.a. | n.a. | n.a. |
| white, fluffy .......... | 1 | n.a. | 0 | 1 | 20 | n.a. | n.a. | n.a. |
| **Frosting mix, prepared:** | | | | | | | | |
| chocolate: | | | | | | | | |
| 1 cup ............ | 50 | 3.10 | n.a. | 205 | 195 | n.a. | n.a. | n.a. |
| creamy, 1/12 pkg. .... | 3 | .54 | 8 | 30 | 74 | .11 | .08 | .09 |
| creamy[1], 1 cup ..... | 96 | 2.70 | n.a. | 218 | 238 | n.a. | n.a. | n.a. |
| creamy[2], 1 cup ..... | 91 | 2.50 | n.a. | 198 | 218 | n.a. | n.a. | n.a. |
| cream cheese, 1/12 pkg. .. | 1 | .06 | 1 | 1 | 13 | 0 | .01 | n.a. |
| sour cream, 1/12 pkg. .... | 1 | .03 | 1 | 1 | 74 | 0 | tr. | n.a. |
| vanilla, creamy, | | | | | | | | |
| 1/12 pkg............. | 1 | .04 | 0 | .15 | 14 | 0 | tr. | n.a. |
| **Fruit,** see specific listings | | | | | | | | |
| **Fruit, mixed** (see also "Fruit cocktail" and "Fruit salad"): | | | | | | | | |
| canned, in heavy syrup, | | | | | | | | |
| 1/2 cup............. | 1 | .46 | 6 | 13 | 100 | .09 | .07 | n.a. |
| dried, pitted, 1 oz....... | 11 | .77 | 11 | 22 | 226 | .14 | .11 | .06 |
| frozen, sweetened, | | | | | | | | |
| 1/2 cup............. | 9 | .35 | 7 | 15 | 164 | .06 | .04 | .08 |
| **Fruit cocktail,** canned: | | | | | | | | |
| in water, 1/2 cup........ | 6 | .31 | 8 | 14 | 115 | .11 | .09 | n.a. |
| in juice, 1/2 cup ........ | 10 | .26 | 9 | 17 | 118 | .11 | .08 | n.a. |
| in light or heavy syrup, | | | | | | | | |
| 1/2 cup............. | 8 | .37 | 7 | 14 | 112 | .11 | .09 | n.a. |
| **Fruit and juice bar,** | | | | | | | | |
| 2.5-fl.-oz. bar........ | 4 | .15 | 3 | 4 | 40 | .04 | 0 | n.a. |
| **Fruit leather:** | | | | | | | | |
| plain, .8-oz. bar........ | 7 | .18 | 5 | 13 | 32 | .04 | .04 | .04 |
| w/cream, .8-oz. bar ..... | 5 | .20 | 3 | 7 | 51 | n.a. | n.a. | n.a. |
| roll, .5-oz. roll ......... | 4 | .14 | 3 | 4 | 41 | .03 | .02 | .03 |
| **Fruit punch drink:** | | | | | | | | |
| canned, 8 fl. oz......... | 20 | .15 | 5 | 2 | 62 | .30 | .13 | .50 |

---

[1] *Prepared with water.*

[2] *Prepared with water and vegetable table fat.*

| | Calcium | Iron | Magnesium | Phosphorus | Potassium | Zinc | Copper | Manganese |
|---|---|---|---|---|---|---|---|---|
| | (Mg) | (Mg) | (Mg) | (Mg) | (Mg) | (Mg) | (Mg) | (Mg) |
| Fruit punch drink, *continued* | | | | | | | | |
| frozen, diluted, 8 fl. oz. | 9 | .22 | 6 | 2 | 31 | .09 | .07 | .25 |
| **Fruit punch flavor drink** | | | | | | | | |
| **mix,** 2 rounded tsp.... | 36 | .13 | 0 | 52 | 1 | .03 | .03 | .01 |
| **Fruit punch juice drink,** | | | | | | | | |
| frozen, diluted, 1 cup | 18 | .57 | 9 | n.a. | 191 | .54 | .06 | .15 |
| **Fruit salad,** canned: | | | | | | | | |
| in water, ½ cup........ | 8 | .36 | 7 | 11 | 95 | .09 | .08 | n.a. |
| in juice, ½ cup ........ | 14 | .31 | 10 | 18 | 144 | .18 | .06 | n.a. |
| in light syrup, ½ cup.... | 8 | .36 | 7 | 11 | 104 | .09 | .08 | n.a. |
| in heavy syrup, ½ cup... | 8 | .36 | 7 | 12 | 103 | .09 | .08 | n.a. |
| tropical, in heavy syrup[1], | | | | | | | | |
| ½ cup............. | 17 | .66 | 17 | 10 | 168 | .14 | .10 | n.a. |
| **Fuki,** see "Butterbur" | | | | | | | | |

---

[1] *With added calcium chloride.*

# G

| | Calcium | Iron | Magnesium | Phosphorus | Potassium | Zinc | Copper | Manganese |
|---|---|---|---|---|---|---|---|---|
| | (Mg) | (Mg) | (Mg) | (Mg) | (Mg) | (Mg) | (Mg) | (Mg) |
| **Garbanzo beans,** see "Chickpeas" | | | | | | | | |
| **Garlic,** raw: | | | | | | | | |
| 1 oz.............. | 64 | .48 | 7 | 43 | 114 | n.a. | n.a. | n.a. |
| 3 cloves, .3 oz........ | 16 | .15 | 2 | 14 | 36 | n.a. | n.a. | n.a. |
| **Garlic herb seasoning** | | | | | | | | |
| (*Tone's Perc*), ¼ tsp. | 2 | .05 | 1 | 3 | 9 | .02 | tr. | .01 |
| **Garlic powder,** 1 tsp. ... | 2 | .08 | 2 | 12 | 31 | .07 | tr. | .02 |
| **Gefilte fish,** in jars, sweet, w/broth, 1.5-oz. piece............. | 10 | 1.04 | 4 | 31 | 38 | .35 | .08 | .03 |
| **Gelatin,** unflavored, dry, 3-oz. pkg.......... | 2 | n.a. | n.a. | n.a. | 6 | .01 | .10 | n.a. |
| **Gelatin bar,** 1 piece .... | n.a. | n.a. | n.a. | 0 | 1 | n.a. | n.a. | n.a. |
| **Ginger,** ground, 1 tsp.... | 2 | .21 | 3 | 3 | 24 | .08 | .01 | .48 |
| **Ginger root,** raw: | | | | | | | | |
| untrimmed, 4 oz........ | 20 | .52 | 45 | 29 | 438 | n.a. | n.a. | n.a. |
| trimmed, sliced, ¼ cup | 4 | .12 | 10 | 7 | 100 | n.a. | n.a. | n.a. |
| **Ginkgo nut:** | | | | | | | | |
| raw, in shell, 1 lb....... | 7 | 3.45 | 93 | 427 | 1760 | 1.18 | .94 | .39 |
| raw, shelled, 1 oz....... | 1 | .28 | 8 | 35 | 145 | .10 | .08 | .03 |
| dried, in shell, 1 lb...... | 69 | 5.52 | 182 | 927 | 3441 | 2.31 | 1.85 | .76 |
| dried, shelled, 1 oz...... | 6 | .45 | 15 | 76 | 283 | .19 | .15 | .06 |
| **Goose,** domesticated: | | | | | | | | |
| roasted[1], meat w/skin, 4 oz.............. | 15 | 3.21 | 25 | 306 | 373 | | .30 | n.a. |
| roasted[1], meat only, 4 oz.............. | 16 | 3.25 | 28 | 350 | 440 | n.a. | .31 | n.a. |
| **Gooseberry:** | | | | | | | | |
| fresh, 1 lb........... | 114 | 1.41 | 45 | 120 | 899 | .56 | .32 | .65 |
| fresh, ½ cup.......... | 19 | .24 | 8 | 20 | 149 | .09 | .05 | .11 |

[1] *Prepared without added ingredients.*

| | Calcium | Iron | Magnesium | Phosphorus | Potassium | Zinc | Copper | Manganese |
|---|---|---|---|---|---|---|---|---|
| | (Mg) | (Mg) | (Mg) | (Mg) | (Mg) | (Mg) | (Mg) | (Mg) |
| **Gooseberry,** *continued* | | | | | | | | |
| canned, in light syrup, | | | | | | | | |
| ½ cup............. | 20 | .42 | 8 | 9 | 97 | .14 | .27 | .22 |
| **Gourd** (see also "Waxgourd"): | | | | | | | | |
| dishcloth: | | | | | | | | |
| raw, untrimmed, | | | | | | | | |
| 1 lb. .......... | 66 | 1.19 | 47 | 106 | 460 | n.a. | n.a. | n.a. |
| raw, trimmed, | | | | | | | | |
| 1" slices, ½ cup... | 10 | .02 | 7 | 15 | 66 | n.a. | n.a. | n.a. |
| boiled, drained, | | | | | | | | |
| 1" slices, ½ cup... | 8 | .32 | 18 | 28 | 403 | n.a. | n.a. | n.a. |
| white-flowered: | | | | | | | | |
| raw, untrimmed, | | | | | | | | |
| 1 lb. .......... | 83 | .64 | 35 | 41 | 475 | 2.22 | n.a. | n.a. |
| raw, 1" cubes, ½ cup | 15 | .12 | 6 | 7 | 87 | .41 | n.a. | n.a. |
| boiled, drained, | | | | | | | | |
| 1" cubes, ½ cup .. | 18 | .18 | 8 | 9 | 124 | n.a. | n.a. | n.a. |
| **Gourd, dried,** strips, see "Kanpyo" | | | | | | | | |
| **Grain,** see specific listings | | | | | | | | |
| **Granola and cereal bars:** | | | | | | | | |
| plain, hard, 1-oz. bar .... | 17 | .84 | 28 | 79 | 95 | .58 | .11 | .50 |
| plain, soft, uncoated, | | | | | | | | |
| 1-oz. bar ........... | 30 | .73 | 21 | 65 | 92 | .43 | .08 | .43 |
| almond, hard, 1-oz. bar | 9 | .71 | 23 | 65 | 77 | n.a. | n.a. | n.a. |
| all varieties (*Kellogg's Nutri-Grain*), 1 bar .... | 16 | 1.80 | 10 | 37 | 75 | 1.50 | .02 | n.a. |
| chocolate chip, hard, | | | | | | | | |
| 1-oz. bar ........... | 22 | .86 | n.a. | n.a. | 71 | n.a. | n.a. | n.a. |
| chocolate chip, soft, | | | | | | | | |
| uncoated, 1-oz. bar ... | 26 | .72 | 22 | 65 | 96 | .43 | .11 | .37 |
| milk chocolate coated, | | | | | | | | |
| soft, 1-oz. bar ....... | 29 | .66 | 19 | 56 | 89 | .37 | .10 | .26 |
| milk chocolate coated, | | | | | | | | |
| soft, w/peanut butter, | | | | | | | | |
| 1-oz. bar ........... | 31 | .41 | n.a. | n.a. | 96 | n.a. | n.a. | n.a. |

| | Calcium | Iron | Magnesium | Phosphorus | Potassium | Zinc | Copper | Manganese |
|---|---|---|---|---|---|---|---|---|
| | (Mg) | (Mg) | (Mg) | (Mg) | (Mg) | (Mg) | (Mg) | (Mg) |
| nut and raisin, soft, | | | | | | | | |
| uncoated, 1-oz. bar . . . | 24 | .62 | 26 | 68 | 111 | .45 | .11 | .34 |
| peanut, hard, 1-oz. bar. . . | 11 | .71 | 31 | 85 | 86 | n.a. | n.a. | n.a. |
| peanut butter, hard, 1-oz. | | | | | | | | |
| bar . . . . . . . . . . . . . . | 12 | .68 | n.a. | n.a. | 82 | n.a. | n.a. | n.a. |
| peanut butter, soft, | | | | | | | | |
| uncoated, 1-oz. bar . . . | 26 | .60 | 24 | 71 | 83 | .53 | .19 | .40 |
| raisin, soft, uncoated, | | | | | | | | |
| 1-oz. bar . . . . . . . . . . | 29 | .69 | 20 | 62 | 103 | .37 | .08 | .36 |
| **Grape:** | | | | | | | | |
| fresh, American type (slip skin): | | | | | | | | |
| untrimmed, 1 lb. . . . . | 36 | .76 | 14 | 25 | 502 | .11 | .11 | 1.89 |
| 10 medium, approx. | | | | | | | | |
| 1.5 oz. . . . . . . . . . . | 3 | .07 | 1 | 2 | 46 | .01 | .01 | .17 |
| peeled and seeded, | | | | | | | | |
| ½ cup . . . . . . . . . . | 7 | .14 | 3 | 5 | 88 | .02 | .02 | .33 |
| fresh, European type (adherent skin), seeded or seedless: | | | | | | | | |
| untrimmed, 1 lb. . . . . | 46 | 1.12 | 28 | 56 | 807 | .24 | .39 | .25 |
| 10 medium, 1.75 oz. | 5 | .13 | 3 | 6 | 93 | .03 | .05 | .03 |
| trimmed, ½ cup. . . . . | 9 | .21 | 5 | 11 | 148 | .05 | .07 | .05 |
| canned, Thompson | | | | | | | | |
| seedless, in water or | | | | | | | | |
| heavy syrup, ½ cup . . . | 13 | 1.20 | 8 | 22 | 132 | .06 | .07 | .05 |
| **Grape juice**, 6 fl. oz.: | | | | | | | | |
| canned or bottled. . . . . . . | 18 | .48 | 18 | 18 | 252 | .12 | .05 | .68 |
| frozen, diluted . . . . . . . . | 6 | .18 | 6 | 6 | 42 | .06 | .02 | .33 |
| **Grapefruit:** | | | | | | | | |
| fresh, pink and red, all areas: | | | | | | | | |
| untrimmed, 1 lb. . . . . | 25 | .28 | 18 | 20 | 297 | .16 | .10 | .02 |
| ½ of 3¾"-diam. fruit, | | | | | | | | |
| 8.5 oz. . . . . . . . . . . | 13 | .15 | 10 | 11 | 158 | .09 | .05 | .01 |
| sections, w/juice, | | | | | | | | |
| ½ cup . . . . . . . . . . | 13 | .14 | 9 | 10 | 148 | .08 | .05 | .01 |
| fresh, white, all areas: | | | | | | | | |
| untrimmed, 1 lb. . . . . | 27 | .13 | 20 | 18 | 329 | .10 | .11 | .03 |

| | Calcium | Iron | Magnesium | Phosphorus | Potassium | Zinc | Copper | Manganese |
|---|---|---|---|---|---|---|---|---|
| | (Mg) | (Mg) | (Mg) | (Mg) | (Mg) | (Mg) | (Mg) | (Mg) |
| **Grapefruit, fresh, white,** *continued* | | | | | | | | |
| ½ of 3¾"-diam. fruit, | | | | | | | | |
| 8.5 oz. . . . . . . . . | 14 | .07 | 11 | 9 | 175 | .08 | .06 | .02 |
| sections, w/juice, | | | | | | | | |
| ½ cup . . . . . . . . . | 14 | .07 | 11 | 9 | 170 | .08 | .06 | .02 |
| canned or in jars: | | | | | | | | |
| in water, ½ cup . . . . . | 18 | .50 | 12 | 12 | 161 | .11 | .08 | .01 |
| in juice, ½ cup . . . . . | 19 | .26 | 13 | .15 | 209 | .09 | .05 | .01 |
| in light syrup, ½ cup | 18 | .51 | 13 | 13 | 164 | .11 | .08 | .01 |
| **Grapefruit juice:** | | | | | | | | |
| fresh, juice from | | | | | | | | |
| 1 average fruit . . . . . . . | 18 | .39 | 24 | 29 | 318 | .10 | .07 | .04 |
| fresh, 6 fl. oz. | 17 | .37 | 23 | 28 | 300 | .10 | .06 | .04 |
| canned, unsweetened, | | | | | | | | |
| 6 fl. oz. . . . . . . . . . . . | 12 | .36 | 18 | 18 | 282 | .18 | .07 | .04 |
| canned, sweetened, | | | | | | | | |
| 6 fl. oz. . . . . . . . . . . . | 12 | .66 | 18 | 18 | 306 | .12 | .09 | .04 |
| frozen, diluted, 6 fl. oz. . . | 12 | .24 | 18 | 24 | 252 | .12 | .06 | .04 |
| **Great northern beans:** | | | | | | | | |
| uncooked, 1 lb. . . . . . . . | 793 | 24.81 | 859 | 2028 | 6291 | 10.46 | 3.80 | 6.46 |
| uncooked, ½ cup. . . . . . . | 159 | 4.98 | 172 | 407 | 1262 | 2.10 | .76 | 1.30 |
| boiled, ½ cup . . . . . . . . | 60 | 1.87 | 44 | 145 | 344 | .77 | .22 | .46 |
| canned, w/liquid, 8 oz. . . . | 121 | 3.56 | 116 | 308 | 796 | 1.48 | .73 | .93 |
| canned, w/liquid, | | | | | | | | |
| ½ cup . . . . . . . . . . . . . | 69 | 2.05 | 67 | 178 | 459 | .85 | .21 | .53 |
| **Green beans:** | | | | | | | | |
| fresh: | | | | | | | | |
| raw, untrimmed, | | | | | | | | |
| 1 lb. . . . . . . . . . . | 149 | 4.14 | 98 | 153 | 833 | .95 | .28 | .85 |
| trimmed, raw, ½ cup | 21 | .57 | 14 | 21 | 115 | .13 | .04 | .12 |
| boiled, drained, | | | | | | | | |
| ½ cup . . . . . . . . . | 29 | .79 | 16 | 24 | 185 | .23 | .06 | .18 |
| canned: | | | | | | | | |
| w/liquid, ½ cup . . . . . | 29 | 1.05 | 15 | 23 | 117 | .24 | .08 | .40 |
| drained, ½ cup . . . . . | 18 | .61 | 9 | 13 | 74 | .20 | .03 | .14 |

| | Calcium | Iron | Magnesium | Phosphorus | Potassium | Zinc | Copper | Manganese |
|---|---|---|---|---|---|---|---|---|
| | (Mg) | (Mg) | (Mg) | (Mg) | (Mg) | (Mg) | (Mg) | (Mg) |
| w/onion and peppers, seasoned, w/liquid, ½ cup . . . . . . . . . | 25 | .54 | 15 | 18 | 106 | .16 | .07 | n.a. |
| frozen, 10-oz. pkg. . . . . . . | 118 | 2.45 | 61 | 91 | 529 | .75 | .14 | 1.09 |
| frozen, boiled, drained, ½ cup . . . . . . . . . . . . | 33 | .60 | 16 | 21 | 86 | .33 | .04 | .22 |
| **Grouper,** mixed species, meat only: | | | | | | | | |
| raw, 1 lb. . . . . . . . . . . . | 123 | 4.01 | 139 | 737 | 2189 | 2.20 | .09 | .06 |
| baked, broiled, or microwaved[1], 4 oz. . . . | 24 | 1.29 | 42 | 162 | 539 | .58 | .05 | .01 |
| **Guava:** | | | | | | | | |
| common: | | | | | | | | |
| untrimmed, 1 lb. . . . . | 72 | 1.12 | 37 | 91 | 1032 | .83 | .37 | .52 |
| 1 fruit, approx. 4 oz. | 18 | .28 | 9 | 23 | 256 | .21 | .09 | .13 |
| trimmed, ½ cup. . . . . | 17 | .09 | 9 | 21 | 235 | .19 | .09 | .12 |
| strawberry, untrimmed, 1 lb. . . . . . . . . . . . . | 82 | .84 | 64 | 105 | 1127 | n.a. | n.a. | n.a. |
| strawberry, trimmed, ½ cup . . . . . . . . . . . | 26 | .27 | 21 | 34 | 357 | n.a. | n.a. | n.a. |
| **Guava sauce,** cooked, ½ cup . . . . . . . . . . . . | 8 | .21 | 8 | 13 | 268 | .20 | .09 | .13 |

---

[1] *Prepared without added ingredients.*

# H

| | Calcium | Iron | Magnesium | Phosphorus | Potassium | Zinc | Copper | Manganese |
|---|---|---|---|---|---|---|---|---|
| | (Mg) | (Mg) | (Mg) | (Mg) | (Mg) | (Mg) | (Mg) | (Mg) |
| **Haddock,** meat only: | | | | | | | | |
| raw, 1 lb.............. | 150 | 4.76 | 177 | 851 | 1411 | 1.69 | .12 | .11 |
| baked, broiled, or | | | | | | | | |
| microwaved[1], 4 oz. ... | 48 | 1.53 | 57 | 273 | 452 | .54 | .04 | (0) |
| smoked, 4 oz. ......... | 56 | 1.59 | 61 | 285 | 471 | .57 | .05 | (0) |
| **Hake,** see "Whiting" | | | | | | | | |
| **Halibut,** meat only: | | | | | | | | |
| Atlantic and Pacific: | | | | | | | | |
| raw, 1 lb........... | 212 | 3.81 | 377 | 1009 | 2039 | 1.89 | .12 | .07 |
| baked, broiled, or | | | | | | | | |
| microwaved[1], 4 oz. | 68 | 1.21 | 121 | 323 | 653 | .60 | .04 | n.a. |
| Greenland: | | | | | | | | |
| raw, 1 lb.......... | 14 | 2.99 | n.a. | 744 | 363 | n.a. | n.a. | n.a. |
| baked, broiled, or | | | | | | | | |
| microwaved[1], 4 oz. | 5 | .96 | n.a. | 238 | 390 | n.a. | n.a. | n.a. |
| **Ham, canned**[2], precooked: | | | | | | | | |
| regular (approx. 13% fat): | | | | | | | | |
| unheated, 1 oz. ..... | 2 | .23 | 4 | 49 | 90 | .47 | .02 | .01 |
| roasted, 4 oz. ...... | 9 | 1.55 | 19 | 276 | 405 | 2.84 | .15 | .03 |
| extra lean and regular: | | | | | | | | |
| unheated, 1 oz. ..... | 2 | .26 | 5 | 59 | 95 | .52 | .02 | .01 |
| roasted, 4 oz. ...... | 8 | 1.21 | 23 | 251 | 398 | 2.63 | .09 | .03 |
| extra lean (approx. 4% fat): | | | | | | | | |
| unheated, 1 oz. ..... | 2 | .27 | 5 | 63 | 103 | .55 | .02 | .01 |
| roasted, 4 oz. ...... | 7 | 1.04 | 24 | 237 | 395 | 2.53 | .06 | .03 |
| chopped, 1 oz......... | 2 | .27 | 4 | 39 | 81 | .52 | .01 | .01 |
| **Ham, cured**[2], whole: | | | | | | | | |
| lean and fat, unheated, | | | | | | | | |
| 1 oz............... | 2 | .20 | 4 | 57 | 88 | .50 | .02 | .01 |

[1] Prepared without added ingredients.
[2] Roasted meats are prepared without added ingredients.

| | Calcium | Iron | Magnesium | Phosphorus | Potassium | Zinc | Copper | Manganese |
|---|---|---|---|---|---|---|---|---|
| | (Mg) | (Mg) | (Mg) | (Mg) | (Mg) | (Mg) | (Mg) | (Mg) |
| lean and fat, roasted, 4 oz. | 8 | .99 | 22 | 243 | 324 | 2.63 | .09 | .02 |
| lean only, unheated, 1 oz. | 2 | .23 | 5 | 66 | 105 | .58 | .02 | .01 |
| lean only, roasted, 4 oz. | 8 | 1.07 | 25 | 257 | 358 | 2.91 | .10 | .02 |
| **Ham, cured, boneless[1]:** | | | | | | | | |
| regular (approx. 11% fat): | | | | | | | | |
|   unheated, 1-oz. slice | 2 | .28 | 5 | 70 | 94 | .61 | .03 | .01 |
|   roasted, 4 oz. | 9 | 1.52 | 25 | 319 | 464 | 2.80 | .16 | .05 |
| extra lean and regular: | | | | | | | | |
|   unheated, 1-oz. slice | 2 | .26 | 5 | 67 | 84 | .58 | .03 | .01 |
|   roasted, 4 oz. | 9 | 1.59 | 22 | 281 | 411 | 2.98 | .13 | .05 |
| extra lean (approx. 5% fat): | | | | | | | | |
|   unheated, 1-oz. slice | 2 | .22 | 5 | 62 | 99 | .55 | .02 | .01 |
|   roasted, 4 oz. | 9 | 1.68 | 16 | 222 | 325 | 3.27 | .09 | .06 |
| steak, extra lean, unheated, 1 oz. | 1 | .28 | 5 | 74 | 92 | .57 | .28 | .01 |
| **Ham, fresh, roasted[1]** (see also "Ham, cured"), 4 oz.: | | | | | | | | |
| whole leg, lean and fat | 7 | 1.13 | 25 | 280 | 373 | 3.24 | .11 | .04 |
| whole leg, lean only | 8 | 1.27 | 28 | 319 | 423 | 3.70 | .12 | .04 |
| rump half, lean and fat | 8 | 1.19 | 29 | 295 | 404 | 3.11 | .12 | .03 |
| rump half, lean only | 8 | 1.29 | 33 | 323 | 443 | 3.41 | .12 | .03 |
| shank half, lean and fat | 7 | 1.10 | 24 | 271 | 352 | 3.32 | .11 | .03 |
| shank half, lean only | 8 | 1.26 | 28 | 315 | 408 | 3.91 | .12 | .04 |
| **"Ham," vegetarian,** frozen (*Worthington Wham*), 1.6 oz. | 5 | 1.10 | n.a. | n.a. | 88 | .14 | n.a. | n.a. |
| **Ham luncheon meat:** | | | | | | | | |
| chopped, 1-oz. slice | 2 | .24 | 4 | 44 | 91 | .55 | .02 | .01 |

---

[1] *Roasted meats are prepared without added ingredients.*

| | Calcium | Iron | Magnesium | Phosphorus | Potassium | Zinc | Copper | Manganese |
|---|---|---|---|---|---|---|---|---|
| | (Mg) | (Mg) | (Mg) | (Mg) | (Mg) | (Mg) | (Mg) | (Mg) |
| Ham luncheon meat, *continued* | | | | | | | | |
| cooked, sliced, extra lean | | | | | | | | |
| (5% fat), 1-oz. slice... | 2 | .22 | 5 | 62 | 99 | .55 | .02 | .01 |
| cooked, sliced, regular | | | | | | | | |
| (11% fat), 1-oz. slice | 2 | .28 | 5 | 70 | 94 | .61 | .03 | .01 |
| minced, 1 oz.......... | 3 | .22 | 5 | 44 | 88 | .54 | .02 | .01 |
| **Ham patty**[1], grilled, 4 oz. | 10 | 1.83 | 11 | 115 | 227 | 2.15 | .11 | n.a. |
| **Ham salad spread,** | | | | | | | | |
| 1 tbsp. ............ | 1 | .09 | 1 | 18 | 22 | .17 | .01 | (0) |
| **Ham and cheese loaf or** | | | | | | | | |
| **roll,** 1 oz. .......... | 16 | .26 | 5 | 72 | 83 | .57 | .02 | .01 |
| **Ham and cheese spread,** | | | | | | | | |
| 1 tbsp. ............. | 33 | .11 | 3 | 74 | 24 | .34 | .01 | .01 |
| **"Hamburger," vegetarian:** | | | | | | | | |
| canned: | | | | | | | | |
| (*Loma Linda Redi-Burger*), 2 slices, 3 oz............ | 12 | 1.06 | n.a. | 136 | 121 | 1.11 | n.a. | n.a. |
| (*Loma Linda Vege-Burger*), ¼ cup, 1.9 oz.......... | 8 | .50 | n.a. | 62 | 30 | .58 | n.a. | n.a. |
| (*Worthington Vegetarian Burger*), ¼ cup, 1.9 oz..... | 4 | 1.73 | n.a. | n.a. | 25 | .39 | n.a. | n.a. |
| frozen, patty: | | | | | | | | |
| (*Loma Linda Sizzle Burger*), 2.5 oz. ... | 61 | 1.85 | n.a. | 200 | 211 | .74 | n.a. | n.a. |
| (*Morningstar Farms Grillers*), 2.3 oz.... | 43 | 1.16 | n.a. | 102 | 127 | .49 | n.a. | n.a. |
| (*Morningstar Farms Prime*), 2.3 oz..... | 46 | 2.14 | n.a. | 102 | 151 | .74 | n.a. | n.a. |
| (*Worthington Fri-Pats*), 2.3 oz...... | 63 | .95 | n.a. | n.a. | 126 | .61 | n.a. | n.a. |

[1] *Fully cooked as purchased.*

| | Calcium (Mg) | Iron (Mg) | Magnesium (Mg) | Phosphorus (Mg) | Potassium (Mg) | Zinc (Mg) | Copper (Mg) | Manganese (Mg) |
|---|---|---|---|---|---|---|---|---|
| garden vegetable (*Morningstar Farms*), 2.4 oz. . . . | 34 | .72 | n.a. | 90 | 180 | .59 | n.a. | n.a. |
| **"Hamburger" mix,** vegetarian, dry: | | | | | | | | |
| (*Loma Linda* Patty Mix), ⅓ cup, .9 oz. . . . . . . . | 22 | 1.38 | n.a. | n.a. | 405 | .12 | n.a. | n.a. |
| (*Worthington GranBurger*), 3 tbsp., .6 oz. . . . . . . . . . . . . | 35 | 2.92 | n.a. | 114 | 219 | .46 | n.a. | n.a. |
| chunk or granules (*Loma Linda Vita-Burger*), .7 oz. . . . . . . . . . . . . | 27 | 1.83 | n.a. | n.a. | 499 | 4.79 | n.a. | n.a. |
| **Hazelnut,** see "Filbert" | | | | | | | | |
| **Head cheese,** pork, 1-oz. slice . . . . . . . . . | 5 | .33 | 3 | 17 | 9 | .37 | .04 | .01 |
| **Heart**[1], 4 oz.: | | | | | | | | |
| beef, simmered . . . . . . . . | 7 | 8.52 | 28 | 284 | 264 | 3.55 | .84 | .07 |
| chicken, simmered. . . . . . | 22 | 10.24 | 23 | 226 | 150 | 8.28 | .57 | .12 |
| lamb, braised. . . . . . . . . | 16 | 6.26 | 27 | 288 | 213 | 4.17 | .69 | .06 |
| pork, braised . . . . . . . . . | 8 | 6.61 | 27 | 202 | 234 | 3.50 | .58 | .08 |
| turkey, simmered . . . . . . . | 15 | 7.81 | 25 | 232 | 208 | 5.98 | .71 | .10 |
| veal, braised . . . . . . . . . | 9 | 4.90 | 20 | 284 | 226 | 2.54 | .49 | n.a. |
| **Hearts of palm,** see "Palm, hearts of" | | | | | | | | |
| **Herring,** meat only: | | | | | | | | |
| Atlantic: | | | | | | | | |
| raw, 1 lb.. . . . . . . . . . | 260 | 4.99 | 144 | 1072 | 1481 | 4.51 | .42 | .16 |
| baked, broiled, or microwaved[1], 4 oz. | 84 | 1.60 | 46 | 344 | 475 | 1.44 | .13 | n.a. |
| kippered, 4 oz. . . . . . . | 95 | 1.71 | 52 | 369 | 507 | 1.54 | .15 | n.a. |
| kippered, 1 fillet, 4⅜", 1.4 oz.. . . . . . . | 33 | .60 | 18 | 130 | 179 | .54 | .05 | n.a. |

[1] *Prepared without added ingredients.*

| | Calcium | Iron | Magnesium | Phosphorus | Potassium | Zinc | Copper | Manganese |
|---|---|---|---|---|---|---|---|---|
| | (Mg) | (Mg) | (Mg) | (Mg) | (Mg) | (Mg) | (Mg) | (Mg) |
| **Herring, Atlantic,** *continued* | | | | | | | | |
| pickled, 4 oz........ | 87 | 1.38 | 9 | 101 | 78 | .60 | .12 | .05 |
| pickled, 1 fillet, 1¾", .5 oz........... | 12 | .18 | 1 | 13 | 10 | .08 | .01 | .01 |
| Pacific: | | | | | | | | |
| raw, 1 lb.......... | n.a. | 5.08 | n.a. | n.a. | 1918 | 2.41 | .35 | .20 |
| baked, broiled, or microwaved[1], 4 oz. | n.a. | 1.63 | n.a. | n.a. | 615 | .77 | .11 | .66 |
| **Herring, canned,** see "Sardines" | | | | | | | | |
| **Hickory nut,** dried: | | | | | | | | |
| in shell, 1 lb........... | 88 | 3.08 | 251 | 488 | 633 | 6.26 | 1.07 | n.a. |
| shelled, 1 oz........... | 17 | .60 | 49 | 95 | 124 | 1.22 | .21 | n.a. |
| **Hominy,** canned, white or yellow, ½ cup ....... | 8 | .50 | 13 | 28 | 7 | .84 | .02 | .06 |
| **Hominy grits,** see "Corn grits" | | | | | | | | |
| **Honey,** 1 tbsp. ........ | 1 | .10 | n.a. | 1 | 11 | n.a. | n.a. | n.a. |
| **Honey loaf,** pork and beef, 1-oz. slice ...... | 5 | .38 | 5 | 41 | 97 | .69 | .02 | .01 |
| **Honey roll sausage,** beef, 1 oz........... | 3 | .62 | 4 | 39 | 83 | .92 | .03 | .01 |
| **Honeydew melon:** | | | | | | | | |
| untrimmed, 1 lb........ | 13 | .15 | 14 | 21 | 566 | n.a. | .09 | .04 |
| ⅒ of 7"-diam. melon, 2" slice, approx. 8 oz. | 8 | .09 | 9 | 13 | 350 | n.a. | .05 | .02 |
| pulp, cubed, ½ cup ..... | 5 | .06 | 6 | 9 | 231 | n.a. | .04 | .02 |
| **Horseradish-tree,** fresh: | | | | | | | | |
| leafy tips: | | | | | | | | |
| raw, untrimmed, 1 lb. ........... | n.a. | 11.25 | 413 | 315 | 947 | n.a. | n.a. | n.a. |
| raw, trimmed, chopped, ½ cup .. | n.a. | .40 | 15 | 11 | 34 | n.a. | n.a. | n.a. |
| boiled, drained, chopped, ½ cup .. | n.a. | .49 | 32 | 14 | 72 | n.a. | n.a. | n.a. |

[1] *Prepared without added ingredients.*

| | Calcium | Iron | Magnesium | Phosphorus | Potassium | Zinc | Copper | Manganese |
|---|---|---|---|---|---|---|---|---|
| | (Mg) | (Mg) | (Mg) | (Mg) | (Mg) | (Mg) | (Mg) | (Mg) |
| **pods:** | | | | | | | | |
| raw, untrimmed, 1 lb. | 71 | .85 | 106 | 118 | 1087 | n.a. | n.a. | n.a. |
| raw, trimmed, sliced, ½ cup | 15 | .18 | 23 | 25 | 231 | n.a. | n.a. | n.a. |
| boiled, drained, sliced, ½ cup | 12 | .27 | 25 | 29 | 270 | n.a. | n.a. | n.a. |
| **Hubbard squash:** | | | | | | | | |
| raw, untrimmed, 1 lb. | 41 | 1.16 | 55 | 61 | 929 | .37 | .19 | n.a. |
| raw, cubed, ½ cup | 8 | .23 | 11 | 12 | 186 | .07 | .04 | n.a. |
| boiled, drained, cubed, ½ cup | 17 | .48 | 22 | 23 | 365 | .15 | .05 | n.a. |
| boiled, drained, mashed, ½ cup | 12 | .33 | 16 | 17 | 252 | .11 | .06 | n.a. |
| **Hummus[1]:** | | | | | | | | |
| 1 lb. | 228 | 7.13 | 131 | 506 | 787 | 4.98 | 1.03 | 2.58 |
| 1 cup | 124 | 3.87 | 71 | 275 | 427 | 2.70 | .56 | 1.40 |
| **Hyacinth beans, fresh:** | | | | | | | | |
| raw, untrimmed, 1 lb. | 209 | 3.12 | 170 | 205 | 1061 | n.a. | n.a. | n.a. |
| raw, ½ cup | 20 | .30 | 16 | 19 | 101 | n.a. | n.a. | n.a. |
| boiled, drained, ½ cup | 18 | .33 | 18 | 22 | 115 | n.a. | n.a. | n.a. |
| **Hyacinth beans, dried:** | | | | | | | | |
| uncooked, 1 lb. | 590 | 23.12 | 1285 | 1685 | 5603 | 42.18 | 6.06 | n.a. |
| uncooked, ½ cup | 137 | 5.36 | 297 | 390 | 1297 | 9.77 | 1.40 | n.a. |
| boiled, ½ cup | 39 | 4.44 | 80 | 117 | 327 | 2.77 | .33 | n.a. |

[1] *Recipe: chickpeas, lemon juice, tahini, olive oil, and garlic.*

| | Calcium | Iron | Magnesium | Phosphorus | Potassium | Zinc | Copper | Manganese |
|---|---|---|---|---|---|---|---|---|
| | (Mg) | (Mg) | (Mg) | (Mg) | (Mg) | (Mg) | (Mg) | (Mg) |
| **Ice, Italian,** lime, 1/2 cup | n.a. | n.a. | n.a. | n.a. | 3 | n.a. | n.a. | n.a. |
| **Ice bar:** | | | | | | | | |
| 2-fl.-oz. bar............ | 0 | 0 | n.a. | 0 | 2 | n.a. | n.a. | n.a. |
| fruit, reduced calorie, | | | | | | | | |
| 1.8-oz. bar......... | 1 | .07 | n.a. | 0 | 13 | n.a. | n.a. | n.a. |
| **Ice cream,** 1/2 cup: | | | | | | | | |
| chocolate............. | 72 | .61 | 19 | 70 | 164 | .38 | .09 | .09 |
| strawberry............ | 79 | .14 | 9 | 66 | 124 | .23 | .02 | .05 |
| vanilla: | | | | | | | | |
| hardened, 16% fat .... | 87 | .04 | 8 | 71 | 118 | .30 | .02 | .01 |
| hardened, 10% fat .... | 85 | .06 | 9 | 69 | 131 | .45 | .02 | .01 |
| French, soft serve .... | 113 | .18 | 11 | 99 | 152 | .45 | .03 | tr. |
| **Ice cream cone,** unfilled: | | | | | | | | |
| plain, wafer type, | | | | | | | | |
| 1 piece ............ | 1 | .14 | 1 | 4 | 4 | .03 | .01 | .02 |
| sugar type, 1 piece ..... | 4 | .44 | 3 | 10 | 14 | .07 | .03 | .07 |
| **Ice cream nuggets,** chocolate coated: | | | | | | | | |
| dark chocolate (*Carnation* | | | | | | | | |
| *Bon Bons*), 5 pieces .. | 55 | .10 | n.a. | 49 | 80 | n.a. | n.a. | n.a. |
| milk chocolate (*Carnation* | | | | | | | | |
| *Bon Bons*), 5 pieces .. | 75 | .22 | n.a. | 65 | 110 | n.a. | n.a. | n.a. |
| **Ice milk,** 1/2 cup: | | | | | | | | |
| vanilla, hardened ....... | 92 | .07 | 10 | 72 | 139 | .29 | .01 | tr. |
| vanilla, soft serve....... | 138 | .05 | 13 | 106 | 194 | .47 | .02 | .01 |
| **Italian sausage,** pork, | | | | | | | | |
| cooked, 1 link, approx. | | | | | | | | |
| 3 oz. (4 oz. raw) ..... | 20 | 1.24 | 15 | 141 | 253 | 1.98 | .06 | .07 |
| **Italian seasoning** (*Tone's* | | | | | | | | |
| *Perc*), 1/4 tsp......... | 4 | .16 | 1 | 1 | 4 | .01 | tr. | .01 |

# J

| | Calcium | Iron | Magnesium | Phosphorus | Potassium | Zinc | Copper | Manganese |
|---|---|---|---|---|---|---|---|---|
| | (Mg) | (Mg) | (Mg) | (Mg) | (Mg) | (Mg) | (Mg) | (Mg) |
| **Jackfruit:** | | | | | | | | |
| untrimmed, 1 lb. . . . . . . | 43 | .76 | 47 | 45 | 385 | .53 | .24 | .25 |
| trimmed, 1 oz. . . . . . . . . | 10 | .17 | 10 | 10 | 86 | .12 | .05 | .06 |
| **Jam and preserves,** all | | | | | | | | |
| flavors, 1 tbsp. . . . . . . | 4 | .20 | n.a. | 2 | 18 | n.a. | n.a. | n.a. |
| **Java plum:** | | | | | | | | |
| untrimmed, 1 lb. . . . . . . | 69 | .68 | 57 | 63 | 289 | n.a. | n.a. | n.a. |
| seeded, ½ cup. . . . . . . . | 13 | .13 | 11 | 12 | 53 | n.a. | n.a. | n.a. |
| **Jelly,** all flavors, 1 tbsp. | 4 | .30 | tr. | 1 | 14 | n.a. | n.a. | n.a. |
| **Jerusalem artichoke:** | | | | | | | | |
| raw, untrimmed, 1 lb. . . . | 44 | 10.64 | 54 | 244 | n.a. | n.a. | n.a. | n.a. |
| raw, sliced, ½ cup. . . . . . | 10 | 2.55 | 13 | 58 | n.a. | n.a. | n.a. | n.a. |
| **Jujube:** | | | | | | | | |
| raw, untrimmed, 1 lb. . . . | 88 | 2.04 | 43 | 96 | 1054 | .22 | .31 | .35 |
| raw, seeded, 1 oz. . . . . . . | 6 | .14 | 3 | 7 | 71 | .01 | .02 | .02 |
| dried, untrimmed, 1 lb. . . | 319 | 7.27 | 149 | 404 | 2144 | .75 | 1.07 | 1.23 |
| dried, 1 oz. . . . . . . . . . . | 22 | .51 | 10 | 28 | 151 | .05 | .08 | .09 |
| **Jute,** potherb: | | | | | | | | |
| raw, untrimmed, 1 lb. . . . | 585 | 13.39 | 179 | 233 | 1572 | n.a. | n.a. | n.a. |
| raw, trimmed, ½ cup. . . . | 29 | .67 | 9 | 12 | 78 | n.a. | n.a. | n.a. |
| boiled, drained, ½ cup. . . | 91 | 1.35 | 27 | 31 | 237 | n.a. | n.a. | n.a. |

# K

|  | Vitamin A (IU) | Vitamin C (Mg) | Thiamin (Mg) | Riboflavin (Mg) | Niacin (Mg) | B6 (Mg) | Folacin (Mcg) | B12 (Mcg) |
|---|---|---|---|---|---|---|---|---|
| **Kale:** | | | | | | | | |
| fresh: | | | | | | | | |
| raw, untrimmed, 1 lb. . . . . . . . . . | 374 | 4.70 | 94 | 155 | 1236 | 1.22 | .80 | 2.19 |
| raw, trimmed, chopped, ½ cup . . | 46 | .58 | 12 | 19 | 152 | .15 | .10 | .26 |
| boiled, drained, chopped, ½ cup . . | 47 | .59 | 12 | 18 | 148 | .15 | .10 | .27 |
| frozen, 10-oz. pkg. . . . . . . | 385 | 2.63 | 50 | 81 | 947 | .50 | .13 | 1.26 |
| frozen, boiled, drained, chopped, ½ cup . . . . . | 90 | .61 | 12 | 18 | 209 | .12 | .03 | .29 |
| **Kale, Scotch, fresh:** | | | | | | | | |
| raw, untrimmed, 1 lb. . . . . | 567 | 8.30 | 243 | 172 | 1245 | 1.02 | .67 | 1.79 |
| raw, trimmed, chopped, ½ cup . . . . . . . . . . . . | 70 | 1.02 | 30 | 21 | 153 | .13 | .08 | .22 |
| boiled, drained, chopped, ½ cup . . . . . . . . . . . . | 86 | 1.25 | 37 | 25 | 178 | .15 | .10 | .27 |
| **Kanpyo, dried:** | | | | | | | | |
| 3 strips, approx. .75 oz. . . . . . . . . . . . . | 53 | .97 | 24 | 36 | 301 | 1.11 | n.a. | n.a. |
| ½ cup . . . . . . . . . . . . . . | 76 | 1.38 | 34 | 51 | 427 | 1.58 | n.a. | n.a. |
| **Kelp,** see "Seaweed" | | | | | | | | |
| **Kidney[1]:** | | | | | | | | |
| beef, simmered, 4 oz. . . . | 19 | 8.29 | 20 | 347 | 203 | 4.79 | .77 | .21 |
| lamb, braised, 4 oz. . . . . . . | 20 | 14.06 | 23 | 329 | 202 | 4.31 | .42 | .16 |
| pork, braised, 4 oz. . . . . . . | 15 | 6.00 | 20 | 272 | 162 | 4.71 | .77 | .17 |
| veal, braised, 4 oz. . . . . . . . | 33 | 3.45 | 27 | 422 | 180 | 4.82 | .41 | .14 |
| **Kidney beans, red, dried:** | | | | | | | | |
| uncooked, 1 lb. . . . . . . . . | 376 | 30.35 | 627 | 1843 | 6163 | 12.63 | 3.17 | 5.04 |
| uncooked, ½ cup . . . . . . . | 76 | 6.16 | 127 | 374 | 1250 | 2.56 | .64 | 1.02 |
| boiled, ½ cup . . . . . . . . . | 25 | 2.58 | 40 | 125 | 355 | .94 | .21 | .42 |
| canned, w/liquid, 8 oz. | 55 | 2.86 | 65 | 213 | 583 | 1.25 | .34 | .55 |

---

[1] Prepared without added ingredients.

| | Calcium | Iron | Magnesium | Phosphorus | Potassium | Zinc | Copper | Manganese |
|---|---|---|---|---|---|---|---|---|
| | (Mg) | (Mg) | (Mg) | (Mg) | (Mg) | (Mg) | (Mg) | (Mg) |
| canned, w/liquid, ½ cup | 31 | 1.61 | 36 | 120 | 329 | .70 | .19 | .31 |
| **Kidney beans, sprouted,** mature seeds: | | | | | | | | |
| raw, 1 lb. | 77 | 3.67 | 95 | 168 | 848 | n.a. | n.a. | n.a. |
| raw, 1 cup | 31 | 1.49 | 39 | 68 | 344 | n.a. | n.a. | n.a. |
| **Kielbasa[1] (see also "Polish sausage"),** pork and beef, 1 oz. | 12 | .41 | 5 | 42 | 77 | .57 | .03 | .01 |
| **Kiwifruit:** | | | | | | | | |
| untrimmed, 1 lb. | 103 | 1.58 | 117 | 157 | 1295 | n.a. | n.a. | n.a. |
| 1 medium, 3.1 oz. | 20 | .31 | 23 | 31 | 252 | n.a. | n.a. | n.a. |
| **Knockwurst[1], pork and** beef, 1 oz. | 3 | .26 | 3 | 28 | 57 | .47 | .02 | n.a. |
| **Kohlrabi:** | | | | | | | | |
| raw, untrimmed, 1 lb. | 50 | .83 | 40 | 96 | 730 | n.a. | n.a. | n.a. |
| raw, trimmed, sliced, ½ cup | 17 | .28 | 13 | 32 | 245 | n.a. | n.a. | n.a. |
| boiled, drained, sliced, ½ cup | 20 | .33 | 16 | 37 | 279 | n.a. | n.a. | n.a. |
| **Koyadofu,** see "Tofu, dried-frozen" | | | | | | | | |
| **Kumquat,** fresh: | | | | | | | | |
| untrimmed, 1 lb. | 186 | 1.64 | 53 | 82 | 821 | .34 | .45 | .36 |
| 1 fruit, approx. ¾ oz. | 8 | .07 | 2 | 4 | 37 | .02 | .02 | .02 |
| seeded, 1 oz. | 12 | .11 | 4 | 5 | 55 | .02 | .03 | .02 |

---

[1] *Nonfat dry milk added.*

# L

| | Calcium | Iron | Magnesium | Phosphorus | Potassium | Zinc | Copper | Manganese |
|---|---|---|---|---|---|---|---|---|
| | (Mg) | (Mg) | (Mg) | (Mg) | (Mg) | (Mg) | (Mg) | (Mg) |

**Lamb**[1], domestic, meat only, 4 oz.:

cubed, for stew or kabob, leg and shoulder:

| | | | | | | | | |
|---|---|---|---|---|---|---|---|---|
| braised, lean only.... | 17 | 3.18 | 32 | 232 | 295 | 7.46 | .16 | .04 |
| broiled, lean only.... | 14 | 2.65 | 35 | 254 | 380 | 6.54 | .17 | .03 |

foreshank, braised:

| | | | | | | | | |
|---|---|---|---|---|---|---|---|---|
| lean w/fat ......... | 23 | 2.43 | 25 | 188 | 291 | 8.72 | .14 | .03 |
| lean only .......... | 23 | 2.57 | 26 | 198 | 303 | 9.82 | .15 | .03 |
| ground, broiled ....... | 25 | 2.03 | 27 | 228 | 384 | 5.30 | .15 | .03 |

leg, roasted:

| | | | | | | | | |
|---|---|---|---|---|---|---|---|---|
| whole, lean w/fat .... | 12 | 2.25 | 27 | 217 | 355 | 4.99 | .13 | .03 |
| whole, lean only..... | 9 | 2.40 | 29 | 234 | 383 | 5.60 | .14 | .03 |
| shank half, lean w/fat | 11 | 2.25 | 28 | 225 | 370 | 5.28 | .13 | .03 |
| shank half, lean only | 9 | 2.34 | 29 | 236 | 388 | 5.69 | .14 | .03 |
| sirloin, lean w/fat.... | 12 | 2.27 | 25 | 208 | 341 | 4.68 | .13 | .02 |
| sirloin, lean only .... | 9 | 2.49 | 28 | 230 | 378 | 5.50 | .13 | .03 |

loin:

| | | | | | | | | |
|---|---|---|---|---|---|---|---|---|
| broiled, lean w/fat ... | 23 | 2.05 | 27 | 222 | 371 | 3.95 | .15 | .02 |
| broiled, lean only.... | 22 | 2.27 | 32 | 256 | 426 | 4.68 | .16 | .03 |
| roasted, lean w/fat ... | 20 | 2.40 | 26 | 204 | 279 | 3.87 | .13 | .02 |
| roasted, lean only ... | 19 | 2.77 | 31 | 234 | 303 | 4.60 | .14 | .03 |

rib:

| | | | | | | | | |
|---|---|---|---|---|---|---|---|---|
| broiled, lean w/fat ... | 22 | 2.13 | 26 | 202 | 306 | 4.54 | .14 | .02 |
| broiled, lean only.... | 18 | 2.51 | 33 | 242 | 355 | 5.98 | .16 | .03 |
| roasted, lean w/fat ... | 25 | 1.81 | 23 | 188 | 307 | 3.96 | .13 | .02 |
| roasted, lean only ... | 24 | 2.01 | 34 | 221 | 357 | 5.07 | .15 | .03 |

shoulder, whole:

| | | | | | | | | |
|---|---|---|---|---|---|---|---|---|
| braised, lean w/fat ... | 28 | 2.72 | 27 | 211 | 281 | 7.22 | .14 | .03 |
| braised, lean only.... | 29 | 3.03 | 31 | 231 | 296 | 8.53 | .15 | .04 |
| broiled, lean w/fat ... | 24 | 2.30 | 29 | 225 | 341 | 6.49 | .15 | .03 |
| broiled, lean only.... | 24 | 2.48 | 33 | 246 | 367 | 7.48 | .16 | .03 |
| roasted, lean w/fat ... | 23 | 2.23 | 26 | 209 | 285 | 5.93 | .12 | .02 |
| roasted, lean only ... | 22 | 2.42 | 28 | 227 | 301 | 6.85 | .13 | .03 |

---

[1] *Prepared without added ingredients.*

| | Calcium (Mg) | Iron (Mg) | Magnesium (Mg) | Phosphorus (Mg) | Potassium (Mg) | Zinc (Mg) | Copper (Mg) | Manganese (Mg) |
|---|---|---|---|---|---|---|---|---|
| **shoulder, arm:** | | | | | | | | |
| braised, lean w/fat . . . | 28 | 2.71 | 29 | 234 | 347 | 6.89 | .16 | .03 |
| braised, lean only. . . . | 29 | 3.06 | 33 | 263 | 383 | 8.28 | .17 | .03 |
| broiled, lean w/ fat . . . | 20 | 2.37 | 29 | 223 | 350 | 5.54 | .15 | .03 |
| broiled, lean only . . . . | 19 | 2.62 | 34 | 248 | 386 | 6.50 | .16 | .03 |
| roasted, lean w/fat . . . | 20 | 2.30 | 26 | 208 | 294 | 5.08 | .13 | .02 |
| roasted, lean only . . . | 18 | 2.53 | 29 | 229 | 314 | 5.95 | .14 | .03 |
| **shoulder, blade:** | | | | | | | | |
| braised, lean w/fat . . . | 31 | 2.66 | 27 | 210 | 276 | 7.78 | .14 | .03 |
| braised, lean only. . . . | 32 | 2.95 | 29 | 229 | 288 | 9.14 | .15 | .04 |
| broiled, lean w/fat . . . | 27 | 1.95 | 27 | 225 | 381 | 6.37 | .14 | .03 |
| broiled, lean only . . . . | 27 | 2.05 | 29 | 245 | 417 | 7.35 | .15 | .03 |
| roasted, lean w/fat . . . | 24 | 2.18 | 25 | 208 | 279 | 6.33 | .12 | .02 |
| roasted, lean only . . . | 24 | 2.35 | 28 | 226 | 293 | 7.35 | .12 | .03 |
| **Lavar,** see "Seaweed" | | | | | | | | |
| **Leek,** fresh: | | | | | | | | |
| raw: | | | | | | | | |
| untrimmed, 1 lb. . . . . | 118 | 4.19 | 56 | 70 | 359 | n.a. | n.a. | n.a. |
| trimmed, 1 medium, | | | | | | | | |
| 4.5 oz. . . . . . . . . . | 73 | 2.60 | 35 | 43 | 223 | n.a. | n.a. | n.a. |
| trimmed, chopped, | | | | | | | | |
| ½ cup . . . . . . . . . | 30 | 1.10 | 14 | 18 | 94 | n.a. | na. | n.a. |
| boiled, drained, | | | | | | | | |
| 1 medium . . . . . . . . . | 37 | 1.36 | 18 | 21 | 108 | n.a. | n.a. | n.a. |
| boiled, drained, chopped, | | | | | | | | |
| ½ cup . . . . . . . . . . . . | 16 | .58 | 8 | 8 | 46 | n.a. | n.a. | n.a. |
| **Leek, freeze-dried:** | | | | | | | | |
| ¼ cup . . . . . . . . . . . . . | 3 | .06 | 1 | 3 | 19 | n.a. | n.a. | n.a. |
| 1 tbsp. . . . . . . . . . . . | 1 | .02 | 0 | 1 | 5 | n.a. | n.a. | n.a. |
| **Lemon,** w/peel, except as noted: | | | | | | | | |
| untrimmed, 1 lb. . . . . . . | 271 | 3.11 | 53 | 67 | 645 | .44 | 1.16 | n.a. |
| 2⅛"-diam. fruit, 3.9 oz. . . . | 66 | .76 | 13 | 16 | 157 | .11 | .28 | n.a. |
| 1-oz. wedge, | | | | | | | | |
| ¼ medium. . . . . . . . . | 16 | .19 | 3 | 4 | 39 | .03 | .07 | n.a. |
| pulp from 2⅛"-diam. | | | | | | | | |
| fruit. . . . . . . . . . . . . . . | 15 | .35 | n.a. | 9 | 80 | .04 | .02 | n.a. |

| | Calcium | Iron | Magnesium | Phosphorus | Potassium | Zinc | Copper | Manganese |
|---|---|---|---|---|---|---|---|---|
| | (Mg) | (Mg) | (Mg) | (Mg) | (Mg) | (Mg) | (Mg) | (Mg) |
| **Lemon extract** (*Virginia Dare*), 1 tsp. . . . . . . . | tr. | tr. | tr. | 0 | 0 | tr. | tr. | n.a. |
| **Lemon juice:** | | | | | | | | |
| fresh, 2 tbsp. or 1 fl. oz. . . . . . . . . . . . | 2 | .01 | 2 | 2 | 38 | .02 | .01 | tr. |
| canned or bottled, 1 fl. oz. . . . . . . . . . . . | 3 | .04 | 3 | 3 | 31 | .02 | .01 | .01 |
| frozen, single strength, 1 fl. oz. . . . . . . . . . . . | 2 | .04 | 3 | 3 | 27 | .02 | .01 | .01 |
| **Lemon peel,** fresh, 1 tsp. | 3 | .02 | tr. | tr. | 3 | n.a. | n.a. | n.a. |
| **Lemon seasoning:** | | | | | | | | |
| and pepper (*Tone's Perc*), ¼ tsp. . . . . . . . . . . . | 2 | .15 | 1 | 1 | 7 | .01 | .01 | .03 |
| and spice (*Tone's Perc*), ¼ tsp. . . . . . . . . . . . | 1 | .06 | tr. | 1 | 4 | tr. | tr. | .01 |
| **Lemonade:** | | | | | | | | |
| frozen, diluted, 8 fl. oz. | 8 | .41 | 5 | 5 | 38 | .09 | .05 | .01 |
| mix, 2 tbsp. . . . . . . . . . . | 66 | .14 | 0 | 34 | 33 | .04 | n.a. | n.a. |
| **Lemonade flavor drink mix**[1], dry, 2 tbsp. . . . . . | 24 | .03 | 0 | 3 | 1 | .01 | .01 | n.a. |
| **Lentils,** dried: | | | | | | | | |
| uncooked, 1 lb. . . . . . . . . | 233 | 40.92 | 484 | 2058 | 4106 | 16.38 | 3.87 | 6.48 |
| uncooked, ½ cup. . . . . . . | 49 | 8.66 | 103 | 435 | 869 | 3.47 | .82 | 1.37 |
| boiled, ½ cup . . . . . . . . . | 19 | 3.30 | 35 | 178 | 366 | 1.25 | .25 | .49 |
| **Lentils,** sprouted: | | | | | | | | |
| raw, untrimmed, 1 lb. . . . . | 111 | 14.55 | 166 | 784 | 1461 | 6.85 | 1.60 | 2.30 |
| raw, ½ cup . . . . . . . . . . | 9 | 1.22 | 14 | 66 | 122 | .57 | .13 | .19 |
| stir-fried[2], 4 oz. . . . . . . . . | 16 | 3.50 | 40 | 174 | 322 | 1.81 | .38 | .06 |
| **Lettuce:** | | | | | | | | |
| Bibb, Boston, or butterhead: | | | | | | | | |
| untrimmed, 1 lb. . . . . | n.a. | .99 | n.a. | n.a. | 862 | .57 | .08 | .45 |

[1] With added nutrients.
[2] No fat added in cooking.

| | Calcium | Iron | Magnesium | Phosphorus | Potassium | Zinc | Copper | Manganese |
|---|---|---|---|---|---|---|---|---|
| | (Mg) | (Mg) | (Mg) | (Mg) | (Mg) | (Mg) | (Mg) | (Mg) |
| 5"-diam. head, trimmed, 5.7 oz. . . . | n.a. | .49 | n.a. | n.a. | 416 | .28 | .04 | .22 |
| cos or romaine: | | | | | | | | |
| untrimmed, 1 lb. . . . . | 154 | 4.69 | 26 | 192 | 1235 | n.a. | n.a. | n.a. |
| shredded, ½ cup, approx. 1 oz. . . . . . | 10 | .31 | 2 | 13 | 81 | n.a. | n.a. | n.a. |
| iceberg: | | | | | | | | |
| untrimmed, 1 lb. . . . . | 80 | 2.17 | 37 | 88 | 680 | .94 | .12 | .65 |
| 6"-diam. head, cored, 1.25 lbs. . . . . . . . | 102 | 2.70 | 48 | 108 | 852 | 1.19 | .15 | .81 |
| 1 leaf, .7 oz. . . . . . . . | 4 | .10 | 2 | 4 | 32 | .04 | .01 | .03 |
| loose leaf: | | | | | | | | |
| untrimmed, 1 lb. . . . . | 197 | 4.06 | 32 | 73 | 766 | n.a. | n.a. | n.a. |
| shredded, 1 oz. or ½ cup . . . . . . . . . | 19 | .39 | 3 | 7 | 74 | n.a. | n.a. | n.a. |
| **Lima beans:** | | | | | | | | |
| fresh: | | | | | | | | |
| raw, untrimmed (in pods), 1 lb. . . . . . . | 69 | 6.26 | 116 | 272 | 933 | 1.55 | .64 | 2.45 |
| raw, trimmed, ½ cup | 27 | 2.45 | 45 | 106 | 365 | .60 | .25 | .95 |
| boiled, drained, ½ cup . . . . . . . . . . | 27 | 2.08 | 63 | 111 | 485 | .67 | .26 | 1.06 |
| canned, w/liquid, ½ cup . . . . . . . . . . . . | 35 | 1.97 | 42 | 88 | 334 | .79 | .20 | .87 |
| frozen: | | | | | | | | |
| baby, 10-oz. pkg. . . . . | 98 | 6.28 | 143 | 297 | 1283 | 1.78 | .36 | 1.99 |
| baby, boiled, drained, ½ cup . . . . . . . . . | 25 | 1.76 | 50 | 101 | 370 | .50 | .18 | .73 |
| Fordhook, 10-oz. pkg. . . . . . . . . . . . | 68 | 4.29 | 108 | 211 | 1357 | 1.39 | .18 | .98 |
| Fordhook, boiled, drained, ½ cup . . . | 19 | 1.16 | 29 | 54 | 347 | .37 | .05 | .26 |
| **Lima beans, dried:** | | | | | | | | |
| large: | | | | | | | | |
| uncooked, 1 lb. . . . . . . | 368 | 34.05 | 1016 | 1746 | 7822 | 12.84 | 3.36 | 7.58 |
| uncooked, ½ cup. . . . | 72 | 6.68 | 199 | 343 | 1535 | 2.52 | .66 | 1.49 |

| | Calcium | Iron | Magnesium | Phosphorus | Potassium | Zinc | Copper | Manganese |
|---|---|---|---|---|---|---|---|---|
| | (Mg) | (Mg) | (Mg) | (Mg) | (Mg) | (Mg) | (Mg) | (Mg) |
| Lima beans, dried, large, _continued_ | | | | | | | | |
| boiled, ½ cup . . . . . . | 16 | 2.25 | 41 | 104 | 478 | .89 | .22 | .49 |
| canned, 8 oz. . . . . . . . | 47 | 4.10 | 89 | 168 | 500 | 1.48 | .41 | .82 |
| canned, w/liquid, | | | | | | | | |
| ½ cup . . . . . . . . . . | 25 | 2.17 | 47 | 89 | 264 | .78 | .22 | .44 |
| baby: | | | | | | | | |
| uncooked, 1 lb. . . . . . | 366 | 28.06 | 854 | 1678 | 6364 | 11.80 | 3.02 | 7.65 |
| uncooked, ½ cup. . . . | 81 | 6.25 | 190 | 374 | 1417 | 2.63 | .67 | 1.70 |
| boiled, ½ cup . . . . . . | 26 | 2.18 | 49 | 116 | 365 | .93 | .20 | .53 |
| **Lime:** | | | | | | | | |
| untrimmed, 1 lb. . . . . . . | 126 | 2.29 | n.a. | 69 | 389 | .42 | .25 | n.a. |
| 2"-diam. fruit, approx. | | | | | | | | |
| 2.8 oz. . . . . . . . . . . . . | 22 | .40 | n.a. | 12 | 68 | .07 | .04 | n.a. |
| **Lime juice:** | | | | | | | | |
| fresh, 2 tbsp. or | | | | | | | | |
| 1 fl. oz. . . . . . . . . . . . | 3 | .01 | 2 | 2 | 34 | .02 | .01 | tr. |
| canned or bottled, | | | | | | | | |
| 1 fl. oz. . . . . . . . . . . . | 4 | .07 | 2 | 3 | 23 | .02 | .01 | tr. |
| **Ling,** meat only: | | | | | | | | |
| raw, 1 lb. . . . . . . . . . . . | 153 | 2.95 | 284 | 900 | 1720 | n.a. | n.a. | n.a. |
| baked, broiled, or | | | | | | | | |
| microwaved[1], 4 oz. . . . | 50 | .94 | 92 | 288 | 551 | n.a. | n.a. | n.a. |
| **Ling cod,** meat only: | | | | | | | | |
| raw, 1 lb. . . . . . . . . . . . | 63 | 1.45 | 119 | 56912 | 1982 | 2.05 | .12 | .09 |
| baked, broiled, or | | | | | | | | |
| microwaved[1], 4 oz. . . . | 20 | .46 | 37 | 293 | 635 | .66 | .04 | .03 |
| **Liquor**[2], pure, distilled, | | | | | | | | |
| 1 fl. oz. . . . . . . . . . . . | 0 | .01 | 0 | 1 | 0 | .01 | .01 | .01 |
| **Litchis:** | | | | | | | | |
| fresh, untrimmed, 1 lb. . . | 14 | .85 | 27 | 84 | 466 | .18 | .40 | .15 |
| fresh, shelled and seeded, | | | | | | | | |
| ½ cup . . . . . . . . . . . . | 5 | .30 | 10 | 30 | 163 | .06 | .14 | .05 |

[1] _Prepared without added ingredients._
[2] _Includes gin, rum, vodka, whiskey, and others, with insignificant variations in mineral content depending on type of liquor._

|  | Calcium | Iron | Magnesium | Phosphorus | Potassium | Zinc | Copper | Manganese |
|---|---|---|---|---|---|---|---|---|
|  | (Mg) | (Mg) | (Mg) | (Mg) | (Mg) | (Mg) | (Mg) | (Mg) |
| dried, untrimmed, 1 lb. . . . | 81 | 4.16 | 104 | 443 | 2718 | .68 | 1.54 | .57 |
| dried, 1 oz. . . . . . . . . . . | 9 | .48 | 12 | 51 | 315 | .08 | .18 | .07 |
| **Liver**[1]: |  |  |  |  |  |  |  |  |
| beef, braised, 4 oz. . . . . . | 8 | 7.68 | 23 | 458 | 266 | 6.88 | 5.12 | .47 |
| beef, pan-fried in |  |  |  |  |  |  |  |  |
|   vegetable oil, 4 oz. . . . . | 12 | 7.12 | 26 | 523 | 413 | 6.18 | 5.06 | .48 |
| chicken, simmered, |  |  |  |  |  |  |  |  |
|   4 oz. . . . . . . . . . . . . . | 16 | 9.60 | 24 | 354 | 159 | 4.92 | .42 | .34 |
| goose, raw, |  |  |  |  |  |  |  |  |
|   1 oz. . . . . . . . . . . . . . . | 12 | n.a. | 7 | 74 | 65 | n.a. | 2.13 | n.a. |
| lamb, braised, |  |  |  |  |  |  |  |  |
|   4 oz. . . . . . . . . . . . . . | 9 | 9.39 | 25 | 476 | 251 | 8.95 | 8.02 | .59 |
| lamb, pan-fried in |  |  |  |  |  |  |  |  |
|   vegetable oil, 4 oz. . . . . | 10 | 11.57 | 26 | 484 | 399 | 6.38 | 11.15 | .67 |
| pork, braised, 4 oz. . . . . . | 11 | 20.32 | 16 | 273 | 170 | 7.62 | .72 | .34 |
| turkey, simmered, |  |  |  |  |  |  |  |  |
|   4 oz. . . . . . . . . . . . . . | 12 | 8.85 | 17 | 308 | 220 | 3.50 | .64 | .29 |
| veal (calf), braised, |  |  |  |  |  |  |  |  |
|   4 oz. . . . . . . . . . . . . . | 8 | 2.97 | 22 | 362 | 232 | 10.80 | 9.02 | .13 |
| veal (calf), pan-fried in |  |  |  |  |  |  |  |  |
|   vegetable oil, 4 oz. . . . . | 14 | 5.93 | 29 | 498 | 497 | 8.92 | 11.21 | .23 |
| **Liver cheese,** pork, |  |  |  |  |  |  |  |  |
|   1 oz. . . . . . . . . . . . . . | 2 | 3.07 | 3 | 59 | 64 | 1.05 | .11 | .06 |
| **Liver pâté,** see "Pâté" |  |  |  |  |  |  |  |  |
| **Liverwurst** (see also |  |  |  |  |  |  |  |  |
|   "Braunschweiger"), |  |  |  |  |  |  |  |  |
|   pork, 1 oz. . . . . . . . . . | 7 | 1.81 | n.a. | 65 | n.a. | n.a. | n.a. | n.a. |
| **Lobster,** northern, meat only: |  |  |  |  |  |  |  |  |
| boiled or steamed[1], 4 oz. | 69 | .44 | 40 | 210 | 399 | 3.31 | 2.20 | .07 |
| boiled or steamed[1], |  |  |  |  |  |  |  |  |
|   1 cup . . . . . . . . . . . . . | 88 | .57 | 51 | 268 | 510 | 4.23 | 2.81 | .09 |

---

[1] *Prepared without added ingredients, except as noted.*

| | Calcium | Iron | Magnesium | Phosphorus | Potassium | Zinc | Copper | Manganese |
|---|---|---|---|---|---|---|---|---|
| | (Mg) | (Mg) | (Mg) | (Mg) | (Mg) | (Mg) | (Mg) | (Mg) |
| **Loganberry,** frozen, | | | | | | | | |
| ½ cup . . . . . . . . . . . . | 19 | .47 | 16 | 19 | 107 | .03 | .09 | .92 |
| **Longan:** | | | | | | | | |
| fresh, untrimmed, 1 lb. . . | 3 | .32 | 23 | 50 | 639 | .11 | .41 | .13 |
| fresh, shelled and seeded, | | | | | | | | |
| 1 oz. . . . . . . . . . . . . | <1 | .04 | 3 | 6 | 75 | .01 | .05 | .01 |
| dried, untrimmed, | | | | | | | | |
| 1 lb. . . . . . . . . . . . | 73 | 8.82 | 76 | 320 | 1075 | .36 | 1.32 | .41 |
| dried, shelled and seeded, | | | | | | | | |
| 1 oz. . . . . . . . . . . . . | 13 | 1.53 | 13 | 56 | 187 | .06 | .23 | .07 |
| **Loquat:** | | | | | | | | |
| untrimmed, 1 lb. . . . . . . | 45 | .77 | 37 | 75 | 748 | .13 | .11 | .42 |
| 1 fruit, approx. | | | | | | | | |
| .5 oz. . . . . . . . . . . . | 2 | .03 | 1 | 3 | 26 | .00 | tr. | .02 |
| peeled and seeded, | | | | | | | | |
| 1 oz. . . . . . . . . . . . . | 5 | .08 | 4 | 8 | 75 | .01 | .01 | .04 |
| **Lotus root:** | | | | | | | | |
| raw, 10 slices, | | | | | | | | |
| 2.9 oz. . . . . . . . . . . . | 36 | .94 | 18 | 81 | 450 | n.a. | n.a. | n.a. |
| boiled, drained, | | | | | | | | |
| 10 slices . . . . . . . . . . | 23 | .89 | 20 | 69 | 323 | n.a. | n.a. | n.a. |
| **Luncheon meat** (see also specific listings): | | | | | | | | |
| pork and beef, 1-oz. slice | 3 | .24 | 4 | 24 | 57 | .47 | .01 | .01 |
| pork and beef, sausage, | | | | | | | | |
| 1 oz. . . . . . . . . . . . . | 4 | .40 | 4 | 34 | 70 | .69 | .02 | .01 |
| canned, pork, 1 oz. . . . . . | 2 | .20 | 3 | 23 | 61 | .42 | .01 | .01 |
| **Lung**[1]: | | | | | | | | |
| beef, braised, 4 oz. . . . . . | 12 | 6.12 | 11 | 202 | 196 | 1.86 | .25 | .02 |
| pork, braised, 4 oz. . . . . . | 9 | 18.61 | 14 | 211 | 171 | 2.78 | n.a. | n.a. |
| **Lupines:** | | | | | | | | |
| uncooked, 1 lb. . . . . . . . | 798 | 19.79 | 896 | 1997 | 4596 | 21.52 | 4.64 | n.a. |

---

[1] *Prepared without added ingredients.*

|  | Calcium | Iron | Magnesium | Phosphorus | Potassium | Zinc | Copper | Manganese |
|---|---|---|---|---|---|---|---|---|
|  | (Mg) | (Mg) | (Mg) | (Mg) | (Mg) | (Mg) | (Mg) | (Mg) |
| uncooked, ½ cup....... | 158 | 3.93 | 178 | 396 | 912 | 4.27 | .92 | n.a. |
| boiled, ½ cup ......... | 42 | .99 | 45 | 106 | 204 | 1.14 | .19 | n.a. |
| **Luxury loaf,** pork, 1-oz. slice .............. | 10 | .30 | 6 | 52 | 107 | .86 | .03 | .01 |

**Lychees,** see "Litchis"

# M

| | Calcium (Mg) | Iron (Mg) | Magnesium (Mg) | Phosphorus (Mg) | Potassium (Mg) | Zinc (Mg) | Copper (Mg) | Manganese (Mg) |
|---|---|---|---|---|---|---|---|---|
| **Macadamia nut,** shelled, except as noted: | | | | | | | | |
| dried: | | | | | | | | |
| in shell, 1 lb........ | 98 | 3.39 | 163 | 192 | 517 | 2.40 | .42 | n.a. |
| 1 oz.............. | 20 | .68 | 33 | 39 | 104 | .49 | .08 | n.a. |
| 1 cup ............ | 94 | 3.23 | 155 | 183 | 493 | 2.29 | .40 | n.a. |
| oil-roasted, 1 oz........ | 13 | .51 | 33 | 57 | 94 | .31 | .09 | n.a. |
| oil-roasted, wholes or | | | | | | | | |
| halves, 1 cup........ | 60 | 2.41 | 157 | 268 | 441 | 1.47 | .40 | n.a. |
| **Macaroni** (see also "Pasta"), dry: | | | | | | | | |
| uncooked: | | | | | | | | |
| enriched, 2 oz....... | 10 | 2.20 | 27 | 85 | 92 | .69 | .15 | .40 |
| protein fortified, | | | | | | | | |
| 2 oz............ | 22 | 2.36 | 37 | 93 | 115 | 1.02 | .16 | .52 |
| vegetable (tricolor), | | | | | | | | |
| 2 oz............ | 20 | 2.44 | 26 | 66 | 163 | .43 | .11 | 2.19 |
| whole wheat, 2 oz.... | 23 | 2.07 | 81 | 147 | 123 | 1.35 | .26 | 1.74 |
| cooked: | | | | | | | | |
| enriched, 4 oz....... | 8 | 1.59 | 20 | 61 | 35 | .60 | .11 | .32 |
| elbow, enriched, | | | | | | | | |
| 1 cup .......... | 10 | 1.96 | 25 | 76 | 44 | .74 | .14 | .40 |
| protein fortified, | | | | | | | | |
| 4 oz............ | 11 | .82 | 34 | 57 | 48 | .57 | .10 | .47 |
| vegetable (tricolor), | | | | | | | | |
| 4 oz............ | 12 | .56 | 22 | 57 | 35 | .50 | .10 | 1.12 |
| whole wheat, 4 oz.... | 17 | 1.20 | 34 | 101 | 50 | .92 | .19 | 1.56 |
| **Mace,** ground, 1 tsp..... | 4 | .24 | 3 | 2 | 8 | .04 | .05 | .03 |
| **Mackerel,** meat only: | | | | | | | | |
| Atlantic: | | | | | | | | |
| raw, 1 lb.......... | 54 | 7.38 | 344 | 983 | 1425 | 2.84 | .33 | .07 |
| baked, broiled, or | | | | | | | | |
| microwaved[1], 4 oz. | 17 | 1.78 | 110 | 315 | 455 | 1.07 | .11 | (0) |

---

[1] *Prepared without added ingredients.*

| | Calcium | Iron | Magnesium | Phosphorus | Potassium | Zinc | Copper | Manganese |
|---|---|---|---|---|---|---|---|---|
| | (Mg) | (Mg) | (Mg) | (Mg) | (Mg) | (Mg) | (Mg) | (Mg) |
| king: | | | | | | | | |
| raw, 1 lb.......... | 140 | 8.07 | 147 | 1125 | 1973 | 2.54 | .12 | .02 |
| baked, broiled, or | | | | | | | | |
| microwaved[1], 4 oz. | 45 | 2.59 | 46 | 361 | 633 | .82 | .04 | .02 |
| Pacific or jack: | | | | | | | | |
| raw, 1 lb.......... | 104 | 5.26 | 127 | 567 | 1842 | 3.04 | .42 | .06 |
| baked, broiled, or | | | | | | | | |
| microwaved[1], 4 oz. | 33 | 1.69 | 41 | 181 | 591 | .98 | .13 | .02 |
| Spanish: | | | | | | | | |
| raw, 1 lb.......... | 52 | 2.00 | 151 | 931 | 2022 | 2.22 | .25 | .06 |
| baked, broiled,or | | | | | | | | |
| microwaved[1], 4 oz. | 15 | .84 | 43 | 307 | 628 | .70 | .07 | .01 |
| **Mackerel, canned,** jack, | | | | | | | | |
| drained, 4 oz. ....... | 273 | 2.31 | 42 | 341 | 220 | 1.16 | .17 | .05 |
| **Mahimahi,** see "Dolphinfish" | | | | | | | | |
| **Malted milk:** | | | | | | | | |
| natural flavor: | | | | | | | | |
| powder, ¾ oz. or 2–3 | | | | | | | | |
| heaping tsp....... | 56 | .16 | 20 | 79 | 159 | .21 | .06 | .09 |
| prepared[2]......... | 347 | .29 | 52 | 307 | 529 | 1.14 | .08 | .09 |
| chocolate flavor: | | | | | | | | |
| powder, ¾ oz. or 2–3 | | | | | | | | |
| heaping tsp......... | 13 | .38 | 15 | 37 | 130 | .19 | .13 | .13 |
| prepared[2]......... | 304 | .50 | 48 | 265 | 500 | 1.11 | .16 | .14 |
| **Mango:** | | | | | | | | |
| untrimmed, 1 lb. ....... | 32 | .40 | 28 | 33 | 487 | .11 | .34 | .09 |
| 1 medium, approx. | | | | | | | | |
| 10.5 oz............. | 21 | .26 | 18 | 22 | 322 | .07 | .23 | .06 |
| peeled and seeded, sliced, | | | | | | | | |
| ½ cup............. | 9 | .11 | 8 | 9 | 129 | .03 | .09 | .02 |
| **Maple syrup** (see also | | | | | | | | |
| "Syrup, table blends"), | | | | | | | | |
| 1 tbsp. ............ | 13 | .24 | 3 | 0 | 41 | .83 | .02 | .66 |

[1] *Prepared without added ingredients.*
[2] *One cup whole milk and ¾ oz. powder.*

| | Calcium | Iron | Magnesium | Phosphorus | Potassium | Zinc | Copper | Manganese |
|---|---|---|---|---|---|---|---|---|
| | (Mg) | (Mg) | (Mg) | (Mg) | (Mg) | (Mg) | (Mg) | (Mg) |
| **Margarine:** | | | | | | | | |
| regular: | | | | | | | | |
| stick, 4-oz. stick . . . . . | 34 | n.a. | 3 | 26 | 48 | n.a. | n.a. | n.a. |
| stick, 1 tsp. . . . . . . . . | 1 | n.a. | tr. | 1 | 2 | n.a. | n.a. | n.a. |
| tub, soft, 1 cup . . . . . | 60 | n.a. | 5 | 46 | 86 | n.a. | n.a. | n.a. |
| tub, soft, 1 tsp. . . . . . | 1 | n.a. | tr. | 1 | 2 | n.a. | n.a. | n.a. |
| liquid, 1 cup . . . . . . . | 150 | n.a. | 13 | 116 | 214 | n.a. | n.a. | n.a. |
| liquid, 1 tsp. . . . . . . . | 3 | n.a. | tr. | 2 | 4 | n.a. | n.a. | n.a. |
| blend: | | | | | | | | |
| 40% fat, 1 cup . . . . . | 41 | n.a. | 4 | 32 | 59 | n.a. | n.a. | n.a. |
| 40% fat, 1 tsp. . . . . . | 1 | n.a. | tr. | tr. | 1 | n.a. | n.a. | n.a. |
| 60% corn oil, 40% butter, 4-oz. stick | 31 | .07 | 3 | 26 | 40 | n.a. | n.a. | n.a. |
| 60% corn oil, 40% butter, 1 tsp. . . . . . | 1 | 0 | 0 | 1 | 2 | n.a. | n.a. | n.a. |
| **Marinara sauce,** see "Tomato sauce" | | | | | | | | |
| **Marjoram,** dried, 1 tsp. | 12 | .50 | 2 | 2 | 9 | .02 | .01 | .03 |
| **Marmalade:** | | | | | | | | |
| citrus, 1 tbsp. . . . . . . . . | 7 | .10 | tr. | 2 | 7 | n.a. | n.a. | n.a. |
| orange, 1 tbsp. . . . . . . . | 8 | .03 | 0 | n.a. | 7 | .01 | .02 | tr. |
| **Marshmallow,** see "Candy" | | | | | | | | |
| **Marshmallow creme topping,** 1 oz. . . . . . . . | 1 | .06 | 1 | 2 | 1 | .01 | .03 | tr. |
| **Mayonnaise dressing,** 1 tbsp. . . . . . . . . . . . | 2 | tr. | n.a. | 4 | 1 | n.a. | n.a. | n.a. |
| **Melon,** see specific listings | | | | | | | | |
| **Melon balls** (cantaloupe and honeydew), frozen, ½ cup . . . . . . . . . . . | 9 | .25 | 12 | 11 | 242 | .15 | .05 | .03 |
| **Mexican seasoning** (*Tone's Perc*), ¼ tsp. . . . . . . . . . . . . . | 3 | .24 | 1 | 3 | 15 | .02 | tr. | .01 |
| **Milk,** cow, fluid: | | | | | | | | |
| buttermilk, cultured, 1 cup . . . . . . . . . . . . | 285 | .12 | 27 | 219 | 371 | 1.03 | .03 | .01 |

| | Calcium | Iron | Magnesium | Phosphorus | Potassium | Zinc | Copper | Manganese |
|---|---|---|---|---|---|---|---|---|
| | (Mg) | (Mg) | (Mg) | (Mg) | (Mg) | (Mg) | (Mg) | (Mg) |
| **whole:** | | | | | | | | |
| 3.3% fat, 1 cup . . . . . | 291 | .12 | 33 | 228 | 370 | .93 | .02 | .01 |
| 3.7% fat, producer, | | | | | | | | |
| 1 cup . . . . . . . . . | 290 | .12 | 33 | 227 | 368 | .93 | .02 | .01 |
| low sodium, 1 cup. . . | 246 | n.a. | 12 | 209 | 617 | n.a. | .02 | .01 |
| **low fat 2%:** | | | | | | | | |
| 1 cup . . . . . . . . . . . | 297 | .12 | 33 | 232 | 377 | .95 | .02 | .01 |
| nonfat milk solids | | | | | | | | |
| added, 1 cup . . . . . | 313 | .12 | 35 | 245 | 397 | .98 | .02 | .01 |
| protein fortified, | | | | | | | | |
| 1 cup . . . . . . . . . | 352 | .15 | 40 | 276 | 447 | 1.11 | .02 | .01 |
| **low fat 1%:** | | | | | | | | |
| 1 cup . . . . . . . . . . . | 300 | .12 | 34 | 235 | 381 | .95 | .02 | .01 |
| nonfat milk solids | | | | | | | | |
| added, 1 cup . . . . . | 313 | .12 | 35 | 245 | 397 | .98 | .02 | .01 |
| protein fortified, | | | | | | | | |
| 1 cup . . . . . . . . . | 349 | .15 | 39 | 273 | 444 | 1.11 | .02 | .01 |
| **skim:** | | | | | | | | |
| 1 cup . . . . . . . . . . . | 302 | .10 | 28 | 247 | 406 | .98 | .03 | .01 |
| nonfat milk solids | | | | | | | | |
| added, 1 cup . . . . . | 316 | .12 | 36 | 255 | 418 | 1.00 | .03 | .01 |
| protein fortified, | | | | | | | | |
| 1 cup . . . . . . . . . | 352 | .15 | 40 | 275 | 446 | 1.11 | .03 | .01 |
| **Milk, canned:** | | | | | | | | |
| condensed, sweetened, | | | | | | | | |
| 1 cup . . . . . . . . . . . | 868 | .58 | 78 | 775 | 1136 | 2.88 | .05 | .02 |
| evaporated, whole, | | | | | | | | |
| 1 cup . . . . . . . . . . . | 658 | .48 | 60 | 510 | 764 | 1.94 | .04 | .02 |
| evaporated, skim, | | | | | | | | |
| 1 cup . . . . . . . . . . . | 738 | .74 | 68 | 496 | 846 | 2.30 | .04 | .02 |
| **Milk, dry:** | | | | | | | | |
| buttermilk, sweet cream, | | | | | | | | |
| 1 oz. . . . . . . . . . . . . . | 336 | .09 | 31 | 265 | 451 | 1.14 | .03 | .01 |
| whole, 1 oz. . . . . . . . . . . | 259 | .13 | 24 | 220 | 377 | .94 | .02 | .01 |
| nonfat: | | | | | | | | |
| regular, 1 oz. . . . . . . | 356 | .09 | 31 | 274 | 509 | 1.16 | .01 | .01 |

| | Calcium (Mg) | Iron (Mg) | Magnesium (Mg) | Phosphorus (Mg) | Potassium (Mg) | Zinc (Mg) | Copper (Mg) | Manganese (Mg) |
|---|---|---|---|---|---|---|---|---|
| **Milk, dry, nonfat,** _continued_ | | | | | | | | |
| calcium reduced, | | | | | | | | |
| 1 oz. . . . . . . . . . . | 79 | n.a. | 17 | 287 | 193 | n.a. | .01 | tr. |
| instant, 1 oz. . . . . . . . | 349 | .09 | 33 | 279 | 483 | 1.25 | .01 | .01 |
| **Milk, goat,** fluid, whole, | | | | | | | | |
| 1 cup . . . . . . . . . . . . | 326 | .12 | 34 | 270 | 499 | .73 | .11 | .04 |
| **Milk, human,** fluid, | | | | | | | | |
| whole, 1 cup . . . . . . . . | 79 | .07 | 8 | 34 | 126 | .42 | .13 | .06 |
| **Milk, imitation,** fluid, | | | | | | | | |
| 1 cup . . . . . . . . . . . . | 79 | .95 | 16 | 181 | 279 | 2.88 | .12 | .23 |
| **Milk, Indian buffalo,** | | | | | | | | |
| fluid, whole, 1 cup . . . . | 412 | .29 | 76 | 286 | 434 | .54 | .11 | .04 |
| **Milk, sheep,** fluid, whole, | | | | | | | | |
| 1 cup . . . . . . . . . . . . | 474 | .24 | 45 | 387 | 334 | n.a. | .11 | .04 |
| **Milkfish,** meat only: | | | | | | | | |
| raw, 1 lb.. . . . . . . . . . | 232 | 1.45 | na. | 737 | n.a. | 3.73 | .15 | n.a. |
| baked, broiled, or | | | | | | | | |
| microwaved[1], 4 oz. . . . | 73 | .46 | n.a. | 236 | n.a. | 1.19 | .05 | .04 |
| **Millet:** | | | | | | | | |
| uncooked, 1 oz.. . . . . . . . | 2 | .85 | 32 | 81 | 55 | .48 | .21 | .46 |
| uncooked, ½ cup. . . . . . . | 8 | 3.01 | 114 | 285 | 195 | 1.68 | .75 | 1.63 |
| cooked, 1 cup . . . . . . . . | 8 | 1.51 | 105 | 240 | 148 | 2.18 | .39 | .65 |
| **Miso:** | | | | | | | | |
| 1 lb. . . . . . . . . . . . . . . | 301 | 12.41 | 191 | 692 | 744 | 15.05 | 1.98 | 3.90 |
| ½ cup. . . . . . . . . . . . . . | 92 | 3.78 | 58 | 211 | 226 | 4.58 | .60 | 1.19 |
| **Molasses:** | | | | | | | | |
| 1 tbsp. . . . . . . . . . . . . | 41 | .94 | 48 | 6 | 293 | .06 | .10 | .31 |
| blackstrap, 1 tbsp. . . . . . . | 172 | 3.50 | 43 | 8 | 498 | .20 | .41 | .52 |
| **Molasses,** cane, | | | | | | | | |
| blackstrap, 1 tbsp. . . . . | 137 | 5.05 | n.a. | 17 | 586 | n.a. | n.a. | n.a. |
| **Monkfish,** meat only: | | | | | | | | |
| raw, 1 lb.. . . . . . . . . . | 37 | 1.46 | 95 | n.a. | n.a. | 1.86 | .13 | .11 |
| baked, broiled, or | | | | | | | | |
| microwaved[1], 4 oz. . . . | 11 | .46 | 31 | n.a. | n.a. | .60 | .04 | .04 |

[1] _Prepared without added ingredients._

| | Calcium | Iron | Magnesium | Phosphorus | Potassium | Zinc | Copper | Manganese |
|---|---|---|---|---|---|---|---|---|
| | (Mg) | (Mg) | (Mg) | (Mg) | (Mg) | (Mg) | (Mg) | (Mg) |
| **Mortadella,** beef and pork, 1 oz. . . . . . . . . . | 5 | .40 | 3 | 27 | 46 | .60 | .02 | .01 |
| **Moth beans,** dried: | | | | | | | | |
| uncooked, 1 lb. . . . . . . . | 681 | 49.21 | 1727 | 2219 | 5400 | 8.71 | 3.12 | 8.26 |
| uncooked, ½ cup. . . . . . . | 147 | 10.63 | 373 | 479 | 1167 | 1.88 | .67 | 1.78 |
| boiled, ½ cup . . . . . . . . | 3 | 2.76 | 91 | 132 | 268 | .52 | .14 | .46 |
| **Mother's loaf,** pork, 1 oz. | 12 | .38 | 4 | 37 | 64 | .41 | .03 | .02 |
| **Muffin:** | | | | | | | | |
| blueberry, 2-oz. piece. . . . | 33 | .92 | 9 | 112 | 70 | .28 | .04 | .25 |
| blueberry, toaster type, 1.2-oz. piece . . . . . . . . | 4 | .17 | n.a. | n.a. | 27 | n.a. | n.a. | n.a. |
| blueberry, toaster type, toasted, 1.1-oz. piece | 4 | .17 | n.a. | n.a. | 27 | n.a. | n.a. | n.a. |
| corn, 2-oz. piece . . . . . . . | 42 | 1.60 | n.a. | 162 | 39 | n.a. | n.a. | n.a. |
| corn, toaster type, 1.2-oz. piece . . . . . . . . | 6 | .49 | n.a. | n.a. | 30 | n.a. | n.a. | n.a. |
| corn, toaster type, toasted, 1.1-oz. piece | 6 | .48 | n.a. | n.a. | 30 | n.a. | n.a. | n.a. |
| English: | | | | | | | | |
| plain, 2-oz. piece . . . . | 99 | 1.42 | 12 | 76 | 75 | .40 | .07 | .20 |
| plain, toasted, 1.8-oz. piece . . . . . | 99 | 1.41 | 12 | 75 | 74 | .40 | .07 | .20 |
| mixed grain, 2.3-oz. piece . . . . . | 129 | 2.00 | n.a. | n.a. | 103 | n.a. | n.a. | n.a. |
| mixed grain, toasted, 2.2-oz. piece . . . . . | 130 | 2.00 | n.a. | n.a. | 103 | n.a. | n.a. | n.a. |
| raisin-cinnamon, 2-oz. piece. . . . . . . | 84 | 1.38 | 9 | n.a. | 119 | .57 | n.a. | n.a. |
| raisin-cinnamon, toasted, 1.8-oz. piece . . . . . | 83 | 1.37 | 9 | n.a. | 118 | .57 | n.a. | n.a. |
| wheat, 2-oz. piece . . . | 101 | 1.63 | n.a. | n.a. | 106 | n.a. | n.a. | n.a. |
| wheat, toasted, 1.8-oz. piece . . . . . | 100 | 1.62 | n.a. | n.a. | 105 | n.a. | n.a. | n.a. |
| whole wheat, 2.3-oz. piece . . . . . . . . . . | 175 | 1.62 | 47 | 186 | 139 | 1.06 | n.a. | 1.18 |

|  | Calcium | Iron | Magnesium | Phosphorus | Potassium | Zinc | Copper | Manganese |
|---|---|---|---|---|---|---|---|---|
|  | (Mg) | (Mg) | (Mg) | (Mg) | (Mg) | (Mg) | (Mg) | (Mg) |
| **Muffin, English,** *continued* | | | | | | | | |
| whole wheat, toasted, 2.2-oz. piece . . . . . | 176 | 1.62 | 47 | 187 | 1.39 | 1.06 | n.a. | 1.19 |
| oat bran, 2-oz. piece . . . . | 36 | 2.39 | 89 | 214 | 289 | 1.05 | .19 | 1.5 |
| wheat bran, toaster type w/raisins, 1.3-oz. piece . . . . . . . . . . . . . | 13 | .96 | n.a. | n.a. | 60 | n.a. | n.a. | n.a. |
| wheat bran, toaster type w/raisins, toasted, 1.2-oz. piece . . . . . . . . | 13 | .96 | n.a. | n.a. | 60 | n.a. | n.a. | n.a. |
| **Muffin mix**[1]: | | | | | | | | |
| blueberry, 1.6-oz. piece | 15 | .90 | n.a. | 90 | 54 | n.a. | n.a. | n.a. |
| bran, 1.6-oz. piece . . . . . . | 27 | 1.70 | n.a. | 182 | 50 | n.a. | n.a. | n.a. |
| corn, 1.6-oz. piece . . . . . . | 30 | 1.30 | n.a. | 128 | 31 | n.a. | n.a. | n.a. |
| **Mulberry,** fresh: | | | | | | | | |
| untrimmed, 1 lb. . . . . . . . | 179 | 8.39 | 83 | 172 | 879 | n.a. | n.a. | n.a. |
| trimmed, ½ cup. . . . . . . . | 28 | 1.30 | 13 | 27 | 136 | n.a. | n.a. | n.a. |
| **Mullet,** striped, meat only: | | | | | | | | |
| raw, 1 lb. . . . . . . . . . . . . | 184 | 4.64 | 130 | 1004 | 1620 | 2.37 | .02 | .07 |
| baked, broiled, or microwaved[2], 4 oz. . . . | 35 | 1.60 | 37 | 277 | 519 | 1.00 | .16 | .02 |
| **Mung beans,** dried: | | | | | | | | |
| uncooked, 1 lb. . . . . . . . . | 599 | 30.55 | 867 | 1663 | 5652 | 12.13 | 4.27 | 4.70 |
| uncooked, ½ cup. . . . . . . | 137 | 7.01 | 196 | 381 | 1296 | 2.78 | .98 | 1.08 |
| boiled, ½ cup . . . . . . . . . | 27 | 1.42 | 48 | 100 | 268 | .85 | .16 | .30 |
| **Mung beans, sprouted,** mature seeds: | | | | | | | | |
| raw: | | | | | | | | |
| 1 lb. . . . . . . . . . . . . | 57 | 4.11 | 96 | 246 | 674 | 1.85 | .74 | .85 |
| 12-oz. pkg. . . . . . . . . | 43 | 3.08 | 72 | 184 | 505 | 1.39 | .56 | .64 |
| ½ cup . . . . . . . . . . . | 7 | .47 | 11 | 28 | 77 | .21 | .09 | .10 |
| boiled, drained, ½ cup . . . | 7 | .40 | 9 | 17 | 63 | .29 | .08 | .09 |
| canned, drained, ½ cup | 9 | .27 | 5 | 20 | 17 | n.a. | .10 | .05 |

---

[1] *Prepared according to package directions, with eggs and water.*
[2] *Prepared without added ingredients.*

| | Calcium | Iron | Magnesium | Phosphorus | Potassium | Zinc | Copper | Manganese |
|---|---|---|---|---|---|---|---|---|
| | (Mg) | (Mg) | (Mg) | (Mg) | (Mg) | (Mg) | (Mg) | (Mg) |
| **Mungo beans,** dried: | | | | | | | | |
| uncooked, 1 lb......... | 889 | 31.01 | 1181 | 2610 | 4647 | 13.97 | 2.99 | 7.32 |
| uncooked, ½ cup....... | 204 | 7.11 | 271 | 598 | 1065 | 3.20 | .69 | 1.68 |
| boiled, ½ cup ......... | 48 | 1.57 | 56 | 140 | 208 | .75 | .13 | .37 |
| **Mushroom:** | | | | | | | | |
| raw: | | | | | | | | |
| untrimmed, 1 lb. .... | 24 | 5.44 | .46 | 457 | 1629 | 3.21 | 2.17 | .49 |
| 1 medium, approx. | | | | | | | | |
| .7 oz............ | 1 | .22 | 2 | 19 | 67 | .13 | .09 | .02 |
| trimmed, pieces, | | | | | | | | |
| ½ cup.......... | 2 | .43 | 4 | 36 | 130 | .17 | .04 | .04 |
| boiled, drained, pieces, | | | | | | | | |
| ½ cup ............. | 4 | 1.36 | 10 | 68 | 277 | .68 | .39 | .09 |
| canned, drained, pieces, | | | | | | | | |
| ½ cup............. | 0 | .62 | n.a. | n.a. | n.a. | .56 | .18 | .07 |
| **Mushroom, enoki,** raw: | | | | | | | | |
| untrimmed, 1 lb........ | 3 | n.a. | 61 | 429 | 1452 | 2.16 | .26 | .31 |
| 1 medium, .1 oz........ | 0 | n.a. | 0 | 3 | 11 | .02 | tr. | tr. |
| **Mushroom, shiitake:** | | | | | | | | |
| dried, 4 oz. ........... | 12 | 1.95 | 150 | 333 | 1740 | n.a. | n.a. | n.a. |
| dried, 1 medium, approx. | | | | | | | | |
| .1 oz............... | 0 | .06 | 5 | 11 | 55 | n.a. | n.a. | n.a. |
| cooked, pieces, 1 cup ... | 4 | .64 | 20 | 43 | 170 | n.a. | n.a. | n.a. |
| **Mushroom gravy:** | | | | | | | | |
| canned, ¼ cup ........ | 4 | .39 | n.a. | 9 | 63 | .42 | .06 | .18 |
| mix, vegetarian (*Loma Linda Gravy Quik*), | | | | | | | | |
| 1 tbsp., .2 oz. ....... | 1 | .29 | n.a. | n.a. | 31 | .05 | n.a. | n.a. |
| **Mussels,** blue, meat only: | | | | | | | | |
| raw, 1 lb.............. | 119 | 17.91 | 153 | 895 | 1450 | 7.25 | .43 | n.a. |
| raw, 1 cup............ | 39 | 5.92 | 51 | 296 | 479 | 2.40 | .14 | n.a. |
| boiled, poached, or | | | | | | | | |
| steamed[1], 4 oz. ...... | 37 | 7.62 | 42 | 323 | 304 | 3.03 | .17 | n.a. |

[1] *Prepared without added ingredients.*

| | Calcium | Iron | Magnesium | Phosphorus | Potassium | Zinc | Copper | Manganese |
|---|---|---|---|---|---|---|---|---|
| | (Mg) | (Mg) | (Mg) | (Mg) | (Mg) | (Mg) | (Mg) | (Mg) |
| **Mustard,** prepared, | | | | | | | | |
| yellow, 1 tsp......... | 4 | .10 | n.a. | 4 | 7 | n.a. | n.a. | n.a. |
| **Mustard greens:** | | | | | | | | |
| fresh: | | | | | | | | |
| raw, untrimmed, 1 lb. | 436 | 6.16 | 133 | 180 | 1495 | n.a. | n.a. | n.a. |
| raw, trimmed, | | | | | | | | |
| chopped, ½ cup .. | 29 | .41 | 9 | 12 | 99 | n.a. | n.a. | n.a. |
| boiled, drained, | | | | | | | | |
| chopped, ½ cup .. | 52 | .49 | 10 | 29 | 141 | n.a. | n.a. | n.a. |
| frozen, chopped: | | | | | | | | |
| 10-oz. pkg. ........ | 329 | 3.67 | 42 | 84 | 481 | .65 | .19 | .96 |
| boiled, drained, ⅓ of | | | | | | | | |
| 10-oz. pkg. ...... | 71 | .79 | 9 | 17 | 98 | .14 | .04 | .21 |
| boiled, drained, | | | | | | | | |
| ½ cup.......... | 75 | .84 | 10 | 18 | 104 | .15 | .04 | .22 |
| **Mustard seeds,** yellow, | | | | | | | | |
| 1 tsp. ............. | 17 | .33 | 10 | 28 | 23 | .19 | .01 | .06 |

# N

| | Calcium (Mg) | Iron (Mg) | Magnesium (Mg) | Phosphorus (Mg) | Potassium (Mg) | Zinc (Mg) | Copper (Mg) | Manganese (Mg) |
|---|---|---|---|---|---|---|---|---|
| **Natto:** | | | | | | | | |
| 1 lb. . . . . . . . . . . . . . . . | 984 | 39.01 | 521 | 789 | 3309 | 13.74 | 3.03 | 6.93 |
| ½ cup . . . . . . . . . . . . . . | 191 | 7.57 | 101 | 153 | 642 | 2.67 | .59 | 1.35 |
| **Navy beans,** dried: | | | | | | | | |
| uncooked, 1 lb. . . . . . . . . | 702 | 29.21 | 783 | 2009 | 5172 | 11.51 | 3.99 | 5.94 |
| uncooked, ½ cup. . . . . . . | 161 | 6.70 | 180 | 461 | 1186 | 2.64 | .91 | 1.36 |
| boiled, ½ cup . . . . . . . . . | 64 | 2.25 | 53 | 143 | 335 | .97 | .27 | .51 |
| canned, w/liquid, 8 oz. . . . | 107 | 4.19 | 106 | 305 | 654 | 1.75 | .47 | .85 |
| canned, w/liquid, | | | | | | | | |
| ½ cup . . . . . . . . . . . . . | 62 | 2.42 | 61 | 176 | 378 | 1.01 | .27 | .49 |
| **Nectarine:** | | | | | | | | |
| untrimmed, 1 lb. . . . . . . . | 19 | .63 | 32 | 66 | 874 | .35 | .30 | .18 |
| 1 medium, 2½" diam., | | | | | | | | |
| 5.3 oz. . . . . . . . . . . . . | 6 | .21 | 11 | 22 | 288 | .12 | .10 | .06 |
| pitted, sliced, ½ cup . . . . | 3 | .11 | 6 | 11 | 146 | .06 | .05 | .03 |
| **New England brand** | | | | | | | | |
| **sausage,** | | | | | | | | |
| pork and beef, 1 oz. . . . . . | 2 | .27 | 4 | 39 | 91 | .77 | .03 | .01 |
| **New Zealand spinach:** | | | | | | | | |
| raw, untrimmed, 1 lb. . . . | 189 | 2.61 | 127 | 91 | 425 | n.a. | n.a. | n.a. |
| raw, chopped, ½ cup. . . . | 16 | .22 | 11 | 8 | 36 | n.a. | n.a. | n.a. |
| boiled, drained, chopped, | | | | | | | | |
| ½ cup . . . . . . . . . . . . . | 43 | .59 | 29 | 20 | 92 | n.a. | n.a. | n.a. |
| **Noodle,** egg, enriched, dry: | | | | | | | | |
| uncooked, plain 2 oz. . . . . | 17 | 2.59 | 34 | 122 | 133 | .91 | .17 | .41 |
| uncooked, spinach, | | | | | | | | |
| 2 oz. . . . . . . . . . . . . . . | 32 | 2.40 | 47 | 110 | 203 | 1.04 | .15 | .58 |
| cooked, plain, 1 cup . . . . | 19 | 2.55 | 31 | 110 | 45 | 1.00 | .14 | .42 |
| cooked, spinach, 1 cup . . . | 30 | 1.74 | 38 | 91 | 59 | 1.01 | .13 | .51 |
| **Noodle, Chinese,** dehydrated: | | | | | | | | |
| chow mein, 1 cup . . . . . . | 9 | 2.13 | 23 | 72 | 54 | .63 | .08 | .61 |
| long rice or cellophane, | | | | | | | | |
| uncooked, 2 oz. . . . . . . . | 14 | 1.23 | 2 | 18 | 6 | n.a. | n.a. | n.a. |

| | Calcium | Iron | Magnesium | Phosphorus | Potassium | Zinc | Copper | Manganese |
|---|---|---|---|---|---|---|---|---|
| | (Mg) | (Mg) | (Mg) | (Mg) | (Mg) | (Mg) | (Mg) | (Mg) |
| **Noodle, Chinese,** *continued* | | | | | | | | |
| long rice, mung bean, | | | | | | | | |
| uncooked, ½ cup..... | 17 | 1.52 | 2 | 22 | 7 | n.a. | n.a. | n.a. |
| **Noodle, Japanese,** dry: | | | | | | | | |
| soba, uncooked, 2 oz. ... | 20 | 1.54 | 54 | 145 | 143 | .97 | .13 | n.a. |
| soba, cooked, 1 cup, | | | | | | | | |
| approx. 4 oz........ | 4 | .55 | 11 | 29 | 40 | .14 | .01 | n.a. |
| somen, uncooked, 2 oz. | 13 | .75 | 16 | 46 | 94 | .26 | .08 | .27 |
| somen, cooked, 1 cup | 14 | .92 | 4 | 47 | 51 | .39 | .05 | .44 |
| **Nopal:** | | | | | | | | |
| raw, untrimmed, 1 lb. | 710 | 2.95 | 251 | 74 | 1390 | 1.28 | .25 | 2.20 |
| raw, trimmed, sliced, | | | | | | | | |
| ½ cup............. | 70 | .29 | 25 | 7 | 137 | .13 | .02 | .22 |
| boiled, drained, 1 cup ... | 245 | .74 | 70 | 23 | 290 | .32 | .07 | .61 |
| **Nutmeg,** ground, | | | | | | | | |
| 1 tsp. ............. | 4 | .07 | 4 | 5 | 8 | .05 | .02 | .06 |
| **Nuts,** see specific listings | | | | | | | | |
| **Nuts, mixed:** | | | | | | | | |
| w/peanuts[1]: | | | | | | | | |
| dry-roasted, 1 oz. ... | 20 | 1.05 | 64 | 124 | 169 | 1.08 | .36 | .55 |
| dry-roasted, 1 cup ... | 96 | 5.07 | 308 | 596 | 817 | 5.21 | 1.75 | 2.65 |
| oil-roasted, 1 oz..... | 31 | .91 | 67 | 132 | 165 | 1.44 | .47 | .54 |
| oil-roasted, 1 cup.... | 153 | 4.56 | 333 | 659 | 825 | 7.22 | 2.36 | 2.69 |
| w/out peanuts[2], oil- | | | | | | | | |
| roasted, 1 oz. ....... | 30 | .73 | 71 | 127 | 154 | 1.32 | .51 | .44 |
| w/out peanuts[2], oil- | | | | | | | | |
| roasted, 1 cup ....... | 153 | 3.70 | 361 | 646 | 783 | 6.71 | 2.59 | 2.23 |

[1] *Mixture of cashews, peanuts, Brazil nuts, filberts, almonds, and pecans.*
[2] *Mixture of cashews, almonds, Brazil nuts, pecans, and filberts.*

# O

| | Calcium | Iron | Magnesium | Phosphorus | Potassium | Zinc | Copper | Manganese |
|---|---|---|---|---|---|---|---|---|
| | (Mg) | (Mg) | (Mg) | (Mg) | (Mg) | (Mg) | (Mg) | (Mg) |
| **Oat** (see also "Cereal"): | | | | | | | | |
| whole grain, 1 cup...... | 84 | 7.37 | 276 | 816 | 669 | 6.19 | .98 | 7.67 |
| rolled or oatmeal: | | | | | | | | |
|    uncooked, 1 oz...... | 15 | 1.19 | 42 | 134 | 99 | .87 | .10 | 1.03 |
|    uncooked, 1 cup .... | 42 | 3.41 | 120 | 384 | 284 | 2.48 | .28 | 2.94 |
|    cooked, 1 cup ...... | 20 | 1.59 | 56 | 178 | 132 | 1.15 | .13 | 1.37 |
| **Oat bran** (see also "Cereal"): | | | | | | | | |
| raw, 1 oz. ............ | 16 | 1.53 | 67 | 208 | 160 | .88 | .11 | 1.60 |
| raw, ½ cup ........... | 27 | 2.54 | 110 | 345 | 266 | 1.46 | .19 | 2.65 |
| cooked, 1 cup ........ | 22 | 1.93 | 88 | 262 | 202 | 1.17 | .14 | 2.11 |
| **Ocean perch,** Atlantic, meat only: | | | | | | | | |
| raw, 1 lb............. | 486 | 4.18 | 138 | 979 | 1240 | 2.17 | .12 | .07 |
| baked, broiled, or | | | | | | | | |
|   microwaved[1], 4 oz. .... | 155 | 1.34 | 44 | 314 | 397 | .69 | .04 | n.a. |
| **Octopus,** meat only: | | | | | | | | |
| raw, 1 lb.............. | 243 | 24.04 | n.a. | 844 | n.a. | 7.63 | 1.97 | .11 |
| boiled, poached, or | | | | | | | | |
|   steamed[1], 4 oz....... | 120 | 10.82 | n.a. | 316 | n.a. | 3.81 | .84 | .05 |
| **Oheloberry,** fresh, 1 cup | 10 | .13 | 9 | 14 | 54 | n.a. | n.a. | n.a. |
| **Oil,** corn, olive, peanut, | | | | | | | | |
|   safflower, soybean | | | | | | | | |
|   (hydrogenated), | | | | | | | | |
|   soybean-cottonseed | | | | | | | | |
|   blend (hydrogenated), | | | | | | | | |
|   or sunflower, 1 tbsp. | 0 | 0 | (0) | 0 | 0 | n.a. | n.a. | n.a. |
| **Okra:** | | | | | | | | |
| fresh: | | | | | | | | |
|   raw, untrimmed, | | | | | | | | |
|     1 lb. .......... | 316 | 3.12 | 2.20 | 246 | 1180 | 2.32 | .37 | 3.86 |
|   raw, trimmed, sliced, | | | | | | | | |
|     ½ cup .......... | 41 | .40 | 28 | 32 | 151 | .30 | .05 | .50 |

---

[1] *Prepared without added ingredients.*

| | Calcium (Mg) | Iron (Mg) | Magnesium (Mg) | Phosphorus (Mg) | Potassium (Mg) | Zinc (Mg) | Copper (Mg) | Manganese (Mg) |
|---|---|---|---|---|---|---|---|---|
| Okra, fresh, *continued* | | | | | | | | |
| boiled, drained, | | | | | | | | |
| sliced, ½ cup . . . . . | 50 | .36 | 46 | 45 | 257 | .44 | .07 | .73 |
| frozen: | | | | | | | | |
| 10-oz. pkg. . . . . . . . | 231 | 1.62 | 123 | 119 | 600 | 1.49 | .24 | 2.48 |
| boiled, drained, ⅓ of | | | | | | | | |
| 10-oz. pkg. . . . . . | 82 | .57 | 43 | 39 | 199 | .53 | .08 | 86 |
| boiled, drained, | | | | | | | | |
| sliced, ½ cup . . . . . | 88 | .62 | 47 | 42 | 215 | .57 | .09 | .94 |
| **Olive,** ripe, pitted, canned: | | | | | | | | |
| Mission and Manzanilla: | | | | | | | | |
| all sizes, 1 oz. . . . . . . | 25 | .94 | 1 | 1 | 2 | .06 | .07 | tr. |
| 10 small, 1.1 oz. . . . . | 28 | 1.06 | 1 | 1 | 3 | .07 | .08 | tr. |
| 10 large, 1.6 oz. . . . . | 39 | 1.45 | 2 | 1 | 4 | .10 | .11 | .01 |
| Sevillano and Ascolano: | | | | | | | | |
| all sizes, 1 oz. . . . . . . | 27 | .94 | n.a. | n.a. | 3 | n.a. | .06 | n.a. |
| 10 jumbo, 2.9 oz. . . . | 78 | 2.76 | n.a. | n.a. | 7 | n.a. | .19 | n.a. |
| 10 supercolossal, | | | | | | | | |
| 5.4 oz. . . . . . . . . . . | 143 | 5.05 | n.a. | n.a. | 14 | n.a. | .34 | n.a. |
| **Olive loaf,** pork, 1-oz. | | | | | | | | |
| slice . . . . . . . . . . . . . | 31 | .15 | 5 | 36 | 84 | .39 | .01 | .01 |
| **Onion,** mature: | | | | | | | | |
| fresh: | | | | | | | | |
| raw, untrimmed, 1 lb. . . | 81 | .89 | 39 | 135 | 640 | .77 | .25 | .56 |
| raw, trimmed, | | | | | | | | |
| chopped, ½ cup . . | 16 | .17 | 8 | 27 | 125 | .15 | .05 | .11 |
| boiled, drained, | | | | | | | | |
| chopped, ½ cup . . | 23 | .26 | 11 | 37 | 174 | .22 | .07 | .16 |
| canned, w/liquid, | | | | | | | | |
| chopped, ½ cup . . . . . | 51 | .15 | 6 | 31 | 124 | .32 | .06 | .11 |
| frozen: | | | | | | | | |
| whole, 10-oz. | | | | | | | | |
| pkg. . . . . . . . . . . . | 102 | 1.29 | 29 | 66 | 402 | .33 | .14 | .36 |
| chopped, 10-oz. | | | | | | | | |
| pkg. . . . . . . . . . . . | 50 | .93 | 20 | 61 | 353 | .19 | .05 | .21 |

| | Calcium | Iron | Magnesium | Phosphorus | Potassium | Zinc | Copper | Manganese |
|---|---|---|---|---|---|---|---|---|
| | (Mg) | (Mg) | (Mg) | (Mg) | (Mg) | (Mg) | (Mg) | (Mg) |
| boiled, drained, chopped, ½ cup .. | 17 | .32 | 7 | 20 | 114 | .07 | .02 | .08 |
| **Onion, green** (scallion), w/top, raw: | | | | | | | | |
| untrimmed, 1 lb. . . . . . . | 314 | 645 | 88 | 161 | 1202 | 1.72 | .36 | .70 |
| chopped, ½ cup . . . . . . . | 36 | .74 | 10 | 18 | 138 | .20 | .04 | .08 |
| chopped, 1 tbsp. . . . . . . . | 4 | .09 | 1 | 2 | 17 | .02 | .01 | .01 |
| **Onion flakes,** dehydrated, 1 tbsp. . . . . . . . . . . . | 13 | .08 | 5 | 15 | 81 | .09 | .02 | .07 |
| **Onion gravy mix** (*Loma Linda Gravy Quik*), 1 tbsp., .2 oz. . . . . . . . | 1 | .10 | n.a. | n.a. | 25 | .04 | n.a. | n.a. |
| **Onion powder,** 1 tsp. . . . | 8 | .05 | 3 | 7 | 20 | .05 | .04 | .01 |
| **Onion rings**[1], frozen: | | | | | | | | |
| 9-oz. pkg. . . . . . . . . . . . | 117 | 2.37 | n.a. | n.a. | 483 | n.a. | n.a. | n.a. |
| oven heated, 2 rings, .75 oz. . . . . . . . . . . . . | 6 | .34 | 4 | 16 | 26 | .08 | .02 | .08 |
| **Orange,** fresh: | | | | | | | | |
| all varieties: | | | | | | | | |
| untrimmed, 1 lb. . . . . | 132 | .33 | 33 | 46 | 599 | .23 | .15 | .08 |
| 1 medium, 2⅝" diam., 6.3 oz. . . . . . . . . . | 52 | .13 | 13 | 18 | 237 | .09 | .06 | .03 |
| sections, w/out membrane, ½ cup | 72 | .18 | 18 | 25 | 326 | .13 | .08 | .05 |
| California navel: | | | | | | | | |
| untrimmed, 1 lb. . . . . | 123 | .37 | 32 | 59 | 550 | .19 | .17 | .08 |
| 1 medium, 2⅞" diam., 7.3 oz. . . . . . . . . . | 56 | .17 | 15 | 27 | 250 | .08 | .08 | .04 |
| sections, w/out membrane, ½ cup | 33 | .10 | 9 | 16 | 147 | .05 | .05 | .02 |
| California Valencia: | | | | | | | | |
| untrimmed, 1 lb. . . . . | 136 | .31 | 34 | 58 | 609 | .20 | .13 | .08 |
| 1 medium, 2⅝" diam., 5.7 oz. . . . . . . . . . | 48 | .11 | 12 | 21 | 217 | .07 | .05 | .03 |

---

[1] *Breaded and par-fried in vegetable oil.*

| | Calcium (Mg) | Iron (Mg) | Magnesium (Mg) | Phosphorus (Mg) | Potassium (Mg) | Zinc (Mg) | Copper (Mg) | Manganese (Mg) |
|---|---|---|---|---|---|---|---|---|
| **Orange, California Valencia,** *continued* | | | | | | | | |
| sections, w/out membrane, | | | | | | | | |
| ½ cup . . . . . . . . . | 36 | .08 | 9 | 16 | 161 | .06 | .03 | .02 |
| Florida: | | | | | | | | |
| untrimmed, 1 lb. . . . . | 144 | .30 | 34 | 39 | 566 | .27 | .13 | .08 |
| 1 medium, 2¹¹⁄₁₆" | | | | | | | | |
| diam., 7.2 oz. . . . . | 65 | .13 | 15 | 18 | 254 | .12 | .06 | .04 |
| sections, w/out membrane, ½ cup . . . . . | 40 | .08 | 10 | 11 | 156 | .08 | .04 | .02 |
| **Orange, canned,** see "Tangerine" | | | | | | | | |
| **Orange drink,** canned, | | | | | | | | |
| 8 fl. oz. . . . . . . . . . . . | 15 | .69 | 5 | 2 | 45 | .22 | .01 | .04 |
| **Orange extract** (*Virginia Dare*), 1 tsp. . . . . . . . | tr. | tr. | tr. | 0 | 0 | tr. | tr. | n.a. |
| **Orange flavor drink mix,** breakfast, | | | | | | | | |
| 3 rounded tsp. . . . . . . | 46 | .16 | 0 | 31 | 40 | .04 | .02 | .01 |
| **Orange juice:** | | | | | | | | |
| fresh, juice from 1 average fruit . . . . . . | 9 | .17 | 9 | 15 | 172 | .04 | .04 | .01 |
| fresh, 6 fl. oz. . . . . . . . . | 20 | .38 | 20 | 32 | 372 | .10 | .08 | .03 |
| canned, 6 fl. oz. . . . . . . . | 18 | .84 | 18 | 24 | 324 | .12 | .11 | .02 |
| chilled, 6 fl. oz. . . . . . . . | 18 | .30 | 18 | 24 | 354 | .06 | .07 | .04 |
| frozen, diluted, 6 fl. oz. | 18 | .18 | 18 | 30 | 354 | .12 | .08 | .02 |
| **Orange peel,** fresh, 1 tsp. . . . . . . . . . | 3 | .02 | tr. | tr. | 4 | n.a. | n.a. | n.a. |
| **Orange-grapefruit juice,** canned, 6 fl. oz. . . . . . . | 18 | .84 | 18 | 24 | 294 | .12 | .14 | .03 |
| **Oregano,** ground, 1 tsp. . . . . . . . . . | 24 | .66 | 4 | 3 | 25 | .07 | .01 | .07 |
| **Oriental seasoning** (*Tone's Perc*), ¼ tsp. . . . . . . . . . . . | 1 | .47 | tr. | 1 | 11 | .01 | tr. | tr. |

| | Calcium | Iron | Magnesium | Phosphorus | Potassium | Zinc | Copper | Manganese |
|---|---|---|---|---|---|---|---|---|
| | (Mg) | (Mg) | (Mg) | (Mg) | (Mg) | (Mg) | (Mg) | (Mg) |
| **Oyster, Eastern,** meat only: wild: | | | | | | | | |
| raw, 1 lb.......... | 204 | 30.22 | 215 | 614 | 709 | 411.90 | 20.20 | 1.67 |
| raw, 6 medium, approx. 3 oz...... | 38 | 5.60 | 40 | 114 | 131 | 76.28 | 3.74 | .31 |
| raw, 1 cup......... | 112 | 16.54 | 118 | 336 | 387 | 225.20 | 11.04 | .91 |
| baked, broiled,or microwaved[1], 4 oz. | n.a. | 4.91 | 52 | 154 | 191 | 83.46 | 3.92 | .33 |
| baked, broiled, or microwaved[1], 6 medium ....... | n.a. | 2.56 | 27 | 80 | 99 | 43.42 | 2.04 | .17 |
| boiled or steamed[1], 4 oz. ........... | 102 | 13.60 | 108 | 230 | 319 | 205.95 | 8.58 | .79 |
| boiled or steamed[1], 6 medium ....... | 38 | 5.04 | 40 | 85 | 118 | 76.28 | 3.18 | .29 |
| farmed: | | | | | | | | |
| raw, 1 lb.......... | n.a. | 26.22 | 151 | 422 | 564 | 172.03 | 3.35 | 1.79 |
| raw, 6 medium, approx. 3 oz...... | n.a. | 4.86 | 28 | 78 | 104 | 31.86 | .62 | .33 |
| baked, broiled, or microwaved[1], 4 oz. | n.a. | 8.81 | 37 | 130 | 172 | 51.20 | 1.63 | .48 |
| baked, broiled,or microwaved[1], 6 medium ....... | n.a. | 4.59 | 19 | 68 | 90 | 26.64 | .85 | .25 |
| **Oyster, Eastern, canned:** | | | | | | | | |
| w/liquid, 4 oz. ......... | 51 | 7.60 | 61 | 158 | 260 | 103.14 | 5.06 | n.a. |
| w/liquid, 1 cup. ........ | 111 | 16.62 | 135 | 344 | 568 | 225.56 | 11.06 | n.a. |
| **Oyster, Pacific,** meat only: | | | | | | | | |
| raw, 1 lb............. | 38 | 23.18 | 101 | 735 | 762 | 75.40 | 7.15 | 2.92 |
| raw, 1 medium, approx. 1.75 oz......... | 4 | 2.56 | 11 | 81 | 84 | 8.31 | .79 | .32 |
| boiled or steamed[1], 4 oz. .............. | 18 | 10.43 | 50 | 276 | 342 | 37.69 | 3.04 | 1.39 |

[1] Prepared without added ingredients.

| | Calcium | Iron | Magnesium | Phosphorus | Potassium | Zinc | Copper | Manganese |
|---|---|---|---|---|---|---|---|---|
| | (Mg) | (Mg) | (Mg) | (Mg) | (Mg) | (Mg) | (Mg) | (Mg) |

Oyster, Pacific, *continued*
boiled or steamed[1],
  1 medium . . . . . . . . . . 4   2.30   11   61   76   8.31   .67   .31

**Oyster plant,** see "Salsify"

**Oyster stew,** see "Soup, canned, condensed"

---

[1] *Prepared without added ingredients.*

# P

| | Calcium | Iron | Magnesium | Phosphorus | Potassium | Zinc | Copper | Manganese |
|---|---|---|---|---|---|---|---|---|
| | (Mg) | (Mg) | (Mg) | (Mg) | (Mg) | (Mg) | (Mg) | (Mg) |
| **Palm, hearts of,** canned: | | | | | | | | |
| 1 cup .............. | 84 | 4.58 | 55 | 95 | 259 | 1.67 | .19 | 2.04 |
| 1 heart, 1.1 oz. ........ | 19 | 1.03 | 12 | 21 | 58 | .38 | .44 | .48 |
| **Pancake,** frozen, microwaved, 4" cake, 1.3 oz. ............ | 22 | 1.25 | 5 | 134 | 26 | .24 | .01 | n.a. |
| **Pancake mix,** prepared, 4"-diam. cake, 1.3 oz. | 48 | .59 | 7 | 127 | 67 | .15 | .04 | .10 |
| **Pancake syrup,** see "Syrup, table blends" | | | | | | | | |
| **Pancreas,** braised[1]: | | | | | | | | |
| beef, 4 oz. ............ | 18 | 2.60 | 24 | 514 | 279 | 5.22 | .10 | .24 |
| lamb, 4 oz. ........... | 14 | 2.40 | 22 | 489 | 330 | 3.04 | n.a. | .05 |
| pork, 4 oz. ............ | 18 | 3.05 | 26 | 330 | 191 | 4.86 | .12 | .22 |
| **Papaya:** | | | | | | | | |
| untrimmed, 1-lb. fruit, 3½" × 5⅛" ........ | 72 | .30 | 31 | 16 | 780 | .22 | .05 | .03 |
| peeled and seeded, cubed, ½ cup ....... | 17 | .07 | 7 | 4 | 180 | .05 | .01 | .01 |
| **Papaya nectar,** canned, 6 fl. oz. ........... | 18 | .66 | 6 | 1 | 60 | .30 | .02 | .02 |
| **Paprika,** 1 tsp. ........ | 4 | .50 | 4 | 7 | 49 | .08 | .01 | .02 |
| **Parsley,** fresh, raw: | | | | | | | | |
| untrimmed, 1 lb. ....... | 594 | 26.72 | 217 | 249 | 2388 | 4.60 | .64 | .69 |
| trimmed, 10 sprigs ..... | 14 | .62 | 5 | 6 | 55 | .11 | .02 | .02 |
| trimmed, chopped, ½ cup ............. | 41 | 1.86 | 15 | 17 | 166 | .32 | .05 | .05 |
| **Parsley, Chinese,** see "Coriander" | | | | | | | | |
| **Parsley, dried:** | | | | | | | | |
| 1 tsp. ............... | 4 | .29 | 1 | 1 | 11 | .01 | tr. | .03 |
| freeze-dried, ¼ cup ..... | 2 | .75 | 5 | 8 | 88 | .09 | .01 | .02 |
| freeze-dried, 1 tbsp. ..... | 1 | .22 | 1 | 2 | 25 | .02 | tr. | 01 |

[1] Prepared without added ingredients.

| | Calcium | Iron | Magnesium | Phosphorus | Potassium | Zinc | Copper | Manganese |
|---|---|---|---|---|---|---|---|---|
| | (Mg) | (Mg) | (Mg) | (Mg) | (Mg) | (Mg) | (Mg) | (Mg) |
| **Parsnip:** | | | | | | | | |
| raw, untrimmed, 1 lb. | 137 | 2.26 | 110 | 272 | 1446 | 2.28 | .46 | 2.16 |
| raw, sliced, ½ cup...... | 24 | .39 | 19 | 47 | 251 | .40 | .08 | .38 |
| boiled, drained, sliced, | | | | | | | | |
| ½ cup............. | 29 | .45 | 23 | 54 | 287 | .20 | .11 | .23 |
| **Passion fruit,** purple: | | | | | | | | |
| untrimmed, 1 lb. ....... | 28 | 3.77 | 68 | 160 | 821 | n.a. | n.a. | n.a. |
| trimmed, 1 oz.......... | 3 | .45 | 8 | 19 | 99 | n.a. | n.a. | n.a. |
| **Passion fruit juice,** fresh, | | | | | | | | |
| yellow, 6 fl. oz. ...... | 6 | .66 | 30 | 48 | 516 | n.a. | n.a. | n.a. |
| **Pasta** (see also "Macaroni"), dry: | | | | | | | | |
| uncooked: | | | | | | | | |
| plain, spaghetti, | | | | | | | | |
| enriched, 2 oz..... | 10 | 2.20 | 27 | 85 | 92 | .69 | .15 | .40 |
| plain, spaghetti, protein | | | | | | | | |
| fortified, 2 oz. | 22 | 2.36 | 37 | 93 | 115 | 1.02 | .16 | .52 |
| corn, 2 oz.......... | 2 | .53 | 68 | 144 | 168 | 1.02 | .12 | .28 |
| spinach, 2 oz. ...... | 33 | 1.21 | 99 | 189 | 215 | 1.57 | .28 | 1.51 |
| whole wheat, 2 oz.... | 23 | 2.07 | 81 | 147 | 123 | 1.35 | .26 | 1.74 |
| cooked: | | | | | | | | |
| plain, spaghetti, 1 cup | 10 | 1.96 | 25 | 76 | 44 | .74 | .14 | .40 |
| plain, spaghetti, protein | | | | | | | | |
| fortified, 1 cup .... | 14 | 1.01 | 42 | 70 | 58 | .70 | .12 | .58 |
| corn, 1 cup ........ | 2 | .34 | 50 | 106 | 43 | .88 | .09 | .21 |
| spinach, 1 cup...... | 42 | 1.46 | 87 | 151 | 81 | 1.51 | .29 | 2.11 |
| whole wheat, 1 cup | 21 | 1.49 | 42 | 124 | 61 | 1.13 | .23 | 1.93 |
| **Pasta, refrigerated, fresh,** w/egg: | | | | | | | | |
| uncooked, 4.5 oz. ...... | 19 | 4.29 | 59 | 209 | 229 | 1.56 | .29 | .20 |
| uncooked, spinach, | | | | | | | | |
| 4.5 oz............. | 55 | 4.22 | 80 | 190 | 348 | 1.79 | .25 | 1.00 |
| cooked, 4 oz.......... | 7 | 1.29 | 20 | 71 | 27 | .64 | .11 | .25 |
| cooked, spinach, 4 oz.... | 20 | 1.26 | 27 | 65 | 42 | .71 | .09 | .36 |
| **Pasta sauce,** see "Tomato sauce" | | | | | | | | |
| **Pâté,** liver, canned, | | | | | | | | |
| 1 tbsp. ............. | 9 | .72 | 2 | 26 | 18 | n.a. | .05 | .02. |

| | Calcium | Iron | Magnesium | Phosphorus | Potassium | Zinc | Copper | Manganese |
|---|---|---|---|---|---|---|---|---|
| | (Mg) | (Mg) | (Mg) | (Mg) | (Mg) | (Mg) | (Mg) | (Mg) |
| **Peach:** | | | | | | | | |
| fresh: | | | | | | | | |
| untrimmed, 1 lb. . . . . | 18 | .38 | 23 | 43 | 677 | .47 | .23 | .16 |
| 1 medium, 2½" diam., | | | | | | | | |
| approx. 4 per lb. . . . | 5 | .10 | 6 | 11 | 171 | .12 | .06 | .04 |
| pulp, sliced, ½ cup . . | 5 | .10 | 6 | 11 | 167 | .12 | .06 | .04 |
| canned, halves or slices: | | | | | | | | |
| in water, clingstone, | | | | | | | | |
| ½ cup. . . . . . . . . | 3 | .39 | 6 | 13 | 121 | .11 | .07 | .06 |
| in juice, clingstone or | | | | | | | | |
| freestone, ½ cup | 8 | .33 | 9 | 22 | 159 | .13 | .06 | n.a. |
| in light syrup, | | | | | | | | |
| clingstone, ½ cup | 5 | .45 | 6 | 14 | 122 | .11 | .07 | .06 |
| in heavy syrup, | | | | | | | | |
| clingstone or | | | | | | | | |
| freestone, ½ cup | 4 | .35 | 7 | 15 | 118 | .11 | .07 | .06 |
| canned, spiced, whole, in | | | | | | | | |
| heavy syrup, ½ cup. . . | 8 | .35 | 8 | 12 | 103 | .10 | .12 | n.a. |
| dehydrated, sulfured, | | | | | | | | |
| uncooked, ½ cup. . . . . | 22 | 3.20 | 33 | 94 | 783 | .45 | .29 | .24 |
| dehydrated, sulfured, | | | | | | | | |
| cooked, ½ cup . . . . . . | 19 | 2.74 | 28 | 80 | 671 | .39 | .24 | .21 |
| dried, sulfured, halves: | | | | | | | | |
| uncooked, 1 lb. . . . . . | 128 | 18.43 | 189 | 541 | 4518 | 2.60 | 1.65 | 1.38 |
| uncooked, 10 halves, | | | | | | | | |
| approx. 4.5 oz. . . . | 37 | 5.28 | 54 | 155 | 1295 | .75 | .47 | .40 |
| uncooked, ½ cup. . . . | 23 | 3.25 | 34 | 96 | 797 | .46 | .29 | .24 |
| cooked, unsweetened, | | | | | | | | |
| ½ cup. . . . . . . . . | 12 | 1.69 | 18 | 50 | 413 | .24 | .15 | .13 |
| cooked, sweetened, | | | | | | | | |
| ½ cup. . . . . . . . . | 11 | 1.62 | 17 | 47 | 395 | .23 | .14 | .12 |
| frozen, 10-oz. pkg. . . . . . . | 7 | 1.06 | 14 | 32 | 370 | .14 | .07 | .08 |
| frozen, sweetened, sliced, | | | | | | | | |
| ½ cup. . . . . . . . . . . . | 3 | .47 | 6 | 14 | 163 | .07 | .03 | .04 |
| **Peach nectar,** canned, | | | | | | | | |
| 6 fl. oz. . . . . . . . . . . . . | 12 | .36 | 6 | 12 | 78 | .12 | .13 | .04 |

| | Calcium | Iron | Magnesium | Phosphorus | Potassium | Zinc | Copper | Manganese |
|---|---|---|---|---|---|---|---|---|
| | (Mg) | (Mg) | (Mg) | (Mg) | (Mg) | (Mg) | (Mg) | (Mg) |

**Peanut,** shelled, except as noted:

all types:

| | Calcium | Iron | Magnesium | Phosphorus | Potassium | Zinc | Copper | Manganese |
|---|---|---|---|---|---|---|---|---|
| in shell, 1 lb........ | 304 | 15.17 | 558 | 1244 | 2333 | 10.81 | 3.78 | 6.40 |
| raw, 1 oz. ......... | 26 | 1.28 | 47 | 105 | 197 | .91 | .32 | .54 |
| raw, 1 cup......... | 134 | 6.69 | 246 | 548 | 1029 | 4.77 | 1.67 | 2.82 |
| boiled, 1 oz. ....... | 18 | .32 | 33 | 63 | 58 | .59 | .16 | .33 |
| boiled, 1 cup ...... | 35 | .64 | 64 | 124 | 113 | 1.15 | .31 | .64 |
| dry-roasted, 1 oz. ... | 15 | .63 | 49 | 100 | 184 | .93 | .19 | .58 |
| dry-roasted, 1 cup ... | 79 | 3.30 | 257 | 523 | 960 | 4.83 | .98 | 3.04 |
| oil-roasted, 1 oz. ..... | 25 | .51 | 52 | 145 | 191 | 1.86 | .36 | .58 |
| oil-roasted, 1 cup.... | 126 | 2.63 | 266 | 744 | 982 | 9.55 | 1.87 | 2.97 |

Spanish:

| | Calcium | Iron | Magnesium | Phosphorus | Potassium | Zinc | Copper | Manganese |
|---|---|---|---|---|---|---|---|---|
| raw, 1 oz. ......... | 30 | 1.09 | 53 | 109 | 208 | .59 | .25 | .74 |
| raw, 1 cup......... | 155 | 5.71 | 274 | 566 | 1086 | 3.10 | 1.31 | 3.85 |
| oil-roasted, 1 oz. ..... | 28 | .64 | 47 | 108 | 217 | .56 | .19 | .66 |
| oil-roasted, 1 cup.... | 147 | 3.35 | 246 | 569 | 1141 | 2.94 | .97 | 3.46 |

Valencia:

| | Calcium | Iron | Magnesium | Phosphorus | Potassium | Zinc | Copper | Manganese |
|---|---|---|---|---|---|---|---|---|
| raw, 1 oz. ......... | 17 | .59 | 52 | 94 | 93 | .94 | .33 | .55 |
| raw, 1 cup......... | 90 | 3.05 | 269 | 491 | 485 | 4.88 | 1.71 | 2.89 |
| oil-roasted, 1 oz. ..... | 15 | .46 | 45 | 89 | 171 | .86 | .24 | .48 |
| oil-roasted, 1 cup.... | 78 | 2.38 | 230 | 460 | 881 | 4.43 | 1.21 | 2.48 |

Virginia:

| | Calcium | Iron | Magnesium | Phosphorus | Potassium | Zinc | Copper | Manganese |
|---|---|---|---|---|---|---|---|---|
| raw, 1 oz. ......... | 25 | .71 | 48 | 106 | 193 | 1.24 | .31 | .48 |
| raw, 1 cup......... | 130 | 3.72 | 250 | 554 | 1008 | 6.47 | 1.62 | 2.48 |
| oil-roasted, 1 oz. ..... | 24 | .47 | 53 | 142 | 183 | 1.85 | .36 | .56 |
| oil-roasted, 1 cup.... | 123 | 2.38 | 269 | 723 | 933 | 9.47 | 1.82 | 2.87 |

**Peanut butter:**

| | Calcium | Iron | Magnesium | Phosphorus | Potassium | Zinc | Copper | Manganese |
|---|---|---|---|---|---|---|---|---|
| chunk style, 2 tbsp...... | 13 | .61 | 51 | 101 | 239 | .89 | .17 | .60 |
| smooth style, 2 tbsp..... | 12 | .59 | 51 | 118 | 214 | .93 | .04 | .14 |

**Peanut flour:**

| | Calcium | Iron | Magnesium | Phosphorus | Potassium | Zinc | Copper | Manganese |
|---|---|---|---|---|---|---|---|---|
| defatted, 1 oz. ......... | 39 | .59 | 104 | 213 | 361 | 1.43 | .50 | 1.37 |
| defatted, 1 cup ........ | 84 | 1.26 | 222 | 456 | 774 | 3.06 | 1.08 | 2.94 |
| low fat, 1 oz............ | 36 | 1.33 | 13 | n.a. | 380 | 1.68 | .57 | 1.19 |
| low fat, 1 cup ......... | 78 | 2.84 | 29 | n.a. | 815 | 3.59 | 1.22 | 2.54 |

**Pear:**

fresh:

| | Calcium | Iron | Magnesium | Phosphorus | Potassium | Zinc | Copper | Manganese |
|---|---|---|---|---|---|---|---|---|
| untrimmed, 1 lb. ..... | 47 | 1.03 | 24 | 44 | 523 | .51 | .47 | .32 |

| | Calcium | Iron | Magnesium | Phosphorus | Potassium | Zinc | Copper | Manganese |
|---|---|---|---|---|---|---|---|---|
| | (Mg) | (Mg) | (Mg) | (Mg) | (Mg) | (Mg) | (Mg) | (Mg) |
| Bartlett, 2½" diam. × 3½", approx. | | | | | | | | |
| 2½ per lb........ | 19 | .41 | 9 | 18 | 208 | .20 | .19 | .13 |
| trimmed, w/skin, sliced, ½ cup..... | 10 | .21 | 5 | 9 | 104 | .10 | .09 | .06 |
| canned, halves: | | | | | | | | |
| in water, ½ cup..... | 5 | .26 | 5 | 9 | 65 | .11 | .06 | .04 |
| in juice, ½ cup ..... | 11 | .36 | 9 | 15 | 119 | .11 | .07 | n.a. |
| in light syrup, ½ cup.......... | 7 | .35 | 6 | 9 | 83 | .11 | .06 | .04 |
| in heavy or extra heavy syrup, ½ cup.......... | 6 | .28 | 6 | 9 | 83 | .11 | .06 | .04 |
| dried, sulfured, halves: | | | | | | | | |
| uncooked, 1 lb...... | 152 | 9.53 | 150 | 266 | 2416 | 1.77 | 1.68 | 1.48 |
| uncooked, 10 halves, 6.2 oz.......... | 59 | 3.68 | 58 | 103 | 932 | .68 | .65 | .57 |
| uncooked, ½ cup.... | 30 | 1.89 | 30 | 53 | 480 | .35 | .33 | .29 |
| cooked, unsweetened, ½ cup.......... | 21 | 1.30 | 21 | 37 | 330 | .24 | .23 | .20 |
| cooked, sweetened, ½ cup.......... | 22 | 1.36 | 22 | 38 | 344 | .25 | .24 | .21 |
| **Pear, Asian,** fresh: | | | | | | | | |
| untrimmed, 1 lb...... | 17 | n.a. | 35 | 44 | 499 | .08 | .21 | .25 |
| 1 fruit, 2½" diam., 4.3 oz............. | 5 | n.a. | 10 | 13 | 148 | .02 | .06 | .07 |
| **Pear nectar,** canned, 6 fl. oz............ | 6 | .48 | 6 | 6 | 24 | .12 | .13 | .05 |
| **Peas, edible-podded:** | | | | | | | | |
| fresh: | | | | | | | | |
| raw, untrimmed, 1 lb. | 183 | 8.87 | 103 | 226 | 852 | n.a. | n.a. | n.a. |
| raw, trimmed, ½ cup | 31 | 1.50 | 17 | 38 | 144 | n.a. | n.a. | n.a. |
| boiled, drained, ½ cup | 33 | 1.58 | 21 | 44 | 192 | .30 | .06 | .13 |
| frozen: | | | | | | | | |
| 10-oz. pkg. ........ | 142 | 5.68 | 66 | 145 | 546 | 1.16 | n.a. | n.a. |
| boiled, drained, ⅓ of 10-oz. pkg. ....... | 50 | 2.02 | 23 | 48 | 183 | .41 | n.a. | n.a. |

| | Calcium | Iron | Magnesium | Phosphorus | Potassium | Zinc | Copper | Manganese |
|---|---|---|---|---|---|---|---|---|
| | (Mg) | (Mg) | (Mg) | (Mg) | (Mg) | (Mg) | (Mg) | (Mg) |

**Peas, edible-podded, frozen,** *continued*

boiled, drained,
| ½ cup | 48 | 1.92 | 22 | 46 | 173 | .39 | n.a. | n.a. |

**Peas, green** (sweet):

fresh:
| raw, in pods, 1 lb. | 42 | 2.53 | 57 | 1186 | 421 | 2.14 | .30 | .71 |
| raw, shelled, ½ cup | 18 | 1.06 | 24 | 77 | 176 | .89 | .13 | .30 |

boiled, drained,
| ½ cup | 22 | 1.24 | 31 | 94 | 217 | .95 | .14 | .42 |

canned:
| w/liquid, ½ cup | 22 | 1.37 | 21 | 66 | 108 | .86 | .13 | .33 |
| drained, ½ cup | 17 | .81 | 15 | 57 | 147 | .60 | .07 | .26 |

seasoned, w/liquid,
| ½ cup | 18 | 1.37 | 17 | 61 | 139 | .74 | .11 | n.a. |

frozen:
| 10-oz. pkg. | 61 | 4.33 | 71 | 227 | 424 | 2.30 | .35 | .96 |

boiled, drained, ⅓ of
| 10-oz. pkg. | 20 | 1.33 | 25 | 76 | 141 | .79 | .12 | .34 |

boiled, drained,
| ½ cup | 19 | 1.26 | 23 | 72 | 134 | .75 | .11 | .33 |

**Peas, snow or Chinese,** see "Peas, edible-podded"

**Peas, split,** dried:
| uncooked, 1 lb. | 249 | 20.07 | 522 | 1662 | 4448 | 13.65 | 3.93 | 6.31 |
| uncooked, ½ cup | 54 | 4.34 | 113 | 359 | 961 | 2.95 | .85 | 1.36 |
| boiled, ½ cup | 13 | 1.26 | 36 | 97 | 355 | .98 | .18 | .39 |

**Peas, sprouted,** mature seeds:
| raw, 1 lb. | 161 | 10.23 | 253 | 746 | 1728 | 4.76 | 1.23 | 1.99 |
| raw, ½ cup | 21 | 1.35 | 34 | 99 | 229 | .63 | .16 | .26 |

**Peas, sweet,** see "Peas, green"

**Peas and carrots:**

canned, w/liquid,
| ½ cup | 29 | .97 | 18 | 58 | 128 | .74 | .13 | .46 |
| frozen, 10-oz. pkg. | 75 | 3.10 | 52 | 171 | 551 | 1.47 | .25 | .68 |

frozen, boiled, drained,
| ½ cup | 18 | .75 | 13 | 39 | 127 | .36 | .06 | .16 |

| | Calcium | Iron | Magnesium | Phosphorus | Potassium | Zinc | Copper | Manganese |
|---|---|---|---|---|---|---|---|---|
| | (Mg) | (Mg) | (Mg) | (Mg) | (Mg) | (Mg) | (Mg) | (Mg) |
| **Peas and onions,** canned, w/liquid, ½ cup | 10 | .52 | 10 | 30 | 57 | .35 | .06 | n.a. |
| **Pecan,** shelled, except as noted: dried: | | | | | | | | |
| in shell, 1 lb. | 87 | 5.11 | 307 | 699 | 942 | 13.15 | 2.84 | 10.83 |
| 1 oz. | 10 | .60 | 36 | 83 | 111 | 1.55 | .34 | 1.28 |
| halves, 1 cup | 39 | 2.30 | 138 | 314 | 423 | 5.91 | 1.28 | 4.87 |
| dry-roasted, 1 oz. | 10 | .62 | 38 | 86 | 105 | 1.61 | .35 | 1.34 |
| oil-roasted, 1 oz. | 10 | .60 | 37 | 84 | 102 | 1.56 | .34 | 1.29 |
| oil-roasted, 1 cup. | 37 | 2.33 | 142 | 324 | 395 | 6.05 | 1.32 | 5.01 |
| **Pecan flour,** 1 cup | 9 | .56 | 34 | 78 | 95 | 1.46 | .32 | 1.21 |
| **Pectin,** unsweetened, dry, 1.75-oz. pkg. | 4 | 1.36 | 1 | 1 | 4 | .23 | .21 | .04 |
| **Pepper, chili, hot,** green or red: raw: | | | | | | | | |
| untrimmed, 1 lb. | 58 | 3.97 | 83 | 151 | 1126 | 1.00 | .58 | .79 |
| trimmed, 1 medium, 1.6 oz. | 8 | .54 | 11 | 20 | 153 | .14 | .08 | .11 |
| trimmed, chopped, ½ cup | 13 | .90 | 19 | 34 | 255 | .23 | .13 | .18 |
| canned, chopped, ½ cup | 5 | .34 | n.a. | 12 | n.a. | n.a. | n.a. | n.a. |
| sun-dried, 10 peppers, .2 oz. | 2 | .33 | 5 | 9 | 101 | .05 | .01 | .04 |
| sun-dried, 1 cup, 1.3 oz. | 16 | 2.23 | 33 | 59 | 692 | .38 | .08 | .30 |
| **Pepper, ground:** | | | | | | | | |
| black, 1 tsp. | 9 | .61 | 4 | 4 | 26 | .03 | .02 | .11 |
| red or cayenne, 1 tsp. | 3 | .14 | 3 | 5 | 36 | .05 | .01 | .04 |
| white, 1 tsp. | 6 | .34 | 2 | 4 | 2 | .03 | .02 | .10 |
| **Pepper, jalapeño,** canned, w/liquid, chopped, ½ cup | 18 | 1.90 | 8 | 12 | 92 | .13 | .10 | n.a. |

| | Calcium (Mg) | Iron (Mg) | Magnesium (Mg) | Phosphorus (Mg) | Potassium (Mg) | Zinc (Mg) | Copper (Mg) | Manganese (Mg) |
|---|---|---|---|---|---|---|---|---|
| **Pepper, sweet** (bell), fresh: | | | | | | | | |
| green or red: | | | | | | | | |
| raw, untrimmed, | | | | | | | | |
| 1 lb. . . . . . . . . . | 34 | 1.72 | 37 | 72 | 660 | .46 | .24 | .43 |
| raw, 1 medium, | | | | | | | | |
| 3.2 oz. . . . . . . . . . | 7 | .34 | 7 | 14 | 131 | .09 | .05 | .09 |
| raw, trimmed, | | | | | | | | |
| chopped, ½ cup . . | 5 | .23 | 5 | 10 | 89 | .06 | .03 | .06 |
| boiled, drained, | | | | | | | | |
| chopped, ½ cup . . | 6 | .31 | 7 | 12 | 113 | .08 | .04 | .08 |
| yellow, raw: | | | | | | | | |
| untrimmed, 1 lb. . . . . | 40 | n.a. | 46 | 87 | 787 | .64 | .40 | .44 |
| 1 large, 6.6 oz. . . . . . | 20 | n.a. | 23 | 44 | 393 | .32 | .20 | .22 |
| 10 strips, 1.8 oz. . . . . | 6 | n.a. | 6 | 12 | 110 | .09 | .06 | .06 |
| **Pepper, sweet, canned** | | | | | | | | |
| (see also "Pimiento"), | | | | | | | | |
| w/liquid, halves, ½ cup | 28 | .56 | 8 | 14 | 102 | .12 | .09 | n.a. |
| **Pepper, sweet, frozen,** | | | | | | | | |
| green or red, chopped, | | | | | | | | |
| 10-oz. pkg. . . . . . . . . | 26 | 1.76 | 23 | 47 | 259 | .17 | .15 | .33 |
| **Pepper, sweet, freeze-dried:** | | | | | | | | |
| green or red, ¼ cup . . . . | 2 | .17 | 3 | 5 | 51 | .04 | .02 | .03 |
| green or red, 1 tbsp. . . . . | 1 | .04 | 1 | 1 | 13 | .01 | .01 | .01 |
| **Pepper sauce, hot:** | | | | | | | | |
| 1 tsp. . . . . . . . . . . . . . | 0 | .02 | 0 | 0 | 7 | .01 | tr. | tr. |
| (*Tabasco*), 1 tsp. . . . . . . . | 1 | .05 | 1 | 1 | 6 | .01 | tr. | .01 |
| **Peppered loaf**, pork and | | | | | | | | |
| beef, 1-oz. slice . . . . . . | 15 | .30 | 6 | 48 | 112 | .92 | .03 | .02 |
| **Pepperoni,** pork and | | | | | | | | |
| beef, 1 oz. . . . . . . . . . . | 3 | .40 | 5 | 34 | 98 | .71 | .02 | n.a. |
| **Perch**, mixed species, meat only: | | | | | | | | |
| raw, 1 lb. . . . . . . . . . . . . | 362 | 4.09 | 136 | 908 | 1219 | 5.05 | .68 | 3.18 |
| baked, broiled, or | | | | | | | | |
| microwaved[1], 4 oz. . . . | 116 | 1.32 | 43 | 291 | 390 | 1.62 | .22 | n.a. |
| **Perch, ocean,** see "Ocean perch" | | | | | | | | |

---

[1] *Prepared without added ingredients.*

| | Calcium | Iron | Magnesium | Phosphorus | Potassium | Zinc | Copper | Manganese |
|---|---|---|---|---|---|---|---|---|
| | (Mg) | (Mg) | (Mg) | (Mg) | (Mg) | (Mg) | (Mg) | (Mg) |
| **Persimmon,** Japanese: | | | | | | | | |
| fresh, untrimmed, 1 lb. | 29 | .59 | 33 | 64 | 612 | .41 | .43 | 1.35 |
| fresh, 1 medium, 2½" × | | | | | | | | |
| 3½", 7.1 oz......... | 13 | .26 | 15 | 28 | 270 | .18 | .19 | .60 |
| dried, 1 oz. ........... | 7 | .21 | 9 | 23 | 227 | .12 | .13 | .39 |
| **Pheasant,** raw, meat | | | | | | | | |
| w/skin, 1 oz. ........ | 3 | .33 | 6 | 61 | 69 | .27 | .02 | tr. |
| **Phyllo dough,** .7-oz. | | | | | | | | |
| sheet.............. | 2 | .61 | 3 | 14 | 14 | .09 | .02 | .09 |
| **Pickle,** cucumber: | | | | | | | | |
| dill, 1 large, 3¾" long, | | | | | | | | |
| 2.3 oz. | 6 | .35 | 7 | 14 | 75 | .09 | .05 | .01 |
| dill, 1 slice, .2 oz. ...... | 1 | .03 | 1 | 1 | 7 | .01 | .01 | tr. |
| sour, 1 medium, | | | | | | | | |
| 3¾" long, 1.2 oz...... | 0 | .14 | 1 | 5 | 8 | .01 | .03 | n.a. |
| sour, 1 slice, .25 oz. .... | 0 | .03 | 0 | 1 | 2 | 0 | .01 | n.a. |
| sweet, 1 large, 3" long, | | | | | | | | |
| 1.2 oz............... | 1 | .21 | 1 | 4 | 11 | .03 | .04 | .01 |
| sweet, 1 slice, .2 oz. .... | 0 | .04 | 0 | 1 | 2 | 0 | .01 | <.01 |
| **Pickle and pimiento loaf,** | | | | | | | | |
| pork, 1-oz. slice...... | 27 | .29 | 5 | 40 | 96 | .40 | .04 | .01 |
| **Picnic loaf,** pork and | | | | | | | | |
| beef, 1-oz. slice...... | 13 | .29 | 4 | 36 | 76 | .62 | .02 | .01 |
| **Pie,** ready-to-serve: | | | | | | | | |
| apple, ⅛ of 9" pie ...... | 13 | .56 | 9 | 29 | 82 | .2 | .06 | .23 |
| blueberry, ⅛ of 9" pie | 10 | .37 | n.a. | n.a. | 63 | n.a. | n.a. | n.a. |
| cherry, ⅛ of 9" pie ..... | 15 | .59 | 10 | 36 | 102 | .22 | .05 | .18 |
| chocolate cream, ⅙ of | | | | | | | | |
| 8" pie ............. | 41 | 1.21 | 24 | 77 | 144 | .26 | .06 | .23 |
| coconut creme, ⅙ of | | | | | | | | |
| 7" pie ............. | 19 | .51 | n.a. | n.a. | 42 | n.a. | n.a. | n.a. |
| coconut custard, ⅙ of | | | | | | | | |
| 8" pie ............. | 84 | .83 | 19 | 127 | 182 | .71 | .07 | .22 |
| custard, ⅙ of 9" pie..... | 146 | 1.50 | n.a. | 172 | 208 | n.a. | n.a. | n.a. |
| egg custard, | | | | | | | | |
| ⅙ of 8" pie ......... | 84 | .61 | 12 | 118 | 112 | .54 | .03 | .06 |

| | Calcium | Iron | Magnesium | Phosphorus | Potassium | Zinc | Copper | Manganese |
|---|---|---|---|---|---|---|---|---|
| | (Mg) | (Mg) | (Mg) | (Mg) | (Mg) | (Mg) | (Mg) | (Mg) |

**Pie,** *continued*

**lemon meringue,** ⅙ of

8" pie . . . . . . . . . . . . | 63 | .69 | 16 | 119 | 100 | .55 | tr. | .07

peach, ⅙ of 8" pie. . . . . . | 9 | .58 | n.a. | n.a. | 146 | .11 | n.a. | n.a.

pecan, ⅙ of 8" pie . . . . . . | 19 | 1.17 | 20 | 87 | 84 | .65 | .22 | .89

pumpkin, ⅙ of 8" pie | 66 | .87 | 16 | 77 | 168 | .50 | .05 | .26

**Pie crust, frozen,**

9" crust . . . . . . . . . . . | 26 | 2.85 | 22 | 75 | 139 | .43 | .10 | .78

**Pie crust mix, prepared,**

9" crust . . . . . . . . . . . | 96 | 3.44 | 24 | 134 | 99 | .62 | .12 | .49

**Pie filling,** canned:

apple, 21-oz. can . . . . . . . | 27 | 1.73 | 14 | 39 | 268 | .24 | 33 | .16

cherry, 21-oz. can . . . . . . | 65 | 1.43 | 39 | 88 | 625 | .33 | .48 | .18

**Pigeon peas,** fresh:

raw, untrimmed (in

pods), 1 lb. . . . . . . . . . | 91 | 3.48 | n.a. | 276 | 1202 | n.a. | n.a. | n.a.

raw, trimmed, ½ cup | 32 | 1.23 | n.a. | 98 | 425 | n.a. | n.a. | n.a.

boiled, drained, ½ cup | 27 | 1.02 | 31 | 81 | 351 | n.a. | n.a. | n.a.

**Pigeon peas, dried,**

boiled, ½ cup . . . . . . . | 36 | .93 | 38 | 100 | 322 | .76 | .23 | .42

**Pignoli nut,** see "Pine nut"

**Pike,** meat only:

northern:

raw, 1 lb. . . . . . . . . . . | 257 | 2.49 | n.a. | 996 | 1173 | 3.03 | .23 | n.a.

baked, broiled, or

microwaved[1], 4 oz. | 83 | .81 | n.a. | 320 | 375 | .98 | .07 | n.a.

walleye:

raw, 1 lb. . . . . . . . . . . | 499 | 5.90 | 136 | 953 | 1766 | 2.81 | .81 | 3.63

baked, broiled, or

microwaved[1],

4 oz. . . . . . . . . . . | 160 | 1.89 | 43 | 305 | 566 | .90 | .26 | 1.16

**Pimiento,** canned:

1 oz. . . . . . . . . . . . . . . . | 2 | .48 | 2 | 5 | 45 | .05 | .01 | .03

1 tbsp. . . . . . . . . . . . . . | 1 | .20 | 1 | 2 | 19 | .02 | .01 | .01

[1] *Prepared without added ingredients.*

| | Calcium | Iron | Magnesium | Phosphorus | Potassium | Zinc | Copper | Manganese |
|---|---|---|---|---|---|---|---|---|
| | (Mg) | (Mg) | (Mg) | (Mg) | (Mg) | (Mg) | (Mg) | (Mg) |
| **Pine nut**, shelled, except as noted: | | | | | | | | |
| pignoli, dried: | | | | | | | | |
| in shell, 1 lb........ | 92 | 32.13 | n.a. | 1774 | 2093 | 14.83 | 3.58 | n.a. |
| 1 oz.............. | 7 | 2.61 | n.a. | 144 | 170 | 1.21 | .29 | n.a. |
| 1 tbsp. ........... | 3 | .92 | n.a. | 51 | 60 | .42 | .10 | n.a. |
| piñon, dried: | | | | | | | | |
| in shell, 1 lb........ | 21 | 7.90 | 606 | 89 | 1624 | 11.07 | 2.68 | n.a. |
| 1 oz.............. | 2 | .87 | 67 | 10 | 178 | 1.22 | .29 | n.a. |
| 10 kernels ......... | 0 | .03 | 2 | 0 | 6 | .04 | .01 | n.a. |
| **Pineapple:** | | | | | | | | |
| fresh: | | | | | | | | |
| untrimmed, 1 lb. ..... | 17 | .87 | 32 | 17 | 267 | .19 | .26 | 3.89 |
| trimmed, 1 slice, 3½" | | | | | | | | |
| diam. × ¾"...... | 6 | .31 | 11 | 6 | 95 | .07 | .09 | 1.39 |
| trimmed, diced, | | | | | | | | |
| ½ cup.......... | 6 | .29 | 11 | 6 | 88 | .06 | .09 | 1.28 |
| canned: | | | | | | | | |
| in water, tidbits, | | | | | | | | |
| ½ cup.......... | 19 | .49 | 22 | 5 | 157 | .15 | .13 | 1.38 |
| in juice, chunks or | | | | | | | | |
| tidbits, ½ cup .... | 17 | .35 | 18 | 8 | 152 | .12 | .11 | n.a. |
| in light syrup, ½ cup | 18 | .49 | 20 | 9 | 133 | .15 | .13 | 1.38 |
| in heavy syrup, | | | | | | | | |
| chunks, tidbits or | | | | | | | | |
| crushed, ½ cup... | 18 | .49 | 20 | 9 | 132 | .15 | .13 | 1.38 |
| frozen, sweetened, | | | | | | | | |
| chunks, ½ cup ...... | 11 | .49 | 12 | 5 | 122 | .14 | .12 | 1.30 |
| **Pineapple juice:** | | | | | | | | |
| canned, 6 fl. oz......... | 30 | .48 | 24 | 12 | 252 | .24 | .17 | 1.86 |
| frozen, diluted, 6 fl. oz. | 18 | .54 | 18 | 12 | 252 | .24 | .17 | 1.85 |
| **Pineapple topping,** | | | | | | | | |
| 2 tbsp. ........... | 9 | .20 | 1 | 3 | 133 | .20 | .01 | n.a. |
| **Pineapple-grapefruit** | | | | | | | | |
| **juice drink,** canned, | | | | | | | | |
| 8 fl. oz............. | 18 | .77 | 15 | 14 | 154 | .15 | .11 | 1.03 |
| **Pineapple-orange juice** | | | | | | | | |
| **drink,** canned, 8 fl. oz. | 13 | .67 | 14 | 10 | 116 | .14 | .10 | .90 |

| | Calcium | Iron | Magnesium | Phosphorus | Potassium | Zinc | Copper | Manganese |
|---|---|---|---|---|---|---|---|---|
| | (Mg) | (Mg) | (Mg) | (Mg) | (Mg) | (Mg) | (Mg) | (Mg) |
| **Pink beans,** dried: | | | | | | | | |
| uncooked, 1 lb. . . . . . . . | 590 | 30.71 | 827 | 1883 | 6638 | 11.58 | 3.67 | 624 |
| uncooked, ½ cup. . . . . . . | 137 | 7.11 | 191 | 436 | 1537 | 2.68 | .85 | 1.45 |
| boiled, ½ cup . . . . . . . . . | 44 | 1.93 | 55 | 139 | 427 | .81 | .23 | .46 |
| **Pinto beans,** dried: | | | | | | | | |
| uncooked, 1 lb. . . . . . . . | 547 | 26.66 | 720 | 1895 | 6023 | 1.50 | 3.51 | 5.13 |
| uncooked, ½ cup. . . . . . . | 116 | 5.64 | 152 | 401 | 1275 | 2.43 | .74 | 1.09 |
| boiled, ½ cup . . . . . . . . . | 41 | 2.22 | 47 | 136 | 398 | .92 | .22 | .47 |
| canned, w/liquid, 8 oz. . . . | 84 | 3.64 | 61 | 208 | 684 | 1.57 | .32 | .52 |
| canned, w/liquid, | | | | | | | | |
| ½ cup . . . . . . . . . . . . . | 44 | 1.93 | 32 | 110 | 362 | .83 | .17 | .28 |
| **Pistachio nut,** shelled, except as noted: | | | | | | | | |
| dried: | | | | | | | | |
| in shell, 1 lb. . . . . . . . | 307 | 15.37 | 359 | 1142 | 2479 | 3.03 | 2.70 | .74 |
| 1 oz. . . . . . . . . . . . . . | 38 | 1.92 | 45 | 143 | 310 | .38 | .34 | .09 |
| 1 cup . . . . . . . . . . . . | 173 | 8.67 | 203 | 644 | 1399 | 1.71 | 1.52 | .42 |
| dry-roasted, 1 oz. . . . . . . | 20 | .90 | 37 | 135 | 275 | .39 | .34 | .10 |
| dry-roasted, 1 cup . . . . . . | 90 | 4.06 | 166 | 609 | 1242 | 1.74 | 1.55 | .43 |
| **Pitanga:** | | | | | | | | |
| untrimmed, 1 lb. . . . . . . . | 36 | .80 | 49 | 44 | 410 | n.a. | n.a. | n.a. |
| trimmed, ½ cup. . . . . . . . | 8 | .18 | 11 | 10 | 89 | n.a. | n.a. | n.a. |
| **Pizza,** see "Fast foods" | | | | | | | | |
| **Plantain,** fresh: | | | | | | | | |
| raw: | | | | | | | | |
| untrimmed, 1 lb. . . . . | 9 | 1.77 | 109 | 100 | 1471 | .41 | .24 | n.a. |
| 1 medium, 9.7 oz. . . . | 5 | 1.07 | 66 | 61 | 893 | .25 | .15 | n.a. |
| trimmed, sliced, | | | | | | | | |
| ½ cup . . . . . . . . . . | 2 | .45 | 28 | 25 | 370 | .11 | .06 | n.a. |
| cooked, sliced, ½ cup . . . | 2 | .45 | 25 | 22 | 358 | .10 | .05 | n.a. |
| **Plum:** | | | | | | | | |
| fresh: | | | | | | | | |
| untrimmed, 1 lb. . . . . | 15 | .43 | 29 | 44 | 733 | .41 | .18 | .21 |
| Japanese or hybrid, | | | | | | | | |
| 1 medium, 2⅛" | | | | | | | | |
| diam., 2.3 oz. . . . . | 2 | .07 | 4 | 7 | 113 | .06 | .03 | .03 |

| | Calcium | Iron | Magnesium | Phosphorus | Potassium | Zinc | Copper | Manganese |
|---|---|---|---|---|---|---|---|---|
| | (Mg) | (Mg) | (Mg) | (Mg) | (Mg) | (Mg) | (Mg) | (Mg) |
| pitted, sliced, ½ cup | 3 | .09 | 2 | 4 | 57 | .03 | .01 | .02 |
| canned, purple: | | | | | | | | |
| in water, ½ cup..... | 9 | .20 | 7 | 17 | 157 | .10 | .05 | .04 |
| in juice, ½ cup ..... | 13 | .42 | 10 | 20 | 195 | .14 | .07 | n.a. |
| in light syrup, | | | | | | | | |
| ½ cup.......... | 12 | 1.08 | 7 | 17 | 117 | .10 | .05 | .04 |
| in heavy syrup, | | | | | | | | |
| ½ cup.......... | 12 | 1.09 | 7 | 17 | 117 | .10 | .05 | .04 |
| **Poi**, ½ cup .......... | 19 | 1.06 | 29 | 47 | 220 | n.a. | n.a. | n.a. |
| **Polish sausage** (see also "Kielbasa"), pork, 1 oz. ............. | 3 | .41 | 4 | 39 | 67 | .55 | .03 | .01 |
| **Pollock**, meat only: | | | | | | | | |
| Atlantic: | | | | | | | | |
| raw, 1 lb.......... | 272 | 2.09 | 304 | 1002 | 1614 | 2.11 | .23 | .07 |
| baked, broiled, or microwaved[1], 4 oz. | 87 | .67 | 98 | 321 | 517 | .68 | .07 | .02 |
| walleye: | | | | | | | | |
| raw, 1 lb.......... | 22 | 1.04 | n.a. | n.a. | 1477 | 1.99 | .20 | .07 |
| baked, broiled, or microwaved[1], 4 oz. | 7 | .32 | n.a. | n.a. | 439 | .68 | .06 | (0) |
| **Pomegranate:** | | | | | | | | |
| untrimmed, 1 lb. ....... | 8 | .76 | n.a. | 20 | 658 | n.a. | n.a. | n.a. |
| 1 medium, 3⅜" × 3¾", 9.7 oz............. | 5 | .46 | n.a. | 12 | 399 | n.a. | n.a. | n.a. |
| **Pompano**, Florida, meat only: | | | | | | | | |
| raw, 1 lb............. | 101 | 2.72 | 121 | 887 | 1728 | 3.26 | .17 | .06 |
| baked, broiled, or microwaved[1], 4 oz. ... | 49 | .76 | 35 | 387 | 721 | .78 | .09 | .03 |
| **Popcorn**, popped: | | | | | | | | |
| air-popped, unsalted, 1 cup ............. | 1 | .21 | 10 | 24 | 24 | .28 | .03 | .08 |
| cheese flavor, 1 cup..... | 12 | .25 | 10 | 40 | 29 | .22 | .02 | .08 |

[1] *Prepared without added ingredients.*

| | Calcium (Mg) | Iron (Mg) | Magnesium (Mg) | Phosphorus (Mg) | Potassium (Mg) | Zinc (Mg) | Copper (Mg) | Manganese (Mg) |
|---|---|---|---|---|---|---|---|---|
| Popcorn, *continued* | | | | | | | | |
| oil-popped, unsalted, | | | | | | | | |
| 1 cup . . . . . . . . . . . . . | 1 | .31 | 12 | 28 | 25 | .29 | .02 | .10 |
| oil-popped, salted, | | | | | | | | |
| 1 cup . . . . . . . . . . . . . | 20 | 0 | .01 | .02 | .10 | n.a. | n.a. | 0 |
| w/caramel coating, | | | | | | | | |
| 1 cup . . . . . . . . . . . . . | 15 | .61 | 12 | 29 | 38 | .20 | .04 | .08 |
| w/caramel coating and | | | | | | | | |
| peanuts, ⅔ cup . . . . . . | 19 | 1.11 | 23 | 36 | 101 | .35 | .08 | .22 |
| **Poppy seeds,** 1 tsp. . . . . | 41 | .26 | 9 | 24 | 20 | .29 | .05 | .19 |
| **Pork**[1] (see also "Ham"), fresh, 4 oz., except as noted: | | | | | | | | |
| loin, whole: | | | | | | | | |
| braised, lean and fat | 9 | 1.32 | 23 | 226 | 391 | 3.44 | .12 | .02 |
| braised, lean only. . . . | 11 | 1.59 | 27 | 271 | 475 | 4.22 | .14 | .02 |
| broiled, lean and fat | 8 | .92 | 28 | 266 | 398 | 2.78 | .10 | .01 |
| broiled, lean only . . . . | 8 | 1.05 | 33 | 316 | 474 | 3.31 | .11 | .01 |
| roasted, lean and fat | 9 | 1.15 | 22 | 251 | 361 | 2.97 | .12 | .02 |
| roasted, lean only . . . | 10 | 1.30 | 25 | 288 | 416 | 3.45 | .11 | .02 |
| loin, blade: | | | | | | | | |
| braised, lean and fat | 16 | 1.47 | 19 | 200 | 379 | 4.37 | .12 | .01 |
| braised, lean only. . . . | 19 | 1.84 | 23 | 243 | 473 | 5.59 | .15 | .02 |
| broiled, lean and fat | 12 | 1.03 | 24 | 229 | 376 | 3.46 | .10 | .01 |
| broiled, lean only . . . . | 15 | 1.22 | 28 | 278 | 463 | 4.30 | .11 | .01 |
| pan-fried[2], lean and fat . . . . . . . . . . . . | 11 | .93 | 22 | 206 | 337 | 3.07 | .09 | .01 |
| pan-fried[2], lean only | 15 | 1.18 | 27 | 269 | 447 | 4.16 | .11 | .01 |
| roasted, lean and fat | 14 | 1.21 | 17 | 196 | 332 | 3.39 | .10 | .01 |
| roasted, lean only . . . | 16 | 1.42 | 19 | 228 | 392 | 4.07 | .11 | .01 |
| loin, center: | | | | | | | | |
| braised, lean and fat | 7 | .94 | 22 | 244 | 359 | 2.80 | .11 | .03 |
| braised, lean only. . . . | 7 | 1.08 | 25 | 285 | 422 | 3.30 | .12 | .04 |
| broiled, lean and fat | 5 | .92 | 28 | 239 | 407 | 2.19 | .09 | .01 |

[1] *Prepared without added ingredients, except as noted.*
[2] *In hydrogenated soybean and cottonseed oils.*

| | Calcium | Iron | Magnesium | Phosphorus | Potassium | Zinc | Copper | Manganese |
|---|---|---|---|---|---|---|---|---|
| | (Mg) | (Mg) | (Mg) | (Mg) | (Mg) | (Mg) | (Mg) | (Mg) |
| broiled, lean only.... | 6 | 1.04 | 34 | 277 | 476 | 2.53 | .09 | .01 |
| pan-fried[1], lean and fat............. | 6 | .95 | 29 | 243 | 412 | 2.22 | .09 | .01 |
| pan-fried[1], lean only | 6 | 1.13 | 36 | 301 | 516 | 2.73 | .10 | .01 |
| roasted, lean and fat | 6 | 1.12 | 22 | 222 | 365 | 2.31 | .09 | .02 |
| roasted, lean only ... | 7 | 1.24 | 24 | 248 | 411 | 2.59 | .09 | .02 |
| **loin, center rib:** | | | | | | | | |
| braised, lean and fat | 11 | 1.21 | 23 | 238 | 468 | 2.66 | .10 | .01 |
| braised, lean only.... | 14 | 1.43 | 26 | 284 | 568 | 3.20 | .11 | .01 |
| broiled, lean and fat | 15 | .82 | 28 | 257 | 421 | 2.30 | .09 | .02 |
| broiled, lean only.... | 17 | .92 | 34 | 302 | 498 | 2.70 | .09 | .02 |
| pan-fried[1], lean and fat............. | 8 | .72 | 24 | 236 | 399 | 1.84 | .08 | .01 |
| pan-fried[1], lean only | 10 | .91 | 32 | 307 | 527 | 2.34 | .09 | .01 |
| roasted, lean and fat | 11 | 1.01 | 22 | 254 | 417 | 2.22 | .08 | .01 |
| roasted, lean only ... | 12 | 1.13 | 24 | 290 | 480 | 2.52 | .09 | .01 |
| **loin, sirloin:** | | | | | | | | |
| braised, lean and fat | 7 | 1.28 | 26 | 222 | 418 | 2.90 | .13 | .02 |
| braised, lean only.... | 8 | 1.51 | 32 | 263 | 502 | 3.48 | .15 | .02 |
| broiled, lean and fat | 6 | .88 | 33 | 256 | 416 | 2.30 | .11 | .01 |
| broiled, lean only.... | 6 | 1.01 | 39 | 301 | 492 | 2.68 | .12 | .01 |
| roasted, lean and fat | 10 | 1.13 | 25 | 260 | 382 | 2.57 | .11 | .03 |
| roasted, lean only ... | 11 | 1.24 | 27 | 286 | 420 | 2.82 | .12 | .03 |
| **loin, top:** | | | | | | | | |
| braised, lean and fat | 11 | 1.17 | 22 | 231 | 452 | 2.59 | .10 | .01 |
| braised, lean only.... | 14 | 1.43 | 26 | 284 | 568 | 3.20 | .11 | .01 |
| broiled, lean and fat | 14 | .79 | 27 | 248 | 405 | 2.23 | .08 | .02 |
| broiled, lean only.... | 17 | .92 | 34 | 302 | 498 | 2.70 | .09 | .02 |
| pan-fried[1], lean and fat............. | 8 | .75 | 24 | 235 | 397 | 1.84 | .08 | .01 |
| pan-fried[1], lean only | 10 | .91 | 32 | 307 | 527 | 2.34 | .09 | .01 |
| roasted, lean and fat | 11 | 1.00 | 20 | 248 | 407 | 2.18 | .08 | .01 |
| roasted, lean only ... | 12 | 1.13 | 24 | 290 | 480 | 2.52 | .09 | .01 |

[1] In hydrogenated soybean and cottonseed oils.

| | Calcium | Iron | Magnesium | Phosphorus | Potassium | Zinc | Copper | Manganese |
|---|---|---|---|---|---|---|---|---|
| | (Mg) | (Mg) | (Mg) | (Mg) | (Mg) | (Mg) | (Mg) | (Mg) |

**Pork,** *continued*

**shoulder, whole:**

| | Calcium | Iron | Magnesium | Phosphorus | Potassium | Zinc | Copper | Manganese |
|---|---|---|---|---|---|---|---|---|
| roasted, lean and fat | 8 | 1.49 | 20 | 227 | 345 | 4.07 | .13 | .02 |
| roasted, lean only ... | 9 | 1.72 | 23 | 262 | 399 | 4.81 | .15 | .03 |
| **shoulder, arm (picnic):** | | | | | | | | |
| braised, lean and fat | 8 | 1.83 | 20 | 217 | 381 | 4.58 | .16 | .02 |
| braised, lean only.... | 9 | 2.21 | 25 | 256 | 459 | 5.64 | .18 | .02 |
| roasted, lean and fat | 9 | 1.35 | 19 | 234 | 332 | 3.75 | .13 | .04 |
| roasted, lean only ... | 10 | 1.61 | 23 | 280 | 398 | 4.62 | .15 | .05 |
| **shoulder, Boston blade:** | | | | | | | | |
| braised, lean and fat | 8 | 1.95 | 22 | 209 | 395 | 5.23 | .16 | .01 |
| braised, lean only.... | 9 | 2.32 | 25 | 243 | 467 | 6.32 | .19 | .02 |
| broiled, lean and fat | 6 | 1.33 | 27 | 239 | 398 | 4.11 | .13 | .01 |
| broiled, lean only.... | 7 | 1.53 | 32 | 277 | 464 | 4.84 | .15 | .01 |
| roasted, lean and fat | 7 | 1.61 | 20 | 221 | 355 | 4.33 | .13 | .01 |
| roasted, lean only ... | 8 | 1.81 | 23 | 248 | 400 | 4.96 | .15 | .02 |
| **spareribs, lean and fat,** | | | | | | | | |
| braised, 6.3 oz. (1 lb. | | | | | | | | |
| raw w/bone) ........ | 38 | 3.28 | 43 | 463 | 566 | 8.15 | .25 | .03 |
| **tenderloin, lean only,** | | | | | | | | |
| roasted ............ | 10 | 1.75 | 28 | 327 | 610 | 3.40 | .18 | .04 |
| **Potato,** fresh or stored: | | | | | | | | |
| **raw, pulp only:** | | | | | | | | |
| untrimmed, 1 lb. .... | 23 | 2.57 | 72 | 158 | 1847 | 1.32 | .88 | .90 |
| 1 medium, | | | | | | | | |
| 2½" diam., | | | | | | | | |
| 5.3 oz. w/skin .... | 8 | .85 | 24 | 52 | 608 | .44 | .29 | .30 |
| diced, ½ cup ....... | 5 | .57 | 16 | 35 | 407 | .29 | .19 | .20 |
| **baked in skin:** | | | | | | | | |
| whole, 1 medium, | | | | | | | | |
| 4¾" × 2⅓" diam., | | | | | | | | |
| 7.1 oz........... | 20 | 2.75 | 55 | 115 | 844 | .65 | .62 | .46 |
| pulp from 4¾"-diam. | | | | | | | | |
| potato .......... | 8 | .55 | 39 | 78 | 610 | .45 | .34 | .25 |
| pulp, ½ cup........ | 3 | .22 | 15 | 30 | 238 | .18 | .13 | .10 |
| skin, 2 oz......... | 19 | 3.94 | 24 | 57 | 321 | .27 | .46 | .34 |

| | Calcium | Iron | Magnesium | Phosphorus | Potassium | Zinc | Copper | Manganese |
|---|---|---|---|---|---|---|---|---|
| | (Mg) | (Mg) | (Mg) | (Mg) | (Mg) | (Mg) | (Mg) | (Mg) |
| boiled: | | | | | | | | |
| in skin, peeled, 1 medium, 2½" diam., 5.3 oz. w/skin .... | 7 | .42 | 30 | 60 | 515 | .41 | .26 | .19 |
| in skin, pulp, ½ cup w/out skin, 2½" diam. | 4 | .24 | 17 | 35 | 295 | .23 | .15 | .11 |
| potato .......... w/out skin, pulp, | 10 | .42 | 26 | 54 | 443 | .37 | .23 | .19 |
| ½ cup .......... | 6 | .24 | 15 | 31 | 256 | .21 | .12 | .11 |
| microwaved in skin: whole, 4¾" × 2½" diam., 7.1 oz. .... | 22 | 2.50 | 54 | 212 | 903 | .73 | .68 | .59 |
| pulp from 4¾"-diam. potato .......... | 8 | .64 | 39 | 170 | 641 | .51 | .37 | .27 |
| pulp, ½ cup. ....... | 4 | .32 | 19 | 85 | 321 | .26 | .18 | .13 |
| skin, 2 oz. ......... | 26 | 3.32 | 21 | 46 | 364 | .29 | .49 | .55 |
| mashed, w/whole milk, ½ cup ............. | 28 | .29 | 19 | 50 | 314 | .30 | .15 | .12 |
| mashed, w/whole milk and margarine, ½ cup | 27 | .28 | 19 | 49 | 303 | .29 | .14 | .12 |
| **Potato, canned, whole:** | | | | | | | | |
| w/liquid, 1-lb. can ...... | 134 | 4.41 | 65 | 98 | 1103 | 1.78 | .32 | .32 |
| 1"-diam. potato, 1.2 oz. | 2 | .44 | 5 | 10 | 80 | .10 | .02 | .03 |
| drained, ½ cup ........ | 5 | 1.13 | 12 | 25 | 206 | .25 | .05 | .09 |
| **Potato, frozen:** | | | | | | | | |
| french-fried[1], heated: | | | | | | | | |
| 9-oz. pkg. ......... | 16 | 2.46 | 43 | 163 | 828 | .80 | .23 | .52 |
| 10 strips, 1.75 oz. | 4 | .62 | 11 | 41 | 209 | .20 | .06 | .13 |
| cottage cut, 9-oz. pkg. ....... | 19 | 2.96 | 44 | 129 | 951 | .82 | .40 | .60 |
| cottage cut, 10 strips, 1.75 oz. ......... | 5 | .75 | 11 | 33 | 240 | .21 | .10 | .15 |
| hash brown: | | | | | | | | |
| 12-oz. pkg. ........ | 34 | 3.34 | 37 | 161 | 968 | .70 | .34 | .50 |

[1] Par-fried in vegetable oil.

| | Calcium (Mg) | Iron (Mg) | Magnesium (Mg) | Phosphorus (Mg) | Potassium (Mg) | Zinc (Mg) | Copper (Mg) | Manganese (Mg) |
|---|---|---|---|---|---|---|---|---|
| Potato, frozen, hash brown, *continued* | | | | | | | | |
| heated[1], 12-oz. pkg. | 31 | 3.09 | 35 | 148 | 894 | .65 | .31 | .46 |
| heated[1], ½ cup . . . . . | 12 | 1.17 | 13 | 56 | 340 | .25 | .12 | .17 |
| puffs[2], 1 piece, .25 oz. . . . | 2 | .11 | 1 | 3 | 27 | .02 | tr. | .02 |
| **Potato chips[3]**, 1 oz.: | | | | | | | | |
| plain . . . . . . . . . . . . . | 7 | .46 | 19 | 47 | 361 | .31 | .09 | .13 |
| plain, light . . . . . . . . . . | 6 | .38 | 25 | 55 | 495 | n.a. | .17 | n.a. |
| barbecue flavor . . . . . . . . | 14 | .55 | 21 | 53 | 358 | .27 | .10 | .14 |
| cheese flavor . . . . . . . . . | 20 | .52 | 21 | 85 | 433 | .26 | .07 | .13 |
| sour cream and onion . . . | 20 | .45 | 21 | 50 | 377 | .28 | .09 | .12 |
| **Potato flour,** ½ cup . . . . . | 30 | 15.98 | n.a. | 160 | 1429 | n.a. | n.a. | n.a. |
| **Potato mix[4]**, ½ cup: | | | | | | | | |
| mashed[5], flakes . . . . . . . | 52 | .23 | 19 | 59 | 245 | .18 | .02 | n.a. |
| mashed[5], granules . . . . . . | 37 | .20 | 20 | 63 | 152 | .26 | .02 | tr. |
| **Potato sticks,** 1-oz. pkg. | 5 | .64 | 18 | 49 | 351 | .28 | .09 | .12 |
| **Poultry,** see specific listings | | | | | | | | |
| **Poultry seasoning,** 1 tsp. . . . . . . . . . . . . | 15 | .53 | 3 | 3 | 10 | .05 | .01 | .10 |
| **Pout,** ocean, meat only: | | | | | | | | |
| raw, 1 lb. . . . . . . . . . . . | 44 | 1.27 | 58 | n.a. | n.a. | .4.68 | .15 | .07 |
| baked, broiled, or microwaved[6], 4 oz. . . . | 15 | .41 | 19 | n.a. | n.a. | 1.50 | .05 | .02 |
| **Pretzels:** | | | | | | | | |
| plain, 1 oz. . . . . . . . . . . | 10 | 1.23 | 10 | 32 | 42 | .24 | .08 | .51 |
| whole wheat, 1 oz. . . . . . . | 8 | .76 | 9 | 35 | 122 | .18 | .08 | n.a. |
| **Prickly pear,** fresh: | | | | | | | | |
| untrimmed, 1 lb. . . . . . . . | 191 | 1.02 | 290 | 83 | 748 | n.a. | n.a. | n.a. |
| 1 medium, 4.8 oz. . . . . . . | 58 | .31 | 88 | 25 | 226 | n.a. | n.a. | n.a. |

---

[1] *Prepared in vegetable oil.*
[2] *Par-fried in vegetable oil.*
[3] *Includes rippled, salt and vinegar, and kettle-cooked varieties.*
[4] *Flakes and granules without milk.*
[5] *Prepared according to package directions, with whole milk and butter.*
[6] *Prepared without added ingredients.*

| | Calcium | Iron | Magnesium | Phosphorus | Potassium | Zinc | Copper | Manganese |
|---|---|---|---|---|---|---|---|---|
| | (Mg) | (Mg) | (Mg) | (Mg) | (Mg) | (Mg) | (Mg) | (Mg) |
| **Prune:** | | | | | | | | |
| canned, in heavy syrup, | | | | | | | | |
| ½ cup............. | 20 | .48 | 17 | 30 | 264 | .22 | .14 | .11 |
| dehydrated: | | | | | | | | |
| uncooked, 1 lb...... | 329 | 15.95 | 291 | 507 | 4801 | 3.41 | 2.77 | 1.42 |
| uncooked, ½ cup.... | 48 | 2.32 | 43 | 74 | 699 | .50 | .40 | .21 |
| cooked, ½ cup ..... | 34 | 1.64 | 30 | 52 | 494 | .35 | .29 | .15 |
| dried, w/pits: | | | | | | | | |
| uncooked, 1 lb...... | 201 | 9.77 | 178 | 311 | 2942 | 2.09 | 1.70 | .87 |
| uncooked, 10 fruits, | | | | | | | | |
| approx. 3.5 oz. ... | 43 | 2.08 | 38 | 66 | 626 | .45 | .36 | .19 |
| uncooked, ½ cup.... | 41 | 2.00 | 37 | 64 | 600 | .43 | .35 | .18 |
| cooked, stewed, un- | | | | | | | | |
| sweetened, ½ cup | 24 | 1.18 | 21 | 37 | 354 | .25 | .21 | .10 |
| cooked, stewed, | | | | | | | | |
| sweetened, ½ cup | 25 | 1.24 | 22 | 39 | 371 | .26 | .21 | .11 |
| dried, pitted: | | | | | | | | |
| uncooked, 4 oz...... | 58 | 2.81 | 51 | 90 | 845 | .60 | .49 | .25 |
| cooked, stewed, | | | | | | | | |
| unsweetened, 4 oz. | 26 | 1.26 | 23 | 40 | 379 | .27 | .22 | .11 |
| cooked, stewed, | | | | | | | | |
| sweetened, 4 oz. ... | 24 | 1.18 | 22 | 37 | 354 | .25 | .20 | .10 |
| **Prune juice,** canned, | | | | | | | | |
| 6 fl. oz............ | 23 | 2.27 | 27 | 48 | 530 | .40 | .13 | .29 |
| **Pudding,** ready-to-serve: | | | | | | | | |
| banana, 5-oz. can ..... | 120 | .18 | 12 | 98 | 156 | .40 | .04 | n.a. |
| chocolate, 5-oz. can..... | 128 | .72 | 30 | 113 | 256 | .6 | .17 | .10 |
| lemon, 5-oz. can ....... | 3 | n.a. | 2 | 7 | 1 | n.a. | n.a. | n.a. |
| rice, 5-oz. can ......... | 73 | n.a. | n.a. | n.a. | 85 | .69 | n.a. | .18 |
| tapioca, 5-oz. can ...... | 119 | .33 | 12 | 113 | 148 | .38 | .04 | n.a. |
| vanilla, 5-oz. can ....... | 99 | .15 | 9 | 77 | 128 | .29 | .03 | n.a. |
| **Pudding,** frozen: | | | | | | | | |
| butterscotch (*Rich's*), | | | | | | | | |
| 3.5 oz.............. | 65 | .04 | 7 | 48 | 121 | .20 | 0 | n.a. |
| chocolate (*Rich's*), | | | | | | | | |
| 3.5 oz.............. | 63 | .26 | 6 | 58 | 128 | .19 | 0 | n.a. |
| vanilla (*Rich's*), 3.5 oz. | 65 | .04 | 7 | 48 | 121 | .20 | 0 | n.a. |

|  | Calcium | Iron | Magnesium | Phosphorus | Potassium | Zinc | Copper | Manganese |
|---|---|---|---|---|---|---|---|---|
|  | (Mg) | (Mg) | (Mg) | (Mg) | (Mg) | (Mg) | (Mg) | (Mg) |
| **Pudding bar:** | | | | | | | | |
| chocolate, 1.7-oz. bar.... | 66 | .21 | 10 | 53 | 105 | .17 | .04 | n.a. |
| vanilla, 1.7-oz. bar...... | 61 | .03 | 5 | 48 | 65 | .16 | .01 | n.a. |
| **Pudding mix[1]:** | | | | | | | | |
| chocolate, ½ cup....... | 146 | .20 | n.a. | 120 | 190 | n.a. | n.a. | n.a. |
| chocolate, instant, | | | | | | | | |
| ½ cup............. | 130 | .30 | n.a. | 329 | 176 | n.a. | n.a. | n.a. |
| raspberry or strawberry, | | | | | | | | |
| ½ cup............. | 296 | tr. | n.a. | 206 | 160 | n.a. | n.a. | n.a. |
| rennet custard: | | | | | | | | |
| caramel, fruit | | | | | | | | |
| flavored, or vanilla, | | | | | | | | |
| ½ cup.......... | 147 | tr. | n.a. | 115 | 160 | n.a. | n.a. | n.a. |
| chocolate, ½ cup.... | 156 | tr. | n.a. | 123 | 160 | n.a. | n.a. | n.a. |
| rice, ½ cup ........... | 133 | .50 | n.a. | 110 | 165 | n.a. | n.a. | n.a. |
| tapioca, ½ cup ........ | 131 | .10 | n.a. | 103 | 167 | n.a. | n.a. | n.a. |
| vanilla, ½ cup ......... | 129 | .10 | n.a. | 273 | 164 | n.a. | n.a. | n.a. |
| vanilla, instant, ½ cup ... | 132 | .10 | n.a. | 102 | 166 | n.a. | n.a. | n.a. |
| **Puff pastry, frozen,** | | | | | | | | |
| 1.7-oz. shell......... | 5 | 1.20 | 7 | 28 | 29 | .25 | .03 | .23 |
| **Pummelo:** | | | | | | | | |
| untrimmed, 1 lb........ | 10 | .29 | 16 | 43 | 549 | .20 | .12 | .04 |
| trimmed, sections, | | | | | | | | |
| ½ cup............. | 4 | .11 | 6 | 16 | 206 | .08 | .05 | .02 |
| **Pumpkin:** | | | | | | | | |
| fresh: | | | | | | | | |
| raw, untrimmed, 1 lb. | 67 | 2.54 | 38 | 140 | 1080 | n.a. | n.a. | n.a. |
| raw, trimmed, cubed, | | | | | | | | |
| ½ cup.......... | 12 | .46 | 7 | 26 | 197 | n.a. | n.a. | n.a. |
| boiled, drained, | | | | | | | | |
| mashed, ½ cup ... | 18 | .70 | 11 | 37 | 281 | n.a. | n.a. | n.a. |
| canned, 8 oz.......... | 60 | 3.16 | 53 | 79 | 466 | .39 | .24 | n.a. |
| canned, ½ cup ....... | 32 | 1.70 | 28 | 42 | 251 | .21 | .13 | n.a. |

[1] *Prepared according to package directions, with whole milk.*

| | Calcium | Iron | Magnesium | Phosphorus | Potassium | Zinc | Copper | Manganese |
|---|---|---|---|---|---|---|---|---|
| | (Mg) | (Mg) | (Mg) | (Mg) | (Mg) | (Mg) | (Mg) | (Mg) |
| **Pumpkin pie mix,** | | | | | | | | |
| canned, ½ cup . . . . . . | 49 | 1.43 | 22 | 60 | 186 | .36 | .09 | n.a. |
| **Pumpkin pie spice,** | | | | | | | | |
| 1 tsp. . . . . . . . . . . . . | 12 | .34 | 2 | 2 | 11 | .04 | .01 | .27 |
| **Pumpkin seeds:** | | | | | | | | |
| whole, roasted, 1 oz. . . . . | 16 | .94 | 74 | 26 | 261 | 2.93 | .20 | n.a. |
| whole, roasted, 1 cup . . . | 35 | 2.12 | 168 | 59 | 588 | 6.59 | .44 | n.a. |
| kernels: | | | | | | | | |
| dried, 1 oz. . . . . . . . . | 12 | 4.25 | 152 | 333 | 229 | 2.12 | .39 | n.a. |
| dried, 1 cup. . . . . . . . | 59 | 20.66 | 738 | 1620 | 1114 | 10.29 | 1.91 | n.a. |
| roasted, 1 oz. . . . . . . | 12 | 4.24 | 152 | 333 | 229 | 2.11 | .39 | n.a. |
| roasted, 1 cup . . . . . . | 97 | 33.92 | 1212 | 2660 | 1829 | 16.89 | 3.14 | n.a. |
| **Purslane:** | | | | | | | | |
| raw, untrimmed, 1 lb. | 224 | 6.86 | 235 | 150 | 1704 | n.a. | n.a. | n.a. |
| raw, ½ cup . . . . . . . . . . | 14 | .43 | 15 | 10 | 107 | n.a. | n.a. | n.a. |
| boiled, drained, ½ cup | 45 | .45 | 39 | 22 | 283 | n.a. | n.a. | n.a. |

# Q

| | Calcium | Iron | Magnesium | Phosphorus | Potassium | Zinc | Copper | Manganese |
|---|---|---|---|---|---|---|---|---|
| | (Mg) | (Mg) | (Mg) | (Mg) | (Mg) | (Mg) | (Mg) | (Mg) |
| **Quail**, raw, meat w/skin, 1 oz. | 4 | 1.13 | n.a. | 78 | 61 | n.a. | .14 | n.a. |
| **Quince:** | | | | | | | | |
| untrimmed, 1 lb. | 30 | 1.94 | 21 | 47 | 545 | n.a. | .36 | n.a. |
| 1 medium, 5.3 oz. | 10 | .64 | 7 | 16 | 181 | n.a. | .12 | n.a. |
| **Quinoa**, uncooked, 1 cup | 102 | 15.73 | 357 | 697 | 1258 | 5.61 | 1.39 | n.a. |

# R

| | Calcium | Iron | Magnesium | Phosphorus | Potassium | Zinc | Copper | Manganese |
|---|---|---|---|---|---|---|---|---|
| | (Mg) | (Mg) | (Mg) | (Mg) | (Mg) | (Mg) | (Mg) | (Mg) |
| **Rabbit[1], domesticated, meat only:** | | | | | | | | |
| roasted, 4 oz. . . . . . . . . | 17 | 2.02 | 19 | 234 | 340 | 2.02 | .17 | .03 |
| stewed, 4 oz. . . . . . . . . . | 23 | 2.69 | 23 | 256 | 340 | 2.69 | .20 | .04 |
| **Radicchio, fresh:** | | | | | | | | |
| untrimmed, 1 lb. . . . . . . | 80 | n.a. | 52 | 165 | 1247 | 2.54 | 1.41 | .57 |
| trimmed, 1 medium leaf, approx. .25 oz. . . . . . . | 2 | n.a. | 1 | 3 | 24 | .05 | .03 | .01 |
| trimmed, shredded, ½ cup . . . . . . . . . . . . | 4 | n.a. | 3 | 8 | 60 | .12 | .07 | .03 |
| **Radish, fresh, raw:** | | | | | | | | |
| untrimmed, 1 lb. . . . . . . | 86 | 1.19 | 36 | 74 | 946 | 1.21 | .16 | .29 |
| trimmed, 10 medium, 1.75 oz. . . . . . . . . . . | 9 | .13 | 4 | 8 | 104 | .13 | .02 | .03 |
| trimmed, sliced, ½ cup | 12 | .17 | 5 | 10 | 134 | .17 | .02 | .04 |
| **Radish, Oriental:** | | | | | | | | |
| fresh: | | | | | | | | |
| raw, untrimmed, 1 lb. . . . . . . . . . . | 97 | 1.43 | 56 | 83 | 813 | n.a. | n.a. | n.a. |
| raw, trimmed, 1 medium, approx. 12 oz. . . . . . . . . . | 91 | 1.35 | 53 | 78 | 767 | n.a. | n.a. | n.a. |
| raw, trimmed, sliced, ½ cup . . . . . . . . . | 12 | .18 | 7 | 10 | 100 | n.a. | n.a. | n.a. |
| boiled, drained, sliced, ½ cup. . . . . | 12 | .11 | 7 | 18 | 211 | n.a. | n.a. | n.a. |
| dried, ½ cup . . . . . . . . . | 365 | 3.90 | 99 | 118 | 2027 | n.a. | n.a. | n.a. |
| **Radish, white icicle, fresh, raw:** | | | | | | | | |
| untrimmed, 1 lb. . . . . . . | 80 | 2.36 | 27 | 83 | 825 | n.a. | n.a. | n.a. |
| trimmed, sliced, ½ cup | 14 | .40 | 5 | 14 | 140 | n.a. | n.a. | n.a. |
| **Radish seeds, sprouted, raw:** | | | | | | | | |
| 1 lb. . . . . . . . . . . . . . . | 230 | 3.90 | 199 | 511 | 389 | 2.54 | .54 | 1.80 |
| ½ cup . . . . . . . . . . . . | 10 | .16 | 8 | 21 | 16 | .11 | .02 | .05 |

[1] Prepared without added ingredients.

|  | Calcium | Iron | Magnesium | Phosphorus | Potassium | Zinc | Copper | Manganese |
|---|---|---|---|---|---|---|---|---|
|  | (Mg) | (Mg) | (Mg) | (Mg) | (Mg) | (Mg) | (Mg) | (Mg) |
| **Raisins:** | | | | | | | | |
| seeded: | | | | | | | | |
| 1 lb. . . . . . . . . . . . . | 127 | 11.73 | 135 | 342 | 3744 | .81 | 1.37 | 1.21 |
| 1 oz. . . . . . . . . . . . . | 8 | .73 | 9 | 21 | 234 | .05 | .09 | .08 |
| ½ cup not packed . . . | 21 | 1.88 | 22 | 55 | 599 | .13 | .22 | .19 |
| seedless: | | | | | | | | |
| 1 lb. . . . . . . . . . . . . | 223 | 9.43 | 150 | 438 | 3406 | 1.20 | 1.40 | 1.40 |
| 1 oz. . . . . . . . . . . . . | 14 | .59 | 9 | 27 | 213 | .08 | .09 | .09 |
| ½ cup not packed . . . | 36 | 1.51 | 24 | 70 | 545 | .19 | .22 | .22 |
| seedless, golden: | | | | | | | | |
| 1 lb. . . . . . . . . . . . . | 238 | 8.11 | 158 | 522 | 3386 | 1.46 | 1.65 | 1.40 |
| 1 oz. . . . . . . . . . . . . | 15 | .51 | 10 | 33 | 211 | .09 | .10 | .09 |
| ½ cup not packed . . . | 38 | 1.30 | 26 | 84 | 541 | .24 | .26 | .22 |
| **Raspberry:** | | | | | | | | |
| fresh: | | | | | | | | |
| untrimmed, 1 lb. . . . . | 96 | 2.49 | 77 | 52 | 662 | 2.00 | .32 | 4.41 |
| untrimmed, 1 pint, | | | | | | | | |
| 11.5 oz. . . . . . . . . . | 69 | 1.78 | 55 | 37 | 474 | 1.44 | .23 | 3.16 |
| trimmed, ½ cup. . . . . | 14 | .35 | 11 | 8 | 94 | .29 | .05 | .62 |
| canned, red, in heavy | | | | | | | | |
| syrup, ½ cup. . . . . . . | 14 | .54 | 16 | 12 | 120 | .20 | .07 | .30 |
| frozen, red, sweetened, | | | | | | | | |
| ½ cup . . . . . . . . . . . . | 19 | .81 | 16 | 21 | 143 | .23 | .13 | .81 |
| **Redfish,** see "Ocean perch" | | | | | | | | |
| **Refried beans,** canned: | | | | | | | | |
| 8 oz. . . . . . . . . . . . . . . . . | 80 | 3.77 | 76 | 195 | 606 | 2.65 | .38 | .36 |
| ½ cup. . . . . . . . . . . . . . . | 45 | 2.09 | 42 | 108 | 336 | 1.47 | .21 | .20 |
| **Relish:** | | | | | | | | |
| hamburger, ½ cup. . . . . . | 5 | 1.40 | 9 | 21 | 93 | .14 | .10 | n.a. |
| hamburger, 1 tbsp. . . . . . | 1 | .17 | 1 | 3 | 11 | .02 | .01 | n.a |
| hot dog, ½ cup . . . . . . . . | 7 | 1.53 | 23 | 49 | 95 | .25 | .10 | n.a. |
| hot dog, 1 tbsp. . . . . . . . . | 1 | .19 | 3 | 6 | 12 | .03 | .01 | n.a. |
| sweet, ½ cup . . . . . . . . . | 4 | 1.06 | 5 | 17 | 30 | .17 | .10 | n.a. |
| sweet, 1 tbsp. . . . . . . . . . | 0 | .13 | 1 | 2 | 4 | .02 | .01 | n.a. |

| | Calcium | Iron | Magnesium | Phosphorus | Potassium | Zinc | Copper | Manganese |
|---|---|---|---|---|---|---|---|---|
| | (Mg) | (Mg) | (Mg) | (Mg) | (Mg) | (Mg) | (Mg) | (Mg) |
| **Rhubarb:** | | | | | | | | |
| fresh, untrimmed, 1 lb. | 293 | .76 | 39 | 49 | 978 | .35 | .07 | .67 |
| fresh, trimmed, diced, | | | | | | | | |
| ½ cup . . . . . . . . . . . . | 52 | .14 | 7 | 9 | 175 | .06 | .01 | .12 |
| frozen, ½ cup . . . . . . . . | 132 | .20 | 12 | 8 | 73 | .07 | .02 | .07 |
| frozen, cooked, | | | | | | | | |
| sweetened, ½ cup . . . . | 174 | .25 | 15 | 10 | 115 | .10 | .03 | .09 |
| **Rice[1]:** | | | | | | | | |
| uncooked, ½ cup: | | | | | | | | |
| brown long grain . . . . | 21 | 1.36 | 131 | 306 | 205 | 1.6 | .26 | 3.44 |
| brown medium grain | 31 | 1.71 | 136 | 250 | 255 | 1.92 | .26 | 3.56 |
| white long grain, | | | | | | | | |
| regular . . . . . . . . . . | 26 | 3.97 | 23 | 106 | 106 | 1.00 | .20 | 1.00 |
| white long grain, | | | | | | | | |
| parboiled . . . . . . . . | 56 | 3.28 | 28 | 125 | 110 | .88 | .18 | .78 |
| white long grain, | | | | | | | | |
| precooked or | | | | | | | | |
| instant . . . . . . . . . | 8 | 2.01 | 6 | 33 | 9 | .46 | .08 | .31 |
| white medium grain | 9 | 4.27 | 34 | 106 | 84 | 1.14 | .11 | 1.08 |
| white short grain . . . . | 3 | 4.23 | 23 | 95 | 76 | 1.10 | .21 | 1.04 |
| cooked, ½ cup: | | | | | | | | |
| brown long grain . . . . | 10 | .41 | 42 | 81 | 42 | .62 | .10 | .89 |
| brown medium grain | 10 | .52 | 43 | 76 | 77 | .61 | .08 | 1.08 |
| white long grain, | | | | | | | | |
| regular . . . . . . . . . . | 8 | .95 | 9 | 34 | 28 | .39 | .05 | .37 |
| white long grain, | | | | | | | | |
| parboiled . . . . . . . . | 17 | .99 | 10 | 37 | 33 | .27 | .08 | .23 |
| white long grain, | | | | | | | | |
| precooked or | | | | | | | | |
| instant . . . . . . . . . | 6 | .52 | 4 | 12 | 3 | .20 | .05 | .19 |
| white medium grain | 3 | 1.39 | 12 | 34 | 27 | .39 | .04 | .35 |
| white short grain . . . . | 1 | 1.36 | 8 | 30 | 24 | .37 | .07 | .33 |
| **Rice, glutinous:** | | | | | | | | |
| uncooked, ½ cup . . . . . . | 10 | 1.47 | 21 | 65 | 71 | 1.10 | .16 | .90 |
| cooked, 1 cup . . . . . . . . | 2 | .17 | 6 | 9 | 12 | .49 | .06 | .31 |
| **Rice, wild,** see "Wild rice" | | | | | | | | |

---

[1] *White rice is enriched.*

| | Calcium | Iron | Magnesium | Phosphorus | Potassium | Zinc | Copper | Manganese |
|---|---|---|---|---|---|---|---|---|
| | (Mg) | (Mg) | (Mg) | (Mg) | (Mg) | (Mg) | (Mg) | (Mg) |
| **Rice bran,** crude, | | | | | | | | |
| 1 cup . . . . . . . . . . . . . | 47 | 15.38 | 648 | 1392 | 1232 | 5.02 | .60 | 11.79 |
| **Rice cakes,** brown rice: | | | | | | | | |
| plain, 1 piece. . . . . . . . . | 1 | .13 | 12 | 32 | 26 | .27 | .04 | n.a. |
| buckwheat, 1 piece . . . . . | 1 | .10 | .14 | 34 | 27 | .22 | .03 | .56 |
| corn, 1 piece. . . . . . . . . . | 1 | .11 | 10 | 29 | 25 | .20 | .04 | .46 |
| multi-grain, 1 piece . . . . . | 2 | .18 | 12 | 33 | 26 | .23 | .04 | .47 |
| rye, 1 piece . . . . . . . . . . . | 2 | .16 | 13 | 34 | 28 | .27 | .04 | n.a. |
| sesame seed, 1 piece. . . . | 1 | .14 | 12 | 34 | 26 | .27 | .04 | n.a. |
| **Rice flour:** | | | | | | | | |
| brown, 1 cup. . . . . . . . . | 18 | 3.13 | 177 | 533 | 456 | 3.87 | .36 | 6.34 |
| white, 1 cup . . . . . . . . . | 16 | .55 | 55 | 155 | 120 | 1.26 | .21 | 1.90 |
| **Rice pudding,** see "Pudding" and "Pudding mix" | | | | | | | | |
| **Rockfish,** Pacific, mixed species, meat only: | | | | | | | | |
| raw, 1 lb.. . . . . . . . . . . . | 42 | 1.86 | 119 | 807 | 1838 | 1.86 | .13 | .07 |
| baked, broiled, or | | | | | | | | |
| microwaved[1], 4 oz. . . . | 14 | .60 | 39 | 259 | 588 | .60 | .04 | (0) |
| **Roll:** | | | | | | | | |
| brown and serve: | | | | | | | | |
| dinner or pan, | | | | | | | | |
| 1-oz. roll . . . . . . . . | 20 | .50 | n.a. | 23 | 25 | n.a. | n.a. | n.a. |
| Parkerhouse, | | | | | | | | |
| 1-oz. roll . . . . . . . . | 9 | .50 | n.a. | 21 | 23 | n.a. | n.a. | n.a. |
| dinner: | | | | | | | | |
| 1-oz. roll . . . . . . . . . . | 34 | .89 | 7 | 33 | 38 | .22 | .04 | .13 |
| egg, 1-oz. roll . . . . . . | 21 | 1.23 | 9 | n.a. | n.a. | n.a. | n.a. | n.a. |
| oat bran, 1-oz. roll. . . | 28 | 1.37 | n.a. | n.a. | n.a. | n.a. | n.a. | n.a. |
| rye, 1-oz. roll. . . . . . . | 9 | .77 | 15 | 45 | 51 | n.a. | n.a. | n.a. |
| wheat, 1-oz. roll. . . . . | 50 | 1.01 | n.a. | n.a. | n.a. | n.a. | n.a. | n.a. |
| whole-wheat, | | | | | | | | |
| 1-oz. roll . . . . . . . . | 30 | .68 | 24 | 63 | 77 | .57 | .07 | .65 |
| French, 1.3-oz. roll. . . . . | 35 | 1.03 | 8 | 32 | 43 | n.a. | n.a. | n.a. |
| hard, 2-oz. roll. . . . . . . . | 54 | 1.87 | 16 | 57 | 61 | .54 | .09 | .26 |

[1] *Prepared without added ingredients.*

| | Calcium | Iron | Magnesium | Phosphorus | Potassium | Zinc | Copper | Manganese |
|---|---|---|---|---|---|---|---|---|
| | (Mg) | (Mg) | (Mg) | (Mg) | (Mg) | (Mg) | (Mg) | (Mg) |
| hoagie or submarine, 11½" long, 4.8-oz. roll......... | 100 | 3.80 | n.a. | 115 | 128 | n.a. | n.a. | n.a. |
| hot dog or hamburger: | | | | | | | | |
| plain, 1.5-oz. roll .... | 60 | 1.36 | 8 | n.a. | 60 | .27 | .05 | .14 |
| light, 1.5-oz. roll .... | 26 | 1.28 | n.a. | n.a. | 34 | n.a. | n.a. | n.a. |
| mixed grain, 1.5-oz. roll....... | 41 | 1.7 | n.a. | n.a. | n.a. | n.a. | n.a. | n.a. |
| **Roll, sweet:** | | | | | | | | |
| cheese, 2.3-oz. roll ..... | 78 | .50 | 12 | 65 | n.a. | .42 | .06 | .14 |
| cinnamon, w/raisin, 2.1-oz. roll.......... | 43 | .96 | 10 | 46 | 67 | .36 | .05 | .18 |
| **Roll, sweet, refrigerated dough,** cinnamon w/frosting, 1.1-oz. roll | 9 | .73 | 3 | 96 | 17 | .09 | .02 | n.a. |
| **Roll mix**[1], cloverleaf, 1.2-oz. roll.......... | 20 | .20 | n.a. | 34 | 43 | n.a. | n.a. | n.a. |
| **Rose apple:** | | | | | | | | |
| untrimmed, 1 lb. ....... | 88 | .20 | 15 | 26 | 374 | .17 | .05 | .09 |
| trimmed, 1 oz.......... | 8 | .02 | 1 | 2 | 35 | .02 | tr. | .01 |
| **Roselle:** | | | | | | | | |
| untrimmed, 1 lb. ....... | 596 | 4.10 | 141 | 103 | 575 | n.a. | n.a. | n.a. |
| trimmed, 1 oz. or ½ cup............. | 62 | .42 | 15 | 11 | 59 | n.a. | n.a. | n.a. |
| **Rosemary,** dried, 1 tsp. | 15 | .35 | 3 | 1 | 11 | .04 | .01 | .02 |
| **Rum extract,** artificial (*Virginia Dare*), 1 tsp. | 1 | .03 | 1 | 1 | 8 | tr. | tr. | n.a. |
| **Rutabaga,** fresh: | | | | | | | | |
| raw, untrimmed, 1 lb. ... | 181 | 2.01 | 89 | 224 | 1299 | 1.31 | .15 | .66 |
| raw, cubed, ½ cup ..... | 33 | .36 | 16 | 41 | 236 | .24 | .03 | .12 |
| boiled, drained, cubed, ½ cup............. | 41 | .45 | 20 | 48 | 277 | .30 | .04 | .15 |
| boiled, drained, mashed, ½ cup............. | 58 | .64 | 28 | 67 | 391 | .42 | .05 | .21 |

[1] *Prepared according to package directions, with water.*

| | Calcium | Iron | Magnesium | Phosphorus | Potassium | Zinc | Copper | Manganese |
|---|---|---|---|---|---|---|---|---|
| | (Mg) | (Mg) | (Mg) | (Mg) | (Mg) | (Mg) | (Mg) | (Mg) |
| **Rye,** whole grain, 1 cup | 56 | 4.51 | 204 | 632 | 446 | 6.30 | .76 | 4.53 |
| **Rye flour:** | | | | | | | | |
| dark, 1 cup . . . . . . . . . . . | 72 | 8.26 | 318 | 809 | 934 | 7.19 | .96 | 8.61 |
| light, 1 cup . . . . . . . . . . . | 21 | 1.84 | 72 | 198 | 238 | 1.78 | .26 | 2.01 |
| medium, 1 cup . . . . . . . . | 24 | 2.16 | 77 | 211 | 347 | 2.03 | .29 | 5.57 |

# S

| | Calcium | Iron | Magnesium | Phosphorus | Potassium | Zinc | Copper | Manganese |
|---|---|---|---|---|---|---|---|---|
| | (Mg) | (Mg) | (Mg) | (Mg) | (Mg) | (Mg) | (Mg) | (Mg) |
| **Sablefish,** meat only: | | | | | | | | |
| raw, 1 lb.............. | n.a. | 5.81 | n.a. | n.a. | 1624 | 1.47 | .10 | .07 |
| baked, broiled, or | | | | | | | | |
| microwaved[1], 4 oz. ... | n.a. | 5.81 | n.a. | n.a. | 521 | .46 | .03 | .02 |
| **Sage,** ground, 1 tsp..... | 12 | .20 | 3 | 1 | 7 | .03 | .01 | .02 |
| **Salad dressing:** | | | | | | | | |
| blue cheese, 1 tbsp...... | 12 | tr. | n.a. | 11 | 6 | n.a. | n.a. | n.a. |
| French, 1 tbsp. ........ | 2 | tr. | 2 | 1 | 2 | n.a. | n.a. | n.a. |
| French, low calorie, | | | | | | | | |
| 1 tbsp. ............ | 6 | tr. | n.a. | 5 | 3 | n.a. | n.a. | n.a. |
| Italian, 1 tbsp......... | 1 | tr. | n.a. | 1 | 5 | n.a. | n.a. | n.a. |
| Italian, low calorie, | | | | | | | | |
| 1 tbsp. ............ | 1 | tr. | n.a. | 1 | 4 | n.a. | n.a. | n.a. |
| mayonnaise type, | | | | | | | | |
| 1 tbsp. ............ | 2 | tr. | n.a. | 4 | 1 | n.a. | n.a. | n.a. |
| Thousand Island, | | | | | | | | |
| 1 tbsp. ............ | 2 | .10 | n.a. | 3 | 18 | n.a. | n.a. | n.a. |
| Thousand Island, low | | | | | | | | |
| calorie, 1 tbsp......... | 2 | .10 | n.a. | 3 | 17 | n.a. | n.a. | n.a. |
| vinegar and oil, 1 tbsp. | 0 | 0 | n.a. | 0 | 1 | n.a. | n.a. | n.a. |
| **Salami:** | | | | | | | | |
| beef, cooked, 1 oz. ..... | 2 | .57 | 4 | 29 | 64 | .61 | .03 | .01 |
| beef and pork, cooked, | | | | | | | | |
| 1 oz............... | 4 | .76 | 4 | 33 | 56 | .61 | .06 | .02 |
| beer, beef, .8 oz........ | 2 | .35 | 3 | 22 | 40 | .56 | .01 | n.a. |
| beer, pork, 1 oz. ....... | 2 | .22 | 4 | 29 | 72 | .49 | .01 | .01 |
| dry or hard, pork, | | | | | | | | |
| 1 oz............... | 4 | .37 | 6 | 65 | n.a. | 1.19 | .05 | .02 |
| dry or hard, pork and | | | | | | | | |
| beef, 1 oz........... | 2 | .43 | 5 | 40 | 107 | .92 | .02 | .01 |
| **"Salami,"** vegetarian | | | | | | | | |
| (*Worthington*), 2 oz. ... | 26 | 1.45 | n.a. | n.a. | 94 | .30 | n.a. | n.a. |

[1] Prepared without added ingredients.

| | Calcium | Iron | Magnesium | Phosphorus | Potassium | Zinc | Copper | Manganese |
|---|---|---|---|---|---|---|---|---|
| | (Mg) | (Mg) | (Mg) | (Mg) | (Mg) | (Mg) | (Mg) | (Mg) |
| **Salmon,** meat only: | | | | | | | | |
| Atlantic: | | | | | | | | |
| wild, 1 lb. . . . . . . . . | 54 | 3.63 | n.a. | 907 | 2223 | n.a. | n.a. | n.a. |
| wild, baked, broiled, or microwaved[1], 4 oz. . . . . . . . . . . . | 17 | 1.17 | n.a. | 290 | 712 | n.a. | n.a. | n.a. |
| farmed, raw, 1 lb. . . . | n.a. | 1.63 | 126 | 1056 | 1644 | 1.80 | .22 | .07 |
| farmed, baked, broiled, or microwaved[1], 4 oz. | n.a. | .39 | 34 | 286 | 435 | .49 | .06 | .02 |
| chinook: | | | | | | | | |
| raw, 1 lb.. . . . . . . . . | 100 | 3.22 | n.a. | n.a. | 1787 | 2.01 | .19 | .07 |
| baked, broiled, or microwaved[1], 4 oz. | 32 | 1.03 | n.a. | n.a. | 573 | .64 | .06 | .02 |
| smoked, 4 oz. . . . . . . | 12 | .96 | 20 | 186 | 198 | .35 | .26 | .02 |
| chum, raw, 1 lb. . . . . . . | 50 | 2.49 | n.a. | 1284 | 1946 | 2.13 | .25 | .82 |
| chum, baked, broiled, or microwaved[1], 4 oz. . . . | 16 | .81 | n.a. | 412 | 624 | .68 | .08 | .02 |
| coho: | | | | | | | | |
| wild, raw, 1 lb. . . . . . | 163 | 2.53 | 139 | 1187 | 1916 | 1.87 | .23 | .06 |
| wild, baked, broiled or microwaved[1], 4 oz. . . . . . . . . . . . | n.a. | .69 | 37 | 365 | 492 | .64 | .08 | .02 |
| wild, poached or steamed[1], 4 oz. . . . | 52 | .81 | 40 | 338 | 516 | .59 | .07 | .02 |
| farmed, raw, 1 lb. . . . | 54 | 1.55 | 141 | 1324 | 2043 | 1.94 | .22 | .06 |
| farmed, baked, broiled, or microwaved[1], 4 oz. | 14 | .44 | 39 | 376 | 522 | .53 | .10 | .02 |
| pink, raw, 1 lb. . . . . . . . | n.a. | 3.49 | n.a. | n.a. | 1463 | 2.48 | .35 | .07 |
| pink, baked, broiled, or microwaved[1], 4 oz. . . . | n.a. | 1.12 | n.a. | n.a. | 469 | .81 | .11 | .02 |
| sockeye (red), raw, 4 oz.. . . . . . . . . . . . | 27 | 2.13 | 109 | 975 | 1774 | 2.45 | .24 | .06 |

[1] *Prepared without added ingredients.*

| | Calcium | Iron | Magnesium | Phosphorus | Potassium | Zinc | Copper | Manganese |
|---|---|---|---|---|---|---|---|---|
| | (Mg) | (Mg) | (Mg) | (Mg) | (Mg) | (Mg) | (Mg) | (Mg) |
| sockeye (red), baked, broiled, or microwaved[1], 4 oz. ... | 8 | .62 | 35 | 313 | 425 | .58 | .08 | .02 |
| **Salmon, canned:** | | | | | | | | |
| pink, w/bone and liquid, 16-oz. can . . . . . . . . . | 969 | 3.83 | 152 | 1492 | 1482 | 4.19 | .46 | n.a. |
| pink, w/bone and liquid, 4 oz. . . . . . . . . . . . . . . | 242 | .95 | 39 | 373 | 370 | 1.04 | .12 | n.a. |
| sockeye (red), w/bone, drained, 13 oz. (16-oz. can w/liquid) . . | 883 | 3.90 | 107 | 1202 | 1392 | 3.75 | .31 | n.a. |
| sockeye (red), w/bone, drained, 4 oz. . . . . . . . | 271 | 1.16 | 33 | 370 | 428 | 1.16 | .10 | n.a. |
| **Salsa,** ½ cup . . . . . . . . . | 60 | .94 | 16 | 30 | 240 | .38 | .09 | .13 |
| **Salsify,** fresh: | | | | | | | | |
| raw, untrimmed, 1 lb. . . . . . . . . . . . . | 237 | 2.76 | 91 | 296 | 1499 | n.a. | n.a. | n.a. |
| raw, trimmed, sliced, ½ cup. . . . . . . . . . . . | 40 | .47 | 15 | 50 | 255 | n.a. | n.a. | n.a. |
| boiled, drained, sliced, ½ cup. . . . . . . . . . . . | 32 | .37 | 12 | 38 | 192 | n.a. | n.a. | n.a. |
| **Salt,** 1 tsp. . . . . . . . . . . . | 1 | .02 | 0 | 0 | 0 | .01 | tr. | .01 |
| **Salt substitute** (*Instead of Salt*), 1 tsp. . . . . . . . | 19 | .77 | 7 | 13 | 40 | .14 | n.a. | n.a. |
| **Sandwich spread:** | | | | | | | | |
| pork and beef, 1 tsp. . . . . . . . . . . . . | 2 | .12 | 1 | 9 | 16 | .15 | .02 | tr. |
| vegetarian (*Loma Linda*), 1.9 oz. . . . . . . . . . . . . . | 20 | 1.30 | n.a. | n.a. | 139 | .41 | n.a. | n.a. |
| **Sapodilla:** | | | | | | | | |
| untrimmed, 1 lb. . . . . . . . | 76 | 2.90 | n.a. | 44 | 700 | n.a. | n.a. | n.a. |
| pulp, ½ cup. . . . . . . . . . . | 26 | .97 | n.a. | 15 | 233 | n.a. | n.a. | n.a. |
| **Sapote:** | | | | | | | | |
| untrimmed, 1 lb. . . . . . . . | 126 | 3.22 | 97 | 90 | 1106 | n.a. | n.a. | n.a. |

[1] *Prepared without added ingredients.*

| | Calcium (Mg) | Iron (Mg) | Magnesium (Mg) | Phosphorus (Mg) | Potassium (Mg) | Zinc (Mg) | Copper (Mg) | Manganese (Mg) |
|---|---|---|---|---|---|---|---|---|
| **Sapote,** *continued* | | | | | | | | |
| 1 medium, approx. | | | | | | | | |
| 11.2 oz.............. | 88 | 2.25 | 68 | 63 | 773 | n.a. | n.a. | n.a. |
| **Sardines,** canned: | | | | | | | | |
| Atlantic, in soybean oil: | | | | | | | | |
| w/bone, drained, | | | | | | | | |
| 4 oz............. | 433 | 3.31 | 44 | 556 | 450 | 1.49 | .21 | .12 |
| w/bone, 2 medium, | | | | | | | | |
| 3" long, .8 oz. .... | 92 | .70 | 9 | 118 | 95 | .31 | .05 | .03 |
| Pacific, in tomato sauce: | | | | | | | | |
| drained, 4 oz. ...... | 272 | 2.61 | 39 | 415 | 387 | 1.59 | .31 | .23 |
| 1 medium, 4¾" long, | | | | | | | | |
| 1.3 oz........... | 91 | .87 | 13 | 139 | 130 | .53 | .10 | .08 |
| **Sauce,** see specific listings | | | | | | | | |
| **Sauerkraut,** canned, | | | | | | | | |
| w/ liquid, ½ cup ..... | 36 | 1.73 | 15 | 23 | 201 | .22 | .11 | n.a. |
| **Sausage** (see also specific listings): | | | | | | | | |
| pork, fresh: | | | | | | | | |
| cooked, 1 link, .5 oz. | | | | | | | | |
| (1-oz. raw link) ... | 4 | .16 | 2 | 24 | 47 | .33 | .02 | .01 |
| cooked, 1 patty, | | | | | | | | |
| approx. 1 oz. | | | | | | | | |
| (2-oz. raw patty) .. | 9 | .34 | 5 | 50 | 97 | .68 | .04 | .02 |
| smoked, 1 link, | | | | | | | | |
| 4" long × 1⅛", | | | | | | | | |
| 2.4 oz........... | 20 | .79 | 13 | 110 | 228 | 1.92 | .05 | n.a. |
| pork and beef, fresh, | | | | | | | | |
| cooked, .5 oz. (1-oz. | | | | | | | | |
| raw link) .......... | n.a. | .15 | 1 | 14 | n.a. | .24 | tr. | n.a. |
| pork and beef, fresh, | | | | | | | | |
| cooked, 1 oz. (2 oz. | | | | | | | | |
| raw patty) ......... | n.a. | .31 | 3 | 29 | n.a. | .50 | .01 | n.a. |
| smoked, pork, 1 link, | | | | | | | | |
| 4" long × 1⅛"....... | 7 | .99 | 8 | 73 | 129 | 1.44 | .04 | .03 |

| | Calcium | Iron | Magnesium | Phosphorus | Potassium | Zinc | Copper | Manganese |
|---|---|---|---|---|---|---|---|---|
| | (Mg) | (Mg) | (Mg) | (Mg) | (Mg) | (Mg) | (Mg) | (Mg) |
| **"Sausage," vegetarian:** | | | | | | | | |
| canned: | | | | | | | | |
| (*Loma Linda Little Links*), 2 links, 1.6 oz.......... | 6 | .46 | n.a. | n.a. | 16 | .56 | n.a. | n.a. |
| (*Worthington Saucettes*), 1.3-oz. link ........... | 9 | 1.15 | n.a. | n.a. | 25 | .26 | n.a. | n.a. |
| frozen: | | | | | | | | |
| (*Morningstar Farms Breakfast Links*), 2 links, 1.6 oz..... | 15 | 2.14 | n.a. | 54 | 59 | .36 | n.a. | n.a. |
| (*Morningstar Farms Breakfast Patties*), 1.3-oz. patty ..... | 15 | 1.67 | n.a. | 107 | 102 | .37 | n.a. | n.a. |
| (*Worthington Prosage Links*), 2 links, 1.6 oz.......... | 15 | 2.14 | n.a. | 54 | 59 | .36 | n.a. | n.a. |
| (*Worthington Prosage Patties*), 1.3-oz. patty ..... | 15 | 1.19 | n.a. | 96 | 78 | .34 | n.a. | n.a. |
| roll (*Worthington Prosage*), ⅝" slice, 1.9 oz.......... | 11 | 1.88 | n.a. | 74 | 82 | .38 | n.a. | n.a. |
| **Savory,** ground, 1 tsp.... | 30 | .53 | 5 | 2 | 15 | .06 | .01 | .09 |
| **Scallion,** see "Onion, green" | | | | | | | | |
| **Scallop,** mixed species, meat only: | | | | | | | | |
| raw, 1 lb.............. | 110 | 1.32 | 254 | 995 | 1460 | 4.33 | .24 | .41 |
| raw, 2 large or 5 small, 1.1 oz.............. | 7 | .09 | 17 | 66 | 97 | .29 | .02 | .03 |
| breaded, fried, 2 large | 13 | .25 | 18 | 73 | 103 | .33 | .02 | n.a. |
| **"Scallop," vegetarian,** canned (*Worthington Skallops*), 3 oz. ...... | 5 | .56 | n.a. | 66 | 10 | .67 | n.a. | n.a. |

| | Calcium | Iron | Magnesium | Phosphorus | Potassium | Zinc | Copper | Manganese |
|---|---|---|---|---|---|---|---|---|
| | (Mg) | (Mg) | (Mg) | (Mg) | (Mg) | (Mg) | (Mg) | (Mg) |
| **Scallop squash:** | | | | | | | | |
| raw, untrimmed, 1 lb. | 84 | 1.78 | 102 | 160 | 808 | 1.31 | .45 | .70 |
| raw, trimmed, sliced, | | | | | | | | |
| ½ cup.............. | 12 | .26 | 15 | 23 | 118 | .19 | .07 | .10 |
| boiled, drained, sliced, | | | | | | | | |
| ½ cup.............. | 14 | .29 | 17 | 25 | 126 | .22 | .08 | .12 |
| **Scrod,** see "Cod" | | | | | | | | |
| **Scup,** meat only: | | | | | | | | |
| raw, 1 lb............. | 183 | 2.40 | 104 | n.a. | 1302 | 2.20 | .23 | .16 |
| baked, broiled, or | | | | | | | | |
| microwaved[1], 4 oz. ... | 58 | .77 | 33 | n.a. | 417 | .70 | .07 | .05 |
| **Sea bass,** mixed species, meat only: | | | | | | | | |
| raw, 1 lb............. | 47 | 1.31 | 188 | 879 | 1161 | 1.83 | .09 | .07 |
| baked, broiled, or | | | | | | | | |
| microwaved[1], 4 oz. ... | 15 | .42 | 60 | 281 | 372 | .59 | .03 | n.a. |
| **Sea trout,** mixed species, meat only: | | | | | | | | |
| raw, 1 lb............. | 78 | 1.20 | 143 | 1132 | 1547 | 2.04 | .14 | .07 |
| baked, broiled, or | | | | | | | | |
| microwaved[1], 4 oz. ... | 25 | .40 | 45 | 364 | 496 | .66 | .04 | .02 |
| **Seasoning mix** (see also specific listings): | | | | | | | | |
| all purpose (*Tone's Perc*), | | | | | | | | |
| ¼ tsp............. | 5 | .14 | 2 | 3 | 10 | .03 | tr. | 02 |
| all purpose, w/herbs, | | | | | | | | |
| (*Tone's Perc*), | | | | | | | | |
| ¼ tsp............. | 3 | .14 | 1 | 1 | 9 | .01 | tr. | .01 |
| garden (*Tone's Perc*), | | | | | | | | |
| ¼ tsp............. | 3 | .14 | 1 | 2 | 10 | .01 | tr. | .01 |
| garden, extra spicy | | | | | | | | |
| (*Tone's Perc*), ¼ tsp. | 2 | .64 | 1 | 1 | 11 | .01 | tr. | .02 |
| spice and herb (*Tone's* | | | | | | | | |
| *Perc*), ¼ tsp........ | 4 | .16 | 1 | 2 | 10 | .02 | tr. | .01 |
| vegetable (*Tone's Perc*), | | | | | | | | |
| ¼ tsp............. | 4 | .05 | 1 | 3 | 10 | .02 | tr. | .01 |

[1] *Prepared without added ingredients.*

| | Calcium | Iron | Magnesium | Phosphorus | Potassium | Zinc | Copper | Manganese |
|---|---|---|---|---|---|---|---|---|
| | (Mg) | (Mg) | (Mg) | (Mg) | (Mg) | (Mg) | (Mg) | (Mg) |
| zesty country (*Tone's Perc*), ¼ tsp......... | 2 | .05 | 1 | 3 | 12 | .02 | tr. | .01 |
| **Seaweed:** | | | | | | | | |
| agar, dried, 1 oz........ | 177 | 6.07 | 218 | 15 | 319 | n.a. | n.a. | 1.20 |
| Irish moss, raw, 1 oz. | 20 | 2.52 | n.a. | 45 | 18 | .55 | .04 | .10 |
| kelp, raw, 1 oz. ........ | 48 | .81 | 34 | 12 | 25 | .35 | .04 | .06 |
| laver, raw, 1 oz......... | 20 | .51 | <1 | 16 | 101 | .30 | .07 | .28 |
| wakame, raw, 1 oz. ..... | 43 | .62 | 30 | 23 | 14 | .11 | .08 | .40 |
| **Semolina,** whole grain, enriched, 1 cup ...... | 29 | 7.28 | 78 | 226 | 311 | 1.75 | .32 | 1.03 |
| **Sesame butter:** | | | | | | | | |
| paste, from whole seeds, 1 oz............... | 273 | 5.45 | 103 | 187 | 165 | 2.07 | 1.20 | .72 |
| paste, from whole seeds, 1 tbsp. ............ | 154 | 3.07 | 58 | 105 | 93 | 1.17 | .67 | .41 |
| tahini: | | | | | | | | |
|   from raw and stoneground kernels, 1 oz...... | 119 | .71 | 27 | 214 | 118 | 1.32 | .46 | n.a. |
|   from raw and stoneground kernels, 1 tbsp. .... | 63 | .38 | 14 | 113 | 62 | .70 | .24 | n.a. |
|   from unroasted kernels[1], 1 oz..... | 40 | 1.80 | 100 | 224 | 130 | 2.97 | n.a. | n.a. |
|   from unroasted kernels[1], 1 tbsp.... | 20 | .89 | 49 | 111 | 64 | .46 | n.a. | n.a. |
|   from roasted and toasted kernels, 1 oz........... | 121 | 2.54 | 27 | 208 | 118 | 1.31 | .46 | n.a. |
|   from roasted and toasted kernels, 1 tbsp. ......... | 64 | 1.34 | 14 | 110 | 62 | .69 | .24 | n.a. |
| **Sesame flour:** | | | | | | | | |
| high fat, 1 oz. ......... | 45 | 4.31 | 102 | 229 | 120 | 3.03 | n.a. | n.a. |

[1] *Nonchemical removal of seed coat.*

| | Calcium (Mg) | Iron (Mg) | Magnesium (Mg) | Phosphorus (Mg) | Potassium (Mg) | Zinc (Mg) | Copper (Mg) | Manganese (Mg) |
|---|---|---|---|---|---|---|---|---|
| **Sesame flour,** *continued* | | | | | | | | |
| partially defatted, 1 oz. | 43 | 4.06 | 103 | 230 | 121 | 3.04 | n.a. | n.a. |
| low fat, 1 oz. | 42 | 4.04 | 96 | 215 | 113 | 2.84 | n.a. | n.a. |
| **Sesame meal,** partially | | | | | | | | |
| defatted, 1 oz. | 43 | 4.13 | 98 | 220 | 115 | 2.91 | n.a. | n.a. |
| **Sesame paste,** see "Sesame butter" | | | | | | | | |
| **Sesame seeds:** | | | | | | | | |
| whole: | | | | | | | | |
| dried, 1 cup | 1404 | 20.95 | 505 | 906 | 674 | 11.16 | 5.88 | 3.54 |
| dried, 1 tbsp. | 88 | 1.31 | 32 | 57 | 42 | .70 | .37 | .22 |
| roasted or toasted, | | | | | | | | |
| 1 oz. | 281 | 4.19 | 101 | 181 | 135 | 2.03 | .70 | .71 |
| kernels: | | | | | | | | |
| dried, 1 cup | 197 | 11.70 | 520 | 1163 | 610 | 15.38 | n.a. | n.a. |
| dried, 1 tbsp. | 10 | .62 | 28 | 62 | 33 | .82 | n.a. | n.a. |
| toasted, 1 oz. | 37 | 2.21 | 98 | 220 | 115 | 2.90 | n.a. | n.a. |
| **Sesbania flower,** raw, | | | | | | | | |
| trimmed, 1 cup | 4 | .17 | 2 | 6 | 37 | n.a. | n.a. | n.a. |
| **Shad,** American, meat only: | | | | | | | | |
| raw, 1 lb. | 214 | 4.38 | 137 | 1234 | 1740 | 1.66 | .29 | .19 |
| baked, broiled, or | | | | | | | | |
| microwaved[1], 4 oz. | 68 | 1.41 | 43 | 396 | 558 | .53 | .09 | .06 |
| **Shallot:** | | | | | | | | |
| raw, chopped, 1 tbsp. | 4 | .12 | n.a. | 6 | 33 | n.a. | n.a. | n.a. |
| freeze-dried, ¼ cup | 7 | .22 | 4 | 11 | 59 | .07 | .02 | .05 |
| freeze-dried, 1 tbsp. | 2 | .05 | 1 | 3 | 15 | .02 | <.01 | .01 |
| **Shark,** mixed species, meat only: | | | | | | | | |
| raw, 1 lb. | 153 | 3.81 | 222 | 955 | 727 | 1.95 | .15 | .07 |
| batter-dipped, fried, | | | | | | | | |
| 4 oz. | 57 | 1.26 | 49 | 220 | 176 | .54 | .05 | n.a. |
| **Sherbet,** orange, ½ cup | 52 | .14 | 7 | 38 | 92 | .46 | .03 | .01 |
| **Sheepshead,** meat only: | | | | | | | | |
| raw, 1 lb. | 95 | 2.09 | 144 | 1418 | 1834 | 1.75 | .14 | .06 |

---

[1] *Prepared without added ingredients.*

| | Calcium | Iron | Magnesium | Phosphorus | Potassium | Zinc | Copper | Manganese |
|---|---|---|---|---|---|---|---|---|
| | (Mg) | (Mg) | (Mg) | (Mg) | (Mg) | (Mg) | (Mg) | (Mg) |
| baked, broiled, or microwaved[1], 4 oz. . . . | 42 | .76 | 40 | 397 | 581 | .71 | .14 | .02 |
| **Shortening**, vegetable, 1 tbsp. . . . . . . . . . . . | 0 | 0 | n.a. | 0 | 0 | n.a. | n.a. | n.a. |
| **Shrimp**, mixed species, meat only: | | | | | | | | |
| raw, 1 lb. . . . . . . . . . . . | 235 | 10.92 | 166 | 932 | 840 | 5.03 | 1.20 | .23 |
| raw, 4 large (32 per lb.), 1 oz. . . . . . . . . . . . . . | 15 | .67 | 10 | 58 | 52 | .31 | .07 | .01 |
| boiled, poached, or steamed[1], 4 oz. . . . . . . | 44 | 3.50 | 38 | 155 | 206 | 1.77 | .22 | .05 |
| boiled, poached, or steamed[1], 4 large. . . . . | 9 | .68 | 7 | 30 | 40 | .34 | .04 | .01 |
| breaded, fried, 4 oz. . . . . . | 76 | 1.43 | 45 | 247 | 255 | 1.56 | .31 | n.a. |
| breaded, fried, 4 large . . . | 20 | .38 | 12 | 65 | 67 | .41 | .08 | n.a. |
| **Shrimp, canned,** drained: | | | | | | | | |
| 4 oz. . . . . . . . . . . . . . . . . | 67 | 3.11 | 46 | 264 | 238 | 1.43 | .34 | n.a. |
| 1 cup . . . . . . . . . . . . . . . | 75 | 3.50 | 53 | 299 | 269 | 1.61 | .38 | n.a. |
| **Sisymbrium seeds,** whole, dried, 1 oz. . . . . | 464 | .03 | 89 | 2 | 605 | .09 | .03 | n.a. |
| **Smelt**, rainbow, meat only: | | | | | | | | |
| raw, 1 lb. . . . . . . . . . . . . | 272 | 4.08 | 136 | 1043 | 1315 | .47 | .04 | .20 |
| baked, broiled, or microwaved[1], 4 oz. . . . | 87 | 1.30 | 43 | 335 | 422 | 2.40 | .20 | n.a. |
| **Snack mix:** | | | | | | | | |
| (*Chex*), ⅔ cup, 1 oz. . . . . | n.a. | 7.00 | 18 | 53 | n.a. | n.a. | n.a. | n.a. |
| (*Doo Dads*), 1 cup, 2 oz. . . . . . . . . . . . . . | 42 | 1.42 | 34 | 168 | 157 | 1.27 | .18 | n.a. |
| **Snail, sea,** see "Whelk" | | | | | | | | |
| **Snap beans,** see "Green beans" | | | | | | | | |
| **Snapper,** mixed species, meat only: | | | | | | | | |
| raw, 1 lb. . . . . . . . . . . . . | 143 | .79 | 146 | 899 | 1894 | 1.61 | .13 | .06 |
| baked, broiled, or microwaved[1], 4 oz. . . . | 45 | .27 | 42 | 228 | 592 | .50 | .05 | .02 |

---

[1] *Prepared without added ingredients.*

| | Calcium | Iron | Magnesium | Phosphorus | Potassium | Zinc | Copper | Manganese |
|---|---|---|---|---|---|---|---|---|
| | (Mg) | (Mg) | (Mg) | (Mg) | (Mg) | (Mg) | (Mg) | (Mg) |
| **Soft drinks and mixers:** | | | | | | | | |
| club soda, 12 fl. oz..... | 17 | n.a. | 4 | 0 | 6 | .36 | n.a. | n.a. |
| cola, 12 fl. oz.......... | 9 | .13 | 3 | 46 | 4 | .05 | .04 | .13 |
| cola, low-calorie[1], | | | | | | | | |
|   12 fl. oz............ | 12 | .11 | 4 | 30 | 0 | .28 | n.a. | n.a. |
| cream soda, 12 fl. oz. ... | 19 | .19 | 3 | 0 | 4 | .24 | .03 | n.a. |
| cream soda (*A & W*), | | | | | | | | |
|   1 fl. oz............. | 1 | .02 | n.a. | tr. | 2 | n.a. | n.a. | n.a. |
| cream soda (*A & W* Diet), | | | | | | | | |
|   1 fl. oz............. | 1 | .01 | n.a. | tr. | 1 | n.a. | n.a. | n.a. |
| ginger ale, 12 fl. oz..... | 12 | .66 | 3 | 1 | 5 | .18 | .07 | n.a. |
| grape, 12 fl. oz......... | 12 | .31 | 4 | 0 | 3 | .26 | .08 | n.a. |
| lemon-lime, 12 fl. oz..... | 9 | .25 | 2 | 1 | 4 | .18 | .04 | .05 |
| mineral water (*Perrier*), | | | | | | | | |
|   8 fl. oz............. | 32 | 0 | 1 | 0 | 0 | 0 | 0 | 0 |
| orange, 12 fl. oz........ | 19 | .23 | 4 | 4 | 9 | .38 | .06 | n.a. |
| pepper type, 12 fl. oz. ... | 12 | .14 | 1 | 41 | 2 | .15 | .02 | n.a. |
| root beer, 12 fl. oz. ..... | 19 | .18 | 4 | 2 | 3 | .26 | .03 | n.a. |
| root beer (*A & W*), | | | | | | | | |
|   1 fl. oz............. | 1 | tr. | n.a. | tr. | 1 | n.a. | n.a. | n.a. |
| root beer (*A & W* Diet), | | | | | | | | |
|   1 fl. oz............. | 1 | tr. | n.a. | tr. | 3 | n.a. | n.a. | n.a. |
| (*Squirt*), 1 fl. oz........ | 1 | tr. | n.a. | tr. | tr. | n.a. | n.a. | n.a. |
| (*Squirt* Low Calorie), | | | | | | | | |
|   1 fl. oz............. | 1 | tr. | n.a. | tr. | 1 | n.a. | n.a. | n.a. |
| (*Vernors*), 1 fl. oz....... | 1 | tr. | n.a. | tr. | <1 | n.a. | n.a. | n.a. |
| (*Vernors* Low Calorie), | | | | | | | | |
|   1 fl. oz............. | 1 | tr. | n.a. | tr. | 1 | n.a. | n.a. | n.a. |
| **Sole,** see "Flatfish" | | | | | | | | |
| **Sorghum,** whole grain, | | | | | | | | |
|   1 cup ............. | 54 | 8.45 | n.a. | 551 | 672 | n.a. | n.a. | n.a. |
| **Sorghum syrup,** 1 tbsp. | 31 | .80 | 21 | 12 | 210 | .09 | .03 | n.a. |

---

[1] *Aspartame sweetened.*

| | Calcium | Iron | Magnesium | Phosphorus | Potassium | Zinc | Copper | Manganese |
|---|---|---|---|---|---|---|---|---|
| | (Mg) | (Mg) | (Mg) | (Mg) | (Mg) | (Mg) | (Mg) | (Mg) |

**Soup, canned,** ready-to-serve, 1 cup:

| | Calcium | Iron | Magnesium | Phosphorus | Potassium | Zinc | Copper | Manganese |
|---|---|---|---|---|---|---|---|---|
| bean (*Grandma Brown's*) | 93 | 2.95 | 73 | 193 | 470 | 1.23 | .32 | .68 |
| beef, chunky | 31 | 2.32 | n.a. | 120 | 336 | 2.64 | .24 | .24 |
| chicken, chunky | 24 | 1.73 | n.a. | 113 | 176 | 1.00 | .25 | .25 |
| clam chowder, | | | | | | | | |
|   Manhattan, chunky | 67 | 2.64 | n.a. | 84 | 384 | 1.68 | .24 | .24 |
| pea (*Grandma Brown's*) | 30 | 2.55 | 56 | 148 | 400 | 3.45 | .18 | .55 |
| pea, split, w/ham, chunky | n.a. | n.a. | n.a. | n.a. | n.a. | n.a. | n.a. | n.a. |
| turkey, chunky | 50 | 1.91 | n.a. | 104 | 361 | 2.12 | .24 | .24 |
| vegetable, chunky | 56 | 1.63 | n.a. | 72 | 396 | 3.12 | .24 | .48 |

**Soup, canned, condensed[1],** 1 cup:

| | Calcium | Iron | Magnesium | Phosphorus | Potassium | Zinc | Copper | Manganese |
|---|---|---|---|---|---|---|---|---|
| asparagus, cream of | 29 | .80 | 4 | 39 | 173 | .88 | .12 | .38 |
| asparagus, cream of[2] | 175 | .87 | 20 | 153 | 359 | .93 | .14 | .38 |
| bean, black | 45 | 2.16 | 42 | 107 | 273 | 1.41 | .39 | .64 |
| bean w/bacon | 81 | 2.05 | 44 | 132 | 403 | 1.03 | .40 | .67 |
| bean w/frankfurters | 86 | 2.34 | 49 | 166 | 477 | 1.18 | .40 | .79 |
| beef noodle | 15 | 1.10 | 6 | 46 | 99 | 1.54 | .14 | .27 |
| celery, cream of | 40 | .62 | 6 | 37 | 123 | .15 | .14 | .25 |
| celery, cream of[2] | 186 | .69 | 22 | 151 | 309 | .20 | .15 | .25 |
| cheese | 142 | .75 | 4 | 136 | 154 | .64 | .13 | .26 |
| cheese[2] | 288 | .81 | 20 | 250 | 340 | .69 | .14 | .26 |
| chicken: | | | | | | | | |
|   broth | 9 | .51 | 2 | 73 | 210 | .25 | .12 | .25 |
|   cream of | 34 | .61 | 3 | 38 | 87 | .63 | .12 | .38 |
|   cream of[2] | 180 | .67 | 18 | 152 | 273 | .68 | .14 | .38 |
|   and dumplings | 15 | .62 | 4 | 61 | 116 | .37 | .12 | .49 |
|   gumbo | 24 | .89 | 4 | 25 | 75 | .38 | .12 | .25 |
|   noodle | 17 | .78 | 5 | 36 | 55 | .40 | .20 | .29 |
|   rice | 17 | .75 | 1 | 21 | 100 | .26 | .12 | .37 |
|   vegetable | 18 | .87 | 6 | 41 | 154 | .37 | .12 | .37 |
| chili beef | 43 | 2.13 | 30 | 148 | 515 | 1.40 | .40 | 1.05 |

---

[1] *Prepared according to package directions, with water, except as noted.*
[2] *Prepared with whole milk.*

|  | Calcium (Mg) | Iron (Mg) | Magnesium (Mg) | Phosphorus (Mg) | Potassium (Mg) | Zinc (Mg) | Copper (Mg) | Manganese (Mg) |
|---|---|---|---|---|---|---|---|---|
| Soup, canned, condensed, *continued* | | | | | | | | |
| clam chowder: | | | | | | | | |
| Manhattan . . . . . . . . . | 26 | 1.64 | 11 | 41 | 188 | .97 | .13 | .38 |
| New England . . . . . . . | 43 | 1.48 | 7 | 54 | 146 | .75 | .12 | .25 |
| New England[1] . . . . . . | 187 | 1.48 | 23 | 157 | 300 | .80 | .14 | .25 |
| consommé, w/gelatin . . . . | 8 | .53 | 0 | 32 | 153 | .37 | .25 | .37 |
| minestrone . . . . . . . . . . | 34 | .92 | 7 | 56 | 312 | .74 | .12 | .37 |
| mushroom: | | | | | | | | |
| w/beef stock . . . . . . . | 10 | .84 | 9 | 36 | 158 | 1.38 | .25 | .38 |
| cream of . . . . . . . . . . | 46 | .51 | 5 | 50 | 101 | .59 | .12 | .25 |
| cream of[1] . . . . . . . . . | 178 | .59 | 20 | 156 | 270 | .64 | .14 | .25 |
| onion. . . . . . . . . . . . . . . | 26 | .67 | 2 | 11 | 69 | .61 | .12 | .25 |
| oyster stew . . . . . . . . . | 22 | .98 | 5 | 48 | 49 | 10.29 | 1.59 | .37 |
| oyster stew[1]. . . . . . . . . . | 167 | 1.04 | 21 | 162 | 235 | 10.34 | 1.61 | .37 |
| pea: | | | | | | | | |
| green. . . . . . . . . . . . . | 27 | 1.95 | 39 | 124 | 190 | 1.71 | .38 | .66 |
| green[1] . . . . . . . . . . . . | 173 | 2.01 | 55 | 238 | 377 | 1.76 | .39 | .66 |
| split, w/or w/out ham | 22 | 2.28 | 48 | 213 | 399 | 1.32 | .37 | .67 |
| pepper pot. . . . . . . . . . . | 23 | .89 | 5 | 42 | 152 | 1.22 | .12 | .61 |
| potato, cream of . . . . . . . | 20 | .48 | 1 | 46 | 137 | .63 | .25 | .38 |
| potato, cream of[1]. . . . . . . | 166 | .54 | 17 | 160 | 323 | .68 | .26 | .38 |
| Scotch broth . . . . . . . . . . | 15 | .83 | 4 | 55 | 159 | 1.59 | .25 | .37 |
| stockpot . . . . . . . . . . . . . | 22 | .87 | 4 | 54 | 238 | 1.16 | .13 | .26 |
| tomato: | | | | | | | | |
| plain . . . . . . . . . . . . . | 13 | 1.76 | 8 | 34 | 263 | .24 | .25 | .25 |
| plain[1]. . . . . . . . . . . . . | 159 | 1.82 | 23 | 148 | 450 | .29 | .26 | .25 |
| beef w/noodle . . . . . . | 18 | 1.12 | 8 | 56 | 221 | .75 | .12 | .25 |
| bisque. . . . . . . . . . . . | 40 | .82 | 9 | 60 | 417 | .59 | .13 | .26 |
| bisque[1] . . . . . . . . . . | 186 | .88 | 25 | 174 | 604 | .63 | .14 | .26 |
| rice . . . . . . . . . . . . . | 23 | .79 | 5 | 33 | 330 | .51 | .13 | .39 |
| turkey noodle. . . . . . . . . | 12 | .94 | 5 | 48 | 75 | .58 | .12 | .25 |
| turkey vegetable. . . . . . . . | 17 | .76 | 4 | 40 | 175 | .61 | .12 | .25 |
| vegetable: | | | | | | | | |
| w/beef. . . . . . . . . . . . | 17 | 1.11 | 6 | 40 | 173 | 1.55 | .18 | .32 |

[1] *Prepared with whole milk.*

| | Calcium | Iron | Magnesium | Phosphorus | Potassium | Zinc | Copper | Manganese |
|---|---|---|---|---|---|---|---|---|
| | (Mg) | (Mg) | (Mg) | (Mg) | (Mg) | (Mg) | (Mg) | (Mg) |
| w/beef broth . . . . . . . | 18 | .97 | 7 | 39 | 192 | .80 | .15 | .34 |
| vegetarian . . . . . . . . . | 21 | 1.08 | 7 | 35 | 209 | .46 | .12 | .46 |
| **Soup mix[1], 1 cup:** | | | | | | | | |
| beef broth or bouillon . . . | 10 | n.a. | 6 | 26 | 36 | n.a. | n.a. | .04 |
| beef noodle . . . . . . . . . . . | 5 | .33 | 9 | 40 | 81 | .10 | n.a. | n.a. |
| chicken noodle. . . . . . . . . | 32 | .50 | 7 | 32 | 31 | .20 | .04 | .02 |
| chicken vegetable. . . . . . . | n.a. | .59 | 21 | 32 | 68 | .21 | .03 | n.a. |
| mushroom. . . . . . . . . . . . | 67 | n.a. | n.a. | 77 | 199 | .09 | .03 | n.a. |
| onion. . . . . . . . . . . . . . . | 13 | .14 | 6 | 31 | 63 | .06 | .02 | .06 |
| pea, green, split or w/ham. . . . . . . . . . . . | 22 | 1.01 | 46 | 134 | 238 | .59 | .19 | .27 |
| tomato, regular or cream of . . . . . . . . . . . . . . . . | 54 | .42 | 15 | 66 | 295 | .21 | .09 | n.a. |
| tomato, vegetable[2] . . . . . . | 8 | .63 | 20 | 29 | 103 | .17 | .03 | n.a. |
| **Sour cream sauce mix[3], ½ cup. . . . . . . . . . . . .** | 273 | .31 | n.a. | n.a. | 367 | .69 | .04 | n.a. |
| **Soursop:** | | | | | | | | |
| untrimmed, 1 lb. . . . . . . . | 43 | 1.82 | 63 | 82 | 845 | n.a. | n.a. | n.a. |
| pulp, ½ cup. . . . . . . . . | 16 | .68 | 23 | 31 | 313 | n.a. | n.a. | n.a. |
| **Soy beverage** (see also "Soy milk"), 8 fl. oz.: | | | | | | | | |
| (*EdenSoy Original* ) . . . . . | 82 | 1.58 | 55 | 143 | 436 | .98 | .32 | n.a. |
| (*EdenSoy* Extra Original), . . . . . . . . . . . | 196 | 1.66 | 54 | 142 | 451 | 1.00 | .34 | n.a. |
| carob (*EdenSoy*) . . . . . . . | 68 | 1.66 | 43 | 105 | 326 | .64 | .21 | n.a. |
| vanilla (*EdenSoy*). . . . . . . | 62 | .84 | 38 | 98 | 292 | .58 | .17 | n.a. |
| vanilla (*EdenSoy* Extra) . . | 196 | .98 | 38 | 92 | 294 | .57 | .18 | n.a. |
| **Soy flour,** stirred: | | | | | | | | |
| full fat, 1 cup. . . . . . . . . | 175 | 5.42 | 364 | 420 | 2138 | 3.33 | 2.48 | 1.93 |

[1] *Prepared according to package directions with water, except as noted.*
[2] *Includes Italian vegetable and spring vegetable.*
[3] *Prepared with whole milk.*

|  | Calcium | Iron | Magnesium | Phosphorus | Potassium | Zinc | Copper | Manganese |
|---|---|---|---|---|---|---|---|---|
|  | (Mg) | (Mg) | (Mg) | (Mg) | (Mg) | (Mg) | (Mg) | (Mg) |
| Soy flour, *continued* | | | | | | | | |
| full-fat, roasted, 1 cup . . . | 160 | 4.94 | 314 | 405 | 1734 | 3.04 | 1.89 | 1.77 |
| defatted, 1 cup . . . . . . . . | 241 | 9.24 | 290 | 674 | 2384 | 2.46 | 4.07 | 3.02 |
| low fat, 1 cup . . . . . . . . . | 165 | 5.27 | 202 | 522 | 2262 | 1.04 | 4.47 | 2.71 |
| Soy meal, defatted, | | | | | | | | |
| 1 cup . . . . . . . . . . . . . | 297 | 16.71 | 373 | 855 | 3038 | 6.17 | 2.44 | 4.64 |
| Soy milk (see also "Soy beverage"), fluid, | | | | | | | | |
| 1 cup . . . . . . . . . . . . . | 10 | 1.38 | 45 | 117 | 338 | .54 | .29 | .41 |
| Soy sauce: | | | | | | | | |
| from soy (tamari), ¼ cup | 12 | 1.38 | 23 | 75 | 123 | .25 | .08 | n.a. |
| from soy (tamari), 1 tbsp. | 4 | .43 | 7 | 23 | 38 | .08 | .02 | n.a. |
| from soy and wheat (shoyu), ¼ cup . . . . . . | 10 | 1.17 | 20 | 64 | 104 | .21 | .07 | n.a. |
| from soy and wheat (shoyu), 1 tbsp. . . . . . . | 3 | .36 | 6 | 20 | 32 | .07 | .02 | n.a. |
| Soybean, green, fresh: | | | | | | | | |
| untrimmed, 1 lb. . . . . . . . | 474 | 8.53 | n.a. | 466 | n.a. | n.a. | n.a. | n.a. |
| raw, trimmed, ½ cup . . . . | 252 | 4.54 | n.a. | 248 | n.a. | n.a. | n.a. | n.a. |
| boiled, drained, ½ cup . . . | 130 | 2.25 | n.a. | 142 | n.a. | n.a. | n.a. | n.a. |
| Soybean, dried: | | | | | | | | |
| uncooked, 1 lb. . . . . . . . . | 1256 | 71.20 | 1271 | 3191 | 8152 | 22.16 | 7.52 | 11.42 |
| uncooked, ½ cup. . . . . . . | 257 | 14.60 | 261 | 654 | 1671 | 4.54 | 1.54 | 2.34 |
| boiled, ½ cup . . . . . . . . . | 88 | 4.42 | 74 | 211 | 443 | .99 | .35 | .71 |
| roasted, 1 lb. . . . . . . . . . . | 626 | 17.69 | 658 | 1647 | 6668 | 14.24 | 3.76 | 9.79 |
| roasted, ½ cup . . . . . . . . | 119 | 3.35 | 125 | 312 | 1264 | 2.70 | .71 | 1.86 |
| dry-roasted, 1 lb. . . . . . . . | 1226 | 17.92 | 1034 | 2942 | 6189 | 21.63 | 4.89 | 9.91 |
| dry-roasted, ½ cup . . . . . | 232 | 3.40 | 196 | 558 | 1173 | 4.10 | .93 | 1.88 |
| Soybean, fermented, see "Miso" and "Natto" | | | | | | | | |
| Soybean, sprouted: | | | | | | | | |
| raw, 1 lb. . . . . . . . . . . . . | 304 | 9.53 | 327 | 744 | 2195 | 5.31 | 1.94 | 3.18 |
| raw, ½ cup . . . . . . . . . . | 23 | .73 | 25 | 57 | 169 | .41 | .15 | .25 |
| steamed, ½ cup. . . . . . . . | 28 | .62 | 28 | 63 | 167 | .49 | .16 | .33 |
| Soybean curd, see "Tofu" | | | | | | | | |

| | Calcium | Iron | Magnesium | Phosphorus | Potassium | Zinc | Copper | Manganese |
|---|---|---|---|---|---|---|---|---|
| | (Mg) | (Mg) | (Mg) | (Mg) | (Mg) | (Mg) | (Mg) | (Mg) |
| **Soybean kernels:** | | | | | | | | |
| roasted and toasted, 1 oz. | 39 | 1.26 | 49 | 103 | 417 | 1.03 | .30 | n.a. |
| roasted and toasted, whole, 1 cup | 149 | 4.81 | 186 | 392 | 1588 | 3.91 | 1.15 | n.a. |
| **Spaghetti,** see "Pasta" | | | | | | | | |
| **Spaghetti sauce,** see "Tomato sauce" | | | | | | | | |
| **Spaghetti squash:** | | | | | | | | |
| raw, untrimmed, 1 lb. | 323 | 8.84 | 258 | 159 | 1824 | 1.74 | .43 | 2.93 |
| raw, trimmed, cubed, ½ cup | 11 | .16 | 6 | 6 | 54 | .09 | .02 | n.a. |
| baked or boiled, drained, ½ cup | 17 | .26 | 8 | 11 | 91 | .16 | .03 | n.a. |
| **Spinach:** | | | | | | | | |
| fresh: | | | | | | | | |
| raw, untrimmed, 1 lb. | 323 | 8.84 | 258 | 159 | 1824 | 1.74 | .43 | 2.93 |
| raw, 10-oz. pkg. | 202 | 5.52 | 161 | 100 | 1139 | 1.09 | .27 | 1.83 |
| raw, trimmed, chopped, ½ cup | 28 | .76 | 22 | 14 | 156 | .15 | .04 | .24 |
| boiled, drained, ½ cup | 122 | 3.21 | 79 | 50 | 419 | .69 | .16 | .84 |
| canned, w/liquid, ½ cup | 97 | 1.85 | 66 | 37 | 269 | .49 | .14 | .58 |
| canned, drained, ½ cup | 135 | 2.46 | 81 | 47 | 370 | .49 | .19 | .64 |
| frozen, leaf, 10-oz. pkg. | 314 | 5.83 | 165 | 116 | 918 | 1.24 | .28 | 2.12 |
| frozen, boiled, drained, leaf, ½ cup | 139 | 1.44 | 65 | 46 | 283 | .66 | .13 | .90 |
| **Spiny lobster,** mixed species, meat only: | | | | | | | | |
| raw, 1 lb. | 221 | 5.54 | n.a. | 1080 | n.a. | 25.74 | 1.73 | .07 |
| raw, 7.4 oz., yield from 2 lb. in shell | 102 | 2.55 | n.a. | 498 | n.a. | 11.86 | .80 | .03 |

| | Calcium | Iron | Magnesium | Phosphorus | Potassium | Zinc | Copper | Manganese |
|---|---|---|---|---|---|---|---|---|
| | (Mg) | (Mg) | (Mg) | (Mg) | (Mg) | (Mg) | (Mg) | (Mg) |

**Spiny lobster,** *continued*
boiled or steamed[1],

| | Calcium | Iron | Magnesium | Phosphorus | Potassium | Zinc | Copper | Manganese |
|---|---|---|---|---|---|---|---|---|
| 4 oz. . . . . . . . . . . . . | 71 | 1.60 | n.a. | 260 | n.a. | 8.24 | .46 | .02 |
| boiled or steamed[1], 5.7 oz. (2 lb. raw in shell) . . . . | 102 | 2.29 | n.a. | 373 | n.a. | 11.85 | .68 | .03 |
| **Spleen,** braised[1]: | | | | | | | | |
| beef, 4 oz. . . . . . . . . . . | 14 | 44.63 | 22 | 346 | 322 | 3.16 | 1.05 | .09 |
| pork, 4 oz. . . . . . . . . . . | 15 | 25.21 | n.a. | 321 | 257 | 4.01 | .15 | .05 |
| **Spot,** meat only: | | | | | | | | |
| raw, 1 lb. . . . . . . . . . . . | 65 | 1.45 | 190 | 844 | 2250 | 2.30 | .21 | .16 |
| baked, broiled, or microwaved[1], 4 oz. . . . | 20 | .46 | 61 | 270 | 721 | .74 | .07 | .05 |
| **Squash,** see specific listings | | | | | | | | |
| **Squash seeds,** see "Pumpkin seeds" | | | | | | | | |
| **Squid,** mixed species, meat only: | | | | | | | | |
| raw, 1 lb. . . . . . . . . . . . | 147 | 3.10 | 148 | 1001 | 1116 | 6.96 | 8.58 | .16 |
| dipped in flour, fried, 4 oz. . . . . . . . . . . . . | 44 | 1.15 | 43 | 285 | 316 | 1.97 | 2.40 | n.a. |
| **Star fruit,** see "Carambola" | | | | | | | | |
| **Steak,** see "Beef" and " 'Beef,' vegetarian" | | | | | | | | |
| **Stomach,** pork, raw, 1 oz. . . . . . . . . . . . . . | 3 | .62 | n.a. | 44 | 57 | .57 | .10 | n.a. |
| **Straightneck squash,** see "Crookneck squash" | | | | | | | | |
| **Strawberry:** | | | | | | | | |
| fresh: | | | | | | | | |
| untrimmed, 1 lb. . . . . | 60 | 1.63 | 45 | 80 | 707 | .54 | .21 | 1.24 |
| untrimmed, 1 pint, approx. 12 oz. . . . . | 45 | 1.23 | 34 | 60 | 530 | .40 | .16 | .93 |
| trimmed, ½ cup . . . . . | 11 | .29 | 8 | 14 | 124 | .10 | .04 | .22 |
| canned, in heavy syrup, ½ cup . . . . . . . . . . . | 16 | .62 | 11 | 15 | 109 | .12 | .08 | .25 |
| frozen: | | | | | | | | |
| unsweetened, ½ cup | 12 | .56 | 8 | 10 | 110 | .10 | .04 | .22 |

[1] *Prepared without added ingredients.*

|  | Calcium | Iron | Magnesium | Phosphorus | Potassium | Zinc | Copper | Manganese |
|---|---|---|---|---|---|---|---|---|
|  | (Mg) | (Mg) | (Mg) | (Mg) | (Mg) | (Mg) | (Mg) | (Mg) |
| sweetened, whole, 10-oz. pkg. | 32 | 1.34 | 18 | 35 | 277 | .15 | .05 | .71 |
| sweetened, whole, ½ cup | 15 | .71 | 8 | 16 | 125 | .07 | .02 | .32 |
| sweetened, sliced, 10-oz. pkg. | 31 | 1.66 | 20 | 36 | 277 | .16 | .06 | .71 |
| sweetened, sliced, ½ cup | 14 | .75 | 9 | 16 | 125 | .07 | .03 | .32 |
| **Strawberry flavor drink mix** (*Carnation* Instant Breakfast), 1 pkt. | 150 | 4.50 | 80 | 150 | 300 | 3.00 | .50 | n.a. |
| **Strawberry topping,** 2 tbsp. | 10 | .41 | 2 | 6 | 31 | .21 | .01 | n.a. |
| **String beans,** see "Green beans" |  |  |  |  |  |  |  |  |
| **Stroganoff sauce mix:** |  |  |  |  |  |  |  |  |
| ½ cup[1] | 261 | .67 | n.a. | 151 | 336 | .55 | .04 | n.a. |
| (*Natural Touch*), 4 tbsp., .8 oz. | 53 | .52 | n.a. | n.a. | 229 | .51 | n.a. | n.a. |
| **Strudel, apple,** 2.5-oz. piece | 11 | .3 | 6 | 24 | n.a. | .13 | .02 | .14 |
| **Stuffing mix,** dry type: |  |  |  |  |  |  |  |  |
| ½ cup prepared | 28 | 1.08 | 11 | 40 | 70 | .26 | .07 | .17 |
| corn bread, ½ cup prepared | 22 | .92 | 12 | 32 | 58 | .21 | .07 | n.a. |
| **Succotash:** |  |  |  |  |  |  |  |  |
| canned: |  |  |  |  |  |  |  |  |
| w/liquid, 8 oz. | 24 | 1.21 | 42 | 126 | 370 | 1.14 | .25 | .83 |
| w/liquid, ½ cup | 14 | .68 | 24 | 71 | 209 | .64 | .14 | .47 |
| w/cream-style corn, 8 oz. | 25 | 1.25 | 2 | 133 | 414 | n.a. | .40 | 1.46 |
| w/cream-style corn, ½ cup | 15 | .73 | 1 | 78 | 243 | n.a. | .24 | .86 |
| frozen, 10-oz. pkg. | 45 | 2.66 | 68 | 220 | 836 | 1.33 | .18 | .84 |

[1] *Prepared according to package directions, with whole milk and water.*

| | Calcium (Mg) | Iron (Mg) | Magnesium (Mg) | Phosphorus (Mg) | Potassium (Mg) | Zinc (Mg) | Copper (Mg) | Manganese (Mg) |
|---|---|---|---|---|---|---|---|---|
| Succotash, *continued* | | | | | | | | |
| frozen, boiled, drained, | | | | | | | | |
| ½ cup . . . . . . . . . . . . | 13 | .76 | 19 | 59 | 225 | .38 | .05 | .24 |
| **Sucker,** white, meat only: | | | | | | | | |
| raw, 1 lb. . . . . . . . . . . | 318 | 5.90 | 136 | 953 | 1724 | 3.40 | .89 | 2.72 |
| baked, broiled, or | | | | | | | | |
| microwaved[1], 4 oz. . . . | 101 | 1.89 | 43 | 305 | 552 | 1.09 | .28 | .87 |
| **Sugar:** | | | | | | | | |
| brown, 1 cup packed . . . . | 187 | 4.80 | n.a. | 56 | 757 | n.a. | n.a. | n.a. |
| granulated or powdered, | | | | | | | | |
| 1 tbsp. . . . . . . . . . . . | tr. | tr. | 0 | tr. | tr. | 0 | n.a. | n.a. |
| **Sugar apple:** | | | | | | | | |
| untrimmed, 1 lb. . . . . . . . | 59 | 1.50 | 53 | 81 | 617 | n.a. | n.a. | n.a. |
| pulp, ½ cup. . . . . . . . . . | 30 | .75 | 27 | 41 | 310 | n.a. | n.a. | n.a. |
| **Summer sausage,** see "Thuringer cervelat" | | | | | | | | |
| **Summer squash,** see specific listings | | | | | | | | |
| **Sunfish,** pumpkinseed, meat only: | | | | | | | | |
| raw, 1 lb. . . . . . . . . . . . . | 363 | 5.44 | 136 | 816 | 1588 | 7.03 | 1.36 | 3.18 |
| baked, broiled, or | | | | | | | | |
| microwaved[1], 4 oz. . . . | 117 | 1.75 | 43 | 262 | 509 | 2.26 | .44 | 1.02 |
| **Sunflower seed butter:** | | | | | | | | |
| 1 oz. . . . . . . . . . . . . . . | 35 | 1.35 | 105 | 209 | 20 | 1.50 | .52 | .60 |
| 1 tbsp. . . . . . . . . . . . . | 19 | .76 | 59 | 118 | 12 | .85 | .29 | .34 |
| **Sunflower seed flour:** | | | | | | | | |
| 1 cup . . . . . . . . . . . . . | 91 | 5.30 | 277 | 551 | 54 | 3.96 | 1.37 | 1.58 |
| 1 tbsp. . . . . . . . . . . . . | 6 | .33 | 17 | 34 | 3 | .25 | .09 | .10 |
| **Sunflower seed kernels,** hulled, except as noted: | | | | | | | | |
| dried: | | | | | | | | |
| in hull, 1 lb. . . . . . . . . | 285 | 16.58 | 866 | 1726 | 1687 | 12.40 | 4.29 | 4.95 |
| 1 oz. . . . . . . . . . . . . | 33 | 1.92 | 100 | 200 | 196 | 1.44 | .50 | .57 |
| 1 cup . . . . . . . . . . . | 168 | 9.75 | 509 | 1015 | 992 | 7.29 | 2.52 | 2.91 |
| dry-roasted, 1 oz. . . . . . | 20 | 1.08 | 37 | 328 | 241 | 1.50 | .52 | .60 |

[1] *Prepared without added ingredients.*

| | Calcium | Iron | Magnesium | Phosphorus | Potassium | Zinc | Copper | Manganese |
|---|---|---|---|---|---|---|---|---|
| | (Mg) | (Mg) | (Mg) | (Mg) | (Mg) | (Mg) | (Mg) | (Mg) |
| dry-roasted, 1 cup . . . . . . | 90 | 487 | 165 | 1479 | 1088 | 6.77 | 2.34 | 2.70 |
| oil-roasted, 1 oz. . . . . . . . | 16 | 1.90 | 36 | 323 | 137 | 1.48 | .51 | .59 |
| oil-roasted, 1 cup. . . . . . . | 76 | 9.05 | 171 | 1538 | 652 | 7.04 | 2.44 | 2.81 |
| toasted, 1 oz. . . . . . . . . . | 16 | 1.93 | 37 | 329 | 139 | 1.50 | .52 | .60 |
| **Swamp cabbage:** | | | | | | | | |
| raw, untrimmed, | | | | | | | | |
| 1 lb. . . . . . . . . . . . . | 268 | 5.83 | 248 | 136 | 1088 | n.a. | n.a. | n.a. |
| raw, trimmed, cupped, | | | | | | | | |
| ½ cup . . . . . . . . . . . . | 43 | .94 | 40 | 22 | 174 | n.a. | n.a. | n.a. |
| boiled, drained, chopped, | | | | | | | | |
| ½ cup . . . . . . . . . . . . | 53 | 1.29 | 30 | 41 | 278 | n.a. | n.a. | n.a. |
| **Sweet potato** (see also "Yam"), fresh: | | | | | | | | |
| raw: | | | | | | | | |
| untrimmed, 1 lb. . . . . | 73 | 1.92 | 34 | 92 | 666 | .91 | .55 | 1.16 |
| 1 medium, 5" long, | | | | | | | | |
| 6.3 oz. . . . . . . . . . . | 29 | .76 | 14 | 37 | 265 | .36 | .22 | .46 |
| peeled, cubed, | | | | | | | | |
| 1 cup . . . . . . . . . | 31 | .80 | 14 | 39 | 279 | .38 | .23 | .49 |
| baked in skin, peeled, | | | | | | | | |
| 1 medium, 5" long, | | | | | | | | |
| 4 oz. . . . . . . . . . . . . | 32 | .52 | 23 | 62 | 397 | .33 | .24 | .64 |
| baked in skin, peeled, | | | | | | | | |
| mashed, ½ cup . . . . . | 28 | .45 | 20 | 55 | 348 | .29 | .21 | .56 |
| boiled w/out skin, | | | | | | | | |
| mashed, ½ cup . . . . . | 35 | .92 | 16 | 44 | 301 | .43 | .26 | .55 |
| **Sweet potato, canned:** | | | | | | | | |
| mashed, ½ cup . . . . . . . . | 38 | 1.70 | 31 | 67 | 268 | .27 | .35 | 1.26 |
| vacuum pack: | | | | | | | | |
| pieces, 8 oz. . . . . . . . | 50 | 2.01 | 55 | 111 | 708 | .41 | .32 | 1.03 |
| pieces, ½ cup . . . . . . | 22 | .89 | 23 | 49 | 313 | .18 | .14 | .46 |
| mashed, ½ cup . . . . . | 28 | 1.13 | 29 | 63 | 398 | .23 | .18 | .08 |
| syrup pack: | | | | | | | | |
| w/liquid, 8 oz. . . . . . . | 35 | 1.82 | 30 | 62 | 421 | .42 | .28 | 1.15 |
| w/liquid, ½ cup . . . . . | 18 | .92 | 15 | 31 | 212 | .21 | .14 | .58 |

| | Calcium | Iron | Magnesium | Phosphorus | Potassium | Zinc | Copper | Manganese |
|---|---|---|---|---|---|---|---|---|
| | (Mg) | (Mg) | (Mg) | (Mg) | (Mg) | (Mg) | (Mg) | (Mg) |
| Sweet potato, canned, syrup pack, *continued* | | | | | | | | |
| drained, ½ cup . . . . . | 16 | .93 | 12 | 25 | 189 | .16 | .16 | .60 |
| **Sweet potato, frozen,** | | | | | | | | |
| baked, cubes, | | | | | | | | |
| ½ cup . . . . . . . . . . . . | 31 | .47 | 18 | 39 | 332 | .26 | .16 | .59 |
| **Sweet potato leaves,** | | | | | | | | |
| trimmed, chopped, | | | | | | | | |
| 1 cup . . . . . . . . . . . . | 13 | .35 | 21 | 33 | 181 | n.a. | n.a. | n.a. |
| **Sweet and sour sauce** | | | | | | | | |
| mix[1], ½ cup . . . . . . . | 21 | .81 | n.a. | n.a. | 33 | .05 | .01 | n.a. |
| **Swiss chard, fresh:** | | | | | | | | |
| raw: | | | | | | | | |
| untrimmed, 1 lb. . . . . | 213 | 7.51 | 340 | 192 | 1583 | n.a. | n.a. | n.a. |
| trimmed, 1 leaf, | | | | | | | | |
| 1.7 oz. . . . . . . . . . | 24 | .86 | 39 | 22 | 182 | n.a. | n.a. | n.a. |
| trimmed, chopped, | | | | | | | | |
| ½ cup . . . . . . . . . | 9 | .32 | 15 | 8 | 68 | n.a. | n.a. | n.a. |
| boiled, drained, | | | | | | | | |
| ½ cup . . . . . . . . . . . . | 51 | 2.00 | 76 | 29 | 483 | n.a. | n.a. | n.a. |
| **Swordfish,** meat only: | | | | | | | | |
| raw, 1 lb. . . . . . . . . . . . | 20 | 3.67 | 122 | 1193 | 1306 | 5.20 | .57 | .09 |
| baked, broiled, or | | | | | | | | |
| microwaved[2], 4 oz. . . . | 7 | 1.18 | 39 | 382 | 4.18 | 1.67 | .18 | (0) |
| **Syrup,** see specific listings | | | | | | | | |
| **Syrup, table blends:** | | | | | | | | |
| corn and maple, | | | | | | | | |
| 2 tbsp. . . . . . . . . . . . | 1 | tr. | n.a. | 4 | 7 | n.a. | n.a. | n.a. |
| cane and 15% maple, | | | | | | | | |
| 1 tbsp. . . . . . . . . . . . | 3 | .16 | 1 | 0 | 7 | .13 | tr. | .11 |
| corn refiners and sugar, | | | | | | | | |
| 1 tbsp. . . . . . . . . . . . | 5 | .15 | 2 | 2 | 13 | .01 | .01 | n.a. |
| pancake, 1 tbsp. . . . . . . . | 0 | .02 | 0 | 2 | 0 | .01 | .04 | n.a. |

---

[1] *Prepared according to package directions, with water and vinegar.*
[2] *Prepared without added ingredients.*

| | Calcium | Iron | Magnesium | Phosphorus | Potassium | Zinc | Copper | Manganese |
|---|---|---|---|---|---|---|---|---|
| | (Mg) | (Mg) | (Mg) | (Mg) | (Mg) | (Mg) | (Mg) | (Mg) |
| pancake, w/butter, 1 tbsp. . . . . . . . . . . . | 0 | .02 | 0 | 2 | 1 | .01 | .04 | n.a. |
| pancake, w/2% maple, 1 tbsp. . . . . . . . . . . . | 1 | .01 | 0 | 2 | 1 | .05 | .01 | .04 |
| pancake, light, 1 oz. . . . . . | 0 | 0 | 0 | 12 | 1 | .01 | tr. | n.a. |

# T

| | Calcium (Mg) | Iron (Mg) | Magnesium (Mg) | Phosphorus (Mg) | Potassium (Mg) | Zinc (Mg) | Copper (Mg) | Manganese (Mg) |
|---|---|---|---|---|---|---|---|---|
| **Taco mix,** vegetarian (*Natural Touch*), 3 tbsp., .6 oz. | 29 | .99 | n.a. | n.a. | 379 | .32 | n.a. | n.a. |
| **Tahini,** see "Sesame butter" | | | | | | | | |
| **Tamari sauce,** see "Soy sauce" | | | | | | | | |
| **Tamarind:** | | | | | | | | |
| untrimmed, 1 lb. | 114 | 4.32 | 141 | 174 | 968 | n.a. | n.a. | n.a. |
| pulp, ½ cup | 45 | 1.68 | 55 | 68 | 377 | n.a. | n.a. | n.a. |
| **Tangerine:** | | | | | | | | |
| fresh: | | | | | | | | |
| untrimmed, 1 lb. | 46 | .34 | 39 | 33 | 511 | n.a. | .09 | .11 |
| 1 medium, 2⅜" diam., approx. 4 oz. | 12 | .09 | .10 | 8 | 132 | n.a. | .02 | .03 |
| sections w/out membrane, ½ cup | 14 | .10 | 12 | 10 | 153 | n.a. | .03 | .03 |
| canned, in juice, ½ cup | 14 | .33 | 14 | 13 | 165 | .63 | .04 | n.a. |
| canned, in light syrup, ½ cup | 9 | .46 | 10 | 12 | 99 | .30 | .06 | n.a. |
| **Tangerine juice:** | | | | | | | | |
| fresh, 6 fl. oz. | 36 | .36 | 12 | 24 | 330 | .06 | .05 | .07 |
| canned, sweetened, 6 fl. oz. | 36 | .36 | 12 | 24 | 330 | .06 | .05 | .07 |
| frozen, sweetened, diluted, 6 fl. oz. | 12 | .18 | 12 | 18 | 204 | .06 | .05 | .07 |
| **Tapioca,** pearl, dry, 1 oz. | 6 | .45 | <1 | 2 | 3 | .03 | .01 | .03 |
| **Taro:** | | | | | | | | |
| raw, untrimmed, 1 lb. | 168 | 2.15 | 128 | 326 | 2306 | n.a. | n.a. | n.a. |
| raw, trimmed, sliced, ½ cup | 22 | .29 | 17 | 43 | 307 | n.a. | n.a. | n.a. |
| cooked, sliced, ½ cup | 12 | .48 | 20 | 50 | 319 | n.a. | n.a. | n.a. |

| | Calcium | Iron | Magnesium | Phosphorus | Potassium | Zinc | Copper | Manganese |
|---|---|---|---|---|---|---|---|---|
| | (Mg) | (Mg) | (Mg) | (Mg) | (Mg) | (Mg) | (Mg) | (Mg) |
| **Taro, Tahitian:** | | | | | | | | |
| raw, trimmed, sliced, ½ cup | 80 | .81 | 29 | 28 | 376 | n.a. | n.a. | n.a. |
| cooked, sliced, ½ cup | 101 | 1.06 | 34 | 45 | 423 | n.a. | n.a. | n.a. |
| **Taro chips:** | | | | | | | | |
| 1 oz. | 17 | .34 | 24 | 37 | 214 | n.a. | n.a. | n.a. |
| 10 chips, .8 oz. | 14 | .28 | 19 | 30 | 174 | n.a. | n.a. | n.a. |
| **Taro leaves:** | | | | | | | | |
| raw, untrimmed, 1 lb. | 292 | 6.12 | 123 | 164 | 1764 | n.a. | n.a. | n.a. |
| raw, trimmed, 1 cup | 30 | .63 | 13 | 17 | 181 | n.a. | n.a. | n.a. |
| steamed, ½ cup | 63 | .87 | 15 | 20 | 341 | n.a. | n.a. | n.a. |
| **Taro shoots:** | | | | | | | | |
| raw, sliced, ½ cup | 5 | .26 | 3 | 12 | 143 | n.a. | n.a. | n.a. |
| cooked, sliced, ½ cup | 9 | .29 | 6 | 28 | 240 | n.a. | n.a. | n.a. |
| **Tarragon,** ground, 1 tsp. | 18 | .52 | 6 | 5 | 48 | .06 | .01 | .13 |
| **Tartar sauce,** 1 tbsp. | 3 | .10 | n.a. | 4 | 11 | n.a. | n.a. | n.a. |
| **Tea:** | | | | | | | | |
| brewed, 6 fl. oz. | 0 | .04 | 5 | 1 | 66 | .04 | .02 | n.a. |
| instant, powder: | | | | | | | | |
| 1 tsp. | 0 | .03 | 3 | 3 | 46 | .02 | .01 | .52 |
| lemon flavor, 1 rounded tsp. | 0 | .01 | 2 | 1 | 48 | .02 | .01 | .43 |
| lemon flavor, saccharin sweetened, 2 tsp. | 0 | .14 | 2 | 2 | 41 | .01 | tr. | .49 |
| lemon flavor, sugar sweetened, 3 rounded tsp. | 1 | .04 | 3 | 3 | 49 | .02 | .01 | .67 |
| **Tea, herbal,** brewed[1], 6 fl. oz. | 4 | .14 | 2 | 0 | 15 | .06 | .03 | .08 |
| **Tempeh:** | | | | | | | | |
| 1 lb. | 422 | 10.25 | 318 | 935 | 1665 | 8.21 | 3.04 | 6.49 |
| ½ cup | 77 | 1.88 | 58 | 171 | 305 | 1.50 | .56 | 1.19 |
| **Teriyaki sauce,** 1 tbsp. | 4 | .31 | 11 | 28 | 41 | .02 | .02 | 0 |

[1] Prepared with distilled water.

| | Calcium (Mg) | Iron (Mg) | Magnesium (Mg) | Phosphorus (Mg) | Potassium (Mg) | Zinc (Mg) | Copper (Mg) | Manganese (Mg) |
|---|---|---|---|---|---|---|---|---|
| **Thirst quencher drink,** bottled, 8 fl. oz....... | 0 | .12 | 1 | 22 | 26 | .05 | .05 | 0 |
| **Thuringer cervelat,** beef and pork, 1 oz. ...... | 2 | .58 | 3 | 28 | 65 | .57 | .02 | .01 |
| **Thyme:** | | | | | | | | |
| fresh, chopped, 1 tsp. ............. | 3 | .14 | 1 | 1 | 5 | .01 | tr. | .01 |
| dried, ground, 1 tsp. ..... | 26 | 1.73 | 3 | 3 | 11 | .09 | .01 | .11 |
| **Tilefish,** meat only: | | | | | | | | |
| raw, 1 lb.............. | 117 | 1.13 | 128 | 850 | 1965 | 1.68 | .19 | .05 |
| baked, broiled, or microwaved[1], 4 oz. ... | 29 | .35 | 37 | 268 | 581 | .60 | .06 | .02 |
| **Toaster pastry:** | | | | | | | | |
| apple cinnamon (*Kellogg's Pop-Tarts*), 1 piece ............ | 12 | 1.80 | 6 | 27 | 50 | .15 | .02 | n.a. |
| blueberry (*Kellogg's Pop-Tarts*), 1 piece ....... | 13 | 1.80 | 8 | 46 | 50 | .30 | .08 | n.a. |
| blueberry, frosted (*Kellogg's Pop-Tarts*), 1 piece ............ | 13 | 1.80 | 8 | 44 | 50 | .29 | .08 | n.a. |
| brown sugar w/cinnamon, 1.8-oz. piece ........ | 17 | 2.01 | 12 | 66 | 57 | .31 | .07 | .16 |
| brown sugar cinnamon (*Kellogg's Pop-Tarts*), 1 piece ............ | 16 | 1.80 | 8 | 32 | 70 | .29 | .04 | n.a. |
| brown sugar cinnamon, frosted (*Kellogg's Pop-Tarts*), 1 piece ....... | 14 | 1.80 | 7 | 46 | 60 | .57 | .04 | n.a. |
| cherry (*Kellogg's Pop-Tarts*), 1 piece ....... | 14 | 1.80 | 8 | 44 | 60 | .29 | .08 | n.a. |

---

[1] *Prepared without added ingredients.*

|  | Calcium (Mg) | Iron (Mg) | Magnesium (Mg) | Phosphorus (Mg) | Potassium (Mg) | Zinc (Mg) | Copper (Mg) | Manganese (Mg) |
|---|---|---|---|---|---|---|---|---|
| cherry, frosted (*Kellogg's Pop-Tarts*), 1 piece . . . . . . . . . . . | 13 | 1.80 | 8 | 42 | 50 | .35 | .10 | n.a. |
| chocolate fudge, frosted (*Kellogg's Pop-Tarts*), 1 piece . . . . . . . . . . . | 20 | 1.80 | 15 | 43 | 80 | .54 | .08 | n.a. |
| chocolate graham (*Kellogg's Pop-Tarts*), 1 piece . . . . . . . . . . . | 18 | 1.80 | 7 | 33 | 65 | .18 | .02 | n.a. |
| chocolate vanilla creme, frosted (*Kellogg's Pop-Tarts*), 1 piece . . . . . . . | 16 | 1.80 | 11 | 36 | 60 | .29 | .06 | n.a. |
| fruit, 1.8-oz. piece . . . . . . | 14 | 1.81 | 10 | 58 | 58 | .34 | .10 | .15 |
| grape, frosted (*Kellogg's Pop-Tarts*), 1 piece . . . . . . . . . . . | 12 | 1.80 | 11 | 46 | 60 | .30 | .05 | n.a. |
| raspberry, frosted (*Kellogg's Pop-Tarts*), 1 piece . . . . . . . . . . . | 11 | 1.80 | 8 | 46 | 60 | .29 | .04 | n.a. |
| strawberry (*Kellogg's Pop-Tarts*), 1 piece . . . | 13 | 1.80 | 8 | 46 | 60 | .35 | .11 | n.a. |
| strawberry, frosted (*Kellogg's Pop-Tarts*), 1 piece . . . . . . . . . . . | 22 | 1.80 | 7 | 42 | 50 | .34 | .07 | n.a. |
| **Tofu**, raw: |  |  |  |  |  |  |  |  |
| firm, 1 lb. . . . . . . . . . . . | 928 | 47.50 | 424 | 861 | 1074 | 7.11 | 1.72 | 5.36 |
| firm, ½ cup. . . . . . . . . . | 258 | 13.19 | 118 | 239 | 298 | 1.98 | .48 | .49 |
| regular, 1 lb. . . . . . . . . . | 475 | 24.33 | 465 | 441 | 550 | 3.64 | .88 | 2.74 |
| regular, ½ cup. . . . . . . . | 130 | 6.65 | 127 | 120 | 150 | 1.00 | .24 | .75 |
| **Tofu, dried-frozen** (koyadofu), 1 lb. . . . . . | 1652 | 44.14 | 268 | 2189 | 88 | 22.21 | 5.35 | 16.73 |
| **Tomatillo**, raw: |  |  |  |  |  |  |  |  |
| 1 lb. . . . . . . . . . . . . . . | 30 | n.a. | 90 | 175 | 1216 | 1.00 | .36 | .69 |
| 1 medium, 1⅝" diam., 1.2 oz. . . . . . . . . . . . | 2 | n.a. | 7 | 13 | 91 | .08 | .03 | .05 |

| | Calcium | Iron | Magnesium | Phosphorus | Potassium | Zinc | Copper | Manganese |
|---|---|---|---|---|---|---|---|---|
| | (Mg) | (Mg) | (Mg) | (Mg) | (Mg) | (Mg) | (Mg) | (Mg) |
| **Tomatillo**, *continued* | | | | | | | | |
| chopped, ½ cup ....... | 4 | n.a. | 13 | 25 | 177 | .15 | .52 | .10 |
| **Tomato, green:** | | | | | | | | |
| raw, untrimmed, | | | | | | | | |
| 1 lb. ............. | 54 | 2.11 | 43 | 117 | 842 | .29 | .37 | .41 |
| raw, 1 medium, | | | | | | | | |
| 2⅗" diam., | | | | | | | | |
| approx. 4.75 oz.. ..... | 16 | .63 | 13 | 35 | 251 | .09 | .11 | .12 |
| **Tomato, red,** ripe: | | | | | | | | |
| fresh: | | | | | | | | |
| raw, untrimmed, | | | | | | | | |
| 1 lb. ........... | 19 | 1.84 | 44 | 101 | 916 | .36 | .31 | .43 |
| raw, 1 medium, 2⅗" | | | | | | | | |
| diam., 4.75 oz.... | 6 | .55 | 13 | 30 | 273 | .11 | .09 | .13 |
| raw, chopped, ½ cup | 4 | .40 | 10 | 22 | 200 | .08 | .07 | .09 |
| boiled, ½ cup ...... | 7 | .67 | 16 | 37 | 335 | .13 | .11 | .16 |
| canned (see also "Tomato paste" and "Tomato puree"): | | | | | | | | |
| whole, 8 oz......... | 60 | 1.37 | 27 | 44 | 501 | .36 | .25 | n.a. |
| whole, ½ cup ...... | 32 | .73 | 14 | 23 | 265 | .19 | .13 | n.a. |
| wedges, in tomato | | | | | | | | |
| juice, 8 oz........ | 59 | 1.05 | 26 | 53 | 569 | .37 | .24 | n.a. |
| wedges, in tomato | | | | | | | | |
| juice, ½ cup ..... | 34 | .61 | 15 | 31 | 329 | .21 | .14 | n.a. |
| stewed, 8 oz........ | 75 | 1.66 | 26 | 45 | 543 | .38 | .25 | n.a. |
| stewed, ½ cup...... | 42 | .93 | 15 | 25 | 307 | .21 | .14 | n.a. |
| w/green chilies, 8 oz. | 45 | .59 | 25 | 32 | 244 | .30 | .20 | n.a. |
| w/green chilies, | | | | | | | | |
| ½ cup.......... | 24 | .31 | 13 | 17 | 129 | .16 | .11 | n.a. |
| dried, see "Tomato, sun-dried" | | | | | | | | |
| **Tomato, stewed,** see "Tomato, red" | | | | | | | | |
| **Tomato, sun-dried:** | | | | | | | | |
| plain: | | | | | | | | |
| 1 lb. ............. | 500 | n.a. | 878 | 1615 | 15,545 | 9.04 | 6.46 | 8.37 |
| 1 cup, approx. | | | | | | | | |
| 32 pieces........ | 60 | n.a. | 105 | 192 | 1851 | 1.08 | .77 | 1.00 |
| 1 piece, .07 oz. ..... | 2 | n.a. | 4 | 7 | 69 | .04 | .03 | .04 |

| | Calcium | Iron | Magnesium | Phosphorus | Potassium | Zinc | Copper | Manganese |
|---|---|---|---|---|---|---|---|---|
| | (Mg) | (Mg) | (Mg) | (Mg) | (Mg) | (Mg) | (Mg) | (Mg) |
| oil-packed, drained: | | | | | | | | |
| 1 lb. . . . . . . . . . . . | 212 | n.a. | 369 | 631 | 7099 | 3.55 | 2.15 | 2.11 |
| 1 cup . . . . . . . . . . | 51 | n.a. | 90 | 153 | 1721 | .86 | .52 | .51 |
| 1 piece, .1 oz. . . . . . | 1 | n.a. | 2 | 4 | 47 | .02 | .01 | .01 |
| **Tomato juice,** canned, | | | | | | | | |
| 6 fl. oz. . . . . . . . . . . | 16 | 1.06 | 20 | 34 | 400 | .26 | .18 | .14 |
| **Tomato paste,** canned: | | | | | | | | |
| 6-oz. can. . . . . . . . . . . | 60 | 5.08 | 87 | 135 | 1585 | .36 | 1.01 | n.a. |
| ½ cup. . . . . . . . . . . . . | 46 | 3.91 | 67 | 104 | 1221 | 1.05 | .78 | n.a. |
| **Tomato puree,** canned: | | | | | | | | |
| 8 oz. . . . . . . . . . . . . . | 34 | 2.10 | 55 | 90 | 953 | .49 | .37 | n.a. |
| ½ cup. . . . . . . . . . . . . | 19 | 1.16 | 30 | 50 | 526 | .54 | .41 | n.a. |
| **Tomato sauce,** canned: | | | | | | | | |
| plain, 8 oz. . . . . . . . . . | 32 | 1.74 | 42 | 73 | 841 | .56 | .44 | n.a. |
| plain, ½ cup . . . . . . . . . | 17 | .94 | 23 | 39 | 452 | .30 | .24 | n.a. |
| marinara sauce, 8 oz. . . . . | 41 | 1.82 | 59 | 80 | 963 | .61 | .32 | n.a. |
| marinara sauce, | | | | | | | | |
| ½ cup . . . . . . . . . . . | 22 | 1.00 | 30 | 44 | 531 | .34 | .18 | n.a. |
| w/mushrooms, 8 oz. . . . . | 29 | 2.01 | 43 | 73 | 863 | .47 | .45 | n.a. |
| w/mushrooms, | | | | | | | | |
| ½ cup. . . . . . . . . . . | 16 | 1.08 | 23 | 39 | 464 | .25 | .24 | n.a. |
| w/onions, 8 oz. . . . . . . . | 38 | 2.11 | 44 | 90 | 937 | .52 | .41 | n.a. |
| w/onions, ½ cup . . . . . . . | 20 | 1.13 | 23 | 48 | 504 | .28 | .22 | n.a. |
| spaghetti or pasta sauce: | | | | | | | | |
| 15.5-oz. jar . . . . . . . . | 124 | 2.85 | 106 | 159 | 1687 | .94 | .50 | n.a. |
| 8 oz. . . . . . . . . . . . . | 64 | 1.48 | 55 | 82 | 872 | .49 | .26 | n.a. |
| ½ cup . . . . . . . . . . . . | 35 | .81 | 30 | 45 | 479 | .27 | .14 | n.a. |
| w/tomato tidbits, 8 oz. . . . | 24 | 1.55 | 46 | 96 | 846 | .44 | .50 | n.a. |
| w/tomato tidbits, | | | | | | | | |
| ½ cup. . . . . . . . . . . . . | 13 | .83 | 24 | 51 | 455 | .23 | .02 | .27 |
| **Tongue**[1]: | | | | | | | | |
| beef, simmered, 4 oz. . . . | 8 | 3.84 | 19 | 161 | 204 | 5.44 | .25 | .03 |
| lamb, braised, 4 oz. . . . . . | 11 | 2.98 | 18 | 152 | 179 | 3.39 | .24 | .04 |
| pork, braised, 4 oz. . . . . . | 22 | 5.66 | 23 | 197 | 269 | 5.14 | n.a. | n.a. |

[1] *Prepared without added ingredients.*

| | Calcium (Mg) | Iron (Mg) | Magnesium (Mg) | Phosphorus (Mg) | Potassium (Mg) | Zinc (Mg) | Copper (Mg) | Manganese (Mg) |
|---|---|---|---|---|---|---|---|---|
| Tongue, *continued* | | | | | | | | |
| veal, braised, 4 oz...... | 10 | 2.37 | 20 | 188 | 184 | 5.11 | .24 | .05 |
| **Toppings,** dessert, see specific listings | | | | | | | | |
| **Tortilla,** ready-to-bake or -fry: | | | | | | | | |
| corn, 7"-diam. piece, | | | | | | | | |
| .9 oz............... | 44 | .35 | 16 | 79 | 39 | .23 | .04 | .10 |
| flour, 8"-diam. piece, | | | | | | | | |
| 1.2 oz............. | 44 | 1.15 | 9 | 44 | 46 | .25 | .09 | .16 |
| **Tortilla chips:** | | | | | | | | |
| (*Buenitos* Regular), | | | | | | | | |
| 1 oz.............. | 6 | .38 | 32 | 55 | 70 | .44 | n.a. | n.a. |
| (*Buenitos* No Salt Added), | | | | | | | | |
| 1 oz.............. | 4 | .38 | 22 | 55 | 70 | .44 | n.a. | n.a. |
| plain, 1 oz. .......... | 44 | .43 | 25 | 58 | 56 | .43 | .03 | .11 |
| nacho flavor, 1 oz...... | 42 | .40 | 23 | 69 | 61 | .34 | .05 | .12 |
| nacho flavor, light, | | | | | | | | |
| 1 oz.............. | 45 | .46 | 28 | 90 | 77 | n.a. | .04 | .12 |
| ranch flavor, 1 oz....... | 40 | .42 | 25 | 68 | 69 | .35 | .03 | .11 |
| taco flavor, 1 oz........ | 44 | .57 | 25 | 68 | 61 | .36 | .05 | .13 |
| **Tortilla flour mix,** see "Wheat flour" | | | | | | | | |
| **Trail mix,** regular, 1 oz. | 22 | .87 | 45 | 98 | 194 | .91 | .28 | .29 |
| **Tree fern,** cooked, | | | | | | | | |
| chopped, ½ cup ..... | 6 | .11 | 4 | 2 | 3 | n.a. | n.a. | n.a. |
| **Tripe,** beef, raw, 1 oz.... | n.a. | .55 | 2 | 22 | 77 | .70 | .03 | n.a. |
| **Triticale,** whole grain, | | | | | | | | |
| 1 cup ............. | 72 | 4.93 | 250 | 686 | 637 | 6.63 | .88 | 6.16 |
| **Triticale flour,** whole | | | | | | | | |
| grain, 1 cup......... | 45 | 3.37 | 199 | 417 | 605 | 3.46 | .73 | 5.44 |
| **Trout,** meat only: | | | | | | | | |
| mixed species: | | | | | | | | |
| raw, 1 lb.......... | 195 | 6.80 | 100 | 1111 | 1637 | 2.99 | .85 | 3.86 |
| baked, broiled, or | | | | | | | | |
| microwaved[1], 4 oz. | 62 | 2.18 | 32 | 356 | 525 | .96 | .27 | 1.24 |

---

[1] *Prepared without added ingredients.*

|  | Calcium | Iron | Magnesium | Phosphorus | Potassium | Zinc | Copper | Manganese |
|---|---|---|---|---|---|---|---|---|
|  | (Mg) | (Mg) | (Mg) | (Mg) | (Mg) | (Mg) | (Mg) | (Mg) |
| rainbow: |  |  |  |  |  |  |  |  |
| wild, raw, 1 lb. . . . . . | 304 | 3.17 | 139 | 1230 | 2183 | 4.88 | .49 | .72 |
| wild, baked, broiled, or microwaved[1], 4 oz. . . . . . . . . . . | n.a. | .43 | 35 | 305 | 508 | .58 | .07 | .02 |
| farmed, raw, 1 lb. . . . | n.a. | 1.25 | 147 | 1277 | 2045 | 1.86 | .21 | .08 |
| farmed, baked, broiled, or microwaved[1], 4 oz. | n.a. | .37 | 36 | 302 | 500 | .56 | .07 | .02 |
| **Trout, sea,** see "Sea trout" |  |  |  |  |  |  |  |  |
| **Tuna,** meat only: |  |  |  |  |  |  |  |  |
| bluefin, raw, 1 lb. . . . . . | n.a. | 4.62 | n.a. | n.a. | 1143 | 2.72 | .39 | .07 |
| bluefin, baked, broiled, or microwaved[1], 4 oz. . . . | n.a. | 1.49 | n.a. | n.a. | 366 | .87 | .12 | (0) |
| skipjack, raw, 1 lb. . . . . . . | 131 | 5.67 | 155 | 1005 | 1846 | 3.72 | .39 | .07 |
| skipjack, baked, broiled, or microwaved[1], 4 oz. | 42 | 1.81 | 50 | 323 | 592 | 1.19 | .12 | .02 |
| yellowfin, raw, 1 lb. . . . . . | 74 | 3.30 | n.a. | 868 | n.a. | 2.38 | .29 | .07 |
| yellowfin, baked, broiled, or microwaved[1], 4 oz. . . . . . . . . . . . . . . | 24 | 1.07 | n.a. | 245 | n.a. | .76 | .09 | .02 |
| **Tuna, canned:** |  |  |  |  |  |  |  |  |
| in soybean oil, drained: |  |  |  |  |  |  |  |  |
| light, 4 oz. . . . . . . . . . | 15 | 1.58 | 35 | 353 | 235 | 1.02 | .08 | .02 |
| light, yield from 6¼-oz. can . . . . . . | 23 | 2.38 | 53 | 532 | 354 | 1.54 | .12 | .03 |
| white, 4 oz. . . . . . . . . | 5 | .74 | 39 | 303 | 378 | .53 | .01 | n.a. |
| white, yield from 6¼-oz. can . . . . . . | 8 | 1.16 | 60 | 475 | 593 | .84 | .23 | n.a. |
| in water, drained: |  |  |  |  |  |  |  |  |
| light, 4 oz. . . . . . . . . | 12 | 1.74 | 31 | 185 | 269 | .87 | .06 | .01 |
| light, yield from 6¼-oz. can . . . . . . | 19 | 2.52 | 45 | 269 | 391 | 1.27 | .09 | .02 |

[1] *Prepared without added ingredients.*

| | Calcium | Iron | Magnesium | Phosphorus | Potassium | Zinc | Copper | Manganese |
|---|---|---|---|---|---|---|---|---|
| | (Mg) | (Mg) | (Mg) | (Mg) | (Mg) | (Mg) | (Mg) | (Mg) |
| **Tuna,** canned, in water, drained, *continued* | | | | | | | | |
| white, 4 oz. . . . . . . . | 24 | 1.67 | 56 | 373 | 408 | .82 | .07 | .03 |
| **"Tuna," vegetarian,** | | | | | | | | |
| frozen (*Worthington* | | | | | | | | |
| *Tuno*), ½ cup drained | 20 | 1.25 | n.a. | 88 | 34 | .40 | n.a. | n.a. |
| **Turbot,** European, meat only: | | | | | | | | |
| raw, 1 lb. . . . . . . . . . . . . | 80 | n.a. | 232 | 583 | 1081 | 1.01 | .17 | n.a. |
| baked, broiled, or | | | | | | | | |
| microwaved[1], 4 oz. | 26 | n.a. | 74 | 187 | 346 | .32 | .05 | n.a. |
| **Turkey,** all classes, roasted[1], 4 oz., except as noted: | | | | | | | | |
| meat w/skin . . . . . . . . . . | 29 | 2.03 | 28 | 230 | 318 | 3.36 | .11 | .02 |
| meat only . . . . . . . . . . . . | 28 | 2.02 | 29 | 242 | 338 | 3.52 | .11 | .02 |
| skin only, 1 oz. . . . . . . . . | 10 | .51 | 5 | 39 | 45 | .59 | .02 | .01 |
| dark meat w/skin . . . . . . . | 37 | 2.57 | 26 | 222 | 311 | 4.72 | .18 | .03 |
| light meat w/skin . . . . . . . | 24 | 1.60 | 29 | 236 | 323 | 2.31 | .05 | .02 |
| back, meat w/skin . . . . . . | 37 | 2.48 | 25 | 214 | 295 | 4.45 | .16 | .03 |
| breast, meat w/skin . . . . . | 24 | 1.59 | 31 | 238 | 327 | 2.30 | .05 | .02 |
| leg, meat w/skin . . . . . . . | 36 | 2.61 | 26 | 226 | 318 | 4.84 | .17 | .03 |
| wing, meat w/skin . . . . . . | 27 | 1.66 | 28 | 223 | 302 | 2.38 | .06 | .02 |
| **Turkey, frozen or refrigerated:** | | | | | | | | |
| breast, whole: | | | | | | | | |
| w/skin (*Norbest* | | | | | | | | |
| Orange Label), | | | | | | | | |
| 3.5 oz. . . . . . . . . . | 12 | n.a. | 16 | 280 | 210 | n.a. | n.a. | n.a. |
| prebrowned, w/skin | | | | | | | | |
| (*Norbest* Orange | | | | | | | | |
| Label), 3.5 oz. . . . . | 11 | n.a. | 17 | 290 | 170 | n.a. | n.a. | n.a. |
| roasted, w/skin, w/ | | | | | | | | |
| broth, 4 oz. . . . . . . | 10 | .75 | 24 | 243 | 281 | 1.74 | .05 | n.a. |
| smoked, w/skin | | | | | | | | |
| (*Norbest* Orange | | | | | | | | |
| Label), 3.5 oz. . . . . | 21 | n.a. | 19 | 300 | 170 | n.a. | n.a. | n.a. |

[1] *Prepared without added ingredients.*

| | Calcium | Iron | Magnesium | Phosphorus | Potassium | Zinc | Copper | Manganese |
|---|---|---|---|---|---|---|---|---|
| | (Mg) | (Mg) | (Mg) | (Mg) | (Mg) | (Mg) | (Mg) | (Mg) |
| skinless (*Norbest* Orange Label), 3.5 oz.......... | 11 | n.a. | 21 | 280 | 210 | n.a. | n.a. | n.a. |
| skinless, salt-free (*Norbest* Blue Label), 3.5 oz..... | 9 | n.a. | 23 | 210 | 260 | n.a. | n.a. | n.a. |
| breast, boneless roast: | | | | | | | | |
| (*Norbest*), 3.5 oz.... | 13 | n.a. | 15 | 250 | 210 | n.a. | n.a. | n.a. |
| (*Norbest* Sweetheart*), 3.5 oz..... | 7 | n.a. | 16 | 240 | 220 | n.a. | n.a. | n.a. |
| breast, steaks: | | | | | | | | |
| cubed (*Norbest*), 3.5 oz.......... | 7 | n.a. | 22 | 243 | 330 | n.a. | n.a. | n.a. |
| cutlets, strips or tips (*Norbest*), 3.5 oz.......... | 9 | n.a. | 18 | 240 | 250 | n.a. | n.a. | n.a. |
| tenders (*Norbest*), 3.5 oz.......... | 7 | n.a. | 18 | 240 | 300 | n.a. | n.a. | n.a. |
| thigh w/skin, roasted, w/ broth, 4 oz.......... | 9 | 1.71 | 19 | 194 | 273 | 4.67 | .16 | n.a. |
| white and dark meat, roasted, seasoned, 4 oz.............. | 6 | 1.85 | 25 | 277 | 338 | 2.88 | .07 | n.a. |
| cured, whole or half (*Norbest* Gourmet), 3.5 oz.............. | 53 | n.a. | 15 | 290 | 450 | n.a. | n.a. | n.a. |
| **Turkey, ground:** | | | | | | | | |
| raw, 4 oz............. | 15 | 1.42 | 22 | 178 | 266 | 2.20 | .10 | .02 |
| raw (*Norbest*), 3.5 oz.... | 72 | n.a. | 15 | 200 | 250 | n.a. | n.a. | n.a. |
| cooked, 4 oz.......... | 20 | 1.58 | 20 | 161 | 221 | 2.35 | .07 | .02 |
| **"Turkey," vegetarian:** | | | | | | | | |
| canned (*Worthington Turkee*), 3 slices, 3.3 oz.............. | 8 | 1.35 | n.a. | n.a. | 46 | .32 | n.a. | n.a. |

| | Calcium | Iron | Magnesium | Phosphorus | Potassium | Zinc | Copper | Manganese |
|---|---|---|---|---|---|---|---|---|
| | (Mg) | (Mg) | (Mg) | (Mg) | (Mg) | (Mg) | (Mg) | (Mg) |
| "Turkey," vegetarian, *continued* | | | | | | | | |
| frozen, smoked (*Worthington*), 3 slices, 2 oz............... | 5 | 1.83 | n.a. | n.a. | 69 | .23 | n.a. | n.a. |
| **Turkey bologna:** | | | | | | | | |
| 1 oz.................. | 24 | .43 | 4 | 37 | 56 | .49 | .01 | n.a. |
| (*Norbest* Deli), 3.5 oz............. | 140 | n.a. | 14 | 131 | 180 | n.a. | n.a. | n.a. |
| **Turkey entree,** frozen, gravy and, 5-oz. pkg. .......... | 20 | 1.31 | 12 | 114 | n.a. | .99 | n.a. | n.a. |
| **Turkey giblets,** simmered[1], 4 oz..... | 15 | 7.61 | 19 | 231 | 227 | 4.17 | .44 | .20 |
| **Turkey gizzard,** simmered[1], 4 oz..... | 17 | 6.17 | 22 | 145 | 239 | 4.72 | .20 | .11 |
| **Turkey ham:** | | | | | | | | |
| (*Norbest*), 3.5 oz. ...... | 13 | n.a. | 15 | 190 | 250 | n.a. | n.a. | n.a. |
| (*Norbest* 95% Fat Free/ *Norbest* Deli), 3.5 oz............. | 13 | n.a. | 15 | 190 | 325 | n.a. | n.a. | n.a. |
| (*Norbest* Tavern), 3.5 oz............. | 9 | n.a. | 16 | 310 | 280 | n.a. | n.a. | n.a. |
| Canadian style (*Norbest*), 3.5 oz............. | 10 | n.a. | 16 | 300 | 280 | n.a. | n.a. | n.a. |
| **Turkey heart,** see "Heart" | | | | | | | | |
| **Turkey liver,** see "Liver" | | | | | | | | |
| **Turkey luncheon meat:** | | | | | | | | |
| breast, 1 oz. .......... | 2 | .11 | 6 | 65 | 79 | .32 | .01 | n.a. |
| breast (*Norbest*), 3.5 oz............. | 10 | n.a. | 21 | 310 | 240 | n.a. | n.a. | n.a. |
| roll, light meat, 1 oz............... | 11 | .36 | 5 | 52 | 71 | .44 | .01 | n.a. |

[1] *Prepared without added ingredients.*

| | Calcium | Iron | Magnesium | Phosphorus | Potassium | Zinc | Copper | Manganese |
|---|---|---|---|---|---|---|---|---|
| | (Mg) | (Mg) | (Mg) | (Mg) | (Mg) | (Mg) | (Mg) | (Mg) |
| roll, light and dark meat, 1 oz. | 9 | .38 | 5 | 48 | 77 | .57 | .02 | n.a. |
| **Turkey pastrami:** | | | | | | | | |
| (*Norbest*), 3.5 oz. | 32 | n.a. | 18 | 310 | 230 | n.a. | n.a. | n.a. |
| (*Norbest* Deli), 3.5 oz. | 52 | n.a. | 18 | 200 | 220 | n.a. | n.a. | n.a. |
| **Turkey salami:** | | | | | | | | |
| cooked, 1 oz. | 6 | .46 | 4 | 30 | 69 | .51 | .01 | n.a. |
| (*Norbest* Deli), 3.5 oz. | 110 | n.a. | 17 | 124 | 240 | n.a. | n.a. | n.a. |
| **Turkey sausage** (*Norbest* Links), 3.5 oz. | 45 | n.a. | 13 | 160 | 230 | n.a. | n.a. | n.a. |
| **Turmeric,** ground, 1 tsp. | 4 | .91 | 4 | 6 | 56 | .10 | .01 | .17 |
| **Turnip,** fresh: | | | | | | | | |
| raw, untrimmed, 1 lb. | 110 | 1.10 | 40 | 99 | 702 | n.a. | n.a. | n.a. |
| raw, trimmed, cubed, ½ cup | 20 | .20 | 7 | 18 | 124 | n.a. | n.a. | n.a. |
| boiled, drained, cubed, ½ cup | 18 | .17 | 6 | 15 | 106 | n.a. | n.a. | n.a. |
| boiled, drained, mashed, ½ cup | 26 | .26 | 9 | 22 | 156 | n.a. | n.a. | n.a. |
| frozen, 10-oz. pkg. | 64 | 1.99 | 29 | 56 | 388 | n.a. | n.a. | n.a. |
| **Turnip greens:** | | | | | | | | |
| fresh: | | | | | | | | |
| raw, untrimmed, 1 lb. | 603 | 3.49 | 98 | 133 | 941 | .61 | 1.11 | 1.48 |
| raw, trimmed, chopped, ½ cup | 53 | .31 | 9 | 12 | 83 | .05 | .10 | .13 |
| boiled, drained, chopped, ½ cup | 99 | .57 | 16 | 21 | 146 | .10 | .18 | .24 |
| canned, w/liquid, ½ cup | 138 | 1.77 | 24 | 24 | 165 | .27 | .10 | .32 |
| frozen, chopped: | | | | | | | | |
| 10-oz. pkg. | 335 | 4.27 | 76 | 78 | 522 | .48 | .16 | 1.05 |

| | Calcium | Iron | Magnesium | Phosphorus | Potassium | Zinc | Copper | Manganese |
|---|---|---|---|---|---|---|---|---|
| | (Mg) | (Mg) | (Mg) | (Mg) | (Mg) | (Mg) | (Mg) | (Mg) |

**Turnip greens, frozen, chopped,** *continued*

boiled, drained, ⅓ of
10-oz. pkg. . . . . . . | 112 | 1.42 | 19 | 25 | 165 | .30 | .11 | .35

boiled, drained,
½ cup . . . . . . . . . | 125 | 1.59 | 21 | 27 | 184 | .34 | .12 | .39

# V

| | Calcium | Iron | Magnesium | Phosphorus | Potassium | Zinc | Copper | Manganese |
|---|---|---|---|---|---|---|---|---|
| | (Mg) | (Mg) | (Mg) | (Mg) | (Mg) | (Mg) | (Mg) | (Mg) |
| **Vanilla flavor drink mix** (*Carnation* Instant Breakfast), 1 pkt. | 150 | 4.50 | 80 | 150 | 300 | 3.00 | .50 | n.a. |
| **Vanilla extract:** | | | | | | | | |
| real, 1 tsp. | 0 | .01 | 0 | 0 | 6 | 0 | tr. | .01 |
| real (*Virginia Dare*), 1 tsp. | tr. | tr. | 1 | 0 | tr. | tr. | tr. | n.a. |
| imitation, 1 tsp. | 0 | .01 | 0 | 1 | 4 | 0 | tr | .02 |
| **Veal**[1], meat only, 4 oz.: | | | | | | | | |
| cubed, for stew, leg and shoulder, braised, lean only | 33 | 1.63 | 32 | 271 | 388 | 6.82 | .17 | .05 |
| ground, broiled | 19 | 1.12 | 27 | 246 | 382 | 4.39 | .12 | .04 |
| leg (top round): | | | | | | | | |
| braised, lean w/fat | 9 | 1.50 | 33 | 282 | 434 | 4.49 | .16 | .04 |
| braised, lean only | 10 | 1.50 | 34 | 286 | 439 | 4.57 | .16 | .05 |
| pan-fried in vegetable oil, lean w/fat | 7 | 1.00 | 35 | 316 | 482 | 3.66 | .07 | .04 |
| pan-fried in vegetable oil, lean only | 8 | 1.00 | 36 | 329 | 501 | 3.83 | .07 | .04 |
| roasted, lean w/fat | 7 | 1.03 | 32 | 265 | 441 | 3.45 | .15 | .03 |
| roasted, lean only | 7 | 1.02 | 32 | 268 | 446 | 3.49 | .15 | .04 |
| loin: | | | | | | | | |
| braised, lean w/fat | 32 | 1.24 | 27 | 249 | 318 | 4.12 | .10 | .04 |
| braised, lean only | 36 | 1.25 | 31 | 269 | 337 | 4.64 | .11 | .04 |
| roasted, lean w/fat | 22 | .99 | 28 | 240 | 369 | 3.44 | .12 | .03 |
| roasted, lean only | 24 | .96 | 29 | 252 | 386 | 3.67 | .13 | .03 |
| rib: | | | | | | | | |
| braised, lean w/fat | 25 | 1.60 | 28 | 238 | 347 | 6.32 | .15 | .04 |
| braised, lean only | 27 | 1.64 | 29 | 247 | 361 | 6.78 | .16 | .05 |
| roasted, lean w/fat | 12 | 1.10 | 25 | 223 | 335 | 4.64 | .11 | .03 |
| roasted, lean only | 14 | 1.09 | 27 | 235 | 353 | 5.09 | .12 | .04 |

[1] *Prepared without added ingredients, except as noted.*

| | Calcium | Iron | Magnesium | Phosphorus | Potassium | Zinc | Copper | Manganese |
|---|---|---|---|---|---|---|---|---|
| | (Mg) | (Mg) | (Mg) | (Mg) | (Mg) | (Mg) | (Mg) | (Mg) |

Veal, *continued*
shoulder, whole:

| | Calcium | Iron | Magnesium | Phosphorus | Potassium | Zinc | Copper | Manganese |
|---|---|---|---|---|---|---|---|---|
| braised, lean w/fat . . . | 40 | 1.61 | 31 | 284 | 350 | 7.47 | .17 | .04 |
| braised, lean only. . . . | 42 | 1.64 | 32 | 295 | 362 | 7.94 | .18 | .04 |
| roasted, lean w/fat . . . | 31 | 1.17 | 28 | 244 | 365 | 5.81 | .16 | .03 |
| roasted, lean only . . . | 31 | 1.17 | 28 | 247 | 371 | 5.95 | .16 | .03 |
| shoulder, arm: | | | | | | | | |
| braised, lean w/fat . . . | 32 | 1.56 | 33 | 298 | 378 | 6.59 | .15 | .04 |
| braised, lean only. . . . | 34 | 1.60 | 34 | 313 | 393 | 7.08 | .15 | .04 |
| roasted, lean w/fat . . . | 29 | 1.30 | 29 | 251 | 395 | 4.74 | .16 | .03 |
| roasted, lean only . . . | 31 | 1.32 | 31 | 356 | 404 | 4.90 | .17 | .03 |
| shoulder, blade: | | | | | | | | |
| braised, lean w/fat . . . | 43 | 1.63 | 29 | 277 | 337 | 7.94 | .19 | .04 |
| braised, lean only. . . . | 45 | 1.67 | 32 | 286 | 346 | 8.38 | .19 | .04 |
| roasted, lean w/fat . . . | 32 | 1.13 | 27 | 240 | 347 | 6.33 | .16 | .03 |
| roasted, lean only . . . | 32 | 1.13 | 27 | 244 | 352 | 6.49 | .16 | .03 |
| sirloin: | | | | | | | | |
| braised, lean w/fat . . . | 19 | 1.36 | 31 | 276 | 364 | 4.90 | .15 | .04 |
| braised, lean only. . . . | 22 | 1.39 | 33 | 294 | 384 | 5.39 | .16 | .04 |
| roasted, lean w/fat . . . | 15 | 1.04 | 29 | 253 | 398 | 3.80 | .15 | .03 |
| roasted, lean only . . . | 16 | 1.03 | 31 | 262 | 414 | 4.01 | .15 | .03 |
| "Veal," vegetarian, frozen (*Worthington Veelets*), 2.5-oz. patty | 36 | .50 | n.a. | n.a. | 121 | .58 | n.a. | n.a. |
| **Vegetable juice cocktail,** canned, 6 fl. oz. . . . . . . | 20 | .77 | 20 | 31 | 351 | .36 | .36 | .18 |
| **Vegetables,** see specific listings | | | | | | | | |
| **Vegetables, mixed:** | | | | | | | | |
| canned, w/liquid, ½ cup . . . . . . . . . . . | 26 | .79 | 19 | 46 | 169 | .63 | .13 | .52 |
| canned, drained, ½ cup . . . . . . . . . . . | 22 | .86 | 13 | 34 | 239 | .34 | .06 | n.a. |
| frozen[1]: 10-oz. pkg. . . . . . . . . | 72 | 2.69 | 67 | 168 | 603 | 1.29 | .27 | .69 |

[1] Includes corn, lima beans, snap beans, green peas, and carrots.

| | Calcium | Iron | Magnesium | Phosphorus | Potassium | Zinc | Copper | Manganese |
|---|---|---|---|---|---|---|---|---|
| | (Mg) | (Mg) | (Mg) | (Mg) | (Mg) | (Mg) | (Mg) | (Mg) |
| boiled, drained, ⅓ of 10-oz. pkg. . . . . . | 22 | .75 | 20 | 46 | 155 | .45 | .08 | .35 |
| boiled, drained, ½ cup . . . . . . . . . | 22 | .75 | 20 | 46 | 154 | .45 | .08 | .35 |

**Vegetarian entree** (see also " 'Beef,' vegetarian" and other specific listings):

| | Calcium | Iron | Magnesium | Phosphorus | Potassium | Zinc | Copper | Manganese |
|---|---|---|---|---|---|---|---|---|
| frozen: | | | | | | | | |
| (*Natural Touch* Dinner Entree), 3-oz. patty | 48 | 1.70 | n.a. | n.a. | 101 | .83 | n.a. | n.a. |
| lentil rice loaf (*Natural Touch*), 3.2-oz. slice . . . . . . | 21 | 1.16 | n.a. | 213 | 161 | 1.04 | n.a. | n.a. |
| nine-bean loaf (*Natural Touch*), 1" slice, 3 oz. . . . . . | 27 | .64 | n.a. | n.a. | 187 | .88 | n.a. | n.a. |
| mix, loaf (*Natural Touch*), 4 tbsp., 1.1 oz. . . . . . . | 41 | 1.70 | n.a. | n.a. | 407 | .53 | n.a. | n.a. |
| mix, savory dinner loaf (*Loma Linda*), ⅓ cup, .9 oz. . . . . . . . . . . . . . | 23 | 1.31 | n.a. | n.a. | 414 | .38 | n.a. | n.a. |
| **Vienna sausage,** canned, beef and pork, 1 oz. . . . | 3 | .25 | 2 | 14 | 29 | .45 | .01 | .01 |
| **Vinegar,** cider, 1 tbsp. . . . | 1 | .10 | n.a. | 1 | 15 | n.a. | n.a. | n.a. |

# W

| | Calcium | Iron | Magnesium | Phosphorus | Potassium | Zinc | Copper | Manganese |
|---|---|---|---|---|---|---|---|---|
| | (Mg) | (Mg) | (Mg) | (Mg) | (Mg) | (Mg) | (Mg) | (Mg) |
| **Waffle,** frozen: | | | | | | | | |
| plain, 1.2 oz.......... | 77 | 1.49 | 7 | 139 | 43 | .19 | .03 | n.a. |
| plain, toasted: | | | | | | | | |
| 1.2 oz.............. | 77 | 1.48 | 7 | 138 | 42 | .19 | .03 | n.a. |
| **Wakame,** see "Seaweed" | | | | | | | | |
| **Walnut:** | | | | | | | | |
| black, dried: | | | | | | | | |
| in shell, 1 lb........ | 63 | 3.34 | 220 | 505 | 570 | 3.72 | 1.11 | 4.65 |
| shelled, 1 oz........ | 16 | .87 | 57 | 132 | 149 | .97 | .29 | 1.21 |
| shelled, chopped, | | | | | | | | |
| 1 cup ......... | 72 | 3.84 | 252 | 580 | 655 | 4.28 | 1.28 | 5.34 |
| English or Persian, dried: | | | | | | | | |
| in shell, 1 lb....... | 191 | 4.98 | 346 | 647 | 1024 | 5.58 | 2.83 | 5.92 |
| shelled, 1 oz........ | 27 | .69 | 48 | 90 | 142 | .78 | .39 | .82 |
| shelled, pieces or | | | | | | | | |
| chips, 1 cup ..... | 113 | 2.93 | 203 | 380 | 602 | 3.28 | 1.66 | 3.48 |
| **Water chestnut, Chinese:** | | | | | | | | |
| raw, sliced, | | | | | | | | |
| ½ cup............. | 7 | .37 | 14 | 39 | 362 | n.a. | n.a. | n.a. |
| canned, 4 medium, | | | | | | | | |
| 1 oz.............. | 1 | .24 | 1 | 5 | 33 | .11 | .03 | n.a. |
| canned, w/liquid, sliced, | | | | | | | | |
| ½ cup............. | 3 | .61 | 3 | 14 | 82 | .27 | .07 | n.a. |
| **Watercress,** raw: | | | | | | | | |
| untrimmed, 1 lb. ....... | 501 | .83 | 87 | 250 | 1376 | n.a. | n.a. | n.a. |
| trimmed, chopped, | | | | | | | | |
| ½ cup............. | 20 | .03 | 4 | 10 | 56 | n.a. | n.a. | n.a. |
| **Watermelon:** | | | | | | | | |
| untrimmed, 1 lb. ....... | 19 | .41 | 25 | 20 | 274 | .17 | .08 | .09 |
| ¹⁄₁₆ of 10"-diam. melon, | | | | | | | | |
| 1"-thick slice, about | | | | | | | | |
| 2 lbs. w/rind ........ | 38 | .83 | 52 | 41 | 560 | .34 | .15 | .18 |
| pulp, diced, ½ cup ..... | 7 | .14 | 9 | 7 | 93 | .06 | .03 | .03 |

| | Calcium (Mg) | Iron (Mg) | Magnesium (Mg) | Phosphorus (Mg) | Potassium (Mg) | Zinc (Mg) | Copper (Mg) | Manganese (Mg) |
|---|---|---|---|---|---|---|---|---|
| **Watermelon seed kernels,** dried, 1 oz. . . . | 15 | 2.07 | 146 | 215 | 184 | n.a. | n.a. | n.a. |
| **Waxgourd:** | | | | | | | | |
| raw, untrimmed, 1 lb. . . . . . . . . . . . . | 61 | 1.29 | n.a. | 61 | 19 | n.a. | n.a. | n.a. |
| raw, trimmed, cubed, ½ cup . . . . . . . . . . . . | 25 | .53 | n.a. | 25 | 8 | n.a. | n.a. | n.a. |
| boiled, drained, cubed, ½ cup . . . . . . . . . . . . | 32 | .67 | n.a. | 30 | 1.0 | n.a. | n.a. | n.a. |
| **Wheat,** whole grain: | | | | | | | | |
| durum, 1 cup . . . . . . . . | 66 | 6.75 | 277 | 975 | 827 | 7.98 | 1.06 | 5.78 |
| hard red spring, 1 cup . . . | 48 | 6.92 | 239 | 638 | 653 | 5.34 | .79 | 7.79 |
| hard red winter, 1 cup . . . | 56 | 6.12 | 243 | 552 | 697 | 5.08 | .83 | 7.65 |
| soft red winter, 1 cup . . . | 46 | 5.39 | 212 | 828 | 667 | 4.41 | .76 | 7.38 |
| hard white, 1 cup . . . . . . | 62 | 8.76 | 178 | 682 | 829 | 6.39 | .70 | 7.34 |
| soft white, 1 cup . . . . . . . | 57 | 9.02 | 151 | 675 | 730 | 5.82 | .72 | 5.72 |
| **Wheat, sprouted,** 1 cup | 30 | 2.32 | 89 | 216 | 182 | 1.79 | .28 | 2.01 |
| **Wheat bran** (see also "Cereal, ready-to-eat"), crude, 1 cup . . . . . . . . | 44 | 6.34 | 366 | 608 | 710 | 4.36 | .60 | 6.90 |
| **Wheat flour:** | | | | | | | | |
| whole grain, 1 cup . . . . . . | 40 | 4.66 | 166 | 415 | 486 | 3.52 | .46 | 4.56 |
| white, enriched: | | | | | | | | |
| all-purpose[1], 1 cup. . . | 18 | 5.80 | 27 | 135 | 134 | .88 | .18 | .85 |
| bread, 1 cup . . . . . . . | 21 | 6.04 | 34 | 133 | 136 | 1.17 | .25 | 1.09 |
| cake, 1 cup . . . . . . . . | 16 | 7.98 | 18 | 93 | 115 | .67 | .15 | .69 |
| self-rising[2], 1 cup . . . | 422 | 5.84 | 24 | 744 | 155 | .78 | .14 | 1.25 |
| tortilla mix, 1 cup . . . | 228 | 7.83 | 23 | 233 | 111 | n.a. | .11 | n.a. |
| **Wheat germ:** | | | | | | | | |
| (*Kretschmer*), 1 oz. or ¼ cup . . . . . . . . . . . . | 14 | 2.30 | 84 | 325 | 327 | 4.62 | .09 | 5.41 |
| crude, 1 oz. . . . . . . . . . . | 11 | 1.77 | 68 | 239 | 253 | 3.48 | .23 | 3.77 |

[1] Not fortified with calcium.
[2] With added nutrients.

| | Calcium | Iron | Magnesium | Phosphorus | Potassium | Zinc | Copper | Manganese |
|---|---|---|---|---|---|---|---|---|
| | (Mg) | (Mg) | (Mg) | (Mg) | (Mg) | (Mg) | (Mg) | (Mg) |
| **Wheat germ,** *continued* | | | | | | | | |
| toasted, 1 oz., approx. | | | | | | | | |
| ¼ cup............. | 13 | 2.58 | 91 | 325 | 269 | 4.73 | .18 | 5.67 |
| **Wheat grass** (*Pines* | | | | | | | | |
| *Instant Vegetable* | | | | | | | | |
| *Nutrition*), 3 tsp. or | | | | | | | | |
| 21 tablets .......... | 52 | 6.00 | 10 | 52 | 320 | tr. | .06 | n.a. |
| **Whelk,** unspecified, meat only: | | | | | | | | |
| raw, 1 lb.............. | 256 | 22.82 | 391 | 640 | 1574 | 7.39 | 4.67 | 2.03 |
| boiled, poached, or | | | | | | | | |
| steamed[1], 4 oz. ...... | 128 | 11.41 | 195 | 320 | 787 | 3.70 | 2.34 | n.a. |
| **Whey:** | | | | | | | | |
| acid, fluid, 1 cup ....... | 253 | .20 | 24 | 191 | 352 | 1.06 | .01 | .01 |
| acid, dry, 1 oz. ........ | 582 | .35 | 56 | 382 | 649 | 1.79 | .01 | tr. |
| sweet, fluid, 1 cup...... | 115 | .15 | 20 | 112 | 396 | 32 | tr. | tr. |
| sweet, dry, 1 oz. ....... | 226 | .25 | 50 | 264 | 590 | .56 | .02 | tr. |
| **Whiskey sour mix,** | | | | | | | | |
| bottled, 1 fl. oz....... | 1 | .04 | 0 | 2 | 9 | .02 | 0 | 0 |
| **White bean:** | | | | | | | | |
| regular: | | | | | | | | |
| uncooked, 1 lb. ..... | 1091 | 47.36 | 862 | 1365 | 8143 | 16.67 | 4.46 | 8.15 |
| uncooked, ½ cup.... | 243 | 10.54 | 192 | 304 | 1813 | 3.71 | .99 | 1.81 |
| boiled, ½ cup ...... | 81 | 3.33 | 57 | 102 | 505 | 1.24 | .26 | .57 |
| canned, w/liquid, | | | | | | | | |
| 8 oz. ........... | 166 | 6.79 | 116 | 207 | 1030 | 2.53 | .53 | 1.17 |
| canned, w/liquid, | | | | | | | | |
| ½ cup .......... | 96 | 3.92 | 67 | 120 | 595 | 1.46 | .30 | .68 |
| small: | | | | | | | | |
| uncooked, 1 lb. ...... | 787 | 35.06 | 828 | 2020 | 6996 | 12.73 | 2.88 | 5.80 |
| uncooked, ½ cup.... | 187 | 8.35 | 197 | 481 | 1666 | 3.03 | .69 | 1.38 |
| boiled, ½ cup ...... | 66 | 2.56 | 61 | 152 | 416 | .98 | .13 | .46 |
| **White sauce,** canned, | | | | | | | | |
| ½ cup............. | 212 | .13 | 132 | 128 | 222 | .27 | .02 | n.a. |

[1] *Prepared without added ingredients.*

| | Calcium | Iron | Magnesium | Phosphorus | Potassium | Zinc | Copper | Manganese |
|---|---|---|---|---|---|---|---|---|
| | (Mg) | (Mg) | (Mg) | (Mg) | (Mg) | (Mg) | (Mg) | (Mg) |
| **Whitefish,** mixed species, meat only: | | | | | | | | |
| raw, 1 lb.............. | n.a. | 1.68 | 94 | n.a. | 1438 | 4.48 | .33 | n.a. |
| baked, broiled, or | | | | | | | | |
| microwaved[1], 4 oz. ... | n.a. | .53 | 48 | n.a. | 460 | 1.44 | 1.04 | n.a. |
| smoked, 4 oz. ......... | 20 | .57 | 26 | 150 | 480 | .56 | .36 | .04 |
| **Whiting,** mixed species, meat only: | | | | | | | | |
| raw, 1 lb.............. | 219 | 1.54 | 94 | 1007 | 1131 | 4.01 | .14 | .47 |
| baked, broiled, or | | | | | | | | |
| microwaved[1], 4 oz. ... | 70 | .48 | 31 | 323 | 492 | .60 | .05 | .15 |
| **Wild rice:** | | | | | | | | |
| uncooked, ½ cup....... | 17 | 1.57 | 142 | 346 | 342 | 4.77 | .42 | 1.06 |
| cooked, ½ cup ........ | 3 | .49 | 26 | 67 | 83 | 1.10 | .10 | .23 |
| **Wine:** | | | | | | | | |
| dessert, 18.8% alcohol, | | | | | | | | |
| 2 fl. oz. ............ | 5 | .14 | 5 | 6 | 54 | .04 | .03 | .07 |
| table, 11.5% alcohol: | | | | | | | | |
| red, 4 fl. oz. ....... | 9 | .51 | 15 | 17 | 132[2] | .11 | .02 | .70 |
| rosé, 4 fl. oz....... | 9 | .45 | 12 | 18 | 117[2] | .07 | .06 | .12 |
| white, 4 fl. oz....... | 11 | .38 | 12 | 17 | 94[2] | .08 | .02 | .54 |
| **Winged beans,** fresh: | | | | | | | | |
| raw, untrimmed, | | | | | | | | |
| 1 lb. .............. | 371 | 6.67 | 152 | 164 | 990 | n.a. | n.a. | n.a. |
| raw, trimmed, sliced, | | | | | | | | |
| ½ cup............. | 16 | .33 | 8 | 8 | 49 | n.a. | n.a. | n.a. |
| boiled, drained, ½ cup | 19 | .34 | 9 | 8 | 85 | n.a. | n.a. | n.a. |
| **Winged beans,** dried: | | | | | | | | |
| uncooked, 1 lb. ........ | 1994 | 60.94 | 812 | 2045 | 4432 | 20.32 | 13.06 | 16.88 |
| uncooked, ½ cup....... | 400 | 12.23 | 163 | 410 | 889 | 4.08 | 2.62 | 3.39 |
| boiled, ½ cup ......... | 122 | 3.72 | 47 | 132 | 241 | 1.24 | .67 | 1.03 |
| **Winter squash,** see specific listings | | | | | | | | |
| **Wolffish,** Atlantic, meat only: | | | | | | | | |
| raw, 1 lb.............. | n.a. | .41 | n.a. | n.a. | n.a. | 3.54 | .13 | .07 |

[1] *Prepared without added ingredients.*
[2] *Average value.*

|  | Calcium | Iron | Magnesium | Phosphorus | Potassium | Zinc | Copper | Manganese |
|---|---|---|---|---|---|---|---|---|
|  | (Mg) | (Mg) | (Mg) | (Mg) | (Mg) | (Mg) | (Mg) | (Mg) |
| Wolffish, *continued* | | | | | | | | |
| baked, broiled, or | | | | | | | | |
| microwaved[1], 4 oz. . . . | n.a. | .14 | n.a. | n.a. | n.a. | 1.13 | .04 | .02 |
| **Wonton wrapper,** | | | | | | | | |
| 1 piece, .3 oz. . . . . . . . | 4 | .27 | 2 | 7 | 7 | .06 | .01 | .05 |

---

[1] *Prepared without added ingredients.*

# Y

| | Calcium (Mg) | Iron (Mg) | Magnesium (Mg) | Phosphorus (Mg) | Potassium (Mg) | Zinc (Mg) | Copper (Mg) | Manganese (Mg) |
|---|---|---|---|---|---|---|---|---|
| **Yam** (see also "Sweet potato"): | | | | | | | | |
| raw, untrimmed, 1 lb. . . . | 64 | 2.12 | 82 | 215 | 3183 | .92 | .69 | n.a. |
| raw, trimmed, cubed, ½ cup . . . . . . . . . . . . | 12 | .41 | 16 | 41 | 612 | .18 | .13 | n.a. |
| boiled, drained, cubed, ½ cup . . . . . . . . . . . . | 9 | .35 | 12 | 33 | 455 | .13 | .10 | n.a. |
| **Yam, canned or frozen,** see "Sweet potato" | | | | | | | | |
| **Yam beans:** | | | | | | | | |
| raw, untrimmed, 1 lb. . . . | 49 | 2.50 | 49 | 73 | 615 | .66 | .20 | .25 |
| raw, trimmed, sliced, 1 cup . . . . . . . . . . . . | 14 | .72 | 14 | 21 | 180 | .19 | .06 | .07 |
| **Yard-long beans,** fresh: | | | | | | | | |
| raw, untrimmed, 1 lb. . . . | 215 | 2.00 | 192 | 254 | 1034 | n.a. | n.a. | n.a. |
| raw, trimmed, sliced, ½ cup . . . . . . . . . . . . | 23 | .21 | 20 | 27 | 109 | n.a. | n.a. | n.a. |
| boiled, drained, sliced, ½ cup . . . . . . . . . . . . | 23 | .51 | 22 | 30 | 151 | n.a. | n.a. | n.a. |
| **Yard-long beans,** dried: | | | | | | | | |
| uncooked, 1 lb. . . . . . . . | 624 | 39.03 | 1531 | 2536 | 5248 | 15.84 | 3.99 | 7.21 |
| uncooked, ½ cup. . . . . . | 116 | 7.23 | 284 | 470 | 972 | 2.94 | .74 | 1.34 |
| boiled, ½ cup . . . . . . . . | 36 | 2.27 | 84 | 156 | 271 | .92 | .19 | .42 |
| **Yeast:** | | | | | | | | |
| baker's active, dry, .2-oz. pkg. . . . . . . . . . . | 5 | 1.16 | 7 | n.a. | 140 | .45 | .04 | .04 |
| baker's, compressed, .6-oz. cake. . . . . . . . . | 3 | .55 | 7 | 57 | 102 | 1.69 | .03 | .03 |
| brewer's[1], dry, 1 tbsp. . . . | 17 | 1.40 | 18 | 140 | 152 | n.a. | n.a. | n.a. |
| **Yellow beans,** dried: | | | | | | | | |
| uncooked, 1 lb. . . . . . . . | 753 | 31.80 | 1007 | 2214 | 4727 | 12.81 | 2.90 | 5.83 |
| uncooked, ½ cup. . . . . . | 163 | 6.87 | 218 | 478 | 1021 | 2.77 | .63 | 1.26 |
| boiled, ½ cup . . . . . . . . | 66 | 2.56 | 61 | 152 | 416 | .98 | .13 | .46 |

[1] *Calcium value may vary from 6 to 60 mg.*

| | Calcium | Iron | Magnesium | Phosphorus | Potassium | Zinc | Copper | Manganese |
|---|---|---|---|---|---|---|---|---|
| | (Mg) | (Mg) | (Mg) | (Mg) | (Mg) | (Mg) | (Mg) | (Mg) |
| **Yellowtail,** meat only: | | | | | | | | |
| raw, 1 lb.. . . . . . . . . . . . | n.a. | 2.20 | n.a. | 712 | n.a. | 2.35 | .20 | .07 |
| baked, broiled, or | | | | | | | | |
| microwaved[1], 4 oz. . . . | n.a. | .71 | n.a. | 228 | n.a. | .76 | .07 | .02 |
| **Yogurt:** | | | | | | | | |
| plain, 8 fl. oz.: | | | | | | | | |
| whole milk. . . . . . . . | 274 | .11 | 26 | 215 | 351 | 1.34 | .02 | .01 |
| lowfat . . . . . . . . . . . | 415 | .18 | 40 | 326 | 531 | 2.02 | .03 | .01 |
| skim . . . . . . . . . . . | 452 | .20 | 43 | 355 | 579 | 2.20 | .03 | .01 |
| coffee or vanilla, low fat, | | | | | | | | |
| 8 fl. oz.. . . . . . . . . . . | 389 | .16 | 37 | 306 | 498 | 1.88 | .03 | .01 |
| **Yogurt, frozen,** soft | | | | | | | | |
| serve: | | | | | | | | |
| chocolate, ½ cup . . . . . . | 106 | n.a. | 19 | 100 | 188 | .36 | .10 | .09 |
| vanilla, ½ cup . . . . . . . . | 103 | .22 | 10 | 93 | 152 | .31 | .03 | n.a. |

---

[1] *Prepared without added ingredients.*

# Z

| | Calcium | Iron | Magnesium | Phosphorus | Potassium | Zinc | Copper | Manganese |
|---|---|---|---|---|---|---|---|---|
| | (Mg) | (Mg) | (Mg) | (Mg) | (Mg) | (Mg) | (Mg) | (Mg) |
| **Zucchini,** w/peel: | | | | | | | | |
| fresh: | | | | | | | | |
| raw, untrimmed, | | | | | | | | |
| 1 lb. . . . . . . . . . | 65 | 1.83 | 94 | 138 | 1068 | .85 | .25 | .55 |
| raw, ends trimmed, | | | | | | | | |
| sliced, ½ cup. . . . . | 10 | .28 | 14 | 21 | 161 | .13 | .04 | .08 |
| raw, boiled, drained, | | | | | | | | |
| sliced, ½ cup. . . . . | 12 | .32 | 19 | 36 | 228 | .16 | .08 | .16 |
| fresh, baby, raw: | | | | | | | | |
| untrimmed, 1 lb. . . . . | 84 | n.a. | 129 | 367 | 1809 | 3.27 | .39 | .78 |
| 1 large, 2⅝" long, | | | | | | | | |
| .6 oz. . . . . . . . . . | 3 | n.a. | 5 | 15 | 73 | .13 | .02 | .03 |
| 1 medium, 3⅛" long, | | | | | | | | |
| .4 oz. . . . . . . . . . | 2 | n.a. | 4 | 10 | 50 | .09 | .01 | .02 |
| canned, Italian style[1], | | | | | | | | |
| 8 oz. . . . . . . . . . . . . | 38 | 1.55 | 31 | 66 | 622 | .58 | 22 | n.a. |
| canned, Italian style[1], | | | | | | | | |
| ½ cup. . . . . . . . . . . . | 19 | .78 | 16 | 33 | 312 | .29 | .11 | n.a. |
| frozen, 10-oz. pkg. . . . . . . | 52 | 1.46 | 38 | 79 | 619 | .59 | .14 | .69 |
| frozen, boiled, drained, | | | | | | | | |
| sliced, ½ cup. . . . . . . . | 19 | .54 | 14 | 28 | 218 | .22 | .05 | .26 |

[1]*Packed in tomato juice.*

# Index

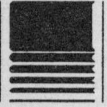